D1461701

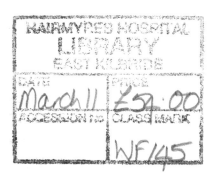

Core Topics in Mechanical Ventilation

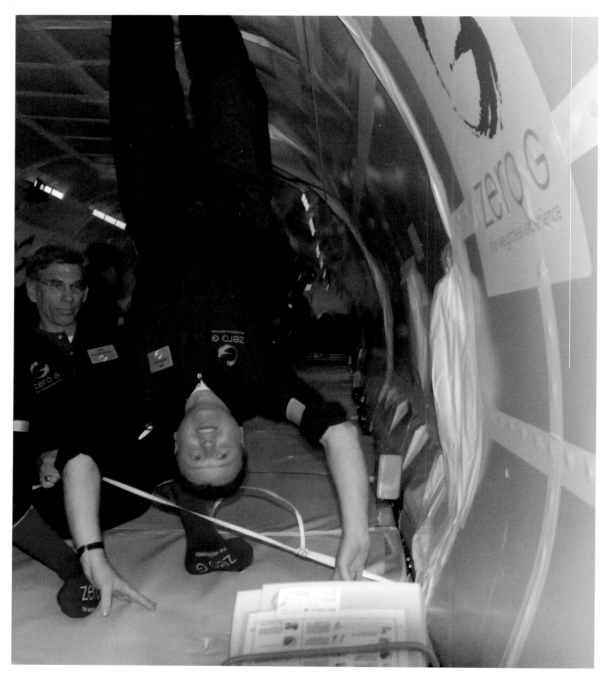

Iain Mackenzie in zero-gravity training for Professor Hawking's flight, April 26, 2007.

Core Topics in Mechanical Ventilation

Edited by

IAIN MACKENZIE
*Consultant in Intensive Care Medicine
and Anaesthesia*

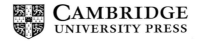

CAMBRIDGE UNIVERSITY PRESS
Cambridge, New York, Melbourne, Madrid, Cape Town, Singapore, São Paulo, Delhi

Cambridge University Press
The Edinburgh Building, Cambridge CB2 8RU, UK

Published in the United States of America by Cambridge University Press, New York

www.cambridge.org
Information on this title: www.cambridge.org/9780521867818

First published 2008

Printed in the United Kingdom at the University Press, Cambridge

A catalogue record for this publication is available from the British Library

Library of Congress Cataloguing in Publication Data

Core topics in mechanical ventilation / [edited by] Iain Mackenzie
 p. ; cm.
Includes bibliographical references and index.
ISBN 978-0-521-86781-8 (hardback)
1. Artificial respiration. I. Mackenzie, Iain, 1961– II. Title.
[DNLM: 1. Respiration, Artificial. WF 145 C7975 2008]

RC87.9.C69 2008
615.8'362 – dc22   2008002984

ISBN 978-0-521-86781-8 hardback

Contents

Contributors

Simon Baudouin, FRCP
Senior Lecturer
Department of Anaesthesia and Critical Care
  Medicine
Royal Victoria Infirmary
Newcastle-upon-Tyne, UK

Andrew Bodenham, FRCA
Consultant in Anaesthesia and Intensive Care
  Medicine
Leeds General Infirmary
Leeds, UK

Ian Clement, PhD MRCP FRCA
Consultant in Anaesthesia and Intensive
  Medicine
Department of Anaesthesia and Critical Care
  Medicine
Royal Victoria Infirmary
Newcastle-upon-Tyne, UK

Craig Davidson, FRCP
Director, Lane Fox Respiratory Unit
Guy's and St. Thomas' NHS Foundation Trust
London, UK

E. Wesley Ely, MD MPH
Professor and Associate Director of Aging
  Research
Division of Allergy, Pulmonary, and Critical Care
  Medicine
Vanderbilt University School of Medicine
Veterans Affairs, Tennessee Valley Geriatric Research,
  Education, and Clinical Center
Nashville, Tennessee, USA

Simon Finney, PhD MRCP FRCA
Consultant in Intensive Care Medicine and
  Anaesthesia
Royal Brompton and Harefield NHS Trust
London, UK

Brian Keogh, FRCA
Consultant in Intensive Care Medicine and
  Anaesthesia
Royal Brompton and Harefield NHS Trust
London, UK

Iain Mackenzie, DM MRCP FRCA
Consultant in Intensive Care Medicine and
  Anaesthesia
John Farman Intensive Care Unit
Addenbrooke's Hospital
Cambridge, UK

Peter Macnaughton, MD MRCP FRCA
Consultant in Intensive Care Medicine and
  Anaesthesia
Plymouth Hospitals NHS Trust
Derriford
Plymouth, UK

Abhiram Mallick, FRCA
Consultant in Anaesthesia and Intensive Care
  Medicine
Leeds General Infirmary
Leeds, UK

Leigh Mansfield
Senior Physiotherapist
Department of Anaesthesia and Critical Care
  Medicine
Royal Victoria Infirmary
Newcastle-upon-Tyne, UK

List of contributors

Terry Martin, MSc FRCS FRCA
Consultant in Anaesthesia and Intensive Care
The Royal Hampshire County Hospital
Winchester, UK

William T. McBride, BSc MD FRCA FFARCS(I)
Consultant Cardiac Anaesthetist
Royal Victoria Hospital
Belfast, UK

Barry McGrattan, FFARCS(I)
Specialist Registrar in Anaesthesia
Royal Victoria Hospital
Belfast, UK

Russell R. Miller III, MD MPH
Assistant Professor
Division of Critical Care and Pulmonary Medicine
LDS and IMC Hospitals
University of Utah School of Medicine
Salt Lake City, Utah, USA

Hugh Montgomery, MD FRCP
Director, Institute for Human Health and
   Performance and Consultant Intensivist
UCL Hospitals
London, UK

Matthew T. Naughton, MD FRACP
Associate Professor of Head, General Respiratory
   and Sleep Medicine
The Alfred Hospital
Prahran
Melbourne, Australia

Mick Nielsen, FRCA
Consultant in Anaesthesia and Intensive Care
Southampton University Hospitals NHS Trust
Southampton, UK

Clare Reid, PhD SRD
Research Dietician
Division of Anaesthesia
University of Cambridge
Addenbrooke's Hospital
Cambridge, UK

Rob Ross Russell, MD FRCPCH
Consultant in Paediatric Intensive Care Medicine
Addenbrooke's Hospital
Cambridge, UK

Sanjoy Shah, MD MRCP EDIC
Consultant in Intensive Care Medicine
University Hospital Wales
Cardiff, UK

Hubert Trübel, MD
Consultant in Paediatrics
Department of Paediatrics
HELIOS Kilinikum Wuppertal
University of Wittenburg/Herdeche
Wuppertal, Germany

Bill Tunnicliffe, FRCA
Consultant in Intensive Care Medicine and
   Anaesthesia
Queen Elizabeth Hospital
Birmingham, UK

David Tuxen, MBBS FRACP MD Dip DHM FJFICM
Associate Professor of Critical Care
The Alfred Hospital
Prahran
Melbourne, Australia

Alain Vuylsteke, MD FRCA
Director of Critical Care
Papworth Hospital NHS Trust
Papworth Everard
Cambridgeshire, UK

Natalie Yeaney, MD FAAP
Consultant Neonatal Intensivist
Addenbrooke's Hospital
Cambridge, UK

Peter Young, MD FRCA
Consultant in Intensive Care and Anaesthesia
The Queen Elizabeth Hospital
King's Lynn, UK

Foreword

Bjorn Ibsen, an anaesthetist and intensivist who practiced for most of his career in Copenhagen, Denmark, died on 7 August 2007. Ibsen is widely regarded as the father of Intensive Care Medicine, the nativity of which occurred in his home city in 1952 during a polio epidemic. Ibsen had trained in radiology, surgery, pathology and gynaecology before travelling to Massachusetts General Hospital in 1949 to gain specialist experience in anaesthesia. He returned to Copenhagen in 1950 and assumed a leading role in managing one of the world's worst polio epidemics that started only two years later. Some 2899 cases developed among the population of two million. Too weak to cough, many patients succumbed to secretion retention with associated carbon dioxide retention. Negative pressure ventilation was effectively the only form of support then available, but Ibsen found that tracheostomy, or endotracheal intubation combined with the careful application of intermittent positive pressure ventilation administered by relays of doctors, medical students and others, was an effective means of overcoming the devastating effects of the disease. In the end, over 1500 practitioners aspirated secretions and performed manual ventilation in shifts. Mortality fell markedly. As a result, the idea that critically ill patients should be supported in centralized facilities by individuals experienced in their care was adopted worldwide.

The new specialty emerged in varying phenotypes according to the history, individual preferences and expertise of those driving the change. In the United States, physicians trained in pulmonary medicine have traditionally also provided critical care. In the United Kingdom, the base specialty of anaesthesia has borne the brunt of intensive care provision over many decades. Only in recent years has the value of bringing varying expertise to intensive care management (ICM) from different clinical base specialties been recognized more formally. Thus in Australia a joint intercollegiate faculty of ICM has been developed, a model that was to an extent copied in the UK. Formal training programmes have been developed, culminating in the UK in ICM being recognized as a specialty in the year 2000. The emergence of diploma and other examinations designed to test competencies in intensive care has been rapid. The strength of national and international specialist societies has grown, with associated academic advancement publicized through congresses and increasingly in highly cited journals.

Against this background, it has given me great pleasure to write the foreword for this exciting volume, expertly conceived and edited by Dr Iain Mackenzie. The contributors to this book come from a wide range of clinical and national backgrounds, thereby reflecting the heterogeneity that is in many senses the strength of the specialty. Moreover, the content reflects the staggering advances that have been made during the past 50 years in the delivery of mechanical ventilatory support. Even those phenomena which would have been easily recognizable to Ibsen, such as the delivery of oxygen therapy, have been subjected to scientific evaluation and technological development. Tracheostomy, used widely in the 1950s polio epidemic, is now performed at the bedside, an innovation of which I suspect Ibsen would have approved. The content of chapters dealing with sedation, paralysis and analgesia might have been more familiar to him, but the agents now employed, the increased understanding of their properties and the clinical benefits attributable to their avoidance, where possible, are evidence of the advances made in this area of pharmacology. The outreach of exper-tise into the wards in pursuit of the 'intensive care without walls' has been greatly facilitated by the advent of non-invasive mechanical ventilatory support.

Finally, the scientific advances in our evaluation of the effects of mechanical ventilation, the recognition that it can do harm if applied inappropriately and the evidence base concerning its use in patients with a wide variety of primary and secondary lung pathologies is a truly outstanding achievement that intensive care medicine can be proud of. I suspect that Bjorn Ibsen, were he privileged to read this volume, would feel the same.

Timothy W. Evans, BSC DSC FRCP FRCA FMedSci
Professor of Intensive Care Medicine
Imperial College
London

Consultant in Intensive Care Medicine
Royal Brompton Hospital
London

Preface

Respiratory support is recognized to be a key component in the resuscitation of acutely ill patients and, as such, the basics are taught to all those who seek to acquire life support skills. Following stabilization, the continued provision of respiratory support, be it in the emergency department, respiratory ward or intensive care unit, is largely taken for granted. However, as the ARDSnet study has recently reminded us, the way we manage mechanical ventilation in the medium and long term actually has a significant impact on patient outcome. Although the literature is full of the evidence necessary to provide optimal respiratory support, synthesizing this evidence into a cohesive and logical approach would be an enormous task for one individual. On the other hand, excellent sections on respiratory support can be found in the major textbooks on critical care and indeed the 'principles and practice of mechanical ventilation' is the sole subject of Martin Tobin's authoritative tome of that name. However, these large reference books are expensive and less than suitable for those who need a more concise and practical overview of the subject. This book therefore seeks to fill the gap between the journals and the major textbooks by bringing together clear, concise and evidence-based accounts of important topics in respiratory support, together with, where necessary, explanations of its physiology and pathology. It is hoped, therefore, that this book will appeal to a very wide audience, and will make a substantial contribution to the interest in,

and teaching of, the art and science of mechanical ventilation. In addition, since many of those who work with patients who require respiratory support do not have an anaesthetic background, knowledge particular to this specialty has not been assumed.

I would welcome any feedback so that future editions of this book can better meet the needs of its readers.

My colleagues in Cambridge, both nursing and medical, must be credited with persuading me of the need for a book such as this, and for that I am grateful. I am also indebted to the contributors from around the world who responded so favourably to my request that they contribute, and then followed through with their chapters. Frank McGinn (GE Healthcare Technologies), Dan Gleeson (Cape Engineering) and John Wines (Cape Engineering) kindly supplied me with information about the histories of their respective companies. I have received assistance in sourcing some of the images from Mr Pyush Jani and Dr Helen Smith. I am very grateful to David Miller for checking the correctness of the English, but must accept any blame for any errors that have crept through. Finally, I would like to thank Diane, my wife, and Katherine, Rebecca, Charlotte and Amy, my daughters, for their unfailing support over the last two years while this book was in production.

Iain Mackenzie

Introductory notes

Physiological notation

Those with a dislike of mathematics will be pleased to know that none of the equations in this book need to be memorized. Having said that, though, understanding the concepts that are encapsulated by the equations presented will help the reader enormously in achieving a significantly deeper level of understanding. As many of the terms in the equations refer to physiological quantities, physiological notation is used, and therefore being able to decipher physiological notation will be helpful

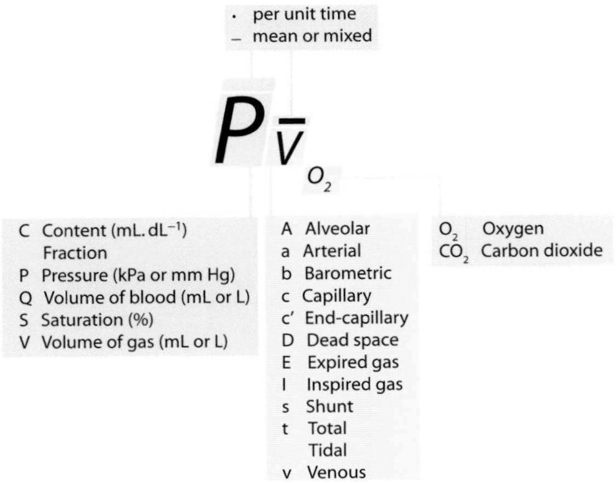

· per unit time
– mean or mixed
$P\bar{V}_{O_2}$
C Content (mL.dL^{-1})
Fraction
P Pressure (kPa or mm Hg)
Q Volume of blood (mL or L)
S Saturation (%)
V Volume of gas (mL or L)
A Alveolar
a Arterial
b Barometric
c Capillary
c′ End-capillary
D Dead space
E Expired gas
I Inspired gas
s Shunt
t Total
Tidal
v Venous
O_2 Oxygen
CO_2 Carbon dioxide

Figure 1 Key to physiological notation.

In the example illustrated, the physiological quantity being referred to is the mixed venous partial pressure of oxygen. Note also that when blood or gas volume, *V* and *Q* respectively, are expressed 'per minute' by placing a dot above the letter, they then refer to volume/time, or flow. Thus *Q*, blood volume, can be converted to $\dot{Q}$, blood flow.

Table 1 In-text notation for commonly used physiological quantities

Quantity	Correct notation	In-text notation
Fractional inspired oxygen concentration	$F_{I_{O_2}}$	FIO_2
Partial pressure of carbon dioxide in alveolar gas	$P_{A_{CO_2}}$	$PACO_2$
Partial pressure of carbon dioxide in arterial blood	$P_{a_{CO_2}}$	$PaCO_2$
Partial pressure of oxygen in alveolar gas	$P_{A_{O_2}}$	PAO_2
Partial pressure of oxygen in arterial blood	$P_{a_{O_2}}$	PaO_2
Partial pressure of carbon dioxide	P_{CO_2}	PCO_2
Partial pressure of oxygen	P_{O_2}	PO_2
Haemoglobin oxygen saturation in arterial blood	$S_{a_{O_2}}$	SaO_2

(Figure 1). The reader may be relieved to hear that formal physiological notation has been completely avoided in the text because it can sometimes extend significantly below the text baseline, as in, for example, the notation representing the partial pressure of oxygen in arterial blood:

$$Pa_{O_2}.$$

However, some quantities are mentioned so often in the text that to refer to these in words would hinder, rather than help, the flow of the text. Therefore, for the most common of these quantities, non-physiological notation has been used for

Table 2 Pressure conversion

	multiply → divide ←	
mm Hg	1.3595	cm H$_2$O
kPa	10.197	cm H$_2$O
kPa	7.5	mm Hg
Atm	101.325	kPa
Bar	100	kPa

in-text references, as it is in many other publications (Table 1).

Units

The European convention on units has been maintained throughout, using kilopascals (kPa) for gas pressures rather than millimetres of mercury (mm Hg), but the conversion factors can be found in Table 2. However, for clarity the symbol for the litre, which is usually abbreviated to the lower case letter 'l', has been substituted by the North American convention of using the capital letter 'L'; thus 'ml' becomes 'mL' and 'dl' becomes 'dL'.

Compound units in clinical practice commonly use the forward slash '/' as the delimiter to denote a denominator unit. For example, 'millilitres per kilogram' would be written 'mL/kg'. In compound units with only two components, this usage is not subject to misunderstanding, but in those with

Table 3 Convention for the use of compound units

Quantity	Common clinical notation	Correct scientific notation
Millilitres **per** kilogram	mL/kg	mL.kg^{-1}
Microgram **per** kilogram **per** hour	μg/kg/hr	μg.kg^{-1}.hr^{-1}
Millilitres **per** minute	mL/min	mL.min^{-1}
Litres **per** minute	L/min	L.min^{-1}
Milliequivalents **per** litre	mEq/L	mEq.L^{-1}
Millimoles **per** litre	mmol/L	mmol.L^{-1}
Kilocalorie **per** milliliter	kcal/mL	kcal.mL^{-1}
Millilitres **per** hour	mL/hr	mL.hr^{-1}
Milligrams **per** kilogram	mg/kg	mg.kg^{-1}
Kilocalories **per** kilogram	kcal/kg	kcal.kg^{-1}
Grams **per** kilogram	g/kg	g.kg^{-1}
Grams **per** deciliter	g/dL	g.dL^{-1}
Micrograms **per** minute	μg/min	μg.min^{-1}
Millilitres **per** kilogram	mL/kg	mL.kg^{-1}
Millilitres **per** day	mL/d	mL.d^{-1}

more than two components, the use of the forward slash is potentially confusing and should be avoided. The convention in this book, therefore, is to use the more correct scientific notation. In this form, the relationship between units is indicated by the superscript power notation, as shown in Table 3.

Chapter 1

Physiology of ventilation and gas exchange

HUGH MONTGOMERY

Among its many functions, the lung has two major ones: it must harvest oxygen to fuel aerobic respiration and it must vent acid-forming carbon dioxide. This chapter will offer a brief overview of how the lung fulfills these functions. It will also discuss some of the mechanisms through which adequate oxygenation can fail. A secure understanding of these principles allows an insight into the way in which mechanical ventilation strategies can be altered in order to enhance oxygenation and carbon dioxide clearance.

Functional anatomy of the lung

The airways

During inspiration, air is drawn into the oropharynx through either the mouth or the nasal airway. Nasal breathing is preferred, as it is associated with enhanced particle removal (by nasal hairs and mucus-laden turbinates) and humidification. However, this route is associated with a fall in pharyngeal pressure. Just as Ohm's law dictates that voltage is the product of current and resistance, so pharyngeal pressure is the product of gas flow and pharyngeal resistance. A 'fat apron' around the pharynx because of obesity may lead to increased pharyngeal compliance, and thus increase the risk of dynamic pharyngeal collapse in such patients. In adults, when pharyngeal flows exceed 30 to 40 litres per minute,

the work of breathing becomes high and the fall in pharyngeal pressure too great for the adequate intake of air: the mouth then becomes the preferred route for breathing.

The larynx remains a protector of the airway, with aryepiglottic and arytenoid muscles able to draw the laryngeal entrance closed like a purse-string and the epiglottis pulled down from above like a trap door. In addition, the arytenoid cartilages can swing inwards to appose the vocal cords themselves, thus offering an effective seal to the entry of particles or gases to the airway beneath. Meanwhile, tight occlusion can be achieved during swallowing or to 'fix' the thorax during heavy lifting, allowing the larynx to resist internal pressures of some 120 cm H_2O. Laryngeal sensitivity to irritation, causing a cough, makes the larynx effective at limiting entry of noxious gases or larger particles, while more intense chemoreceptor stimulation can cause severe laryngeal spasm, preventing any meaningful gas flow. In the anaesthetic room, this can be life-threatening.

When air enters the trachea, it is supported by anterior horse-shoes of cartilage (Figure 1.1). However, these are compliant, and tracheal collapse occurs with extrinsic pressures of only 40 cm H_2O. Ciliated columnar epithelium yields an upward-moving mucus 'escalator'. The trachea then divides into the right and left main bronchi (generation 1 airways), and then into lobar and

Core Topics in Mechanical Ventilation, ed. Iain Mackenzie. Published by Cambridge University Press.
© Cambridge University Press 2008.

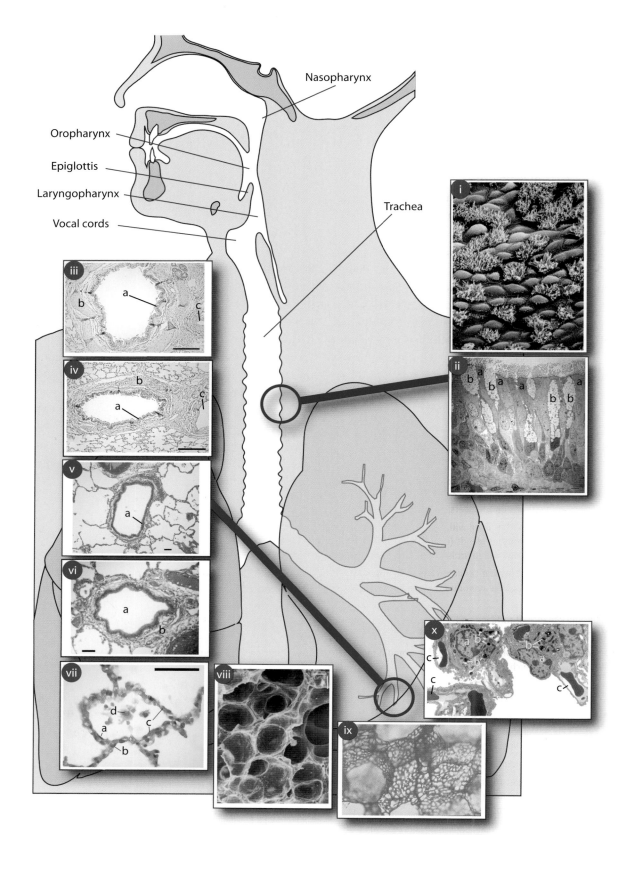

Nasopharynx

Oropharynx

Epiglottis

Laryngopharynx

Vocal cords

Trachea

segmental bronchi (generations 2–4). The right main bronchus is wider and more vertical than the left, and is thus the 'preferred' path for inhaled foreign bodies. Cartilaginous horse-shoe supports in the upper airways give way to plates of cartilage lower down, but all will collapse when exposed to intrathoracic pressures of >50 cm H_2O (or less in situations in which the walls are diseased, such as in chronic obstructive pulmonary disease or bronchomalacia).

Successive division of bronchi (generations 5–11) yield ever-smaller airways (to about 1 mm diameter), all of which are surrounded by lymphatic and pulmonary arterial branch vessels. They are supported by their cartilaginous plates and rarely collapse because intra-bronchial pressure is nearly always positive. So long as there is patency between alveoli and bronchi, even forced expiration allows sufficient gas flow to maintain intra-bronchial pressures to a level above intrathoracic pressures.

Bronchioles (generations 12–16) lack cartilaginous support, but are held open by the elastic recoil of the attached lung parenchyma, making airway collapse more likely at lower lung volumes. The cross-sectional area of these very small distal airways, and their very thin walls, makes airway resistance at this level almost nil in the absence of contraction (bronchoconstriction) of the wall's smooth muscle cells. Subsequent respiratory bronchioles (generations 17–19) have increasing numbers of gas-exchanging alveolar sacs in their walls; these bronchioles are anchored open under tension from surrounding parenchyma. Each of 150 000 or so 'primary lobules' represents the distal airway subtended by a respiratory bronchiole. Distally (generation 20–22), alveolar duct walls give rise to some

---

Figure 1.1 Gross and microscopic anatomy of the respiratory tract.

Inset i: Conventional microscopy view of the surface of the ciliated epithelium of the trachea showing cells bearing cilia adjacent to cells which appear flat, but which in fact bear microvilli. Photomicrograph courtesy of the Ernest Orlando Lawrence Berkeley National Laboratory, California.

Inset ii: Transmission electron microscope image of a thin section cut through the bronchiolar epithelium of the lung showing ciliated columnar cells (a) interspersed by non-ciliated mucous-secreting (goblet) cells (b). Slide courtesy of Dr Susan Wilson, Histochemistry Research Unit, University of Southampton.

Inset iii: Section of bronchus lined with pseudo-stratified columnar epithelium (a), and surrounded by a ring of hyaline cartilage (b). The presence of sero-mucous glands (c) differentiates this from a bronchiole. This section also contains an arteriole (d). Bar = 250 microns. Slide reproduced with permission. Copyright © Department of Anatomy and Cell Biology, University of Kansas.

Inset iv: Tiny islands of hyaline cartilage (a) confirm that this is bronchus rather than bronchiole, and adjacent is a pulmonary vein (b). Bar = 250 microns. Slide reproduced with permission. Copyright © Department of Anatomy and Cell Biology, University of Kansas.

Inset v: The absence of cartilage and sero-mucous glands means that this is a bronchiole, with a surrounding cuff of smooth muscle (a). Bar = 25 microns. Slide courtesy of Dr Susan Wilson, Histochemistry Research Unit, University of Southampton.

Inset vi: A small bronchiole (a) surrounded by smooth muscle (b). Bar = 25 microns. Slide courtesy of Dr Susan Wilson, Histochemistry Research Unit, University of Southampton.

Inset vii: An alveolus lined by thin flat type I pneumocytes (a) and cuboidal, surfactant-secreting type II pneumocytes (b), with an integral network of fine capillaries (c) embedded within the alveolar walls. The lumen of the alveolus contains a large alveolar macrophage (d). Bar = 25 microns. Slide courtesy of Dr Susan Wilson, Histochemistry Research Unit, University of Southampton.

Inset viii: Scanning electron microscope image of the alveolar honeycomb. Photomicrograph courtesy of the Ernest Orlando Lawrence Berkeley National Laboratory, California.

Inset ix: This photomicrograph shows the fine network of capillaries that enmesh the alveoli.

Inset x: Transmission electron microscopic image of alveolar cells, showing large cuboidal type II pneumocytes (a) packed with vesicles containing surfactant (b). Nearby alveolar capillaries containing red blood cells can be seen (c). Photomicrograph courtesy of the Rippel Electron Microscope Facility, Dartmouth College, New Hampshire.

20 alveolar sacs, containing one third of all alveolar gas. The terminal alveolar sacs (generation 23) are blind-ending.

The Alveoli and Their Blood Supply

Each lung may contain up to half a billion alveoli, which are compressed by the weight of overlying lung and are thus progressively smaller in a vertical gradient. Alveolar gas can pass between adjacent alveoli through small holes called 'the pores of Kohn'. The pulmonary capillaries form a rich network enveloping the alveoli, with the alveolar epithelium closely apposed to the capillary endothelium. The other surface of the capillary is embedded in the septal matrix.

Blood delivered into the pulmonary arteries from the right ventricle flows at a pressure less than 20% of that of the systemic circulation. With near identical blood flows, one can infer that pulmonary vascular resistance is correspondingly five- to sixfold lower than systemic. Working at lower pressure, the pulmonary arterial wall is correspondingly thinner, while the pulmonary arteriolar wall contains virtually no smooth muscle cells at all. Capillaries in dependent areas of the lung tend to be better filled than areas higher up (due again to gravitational effects), while lung inflation compresses the capillary bed and increases effective resistance to blood flow. Blood flows across several alveolar units before passing into pulmonary venules and thence to the pulmonary veins.

Pulmonary mechanics

Air enters the lung in response to the generation of a negative[1] intrathoracic pressure (in normal ventilation, or in negative pressure and cuirass mechanical ventilation), or to the application of a positive airway pressure (in positive pressure ventilation modes). Work is thus performed in overcoming both resistance to gas flow and elastic tension in the lung tissue during the thoracic expansion of inspiration. A small quantity of energy is also dissipated in overcoming lung inertia and by the friction of lung deformation.

Elasticity and the lung

The lung's elasticity derives from elastin fibres of the lung parenchyma, which accounts for perhaps one third of elastic recoil, and from the surface tension of the fluid film lining the alveoli. When fully collapsed,[2] the resting volume of the lung is considerably smaller than the volume it occupies when fully expanded in the chest cavity. Fully expanded, the elasticity of the lungs generates a subatmospheric pressure in the pleural space of about -5.5 cm H_2O (Figure 1.2). At peak inspiration, when the thoracic cage is maximally expanded, this pressure may fall to nearly -30 cm H_2O.

It is worth giving some thought to the issue of surface tension forces within the lung. The pressure within a truly spherical alveolus (P_A) would normally be calculated as twice the surface tension (T_s) divided by the alveolar radius (r):

$$P_A = \frac{2 \times T_s}{r}. \tag{1.1}$$

This equation tells us that if surface tension were constant, the alveolar pressure would be inversely proportional to the alveolar radius. In other words, alveolar pressure would be higher in alveoli with a smaller radius (Figure 1.3). If this were the case, it would mean that smaller alveoli would rapidly empty their gaseous content into larger adjacent alveoli and collapse. Taken to its logical conclusion, all of the alveoli in a lung would empty into one huge alveolus.

Fortunately, surface tension is *not* constant because of the presence of a mixture of phospholipids[3] and proteins[4] that floats on the surface of

---

[1] Also referred to as *subatmospheric*.

[2] For example, when removed from the chest at autopsy.
[3] Mainly phosphatidylcholine, commonly referred to as *lecithin*.
[4] Surfactant proteins A to D, often referred to as *SP-A*, *SP-B*, etc.

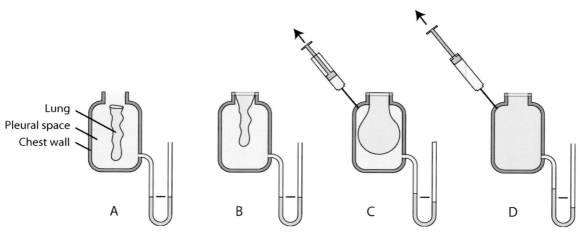

Figure 1.2 Negative pleural pressure.

A: The respiratory system can be compared to a rubber balloon (the lungs) placed inside a glass jar (the chest cavity) with the space between the outside of the balloon and the inside of the jar representing the pleural space.

B: The opening of the glass jar is sealed over by the rubber balloon, sealing the space between the outside of the balloon and the inside of the jar from the atmosphere.

C: As residual gas in this space is evacuated the pressure in the 'pleural space' drops below atmospheric and the balloon expands.

D: Once all the gas in the 'pleural space' is evacuated the 'lung' is completely expanded to fill the 'chest cavity'. The pressure inside the 'lung' remains atmospheric while the pressure in the pleural space is subatmospheric (negative).

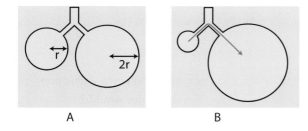

Figure 1.3 Alveolar instability with constant surface tension.

A: With constant surface tension (T_s), the alveolar pressure in the smaller alveolus is $\frac{2 \times T_s}{r}$ and the pressure in the larger alveolus is $\frac{2 \times T_s}{2r}$, which means that whatever the values of T_s and r, the pressure is only half that in the larger alveolus.

B: Under these circumstances, gas flows from the smaller alveolus (higher pressure) to the larger alveolus (lower pressure).

the fluid lining the alveoli (the surfactant; see Figure 1.4), which reduces the surface tension *in proportion to the change in the surface area*: the smaller the surface area of the alveolus, the greater the reduction in surface tension. This means that gas in fact tends to flow from larger to smaller alveoli, producing homogeneity of alveolar volume and stabilizing the lung. One other major advantage of this effect on fluid surface tension is that the lung's compliance is significantly increased, reducing the negative pressure generated by the lung in the pleural space. This consequently reduces the hydrostatic pressure gradient between the inside of the pulmonary capillaries and the pulmonary interstitium, minimizing the rate at which intravascular fluid is drawn from the capillaries. Lack of surfactant, for instance in intensive care patients with acute lung injury, thus tends to cause alveolar collapse and reduce lung compliance, which substantially increases the work of breathing.

As the chest expands during inspiration, intra-alveolar pressure falls to little more than -1 cm H_2O, causing the air to flow down a pressure gradient from the nose and mouth to the alveoli. It is notable just how modest the intra-alveolar pressures have to be to cause gas to flow in and

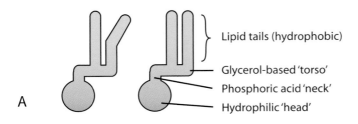

A

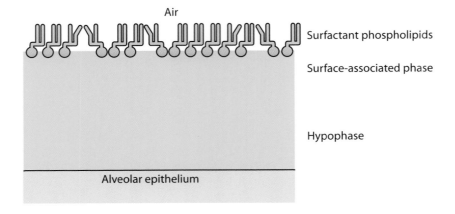

B

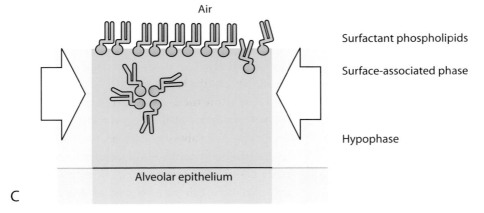

C

Figure 1.4 Surfactant.

A: Surfactant phospholipids are composed of two hydrophobic fatty acid tails joined to a hydrophilic head via glycerol and phosphoric acid. The most common phospholipid in surfactant is phosphatidylcholine, while the hydrophilic head is choline. Fatty acids in which all the bonds between adjacent carbon atoms are single are said to be 'saturated', and are physically flexible, allowing the molecule to pack in closely to its neighbour. Fatty acids in which one or more of the carbon–carbon bonds are double are said to be 'unsaturated'. These double bonds impart an inflexible angulation to the molecule, which prevents it from packing closely. The most effective phosphatidylcholine molecules are ones in which both fatty acid tails are saturated ('di-saturated'), such as dipalmitoyl-phosphatidylcholine.

B: The surfactant phospholipids float on the surface of the fluid lining the alveoli, with their hydrophilic heads in contact with the aqueous phase and their hydrophobic tails sticking in the air.

C: Expiration reduces the surface area of the alveolus, squeezing the bulkier and less effective phospholipids into the surface-associated phase. The remaining phospholipids, being predominantly disaturated, are more effective at reducing the surface tension and, as their concentration is increased, the surface tension is reduced further.

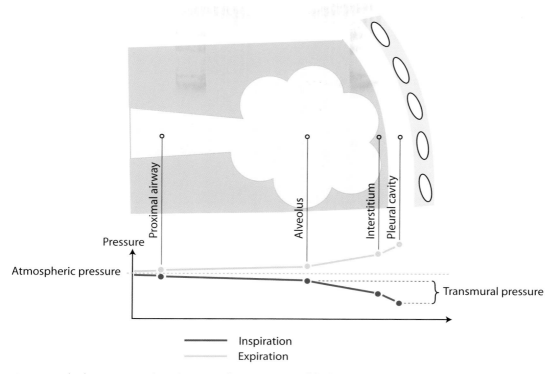

Figure 1.5 Absolute pressures along the airway during inspiration (blue) and expiration (green). During inspiration (blue) there is a pressure gradient between the proximal airway that is at atmospheric pressure at the mouth and the pleural space that is reversed during expiration.

out of the lung during normal breathing, a factor to be considered when comparison is made with mechanical modes of ventilation. Of course, much higher pressures *can* be achieved. Straining against a closed glottis, for example, can raise alveolar pressure to 190 cm H_2O, while maximal inspiratory effort can reduce pressure to as low as -140 cm H_2O.

Transmural pressure is defined as the difference between the pressure in the pleural cavity and that in the alveolus (Figure 1.5). To remain open, alveolar pressure must be greater than that of the surrounding tissue. During inspiration, intra-pleural pressure falls to a greater degree than alveolar pressure, and the transmural pressure gradient thus increases. Over the range of a normal breath, the relationship between transmural pressure gradient and lung volume is almost linear. This relationship holds true for

the alveoli, but the lower down in the lung the alveoli are, the more the distending transmural pressure gradient is counteracted by the weight of lung tissue compressing the alveolus from above. For this reason, dependent alveoli tend to have a smaller radius and are more likely to collapse.

The 'expandability' of the lung is known as its compliance. A high compliance means that the lung expands easily. The compliance of the normal respiratory system (lungs and thoracic cage) in upright humans is about 130 mL.cm H_2O^{-1}, while that of the lungs alone is roughly twice that value, demonstrating that half of the work of breathing during health simply goes into expanding the rib cage. When a positive pressure is applied to the respiratory system, such as during positive pressure ventilation, gas immediately starts to flow into the lungs, which then expand. However, while gas is flowing,

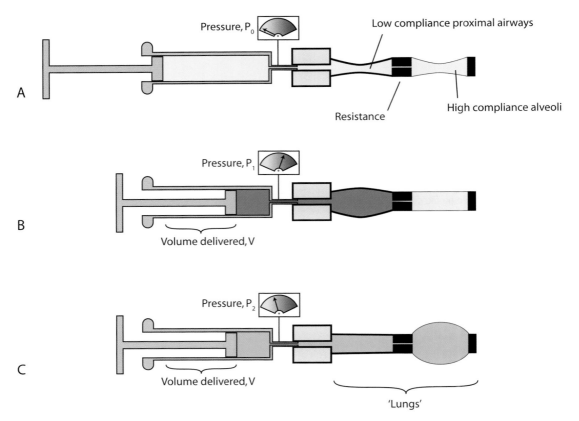

Figure 1.6 Two-compartment model of static and dynamic compliance.

A: In this model the ventilator is represented by the syringe, which is attached to the two-compartment lung model that consists of a low-compliance proximal chamber (the proximal airways) separated from a high-compliance distal chamber (the alveoli) by a fixed resistance. Prior to the onset of gas delivery (inspiration), the whole system is at the same pressure: P_0.

B: Gas is delivered to the lung model with a moderate increase in gas pressure in the syringe (the ventilator) and proximal chamber (the large airways) but with only a small increase in pressure in the distal chamber (the alveoli) as gas seeps through the resistance. Compliance measured just prior to the end of inspiration would be given by V/P_1.

C: Without the delivery of any further gas from the ventilator, the volume of the distal chamber continues to increase until the pressure in both chambers becomes the same. As gas redistributes from the high-pressure proximal chamber to the low-pressure distal chamber, the gas also expands slightly. At equilibrium, the compliance is given by V/P_2, which is larger than that calculated in B because $P_2 < P_1$.

the proximal airway pressure *must* be higher than alveolar pressure,[5] and the steepness of this pressure gradient will depend on the *resistance* to gas flow. Therefore, during inflation the ratio of volume change to inflating pressure (known as *dynamic compliance*) is lowered by the effect of resistance

to gas flow (Figure 1.6). At the end of inspiration, the proximal airway pressure immediately falls as gas delivery ceases (and with it, the resistive contribution to airway pressure) and then falls a little further as gas is redistributed from low-compliance proximal airways to high-compliance alveoli. There is also an associated small increase in total lung volume. The percentage of *total* change in lung volume

---

[5] Otherwise gas would not flow.

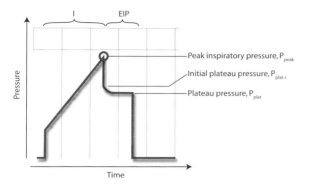

Figure 1.7 A pressure and time profile during volume-targeted constant flow mechanical ventilation.

For a delivered tidal volume of V mL, *dynamic* compliance is given by V/P_{peak} and *static* compliance is given by V/P_{plat}. The difference between P_{peak} and P_{plat-i} is due to airways resistance, while the difference between P_{plat-i} and P_{plat} is due to inter-alveolar gas redistribution (pendelluft) and hysteresis.

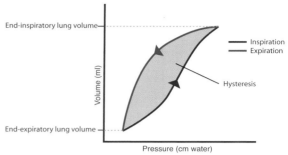

Figure 1.8 Inspiratory and expiratory volume/pressure loop during positive pressure inflation showing the phenomenon of hysteresis.

During inspiration (blue) of the lung, both pressure (x-axis) and volume (y-axis) increase, but this is non-linear. During expiration, the volume/pressure curve traces a different path. The area subtended by the inspiratory and expiratory paths represents the energy consumed by hysteresis.

when held at a set pressure is known as the lung's *static* compliance. Put another way, if a set volume of air is used to inflate a lung, pressure will rise accordingly, but (with lung volume held) will then gradually fall by some 25% or so (Figure 1.7). This effect is one of the contributing factors to a phenomenon known as *hysteresis* in which the lung traces a different path on an expiratory plot of lung pressure (x-axis) against volume (y-axis) than it does during inflation (Figure 1.8). Other contributors to hysteresis include the opening of previously collapsed alveoli during inflation,[6] displacement of lung blood at higher lung volumes, 'stress relaxation' of lung elastic fibres, and perhaps most importantly, the surface-area-dependent effect of surfactant in reducing surface tension. In practice, what this means is that at any given inflation pressure, lung volume will be greater during expiration than inspiration because the lungs are resistant to accepting a new higher volume, and then resistant to giving it up again.

---

[6] Commonly referred to as alveolar 'recruitment'.

LUNG VOLUMES

Total lung capacity (TLC) is the volume of intrapulmonary gas at the end of a maximal inspiration. Functional residual capacity (FRC) is the volume remaining in the lungs at the end of normal expiration that rises with body size (as determined by height) and on assumption of the upright posture. In mechanically ventilated subjects, FRC is also known as the end-expiratory lung volume (EELV). FRC is reduced when the lung is extrinsically compressed (from pleural fluid or abdominal distension), when lung elastic recoil is increased, or when the lungs are fibrosed.

Gas exchange

OXYGEN UPTAKE

Oxygenation is accomplished through the diffusion of oxygen down its partial pressure gradient (Box 1.1) from the alveolus, across the alveolar epithelium, and thence across the closely apposed capillary endothelium to the capillary blood, a distance of $<0.3\ \mu m$. The capacity to transfer oxygen from alveolus to red blood cell is determined by (1) the surface area for diffusion and (2) the ratio

Box 1.1 Diffusion and partial pressures

Diffusion describes the passive movement of a substance from an area of high concentration to one of low concentration. Diffusion also applies to gases, but in this case the motive force is the differential *partial pressure* of the gas. Partial pressure simply refers to the proportion of the total gas pressure that is attributable to the gas in question. As an example, if you have a 1-litre flask containing 800 mL of helium and 200 mL of oxygen at atmospheric pressure (101 kPa), the partial pressure of oxygen in the flask will be

$$\frac{200}{800 + 200} \times 101 = 20.2 \text{ kPa}.$$

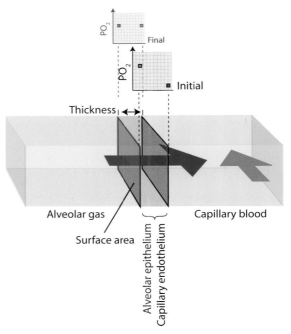

Figure 1.9 Factors that determine the capacity to transfer oxygen from alveolar gas to capillary blood. Oxygen diffusion (blue arrow) proceeds from alveolar gas (shown on the left) to capillary blood (shown on the right) across the intervening barrier of the alveolar epithelium and capillary endothelium, with capillary blood shown flowing away from the observer (red arrow). The capacity to transfer oxygen to red blood cells depends on the surface area for diffusion, and the ratio between the speed of diffusion and the length of time that the red cells spend in contact with the alveolus (referred to as the 'contact time').

The *speed* of diffusion is determined by the (1) initial partial pressure gradient of oxygen between alveolar gas and capillary blood; (2) the thickness of the barrier constituted by the alveolar epithelium, capillary endothelium and any other intervening tissue; and (3) the solubility of oxygen in this barrier.

The contact time is inversely proportional to the cardiac output and at rest is normally 0.75 seconds. Breathing air at sea level, red cells passing the alveolus are normally fully saturated after only 0.25 seconds, leaving a 'reserve' of 0.5 seconds. Diffusion limitation to oxygen transfer is therefore only seen with conditions that reduce the speed of diffusion (low alveolar partial pressure of oxygen or increased barrier thickness), reduce the contact time, or both. In trained athletes at maximum exertion the contact time falls to just over 0.25 seconds.

between the speed of diffusion and the alveolar contact time, which is the length of time the red cell remains in contact with the alveolus (Figure 1.9).

The *speed* of diffusion is determined by the partial pressure gradient of oxygen between alveolar gas and capillary blood, the thickness of the barrier between alveolus and capillary, and the solubility of oxygen in this barrier. Because there are no factors that influence oxygen's solubility under physiological conditions, the only sources of variation in the speed of diffusion are the partial pressure gradient of oxygen and the barrier thickness.

The partial pressure of oxygen in alveolar gas is not the same as the partial pressure of oxygen in inspired gas because alveolar gas contains two other constituents: carbon dioxide and water vapour. Therefore, breathing air at sea level, the alveolus contains four gases: nitrogen, oxygen, carbon dioxide and water vapour. The total pressure of these gases must equal atmospheric pressure (101 kPa):

$$P_{A_{N_2}} + P_{A_{O_2}} + P_{A_{CO_2}} + P_{A_{H_2O}} = 101 \, kPa. \quad (1.2)$$

The saturated vapour pressure of water at body temperature is 6.3 kPa, leaving 94.7 kPa of pressure for nitrogen, oxygen and carbon dioxide. Because nitrogen is not exchanged in the alveoli, it continues to occupy 79% of the remaining gas mixture, and so has an alveolar partial pressure of 74.8 kPa. This leaves the remaining 19.9 kPa for oxygen and carbon dioxide:

$$P_{A_{O_2}} + P_{A_{CO_2}} = 94.7 - 74.8 = 19.9 \ kPa. \quad (1.3)$$

Alveolar carbon dioxide diffuses from mixed venous blood into the alveolus until the partial pressures in the two compartments are the same. The partial pressure of carbon dioxide in arterial blood, about 4.5 kPa, therefore serves as a good estimate of the partial pressure of alveolar carbon dioxide. However, because the metabolism of fats produces less carbon dioxide than the metabolism of carbohydrate per unit volume of oxygen consumed, the alveolar partial pressure of carbon dioxide must be corrected for the respiratory quotient (RQ) when substituted into Equation 1.3:

$$P_{A_{O_2}} + \frac{P_{A_{CO_2}}}{RQ} = 19.9 \ kPa$$
$$\Rightarrow P_{A_{O_2}} + \frac{4.5}{0.8} = 19.9 \ kPa$$
$$\Rightarrow P_{A_{O_2}} = 19.9 - 5.625 = 14.275 \ kPa$$

In general, therefore, the partial pressure of alveolar oxygen is given by the equation:

$$P_{A_{O_2}} = \left[F_{I_{O_2}} \times (P_b - 6.3) \right] - \frac{Pa_{CO_2}}{0.8}. \quad (1.4)$$

When FIO_2 is the fractional concentration of oxygen in the inspired air, P_b is the barometric (atmospheric) pressure, and $PaCO_2$ is the arterial partial pressure of carbon dioxide, all measured in kPa. Oxygen partial pressure in mixed venous blood is roughly 5.3 kPa and, as calculated above, in alveolar gas is about 14.3 kPa. A diffusion gradient of about 8 kPa thus drives oxygen across the alveolar surface and into the blood under normal conditions.

The thickness of the diffusion barrier between the alveolus and the capillary is largely determined by the combined thickness of the alveolar epithelium and capillary endothelium, which is usually less than 0.3 μm. Increases in barrier thickness can be caused by the accumulation of fluid in the space between these two layers of cells, or by the accumulation of other material such as collagen (lung fibrosis) or malignant cells (carcinomatosis). Increased barrier thickness can also be caused by the accumulation of material on the alveolar surface itself, including fluid (pulmonary oedema), blood, pus or protein.

As the blood transits the capillary, it absorbs increasing amounts of oxygen, and the gradient-driving diffusion falls. However, haemoglobin's affinity for oxygen has unique characteristics (Figure 1.10), and blood oxygen tension nearly matches alveolar by the time that only a third of the capillary has been transited, which occurs in about 0.25 seconds at rest. The alveolar contact time is inversely proportional to cardiac output, and in trained athletes can fall to as little as 0.25 seconds, the time normally required for full saturation. Under these conditions, small decreases in the speed of diffusion, such as by exercising at altitude, can result in significant arterial desaturation.

Even when all the blood leaving the alveoli has an oxygen partial pressure that is the same as the alveolar partial pressure, the partial pressure of oxygen in arterial blood leaving the left ventricle is slightly lower because of the presence of an anatomical *shunt*. This shunt is caused by the dilution of arterialized blood that has come from the alveoli by true venous blood that drains into the pulmonary veins from the bronchial circulation (supplying the airways rather than alveoli) or from the left ventricular endocardium via the tiny thebesian veins. Such effects are normally only minor, causing a fall in anticipated arterial partial pressure of oxygen of just 0.5 to 0.8 kPa.

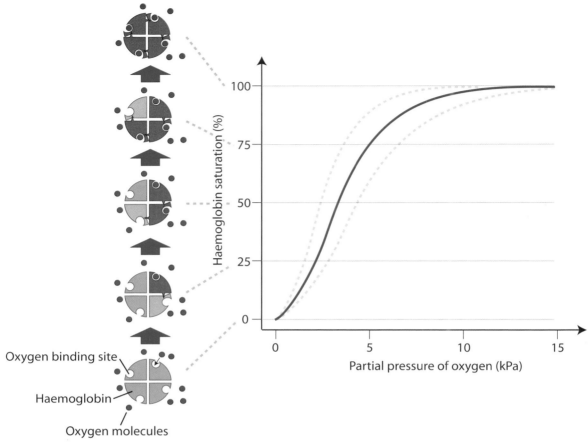

Figure 1.10 Intermolecular co-operation and the oxy-haemoglobin dissociation curve. A haemoglobin molecule consists of four chains, each with one binding site for molecular oxygen (O_2). When a molecule of oxygen occupies its binding site on any one of the chains, it provokes a change in the shape of that chain which *increases* the affinity of its neighbouring chain for oxygen (shown here in amber), making it easier for that chain to bind oxygen. This intermolecular co-operation accounts for the non-linear relationship between haemoglobin oxygen saturation and oxygen partial pressure, often referred to as the 'oxy-haemoglobin dissociation curve' (shown on the right). Haemoglobin's affinity for oxygen can be either increased (blue interrupted line) or decreased (pink interrupted line) by other factors, effects which are often referred to as 'left-shift' or 'right-shift', respectively. Increased temperature and acidosis decrease haemoglobin's affinity for oxygen (right-shift), while decreased temperature and alkalosis do the reverse. Fetal variants of haemoglobin bind oxygen with greater affinity than do adult variants, making it possible for oxygen to be transferred from maternal to fetal haemoglobin in the placenta.

Causes of low arterial partial pressure of oxygen

As described previously, the arterial partial pressure of oxygen is derived from the mixture in the left side of the heart of blood having a range of partial pressures of oxygen, depending on its source. Blood leaving normally ventilated alveoli *with optimal oxygen transfer* will have a partial pressure of oxygen

that is determined by the *alveolar* partial pressure of oxygen, as shown in Equation (1.4) above. This tells us that under these conditions, the principal variables involved in determining PO_2 are (1) the fractional concentration of oxygen in the inspired gas (FIO_2), (2) the barometric pressure of the inspired gas and (3) the alveolar partial pressure of carbon dioxide.

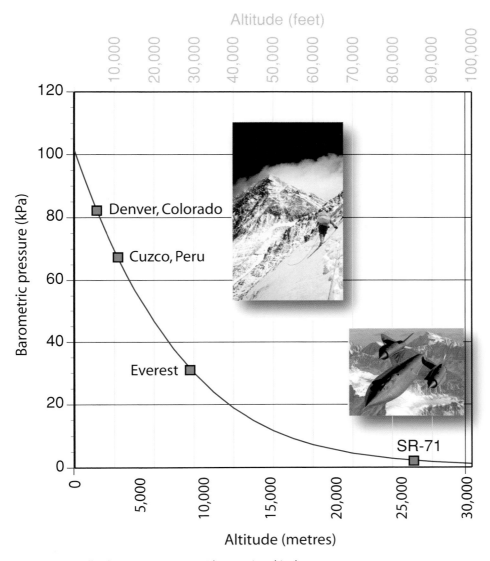

Figure 1.11 A fall in barometric pressure with increasing altitude.

The barometric (atmospheric) pressure falls non-linearly with increasing altitude. The highest permanent human habitation is believed to be La Rinconada, Peru, at 16 700 feet (5100 metres).

FiO_2. Low fractional concentration of inspired oxygen is not usually a problem in patients receiving mechanical ventilation, though it did cause the death of a child in the UK as recently as 2001 when they were ventilated with a hypoxic gas mixture from an old anaesthetic machine. Modern anaesthetic machines and intensive care ventilators are designed to be incapable of delivering hypoxic gas mixtures, though old machines which can do so remain in use in many countries.

Barometric pressure. Low barometric pressure is never a problem in Europe except during aerial transport (see Chapter 16), but in other parts of the world this may be a significant factor (Figure 1.11).

Hypoventilation. If oxygen consumption in peripheral tissues remains constant, so too must the quantity of oxygen extracted from the alveolus. In profound hypoventilation, the amount of oxygen being delivered to the alveolus will fall, as will the ratio of delivery to extraction. As a result, alveolar (and thus arterial) partial pressure of oxygen will fall. This phenomenon will be compounded by a rise in alveolar carbon dioxide tension due to failure of clearance, which will cause a further fall in alveolar PO_2.

Diffusion limitation. The three factors above have all assumed optimal oxygen transfer between alveolar gas and capillary blood, but as discussed above, this assumes a normal ratio between the speed of diffusion and the alveolar contact time. A reduction of contact time (with an increase in cardiac output) or reduction in the speed of diffusion caused by an increased diffusion distance can also cause a low arterial partial pressure of oxygen.

Besides the normal 'anatomical' shunts that contribute venous blood to the arterial pool described above, two other sources of shunt can contribute to arterial hypoxaemia: pathological and alveolar shunts.

Pathological shunts. These are caused by abnormal connections between the right and left sides of the heart, allowing venous blood to join arterial blood in the left ventricle without passing through the lungs. When arising during fetal development, these shunts are usually situated within the heart itself and are caused by failure in the development of midline structures such as the septa between the atria or ventricles.

Similar defects can occasionally arise in adulthood following infarction of the septal tissue or as a consequence of cardiac trauma. Even less commonly, a right-to-left shunt can arise in adulthood when either surgery or pulmonary disease allows blood to pass through a patent foramen ovale. Congenital intra-pulmonary shunts are rare and are usually associated with massive intra-pulmonary arterio-venous malformations. Intra-pulmonary shunts acquired in adulthood are also very uncommon, but can occur in patients with severe liver disease.

Alveolar shunts. So far, the discussion has assumed that blood draining from the alveoli has come from alveoli with completely normal ventilation and perfusion, and is therefore optimally oxygenated. In reality, both alveolar ventilation and perfusion can range from normal to none (Figure 1.12). Thus at one end of the spectrum there are alveoli with normal ventilation but no perfusion (so-called 'dead space'), and at the other end there are alveoli with normal perfusion but no ventilation (a so-called 'true shunt'). With respect to oxygenation, it is the *perfused units with markedly reduced or absent ventilation* which are important, as these act as 'shunts' through which blood can travel from systemic veins to systemic arteries without becoming oxygenated. The impact of a shunt on arterial haemoglobin oxygen saturation is directly proportional to the size of the shunt in terms of blood flow. So, for example, if 80% of pulmonary venous blood comes from ventilated alveoli with an SaO_2 of 98% and 20% comes from non-ventilated alveoli with an SaO_2 of 75%, the resulting SaO_2 is calculated as

$$(0.8 \times 98) + (0.2 \times 75) = 93.4\%. \tag{1.5}$$

This calculation allows the size of the shunt to be estimated (Box 1.2). It is also worth noting that because the blood coming from ventilated alveoli has almost the same PO_2 as alveolar gas, there is almost no capacity for these alveoli to absorb additional oxygen in order to compensate for blood coming from alveoli that are poorly ventilated (low $\dot{V}/\dot{Q}$) or not ventilated at all (a true shunt). In contrast, venous blood only loses 10 to 15% of its carbon dioxide content in passing through ventilated alveoli. In this case, failure to clear carbon dioxide from blood passing through unventilated alveoli is easily compensated by an increase in carbon dioxide elimination from blood passing through ventilated

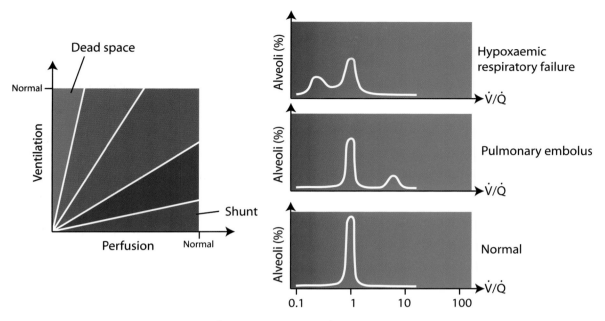

Figure 1.12 Spectrum of alveolar ventilation ($\dot{V}$) to alveolar perfusion ($\dot{Q}$).

The graph on the left represents the possible relationship between ventilation on the y-axis and perfusion on the x-axis for pulmonary alveoli and for convenience identifies five colour-coded zones. These range from alveoli with normal perfusion but little or no perfusion (blue), through those with normal perfusion and normal perfusion (blue-green), to those with little or no perfusion but normal ventilation (green). Using the same colour-code, the distribution of these V/Q ratios is shown on the right for a subject with normal lungs (bottom), a patient with a small pulmonary embolus (middle) and a patient with severe hypoxaemic respiratory failure (top).

alveoli. This explains why patients with acute lung disorders develop arterial hypoxaemia long before developing hypercarbia, if indeed they ever do.

Even in healthy lungs without alveoli that are either unventilated or unperfused, there is a natural variation in ventilation and perfusion due to the effects of gravity.

Ventilation inequality. Prior to the onset of inspiration, alveoli will have varying end-expiratory volumes depending on the local trans-pulmonary pressure. Because of the weight of the lung parenchyma and the blood contained within it, the pleural pressure becomes progressively less negative in a vertical gradient from top to bottom.[7] Consequently the trans-pulmonary pressure, which is the difference between alveolar and pleural pressure, also declines in a vertical gradient from top to bottom. Alveoli in the lowest part of the lung will therefore have the smallest end-expiratory volume, while alveoli in the highest part of the lung will have the largest end-expiratory volume. The relationship we see between pressure and volume for the whole lung also applies to each alveolus. This means that at the start of inspiration there is a vertical compliance gradient, with the most compliant alveoli above and the least compliant below, which means that for a small change in pleural pressure the alveoli above will increase in volume the most, while those at the bottom will increase the least. In the middle of inspiration, with each alveolus having moved up its own volume/pressure curve, the alveoli at the top of the

---

[7] This applies whatever the position of the subject – erect, supine, prone or lying on one side.

Box 1.2 How to estimate total shunt

Total shunt assumes that arterial blood is composed of a mixture of blood from only two sources, blood from 'perfect' alveoli and shunted blood never exposed to alveolar oxygen. If CaO_2 is the oxygen content of arterial blood, $C\bar{v}O_2$ is the oxygen content of mixed venous blood and $Cc'O_2$ is the oxygen content in end-capillary blood from 'perfect' alveoli, which can be estimated from Equation 1.4 and the oxy-haemoglobin dissociation curve (Figure 6.1), then

$$Ca_{O_2} = x\,(Cc'_{O_2}) + y\,(C\bar{v}_{O_2})$$

$$\text{where } x + y = 1.$$

This equation can be re-arranged and solved for x:

$$x = \frac{Cc'_{O_2} - Ca_{O_2}}{Cc'_{O_2} - C\bar{v}_{O_2}} \qquad (1.6)$$

With a patient breathing 40% oxygen at sea level, a PaO_2 of 8 kPa, SaO_2 of 90.6%, $PaCO_2$ of 6.4 kPa, mixed venous PO_2 of 5.2 kPa and mixed venous SO_2 of 73.6%, we calculate the shunt as follows.

First, we calculate the alveolar partial pressure of oxygen from Equation 1.4:

$$P_{A_{O_2}} = [F_{I_{O_2}} \times (Pb - 6.3)] - \frac{P_{a_{CO_2}}}{0.8}$$

$$P_{A_{O_2}} = [0.4 \times (101.325 - 6.3)] - \frac{6.4}{0.8} = 30.$$

From the oxy-haemoglobin dissociation curve, the estimated saturation of this blood would be 99.9%, and therefore the oxygen content (Equation 6.5) would be

$$Cc'_{O_2} = (15 \times 1.34 \times 0.999)$$

$$+ (0.0225 \times 30) = 20.75.$$

Then we substitute this value, and the other calculated values, into Equation 1.6:

$$y = \frac{20.75 - 18.39}{20.75 - 14.91} = 0.404$$

This, based on the assumptions outlined above, puts the shunt in this case at 40.4%.

lung are now *less* compliant, while the alveoli below are *more* compliant. Consequently, in this phase of inspiration the same small change in pleural pressure now causes a much smaller increase in alveolar volume in alveoli above and a much larger increase in alveolar volume in alveoli below. Finally, at the end of inspiration, the very lowest alveoli start to become more compliant and undergo the largest volume change (Figure 1.13).

Perfusion. Blood flow also varies in different regions of the lung. In the upper regions (zone 1),[8] alveolar pressure exceeds arterial pressure and units receive no perfusion (Figure 1.14). In the mid-lung (zone 2), arterial pressure exceeds alveolar, and both are greater than venous pressure. Flow will thus depend on the degree of compression of the pulmonary capillaries by alveolar pressure. The greater the arterial pressure, the wider open the vessels are held, and flow increases. In the lowest parts of the lung (zone 3), both venous and arterial pressure exceed alveolar pressure. The vessel between artery and vein will thus be held wide open, and flow will relate to the A-V pressure difference.

Meanwhile, a number of factors can also cause variation in perfusion. On a macroscopic scale, blood flow turns out to be relatively homogeneous throughout the lung, but will always tend to be greater per unit lung volume in the more dependent part of the lung. This, of course, tends to lead to better ventilation–perfusion matching during spontaneous ventilation as dependent areas also tend to be better ventilated. On a smaller scale, microvascular or macrovascular thrombotic occlusion of vessels, or vasoconstriction as a response to regional hypoxia or to endothelial dysfunction, may all cause regional falls in blood flow.

---

[8] These are sometimes referred to as *West's zones* after Professor John West of the University of California, San Diego, who first described them.

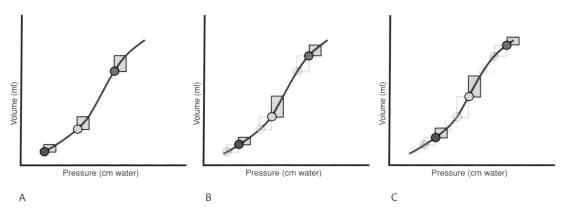

A   B   C

Figure 1.13 Vertical ventilation inequality.

A: Prior to the onset of inspiration, alveoli in different parts of the lung are on different parts of the volume/pressure curve because of the vertical gradient of trans-pulmonary pressure. Alveoli in the highest part of the lung (red), exposed to the largest trans-pulmonary pressure, have the biggest resting volume, with alveoli below (yellow and green) having progressively smaller volumes. At the beginning of inspiration, and following a modest increase in trans-pulmonary pressure, which is the same for all alveoli, the alveoli undergo a volume change that is determined by their position on the volume/pressure curve. Poorly compliant alveoli at the bottom (green) and middle (yellow) of the lung undergo small or moderate increases in volume, while alveoli near the top (red) undergo a significant increase in volume.

B: As inspiration progresses, the compliance of alveoli near the top of the lungs starts to fall, while the compliance of alveoli below starts to increase. Now with a uniform increase in trans-pulmonary pressure, alveoli near the top increase by only a small amount, while alveoli in the middle undergo a much larger increase in volume.

C: Towards the end of inspiration, the compliance of the lowest alveoli now starts to increase while the compliance of alveoli near the top continues to decrease. Now the largest volume changes are in the middle and lower parts of the lung, with only very modest increases in lung volume at the top.

Together, regional differences in the ventilation and perfusion of lung units will lead to some variation in $\dot{V}/\dot{Q}$ across these units, with values being higher towards the apex, and lower towards the bases. However, the fact that nearly all perfused lung units are also ventilated means that there is no significant alveolar shunt, and arterial oxygen tension, when allowing for anatomical shunt, is close to that predicted of a 'perfect lung'. While $\dot{V}/\dot{Q}$ matching may prove near ideal and homogeneous across lung units in health, this is not the case in disease. Here, vascular occlusion, vasoconstriction, endothelial dysfunction and vessel compression by greatly expanded alveolar units may all cause marked inhomogeneity in $\dot{V}/\dot{Q}$ matching. This may cause marked hypoxaemia. Strategies for improving oxygenation are discussed in Chapter 3.

Carbon dioxide clearance

Like oxygen, carbon dioxide, which is continually produced in the tissues and in the lungs, diffuses down a partial pressure gradient but in the opposite direction, from pulmonary arterial blood to alveolar gas. As with oxygen, the blood leaving the alveolus will have the same partial pressure of carbon dioxide as the alveolar gas. In the absence of alveolar ventilation, carbon dioxide accumulates in the blood, with a concentration rising by the rate of production divided by the volume of distribution. To prevent the accumulation of carbon dioxide and maintain a steady arterial concentration, alveolar clearance of carbon dioxide must match systemic production. So, for example, if the body is producing $200 \, mL.min^{-1}$ of carbon dioxide, alveolar ventilation must also eliminate $200 \, mL.min^{-1}$ of carbon

Box 1.3 Calculation of total dead space

As dead space, by definition, does not contribute to the elimination of carbon dioxide, its volume in proportion to the tidal volume can be calculated because we know that

CO_2 eliminated in alveolar gas

= CO_2 eliminated in mixed expired gas.

In other words

$$P_{ACO_2} \times \dot{V}_A = P\bar{E}_{CO_2} \times \dot{V}_T$$

which can be rearranged as follows:

$$P_{ACO_2} \times \dot{V}_A = P\bar{E}_{CO_2} \times \dot{V}_T$$

$$\frac{P_{ACO_2}}{P\bar{E}_{CO_2}} = \frac{\dot{V}_T}{\dot{V}_A},$$

but

$$\dot{V}_T = \dot{V}_A + \dot{V}_D$$

so

$$\frac{\dot{V}_D}{\dot{V}_T} = \frac{P_{ACO_2} - P\bar{E}_{CO_2}}{P_{ACO_2}}.$$

However, because we can assume that the *arterial* partial pressure of carbon dioxide is a reasonable approximation to the *alveolar* partial pressure of carbon dioxide, this becomes

$$\frac{\dot{V}_D}{\dot{V}_T} = \frac{P_{a_{CO_2}} - P\bar{E}_{CO_2}}{P_{a_{CO_2}}}. \qquad (1.7)$$

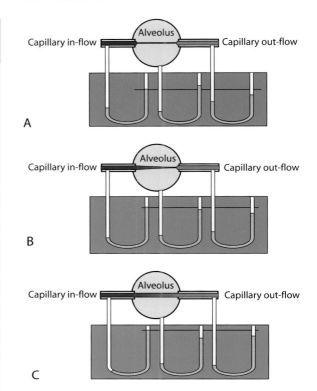

Figure 1.14 West's zones.

A: *Zone 1*. Vertically, at the top of the lung, end-inspiratory alveolar pressure exceeds both pulmonary arteriolar pressure (capillary in-flow) and pulmonary venular (capillary out-flow) pressures, and trans-capillary blood flow only occurs during end-expiration and early inspiration.

B: *Zone 2*. In the middle of the lung, pulmonary arteriolar pressure (capillary in-flow) is greater than end-inspiratory alveolar pressure which is, in turn, greater than pulmonary venular (capillary out-flow) pressure. Here trans-capillary blood flow ceases near end-inspiration and resumes during early expiration.

C: *Zone 3*. In the lung base, both pulmonary arteriolar pressure (capillary in-flow) and pulmonary venular (capillary out-flow) pressure are greater than end-inspiratory alveolar pressure and therefore trans-capillary blood flow occurs throughout the respiratory cycle.

dioxide, and the volume of alveolar gas used to do this determines the alveolar concentration of carbon dioxide as well as the arterial partial pressure of carbon dioxide (Figure 1.15):

$$\frac{CO_2 \text{ Production(mL/min)}}{\text{Alveolar ventilation(mL/min)}}$$
$$\times 101.325 = P_{A_{O_2}} \approx P_{a_{O_2}}. \qquad (1.8)$$

However, not all of the inspired gas contributes to the *alveolar* ventilation. Some of the inspired gas may ventilate alveoli that have no perfusion (that is, physiological dead space), some will occupy parts of the respiratory tract that do not

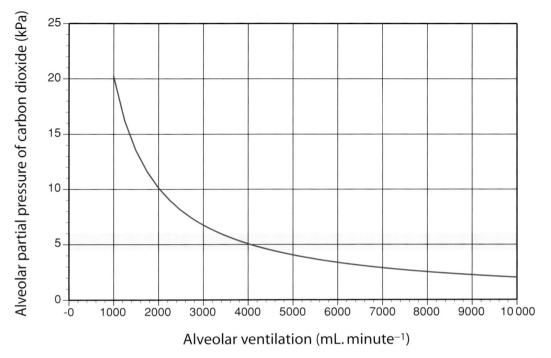

Figure 1.15 Alveolar ventilation and resulting alveolar partial pressure of carbon dioxide. The plot shows alveolar ventilation in mL.min^{-1} (x-axis) and the resulting alveolar partial pressure of carbon dioxide in kPa (y-axis) in someone producing 200 mL.min^{-1} of carbon dioxide, with the normal range of alveolar partial pressure of carbon dioxide shaded in green (4.5 to 6 kPa).

participate in gas exchange[9] (anatomical dead space), and, in patients receiving respiratory support, some will occupy the airway interface (equipment dead space). Because only the alveolar volume (VA) contributes to carbon dioxide clearance, the tidal volume (VT) required will be determined by the size of the total dead space (VD):

$$V_T = V_A + V_{D_A} + V_{D_{anat}} + V_{D_{eqpt}} \qquad (1.9)$$

but

$$V_{D_A} + V_{D_{anat}} + V_{D_{eqpt}} = V_D;$$

therefore

$$V_T = V_A + V_D. \qquad (1.10)$$

Equation 1.10 applies to each breath, but expressed as a rate, both sides of the equation must be multiplied by the respiratory rate:

$$f V_T = f V_A + f V_D, \qquad (1.11)$$

subtracting $f V_D$ from both sides of the equation:

$$f V_T - f V_D = f V_A \qquad (1.12)$$

but

$$f V_A = \dot{V}_A$$

therefore

$$f V_T - f V_D = \dot{V}_A \qquad (1.13)$$
$$f (V_T - V_D) = \dot{V}_A. \qquad (1.14)$$

A number of important observations can be made from these results. First, from Equation 1.8

---

[9] That is, the nose, mouth, pharynx, trachea, bronchi and all the bronchial divisions down to the bronchioles.

we can see that the greater the systemic production of carbon dioxide, the greater the alveolar ventilation required to maintain a constant arterial partial pressure of carbon dioxide. Second, from Equation 1.13 we can see that the greater the dead space (V_D), the greater must be either the tidal volume (V_T) or the respiratory rate (f) so that constant alveolar minute ventilation will be maintained. The ratio of dead space to minute ventilation can be estimated from the $PaCO_2$ and the partial pressure of carbon dioxide in end-expiratory gas (see Box 1.3). Strategies for improving carbon dioxide elimination are discussed in Chapter 4.

SUMMARY

1. The airways must humidify inspired gases and remove particulate pollution.
2. The lungs have a dual role in clearing carbon dioxide and providing oxygen.
3. Lung compliance represents the 'distensibility' of the lung and alters in disease.
4. Compliance may also differ between lung units.
5. Homogeneous and matching ventilation and perfusion of all lung units would offer perfect gas exchange.
6. There is a heterogeneity of ventilation/perfusion matching in normal lungs, and this may worsen in disease.
7. Poor $\dot{V}/\dot{Q}$ matching causes hypoxaemia and may also increase the minute ventilation required for carbon dioxide clearance.

FURTHER READING

- Nunn JF, Lumb AB. *Nunn's Applied Respiratory Physiology*, 6th Edn. Butterworth-Heinemann Ltd, London.

Chapter 2

Assessing the need for ventilatory support

MICK NIELSEN AND IAIN MACKENZIE

Intensive care medicine has its origins in the successful use of positive pressure ventilation to treat acute respiratory failure associated with the poliomyelitis epidemic in Copenhagen in 1952, and mechanical ventilation remains a cornerstone in the provision of modern life support. This chapter will focus on assessing the need for ventilatory support in seriously ill patients in acute wards, emergency departments and critical care units; it will not consider ventilatory support during anaesthesia and surgery.

The need for ventilatory support is probably the commonest reason for patients requiring admission to critical care units, and the provision of mechanical ventilation has major resource implications. It also carries significant complications in the form of ventilator-associated pneumonia, ventilator-induced lung injury, barotrauma and adverse circulatory effects, all of which can contribute to both morbidity and mortality. Any associated requirement for sedative drugs has additional undesirable effects. Although a patient may appear to 'need' ventilatory support, it must also be considered whether, for that individual, it would be appropriate.

Besides those who work in intensive care, there are many others who encounter patients who appear to 'need' mechanical ventilation, such as ambulance crews or staff working in emergency depart-

ments, respiratory wards, or acute medical or surgical wards. However, with the exception of those who work in intensive care, none of these other groups will appreciate the consequences of instituting mechanical ventilation in a patient for whom this option was inappropriate. For those not involved in intensive care, insight into why early involvement of an experienced intensive care clinician is vital will be provided by a brief discussion of the factors that contribute to the decision to offer, or withhold, mechanical ventilation. This insight is important not just for identifying those for whom mechanical ventilation is not an option, but also because early, appropriate intervention may actually avert the need for ventilation entirely. In an emergency situation when there is doubt about the need for ventilation, treatment should be started and then the situation reviewed once the patient is more stable.

The principle of reversibility

For a few patients in a few countries, long-term mechanical ventilation is a service that can be provided either at home, or in an appropriate care setting. When available, it is then up to the patient to make an informed decision and accept or decline this option (see Chapter 19). For the majority, however, long-term ventilatory support is either unavailable or inappropriate, and under these

> ## Box 2.1
>
> A 23-year-old female presented to the haematology ward with severe and rapidly progressive stridor 6 months after a bone marrow transplant for acute lymphoblastic leukaemia. Plain radiography and urgent computed tomography showed massive upper mediastinal lymphadenopathy with severe compression of the mid-portion of the trachea. Although the most likely diagnosis was recurrence of her original disease, it was felt that this could not be confirmed or refuted before the airway compromise became fatal, and a decision was made to intubate and ventilate the patient. Within 48 hours the diagnosis of recurrent leukaemia was made, which was, in the opinion of her haematologists, untreatable and inevitably fatal. Following discussion between the intensive care team, the haematologists and the girl's family, her sedation was lightened. Her prognosis was explained to her by members of the haematology team that she knew and trusted. The patient then requested to see certain members of her family and wrote letters to her friends. After a further 48 hours, she declared that she was ready to die. She was sedated, extubated, and died peacefully.

circumstances mechanical ventilation should be instituted *only* if the condition precipitating the need for mechanical ventilation is reversible.

The principle of quality and length of life after intensive care

A prolonged period of ventilatory support, with all its discomforts and complications, is a price that many, but not all, patients would find worth paying *if* at the end of it they are able to return to a quality of life that they would find acceptable. A minority of patients have the foresight to make their wishes in this regard known, either in the form of a living will, or by making their opinion widely known among their friends and relatives. As quality of life is a uniquely personal experience, it is impossible to make a judgement as to whether someone else would find a particular set of circumstances acceptable. Therefore, in the absence of clear indications from the patient, or absolute certainty about the ultimate extent of a patient's disability, few clinicians would withhold mechanical ventilation purely on the grounds of 'quality of life'. A closely related, but quite distinct, issue is the question of 'quantity' of life, or an estimation of the patient's chances of actually surviving her period of mechanical ventilation and thereafter. For those with an inevitably fatal

disease and a short life expectancy, there are very few circumstances in which mechanical ventilation is appropriate (Box 2.1). More challenging situations occur when mechanical ventilation is deemed futile because the chances of survival are very low. The questions arise, for example, as to how low the chances of survival have to be for mechanical ventilation to be considered futile (under 5%? Under 1%?) or whether it matters that the patient is only 25 years old, or that his injuries are self-inflicted.

The principle of availability

When more people need to travel on a bus than there are seats to accommodate them, there is always the option to stand for the duration of the journey. When there are more patients who need mechanical ventilation than there are mechanical ventilators, someone must go without. Of course, the situation is rarely quite as stark as that, but the principle nevertheless applies. Inevitably, therefore, the intensive care clinician will be, to some extent, balancing the needs of her existing patients with those of the patient for whom mechanical ventilation is being considered.

Which patients need ventilatory support?

Patients requiring ventilatory support fall into two broad categories. First, there are those with

Table 2.1 Indications for mechanical ventilation other than respiratory failure

1. Patients following major surgery with whom:
   a. issues relating to circulatory instability, metabolic acidosis, or hypothermia may need to be addressed.
   b. intra-operative bleeding can only be controlled by physical tamponade with large packs or dressings and who will need to return to theatre for these to be removed.
   c. a number of operative procedures are required over consecutive days.
2. Patients in whom mechanical ventilation is required to assist with the control of raised intracranial pressure, such as following traumatic brain injury or severe hepatic encephalopathy.
3. Patients whose airway needs to be protected from the following:
   a. aspiration, usually in the context of a diminished level of consciousness, such as following deliberate overdose, or who have received large doses of benzodiazepines or barbiturates to control seizures or agitation.
   b. obstruction from soft tissue swelling in the structures that constitute the upper airway or adjacent structures (for example, facial trauma, acute epiglottitis, laryngeal tumours, acute bacterial pharyngitis, compression from an enlarged thyroid or lymph nodes in the upper mediastinum or throat).
4. Patients who need to be kept motionless when:
   a. they are too agitated or confused to co-operate with critical diagnostic imaging (usually computed tomography or magnetic resonance imaging) or diagnostic procedures (for example, lumbar puncture).
   b. they have unstable fractures of the spine prior to surgical stabilization.
   c. in the rare situation a surgical repair is too delicate or could be compromised by coughing or movement.
   d. the even rarer situation of tetanus occurs.

established or impending respiratory failure. This may arise because of failure of the 'ventilatory pump' or of intra-pulmonary gas-exchanging mechanisms, or, more frequently, of both. These will be discussed in more detail below. Second, there are those who need support for reasons not directly related to the respiratory system (Table 2.1).

Figure 2.1 summarizes the mechanisms by which acute respiratory failure can develop. Failure of the ventilatory pump – essentially, the bellows mechanism responsible for moving air into and out of the lungs – causes alveolar hypoventilation and thus hypercapnia and hypoxaemia (type II respiratory failure). Acute respiratory failure can result from interference with any part of the chain of events involved in normal tidal breathing. This may occur in the respiratory centres in the medulla (where respiratory drive originates), in the motor pathways in the spinal cord and lower motor neurones, at the neuromuscular junction, in the inspiratory muscles themselves, in the chest wall or in the airway.

If alveoli collapse or fill with cardiogenic oedema (as in left ventricular failure), or non-cardiogenic oedema (as in acute lung injury or acute respiratory distress syndrome), ventilation-perfusion matching in the lung fails and hypoxaemia results (type I respiratory failure).

In the critically ill, one rarely sees either of these types of respiratory failure in their pure form and patients most often present with a combination of the two. For example, unless rapidly treated, the patient with pure respiratory depression and hypoventilation from an opiate overdose will develop alveolar atelectasis, sputum retention and possibly pneumonia, and hence elements of type I respiratory failure. Correspondingly, if a patient with type I respiratory failure from pneumonia fails to respond to treatment, the reduced lung compliance and increased work of breathing may lead to inspiratory muscle fatigue and elements of type II respiratory failure. In extreme cases, the work of breathing may become unsustainable and, if

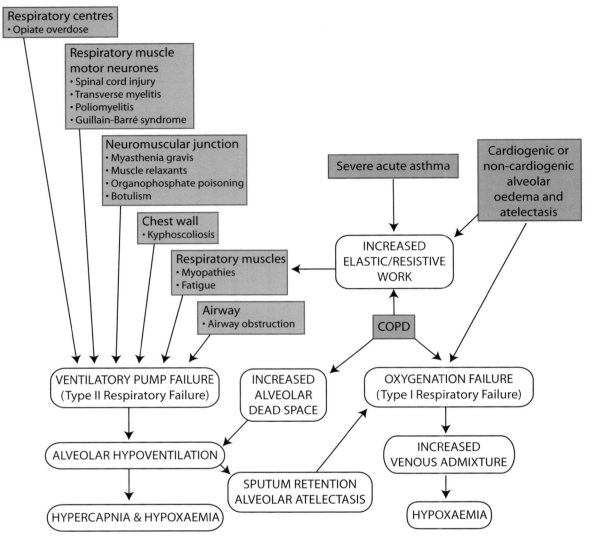

Figure 2.1 Mechanisms producing acute respiratory failure and COPD.

not rapidly relieved, this will result in respiratory arrest.

Muscle fatigue is defined as a condition in which there is loss of the capacity to develop skeletal muscle force or velocity resulting from muscle activity under load and which is reversible with rest.[1] The ability to recover with rest distinguishes muscle fatigue from muscle weakness, in which the capacity of a muscle to generate force is impaired even when rested. In the clinical setting, especially in patients with neurological disorders, it can be difficult to distinguish between respiratory muscle weakness and fatigue because weak muscles are susceptible to fatigue. Both weakness and fatigue may cause respiratory muscle failure.

Patients with chronically high respiratory loads, as well as those with asthma and chronic obstructive pulmonary disease (COPD) who can experience a sudden increase in load, are clearly at risk of respiratory muscle fatigue. In others, fatigue may

Table 2.2 The aims of ventilatory support

- Improve oxygenation and carbon dioxide clearance
- Reduce or eliminate excessive work of breathing
- Minimize the risk of complications

result from failure in the delivery of oxygen and substrate to respiratory muscles, as in septic or cardiogenic shock.

It is important to appreciate that while supplementary oxygen may treat the hypoxaemia associated with either 'pump failure' or 'lung failure', it does nothing to relieve the increased work of breathing in type I respiratory failure or to correct the hypercapnia in type II respiratory failure. The latter can only be accomplished through an increase in alveolar ventilation.

The aims of ventilatory support

In the clinical settings described above, the aims of ventilatory support can be summarized as follows (Table 2.2):

- To improve oxygenation and carbon dioxide clearance through preventing and reversing alveolar atelectasis, reducing venous admixture and enhancing alveolar ventilation.
- To reduce, or eliminate entirely, excessive work in breathing by off-loading the respiratory muscles. This may be achieved by improving lung compliance through alveolar recruitment, by reducing airways resistance with bronchodilators or by assisting or substituting mechanical support for spontaneous respiration. In patients with respiratory muscle fatigue, this off-loading, with a period of rest, may allow time for recovery of function. Whereas normally, at rest, the work of breathing accounts for only around 2% of total oxygen consumption, in some patients with severe lung pathology, the respiratory muscles may account for as much as 50% of metabolic requirements.[2]

In such situations, in which oxygen delivery is compromised, mechanical ventilation may also release significant amounts of oxygen for use by other tissues by reducing the oxygen cost of breathing.

- To minimize the risk of complications, such as ventilator-induced lung injury, ventilator-associated pneumonia, the side effects of sedative or relaxant drugs used to facilitate ventilation, or equipment failure.
- To use, when present, an endotracheal tube or tracheostomy to maintain and protect the airway and allow more effective clearance of secretions.

Clinical assessment

It is impossible to define exactly the point at which ventilatory support should begin. A wide variety of factors must be taken into account, and there is no substitute for an assessment by an experienced clinician. An element of anticipation is important, and the decision to intubate and ventilate should be made before the patient is *in extremis*. Early intubation is preferable to an emergency intervention when the patient will be less stable, more vulnerable to serious hypoxia and hypotension, and more likely to aspirate. If in doubt, the patient should be moved to where he can be closely monitored and where staff with the necessary airway skills are immediately available.

If the patient needs to be transferred between hospitals for further management, then consideration should be given to intubating him/her beforehand rather than having to do it urgently, in transit, in less than ideal circumstances. Similarly, if the patient is due to undergo imaging in an x-ray department, which means rapid access may be difficult, then the case for early intubation is again strengthened.

Given the mechanisms which underlie the two types of respiratory failure, assessment of the need for ventilatory support will focus on the two corresponding areas: the functioning of the ventilatory pump and the efficiency of intrapul-monary gas exchange. This part of the chapter will therefore concentrate on those aspects of the clinical assessment which identify actual or impending respiratory muscle fatigue or weakness and which assess the adequacy of ventilation and gas exchange.

General. When available, the patient's history should give some idea of the underlying pathology and therefore its likely course and rate of progression. Speaking directly to the patient contributes substantially to the assessment by clarifying features such as the level of arousal, cognitive function, the pattern of respiration and the patient's ability to answer in sentences, short phrases, single words or perhaps only non-verbally. Changes in the capacity for speech can be a useful objective sign of improvement or deterioration. Listening to the patient is not, of course, restricted to speech; the sound (or lack) of his breath sounds should be noted. For example, a high-pitched inspiratory noise suggests extrathoracic airway obstruction, while an expiratory wheeze is a sign of the narrowing of the small airway often, but not always, due to bronchospasm. The patient's physical appearance may also contribute to the assessment. Deep central cyanosis is difficult to miss, but a more modest degree of central cyanosis is an unreliable clinical sign. Tremor or involuntary twitches of the hands and arms might suggest hypercapnia, especially if the patient's hands are warm and sweaty. The pulse and its character provide additional information. A rapid, bounding pulse would be consistent with either hypercapnia or sepsis, while a thready or impalpable pulse might suggest shock; with gentle pressure, a pulse that becomes impalpable during inspiration indicates significant respiratory paradox, a sign of severe bronchospasm. The fingers might reveal clubbing or nicotine stains, and evidence of chronic lung disease can be confirmed by a barrel chest, cachexia and signs of premature ageing.

Inspection also reveals the effort the patient is making to breathe and can give the clinician a very good idea of whether he is near, or indeed has reached, his physical limit. Signs of significant respiratory work are easy to spot, with flaring of the nostrils, the use of accessory respiratory muscles, a tracheal tug and marked intercostal recession. As a patient approaches the limits of his respiratory capacity, his behaviour may be influenced by his age and previous experience. Younger patients, for example, may tend to become agitated and combative, while older patients are more likely to become progressively more obtunded.

Respiratory pattern – rate and tidal volume. Respiratory rate is easily measured, and tachypnoea has long been recognized as an extremely sensitive marker of a worsening clinical situation.[3, 4] However, it is a very non-specific sign and other evidence of a respiratory cause should be sought.

Rapid shallow breathing, characterized by a high respiratory rate and low tidal volume, is common in the critically ill and, while it may reflect respiratory muscle fatigue, this is not invariably the case. Such patients are susceptible to many factors simultaneously, and rapid shallow breathing may result from various mechanisms including increased mechanical load, chemoreceptor stimulation, operating lung volume, reflexes originating in the lungs and respiratory muscles, altered respiratory motor neurone discharge patterns, sense of effort and cortical influence.[5] Nonetheless, although the pathophysiology underlying rapid shallow breathing may be uncertain, this does not detract from its value in clinical decision-making.

Using a suitable respirometer, tidal volume can be measured to quantify rapid shallow breathing more accurately. However, such devices, and the associated use of a mouthpiece or facemask in non-intubated patients, can artifactually alter tidal volumes and respiratory patterns, and non-invasive methods such as inductance plethysmography are not widely available. This complication detracts from the value of such a formal measurement, and a simple clinical assessment of tidal volume is normally sufficient.

Respiratory pattern – thoraco-abdominal motion. The analysis of respiratory movements can provide information about the activity of respiratory muscles, particularly the diaphragm, the rib cage's inspiratory muscles and the abdominal muscles. Two abnormal patterns are most commonly seen. First, with abdominal paradox, there is inward movement of the abdominal wall during inspiration, the reverse of the normal pattern. This reflects inefficient, weak, or absent contraction of the diaphragm to the point that it is unable to withstand the negative inspiratory pressure developed in the thorax by the rib cage muscles. The second pattern, respiratory alternans, has breaths with the rib cage clearly predominating, alternating with other breaths in which abdominal movement predominates. Because the diaphragm and rib cage muscles may become separately fatigued,[6] it has been suggested that this pattern of breathing may delay the onset of respiratory muscle failure.[7]

Close observation and palpation for several minutes by an experienced clinician should be sufficient to reveal these abnormal patterns, especially with the patient recumbent. Despite being associated with an increased likelihood of needing ventilatory support,[8] these abnormal patterns are not specific for respiratory muscle fatigue and can appear in healthy subjects immediately after increasing ventilatory load. They are perhaps best regarded as a reflection of increased ventilatory load, which may or may not induce respiratory muscle fatigue.[7]

Lung volumes. In the past, vital capacity measurements have been suggested as an objective indicator of the need for mechanical ventilation,[9] although currently they find limited application. They may be helpful, however, in progressive neurological conditions such as Guillain–Barré syndrome[10] in which, as vital capacity falls, the ability to generate an

effective cough and take deep breaths to prevent progressive collapse of dependent lung zones deteriorates. A value of less than 15 mL.kg^{-1} should strongly suggest a possible need for ventilatory support. In these circumstances, respiratory rate and tidal volume are highly variable, except during the few hours preceding intubation, when rapid shallow breathing occurrs.[10]

Repeated measurements of vital capacity are less helpful in predicting the need for intubation and ventilation in myasthenia gravis.[11] This may be due to the more erratic course of this disease, which sometimes involves sudden deteriorations.

Vital capacity measurements can be made using a close-fitting facemask or mouthpiece and a suitable respirometer, but care is needed to ensure accurate and reproducible values. The patient also has to be encouraged to make a maximal effort.

Maximal inspiratory pressure. Maximal inspiratory pressure has long been used to assess inspiratory muscle strength in the clinical setting. It requires a maximal inspiratory effort against a closed airway and is highly dependent on patient co-operation and coordination. Inspiratory pressures are most easily measured in intubated patients and therefore have mainly found use in the context of weaning from mechanical ventilation when, in the past, the ability to generate a pressure of −25 cm H_2O has been taken to indicate that a patient could be considered for weaning and extubation.

Phrenic nerve stimulation and sniff manoeuvres can be used to assess diaphragmatic function independent of patient volition, but require oesophageal and gastric balloons to measure transdiaphragmatic pressure. These techniques, and measures such as pressure-time indices, maximal relaxation rates and electromyography of inspiratory muscles, are available, but not generally applicable in a clinical setting.

Pulse oximetry. The ability to measure haemoglobin oxygen saturation non-invasively at the bedside is now available in most acute care settings,

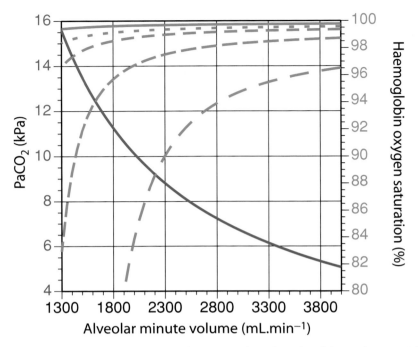
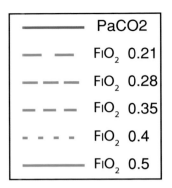

Figure 2.2 Relationship between alveolar minute volume (x-axis) and the resulting arterial partial pressure of carbon dioxide (y-axis, left) and haemoglobin saturation (y-axis, right) when breathing gas with a fractional inspired oxygen concentration between 21% and 50%.

either from dedicated hand-held units, or as part of a monitor that can measure other physiological variables such as blood pressure, the electrocardiogram and the respiratory rate. Although convenient, the interpretation of peripheral saturations can be dangerously reassuring to the unwary in three regards.

First, although the partial pressure of oxygen, and therefore the haemoglobin oxygen saturation, falls with hypoventilation when breathing air, this is easily compensated for by very small increases in the fractional inspired oxygen concentrations (FIO_2, Figure 2.2). If a patient hypoventilates on room air, this is likely to cause alarm when the saturations fall below 90%, at which point the alveolar partial pressure of carbon dioxide ($PaCO_2$) will be high (8.8 kPa), although not dangerously so. In contrast, if the alveolar hypoventilation goes unnoticed and the patient is given supplemental oxygen with an FIO_2 of only 28%, the alveolar minute volume

would have to fall to 1450 mL per minute before the saturations fell to 90%, by which time the $PaCO_2$ would be just under 14 kPa. This degree of hypercapnia would be very likely to cause carbon dioxide narcosis, putting the patient at risk of either airway obstruction or aspiration. It is important to realize, therefore, that just because a patient has a reasonable haemoglobin oxygen saturation, if she is receiving supplemental oxygen, she might still be in considerable danger from hypoventilation.

Second, the haemoglobin saturation should always be assessed in the context of the FIO_2. For example, a patient with a haemoglobin oxygen saturation of 88% might in fact not be as much a cause for concern as another patient with saturations of 94% if the former is breathing room air and the latter is breathing 60% oxygen.

Finally, the clinician should beware the patient who has carbon monoxide poisoning. Pulse oximeters are unable to distinguish between

Table 2.3 Factors to take into account when considering blood gas results
• Normal blood gas values for that patient
• Work of breathing
• Likely course of the disease process
• Degree of cardiovascular stability
• Metabolic requirements
• Presence of any bulbar involvement

Table 2.4 Signs of increased work of breathing
• Increased respiratory rate
• Abnormal respiratory patterns (abdominal paradox, respiratory alternans)
• Use of accessory muscles, intercostal recession
• Reduced capacity for speech

carboxy-haemoglobin and oxy-haemoglobin, which can only be assessed in blood gas analysers equipped with multiple wavelength spectrophotometers or using a co-oximeter. It is therefore quite possible for a patient to be critically hypoxic with oxy-haemoglobin saturations of less than 75%, but to have an apparently normal haemoglobin saturation on a pulse oximeter. Nonetheless, as a general rule, a saturation of less than 90% in a patient breathing 60% oxygen strongly suggests the need for intervention.

Arterial blood gases. The measurement of arterial blood gases plays an important part in assessing these patients. As always, when interpreting the results, it is essential to take into account the inspired oxygen concentration. An arterial oxygen tension (PaO_2) of less than 8 kPa on 60% oxygen strongly suggests the need for ventilatory support, as does a $PaCO_2$ of more than 8 kPa or hypercapnia with an impaired level of consciousness. However, blood gas results on their own are rarely the sole indication for mechanical ventilation. When deciding what action to take on blood gas results, it is important to take various other factors into consideration (Table 2.3). For example, many patients with severe, longstanding respiratory disease are chronically hypoxaemic or hypercapnic, or both, and lead surprisingly normal lives with blood gases that would cause serious concern in someone previously fit and well.

The values must also be taken in the context of the effort being expended to achieve them

(Table 2.4). The harder the patient is having to work, the more urgent the need to intervene. A patient with normal blood gases but who is working to the point of exhaustion needs prompt, active intervention far more than someone with abnormal gases but who is conscious, orientated, speaking full sentences and not distressed. The signs of increased respiratory work described above are important in making this assessment. In general, because of the various compensatory mechanisms that come into play, an increase in $PaCO_2$ is a late sign of respiratory muscle fatigue.

The likely course of the underlying pathology and the intensity of current treatment provide a very good indication of whether the situation is likely to improve or deteriorate. The possibility of a significant improvement within a short time may encourage one to 'watch and wait' rather than intubate and ventilate immediately. Similarly, one might intervene earlier if the patient has an ineffective cough and is likely to deteriorate further through retaining secretions.

The degree of cardiovascular stability is also an important consideration because respiratory muscles are dependent on their blood supply and oxygen delivery for continuing function. If these are jeopardized, respiration is likely to fail rapidly. Also, along with the respiratory system, the cardiovascular system is the other major determinant of tissue oxygen delivery. If the circulation is inadequate or unstable, it is preferable to establish ventilatory support early.

For given blood gas results, one might actively intervene earlier in an agitated, toxic, febrile patient

Table 2.5 Criteria suggesting the need for ventilatory support

- Respiratory rate >35 breaths.min^{-1}
- PaO$_2$ <8 kPa, or SpO$_2$ < 90% on 60% oxygen
- PaCO$_2$ 8 kPa* or hypercapnia with an impaired conscious level
- Vital capacity <15 mL.kg^{-1} in patients with neuromuscular disorders

PaO$_2$: arterial oxygen tension; SpO$_2$: saturation on pulse oximetry; PaCO$_2$: arterial carbon dioxide tension.
* In the absence of chronic hypercapnia.

with increased oxygen consumption and carbon dioxide production than in one whose metabolic needs are low through perhaps mild hypothermia and inactivity.

In patients with neurological disorders, one should intubate and ventilate earlier in the presence of bulbar involvement along with a likelihood of problems maintaining the airway and protecting it from aspirated gastric contents.

Conclusions. In general, when assessing the need for ventilatory support, clinical symptoms and signs are more useful than arterial blood gases or other physiological measurements. There is no substitute for an assessment of the overall clinical picture by an experienced clinician. Nonetheless, some findings strongly suggest a need for ventilatory support (Table 2.5). Any additional evidence of increased respiratory work makes the need for further assessment and possible intervention even more urgent.

Other considerations

Depending on the circumstances, rather than intubating and ventilating a patient, it may be worth undertaking a trial of non-invasive ventilatory support (see Chapter 3). In the situation in which, despite a high inspired oxygen concentration, the patient is hypoxaemic but has not tired to the point of exhaustion, continuous positive airway pressure (CPAP) may be tried and can be applied with a tight-fitting face mask. By recruiting collapsed alveoli and increasing functional residual capacity, CPAP improves arterial oxygenation and also reduces the work of breathing. If the patient is also hypercapnic, non-invasive positive pressure ventilation (NIPPV) may be tried as this will also enhance alveolar ventilation. NIPPV may also have a role when, for whatever reason, invasive ventilation is deemed to be inappropriate.

FURTHER READING

- Roussos C, Koutsoukou A. Respiratory failure. *Eur Respir J.* 2003;22: Suppl 47, 3S–14S.

REFERENCES

1. NHLBI Workshop summary. Respiratory muscle fatigue. Report of the Respiratory Muscle Fatigue Workshop Group. *Am Rev Respir Dis.* 1990;142(2):474–80.
2. Field S, Kelly SM, Macklem PT. The oxygen cost of breathing in patients with cardiorespiratory disease. *Am Rev Respir Dis.* 1982;126(1):9–13.
3. Gravelyn TR, Weg JG. Respiratory rate as an indicator of acute respiratory dysfunction. *JAMA.* 1980;244(10):1123–5.
4. McFadden JP, Price RC, Eastwood HD, Briggs RS. Raised respiratory rate in elderly patients: a valuable physical sign. *Br Med J (Clin Res Ed).* 1982;284(6316):626–7.
5. Tobin MJ, Brochard L, Rossi A. Assessment of respiratory muscle function in the intensive care unit. *Am J Respir Crit Care Med.* 2002; 166(4):610–23.
6. Fitting JW, Bradley TD, Easton PA *et al.* Dissociation between diaphragmatic and rib cage muscle fatigue. *J Appl Physiol.* 1988; 64(3):959–65.
7. Supinski GS, Fitting JW, Bellemare F. Assessment of respiratory muscle fatigue. *Am J Respir Crit Care Med.* 2002;166:571–9.

8. Ashutosh K, Gilbert R, Auchincloss JH, Jr. *et al.* Asynchronous breathing movements in patients with chronic obstructive pulmonary disease. *Chest*. 1975;67(5):553–7.

9. Pontoppidan H, Geffin B, Lowenstein E. Acute respiratory failure in the adult. *Engl J Med*. 1972;287(15):743–52.

10. Chevrolet JC, Deleamont P. Repeated vital capacity measurements as predictive parameters for mechanical ventilation need and weaning success in the Guillain-Barré syndrome. *Am Rev Respir Dis*. 1991;144(4):814–18.

11. Rieder P, Louis M, Jolliet P *et al.* The repeated measurement of vital capacity is a poor predictor of the need for mechanical ventilation in myasthenia gravis. *Intensive Care Med*. 1995;21(8):663–8.

Chapter 3

Oxygen therapy, continuous positive airway pressure and non-invasive ventilation

IAN CLEMENT, LEIGH MANSFIELD AND SIMON BAUDOUIN

It is not surprising, to anyone trained in anaesthesia or critical care, that ventilation can be successfully maintained by non-invasive methods. Following induction of anaesthesia, patients are routinely ventilated non-invasively, using an anaesthetic facemask and 'bag' system before intubation. It is also well known that modern critical care units originated during the paralytic polio epidemics of the 1950s and 1960s (see Chapter 20). Prior to these pandemics, patients with respiratory muscle paralysis were successfully ventilated for prolonged periods using negative pressure non-invasive tank and cuirass ventilators. However, during these particular pandemics the incidence of bulbar paresis was unusually high, and it was the introduction of tracheal intubation and positive pressure ventilation that resulted in a dramatic reduction in mortality. These events, together with the smaller size and lower cost of 'iron lungs', heralded a marked decline in the practice of non-invasive respiratory support during the 1970s.

Interest in non-invasive methods of support was rekindled in the 1980s by the discovery that the beneficial effect of positive end-expiratory pressure (PEEP) could be reproduced using non-invasive delivery systems. The development of more comfortable masks as a result of improvements in plastics technology should also be acknowledged as significantly contributing to this change. It was then a logical, but nevertheless very innovative, step to use the same interface to attempt to deliver ventilatory support.

Successful case reports, followed by case series, began to appear in the literature as it became clear that non-invasive ventilation (NIV) could support certain groups of patients with acute respiratory failure.[1, 2] The 1990s saw a number of important changes to NIV provision. These included the development of improved patient interfaces, the design and manufacture of dedicated NIV machines, and the reporting of several randomized controlled trials (RCTs) on the use of NIV in acute respiratory failure.

NIV is now a standard of care for some patient groups with acute respiratory failure and a number of national and international bodies have produced guidelines.[3] Novel uses of NIV continue to be explored, although not all trials have demonstrated successful outcomes when compared with traditional alternatives. Research in the field continues at a pace with recent reports including possible use in severe acute respiratory syndrome (SARS) and motor neuron disease.

This chapter will present in three parts an overview of three related fields. The first part will discuss the issues of oxygen therapy both alone and in conjunction with non-invasive support. The second part will survey the use and role of

Core Topics in Mechanical Ventilation, ed. Iain Mackenzie. Published by Cambridge University Press.
© Cambridge University Press 2008.

continuous positive airway pressure (CPAP), which remains a valuable alternative to ventilation in some situations. The final part will focus on NIV and will include a summary of the available evidence base and cover some of the more practical issues of machine and patient interfaces.

Oxygen delivery

Since its discovery, supplemental oxygen has been used to alleviate tissue hypoxia caused by respiratory or cardiac insufficiency and is one of the most frequently administered substances in the hospital environment. Tissue oxygenation is dependant upon adequate oxygen delivery and extraction, with early detection and correction of tissue hypoxia being essential if progressive organ dysfunction and death are to be avoided.[4] Supplemental oxygen can be life-saving in some situations, but it cannot reverse the inadequate oxygen delivery caused by a low cardiac output or impaired ventilation. In patients receiving supplemental oxygen, the presence of a normal arterial haemoglobin oxygen saturation (SaO_2) does not exclude the presence of either significant ventilatory failure or tissue hypoxaemia.

Fractional inspired oxygen concentration (FiO_2) and the arterial partial pressure of oxygen (PaO_2)

Room air contains approximately 21% oxygen and therefore has an FiO_2 of 0.21. It is therefore possible to deliver any range of FiO_2 from 0.21 to 1 depending on the air/oxygen mixture used and the characteristics of the delivery device and interface. The relationship between FiO_2 delivered and the PaO_2 achieved cannot be realistically predicted in the ill patient. Oxygen uptake by haemoglobin is determined by the *alveolar* partial pressure of oxygen (PAO_2), which in turn is determined by the FiO_2 and the barometric pressure. This is summarized by the alveolar gas equation (see Equation 1.4). In health, the PAO_2 is about 14 kPa with a resulting PaO_2 of

between 12 and 14 kPa, which demonstrates the normally very low alveolar–arterial gradient and the efficiency of gas transfer. In lung disease, this efficiency is reduced, mostly by increased shunting of deoxygenated blood through lung units with a reduced capacity for gas exchange. In clinical practice, FiO_2 is usually titrated against the peripherally measured arterial haemoglobin oxygen saturation or against the PaO_2 measured in a sample of arterial blood.

Interface

Oxygen is usually administered by face mask or nasal cannulae, and it is essential to appreciate that neither device will deliver 100% oxygen. Nasal cannulae consist of two prongs that sit at the nostril, providing a convenient method of administering pure oxygen at between 1 and 4 mL.min^{-1} (Figure 3.1). However, the resulting inspired oxygen concentration will vary: the higher the patient's inspiratory flow rate, the lower the resulting oxygen concentration because of its dilution with air (Box 3.1). The main advantage of nasal cannulae is their comfort and the ability of patients to tolerate them for long periods of time while still being able to eat, drink and talk. Disadvantages include the inability to deliver high concentrations of supplemental oxygen, the unpredictability of the FiO_2 and the necessity for the patient to breathe through their nose.

Face masks come in numerous designs and are either variable or fixed performance devices (Figure 3.1). Simple variable performance masks may deliver oxygen concentrations between 35% and 70%. To achieve an oxygen concentration towards the higher end of the spectrum, it is necessary to use a device with an attached reservoir bag. The reservoir acts as a 'store' of 100% oxygen and needs to be of sufficient volume that it does not completely empty during each inspiration. It should also be completely filled before the system is attached to the patient. This will be the device of choice in all situations when critical illness is suspected, such as

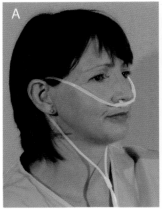
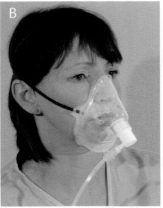
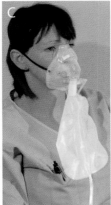
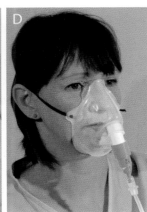

Figure 3.1 Devices for the administration of oxygen.

A: Nasal cannulae

B: Variable performance mask

C: Variable performance mask with reservoir

D: Fixed performance mask

shock, burns and severe hypoxaemia. In the absence of a pressurized circuit, it will deliver the highest oxygen concentration possible to the spontaneously breathing patient. However, in practice it is difficult to achieve oxygen levels close to 100% because, even in a perfectly working system, the interface between device and subject is a source of entrained air. These masks also use relatively low flow rates (4 to 15 L.min^{-1}) to deliver oxygen, and there may be an element of carbon dioxide retention within the mask.

Variable performance face masks are satisfactory when it is not necessary to determine the accuracy of oxygen concentration being delivered, but in some patients it is important to precisely control the FiO$_2$. Fixed performance devices, whose designs are based on the Venturi principle, will allow for the oxygen concentration to be more specifically controlled. Devices delivering an FiO$_2$ of 0.24, 0.28, 0.35, 0.4 and 0.6 are available. The oxygen enters the mask through a narrow jet and as it does so entrains air in a fixed proportion that is determined by the specific dimensions of the device (Figure 3.2). When sup-

plied with 4 to 15 L.min^{-1} of oxygen,[1] a total flow rate of approximately 35 to 45 L.min^{-1} of oxygen-enriched air is delivered to the patient, effectively eliminating the risk of re-breathing. In contrast to variable-performance masks, these devices deliver oxygen concentrations within 2% of their expected concentration, providing they are supplied with the correct oxygen flow rate. A disadvantage of a fixed performance device is often the noise the jet of air creates; however, many patients report that the noise doesn't bother them and they enjoy the 'breeze' from the jets.

Oxygen-induced hypercapnia

Controlled low-concentration oxygen has become an important treatment in the management of patients with acute hypercapnic respiratory failure secondary to chronic obstructive pulmonary disease (COPD). Critical care has correctly focused on the dangers of untreated hypoxaemia. However, uncontrolled oxygen therapy continues to

[1] The required oxygen flow rate is specific to each particular Venturi device and is usually marked on the device itself.

Box 3.1

Although nasal cannulae or a face mask are connected to a supply of pure oxygen, they can only deliver a *relatively* low flow rate that is set at the flow-meter, typically up to a maximum of 10 L.min^{-1}. However, even during normal quiet breathing, the peak inspiratory flow rate, which occurs at the beginning of the breath, can be as high as 20 L.min^{-1}; when respiratory drive is increased, the peak inspiratory flow can rise to 60 L.min^{-1}. Assuming, for the sake of argument, that *all* of the oxygen supplied to the patient is inhaled, the concentration of oxygen in the inspired mixture of air and oxygen will be determined by the ratio at any one instant between the oxygen flow rate and the total inspiratory flow rate. Illustrated in the graph is the resulting inspired oxygen concentration (y-axis) shown for the inspiratory flow rate (x-axis) when inhaling air supplemented by pure oxygen at 5, 10, 20 and 30 L.min^{-1}.

Even when supplied with pure oxygen at 20 L.min^{-1} (which is unusually high), the graph shows that a breathless patient with a peak inspiratory flow rate of 60 L.min^{-1} will be inhaling gas with an F_IO_2 that falls to as low as 47%.

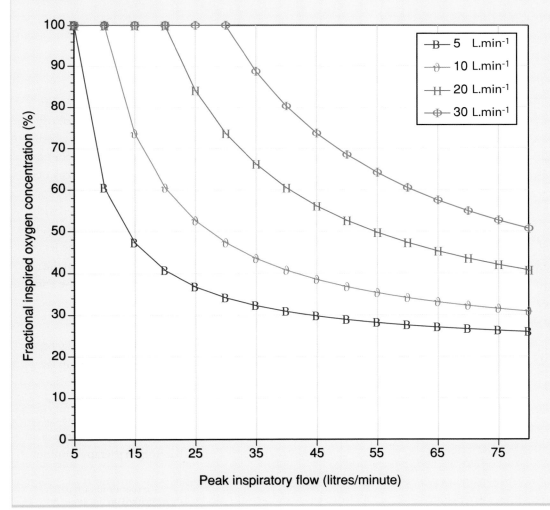

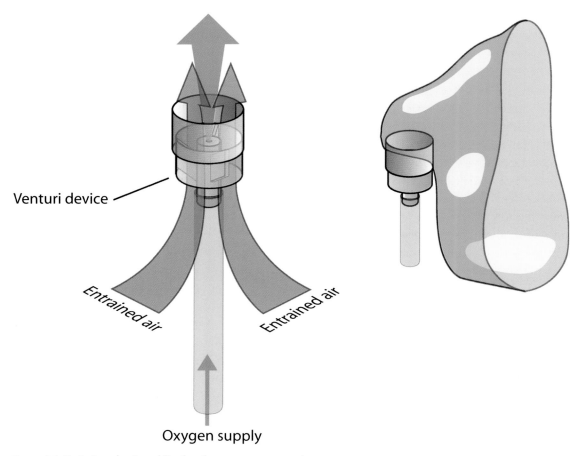

Venturi device

Entrained air

Entrained air

Oxygen supply

Figure 3.2 Venturi mechanism of fixed performance oxygen masks.

If oxygen is supplied to the venturi device at the correct flow rate, air will be entrained through the vents to provide an air/oxygen mixture with a specific oxygen concentration. As the total gas flow to the patient usually exceeds her peak inspiratory flow rate, the patient does not draw air into the device from around the mask and therefore only inhales the air/oxygen mixture supplied. Venturi devices are available that supply 24% (blue, oxygen flow at 2 L.min^{-1}), 28% (white, oxygen flow at 28 L.min^{-1}), 35% (yellow, oxygen flow at 8 L.min^{-1}), 40% (red, oxygen flow at 10 L.min^{-1}) or 60% (green, oxygen flow at 15 L.min^{-1}).

be a problem in some patients with chronic respiratory failure. This was readily confirmed in one large trial of NIV in patients with COPD.[5] In a significant number of patients, hypercapnia was reduced when uncontrolled oxygen therapy was replaced by controlled oxygen therapy.

Oxygen-induced hypercapnia may be caused by increased dead space due to ventilation/perfusion changes resulting from the release of hypoxic vaso-constriction or loss of hypoxic respiratory drive. If the hypoxic stimulation of peripheral chemoreceptors is removed by supplemental oxygen, then the level of ventilation may fall, resulting in carbon dioxide retention. It is important to balance the avoidance of severe hypercapnia with the maintenance of adequate oxygen delivery, and aiming for a haemoglobin oxygen saturation of 88% may be appropriate for these patients.

Target saturations

As with any drug, oxygen should be prescribed, and it appears that target saturations rather than specific oxygen concentration may be the most appropriate route to take. In the past, oxygen was prescribed at a fixed concentration or flow rate. However, several audits have shown that many patients do not receive the prescribed dose of oxygen. Furthermore, a patient's oxygen requirement may vary over time, so the prescribed dose may be too high or too low for a patient even a short time after the prescription is written. For this reason, prescribing a target saturation range rather than prescribing a fixed dose of oxygen may be more appropriate. This method also has the advantage of being safer, because it will give non-medical practitioners the autonomy to alter oxygen therapy as the patient's requirements increase and decrease. Primarily, this will avoid a delay in increasing the FiO_2 when the patient is deteriorating and 'at risk'. Staff on the ward can prevent worsening hypoxaemia while simultaneously informing the relevant clinical team of the patient's deteriorating condition. This has been shown to be an effective strategy in small-scale local audit reports and is likely to be the approach proposed in future national oxygen guidelines.

Safe use of oxygen

High concentrations of oxygen over a prolonged period may damage the lungs, although it is difficult to determine the specific effects in the human population.[6] Progressive decrease in lung compliance can occur, along with haemorrhagic interstitial and intra-alveolar oedema that results in pulmonary fibrosis. Precise details about safe concentrations and acceptable periods of exposure to oxygen therapy remain unknown, and toxicity may occur. While it is important to avoid oxygen toxicity when possible, the resulting hypoxaemia can only be resolved by increasing the oxygen concentration; therefore, being caught in a precarious cycle. Dangers of oxygen therapy should always be consid-

ered but should never prevent oxygen from being given. These issues are considered in more detail in Chapter 14.

Oxygen delivery summary

The ready availability of oxygen in the hospital setting may have led to a degree of complacency in terms of oxygen prescribing. Excessive as well as insufficient uses of oxygen continue to be issues. Many hypoxic patients benefit from high-flow oxygen and, in the emergency situation, high-flow oxygen should always be given initially. However, some patients do develop hypercapnia due to high-flow oxygen and will require more precise titrating of oxygen.

Continuous positive airway pressure

Staff working in anaesthesia and critical care are very familiar with the use of PEEP in patients receiving mechanical ventilation via an endotracheal tube or laryngeal mask airway, referred to as CPAP in patients who are not mechanically ventilated, and *expiratory positive airway pressure* (EPAP) in patients receiving non-invasive mechanical ventilation. Regardless of nomenclature, the principle in each case is the same – namely that between breaths the pressure in the patient's airway instead of being allowed to return to atmospheric pressure, as it would normally, is maintained at a pressure above atmospheric pressure of up to 20 cm H_2O (Figure 3.3). This section examines the role of CPAP as a therapy in its own right.

In the hospital setting, CPAP is generally administered via a full face mask, which is closely applied to the patient's face to minimize leaks. CPAP can also be applied via a nasal mask, helmet or in invasive airways using an endotracheal or tracheostomy tube (Figure 3.4). In addition to the patient interface, a circuit and a high-capacity gas supply are also required. The simplest circuits take the form of a 'T-piece' with a pressure relief valve on the end that maintains the pressure in the circuit and allows

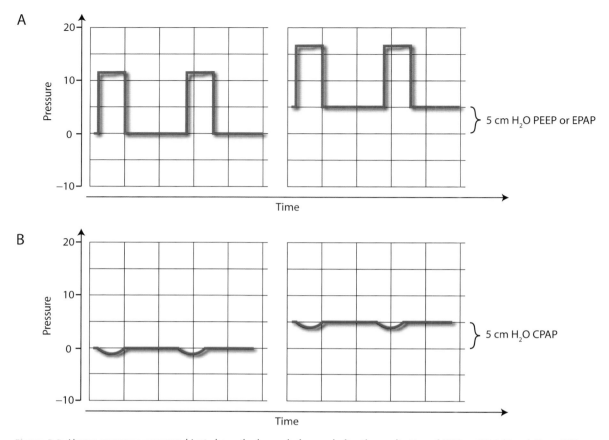

Figure 3.3 Airway pressures measured just above the larynx before and after the application of PEEP or EPAP (Panel A) or CPAP (Panel B).

A: Pressure profile in the upper airway for a patient receiving pressure-targeted (rather than volume-targeted) mechanical ventilation that can be delivered either invasively (via a tracheal tube) or non-invasively (via a tight-fitting mask). On the left, the airway pressures can be seen to return to zero (atmospheric pressure) between breaths, but following the application of 5 cm H_2O of *positive end-expiratory pressure* (PEEP, invasive ventilation) or *expiratory positive airway pressure* (EPAP, non-invasive ventilation), the airway pressure remains elevated between breaths.

B: Pressure profile measured just above the larynx in a patient breathing spontaneously before (left) and after (right) the application of 5 cm H_2O of *continuous positive airway pressure* (CPAP).

The use of the terms PEEP, EPAP and CPAP are by convention, rather than signifying some subtle distinction in mechanism.

expiratory gas to vent out of the system (Figure 3.5). These circuits are simple to set up and use, but they suffer a drawback in that a drop in pressure of some degree within the circuit is inevitable during inspiration, particularly in the hyperventilating patient. High gas flows are required to reduce this effect (Figure 3.6). An alternative system incorporates a large set of bellows into the circuit to act as a reservoir, thus minimizing the fall in circuit pressure during inspiration (Figure 3.7). The ventilators used for invasive or non-invasive ventilation can also provide CPAP.

Because CPAP, in contrast to NIV, does not require a ventilator, it can be provided more cheaply and with relatively little training. However, the types of patient who may require CPAP are likely to need to

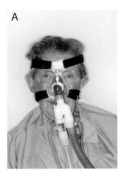
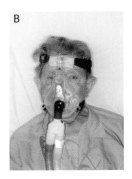
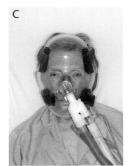
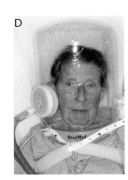

Figure 3.4 Interface devices for the provision of CPAP.

A: Nasal mask.

B: Traditional 'face' mask that covers the mouth and nose. Note the forehead support that reduces the pressure that the mask exerts on the skin over the bridge of the nose.

C: A true face mask that covers the entire face.

D: A hood which covers the patient's head and that seals around the patient's neck. Note the circular access point on the front of the device. This can be opened to allow the patient to eat, drink, or receive mouth care. Note also the pressure gauge which can be seen lateral to the patient's left ear.

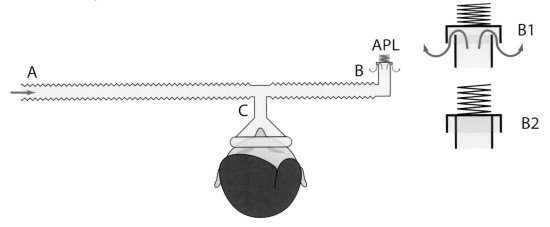

Figure 3.5 Typical circuit arrangement for the provision of CPAP.

Gas is delivered to the circuit at A at the desired oxygen concentration and spills out of the spring-operated airway pressure-limiting (APL) valve at B, which is normally held open by the escaping gas (B1). As the patient inhales, there is the potential for the circuit to lose pressure, especially if the patient's inspiratory flow rate approaches the flow rate at which gas is supplied to the circuit. If the patient's inspiratory flow rate matches or exceeds the flow rate at which gas is supplied to the circuit, the pressure in the circuit will fall, and the APL valve closes (B2). If this is happening, either the flow rate at which gas is supplied to the circuit must be increased, or the circuit must be changed for one that has a reservoir.

be managed in areas of the hospital that can provide higher levels of care. One of the drawbacks of the simple T-piece and valve systems is that the requirement for high gas flows makes it difficult to transfer patients either within or between hospitals without interrupting CPAP therapy. Some of the newer transport ventilators are able to deliver CPAP non-invasively at relatively low flows.

Physiological effects of CPAP

The application of CPAP to a patient will result in an immediate increase in functional residual capacity

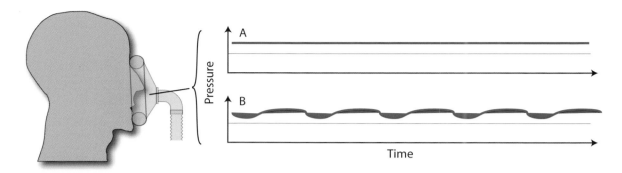

Figure 3.6 Pressure fluctuations within the mask of a CPAP circuit.

A: In this ideal (and non-existent) system, the mask pressure remains constant throughout the respiratory cycle.

B: In practice mask pressures fluctuate during the respiratory cycle, falling during inspiration and rising during expiration. The green shaded areas represent the work performed by the CPAP circuit on the patient; the red areas represent the work performed by the patient on the CPAP circuit. The sum of these two areas (green and red) is always the same, because no net work is performed. However, the work performed by the patient on the CPAP circuit adds to the overall work of breathing. The larger the pressure fluctuations are in the circuit, the higher the additional work of breathing is for the patient.

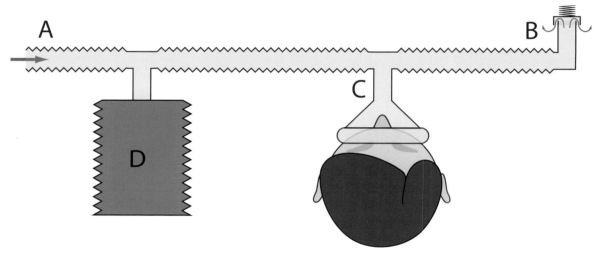

Figure 3.7 CPAP circuit incorporating a reservoir.

These circuits are much less likely to become depressurized even with high peak inspiratory flow rates, and therefore represent less of a burden to the patient in terms of the work of breathing.

(FRC). This may subsequently lead to recruitment of collapsed lung units and a reduction in shunt. This is one reason why CPAP is seen primarily as a treatment for hypoxic (type I) respiratory failure. CPAP may also improve ventilatory mechanics and thus be of some benefit in hypercapnic (type II) respiratory failure. In patients with air trapping and high intrinsic PEEP, the application of CPAP reduces the pressure difference between the proximal airways and the alveoli. This may reduce the work of inspiration and can allow some improvement in ventilation (Figure 3.8). Even in patients without intrinsic PEEP, the increase in FRC may increase pulmonary compliance and reduce the work of

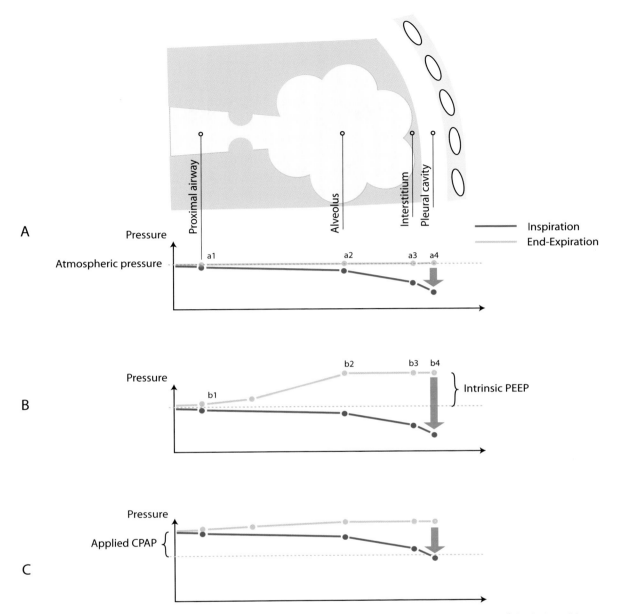

Figure 3.8 The effect of continuous positive airway pressure in reducing the work of breathing in patients with intrinsic positive end-expiratory pressure (intrinsic PEEP).

A: In normal lungs, the pressure all along the airway down to the alveoli falls to atmospheric pressure (a1, a2, a3 and a4) at the end of expiration (green line). This means that a relatively small drop in intrapleural pressure can easily generate a negative pressure gradient between the alveoli and upper airway to draw gas into the lung (blue line).

B: If a patient has significant intrinsic positive end-expiratory pressure (intrinsic PEEP, also known as auto-PEEP) as a result of narrowed airways and gas trapping, the alveolar pressure does not fall to atmospheric pressure before the start of the next breath (b1, b2, b3 and b4). This means that a very significant negative intrapleural pressure must be generated before being able to establish a similar negative pressure gradient between the alveoli and upper airway (blue line).

C: By applying CPAP to match the intrinsic PEEP the end-expiratory pressure gradient between alveoli and upper airway is significantly reduced (green line). This means that a much smaller negative intrapleural pressure has to be generated before gas starts to flow from the upper airway to alveoli, reducing the work of breathing.

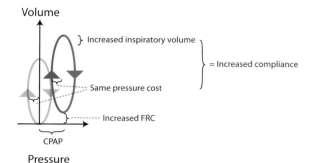

Volume

} Increased inspiratory volume

= Increased compliance

Same pressure cost

Increased FRC

CPAP

Pressure

Figure 3.9 Effect of CPAP on lung compliance.

The relationship between intrapleural pressure and lung volume is shown for inspiration (blue) and expiration (green) both before (light) and after (dark) the application of CPAP. Compared to the inspiratory/expiratory loop at baseline the application of CPAP has shifted the loop to the right, has increased the end-expiratory lung volume (FRC), and has increased the height of the loop (tidal volume) for the same inspiratory pressure gradient, reflecting an increase in pulmonary compliance.

breathing (Figure 3.9). However, the application of CPAP inevitably adds dead space at the mask,[2] and depending on the type of circuit may add substantially to the work of breathing. For these reasons, the benefit of CPAP therapy in type II respiratory failure is unpredictable and NIV is now the preferred treatment option in these patients.

CPAP has a number of haemodynamic effects. The increase in intrathoracic pressure leads to a reduction in both venous return and left ventricular after-load. This probably explains some of the beneficial effects seen from CPAP in cardiogenic pulmonary oedema. In patients who are hypovolaemic, these same effects can lead to profound hypotension.

---

[2] This makes the clearance of carbon dioxide much less efficient, and necessitates an increase in the patient's minute volume if they are to maintain the same arterial partial pressure of carbon dioxide. An increased minute volume requires an increase in either tidal volume, or respiratory rate, or both, and will inevitably increase the work of breathing. However increases in either respiratory rate or tidal volume will additionally increase the peak inspiratory flow rate . . . which *independently* contributes to the work of breathing in a CPAP circuit.

Clinical uses of CPAP

CPAP therapy has been described in a variety of conditions leading to either acute or chronic respiratory failure. The largest body of evidence in support of a role for CPAP exists for its use in acute cardiogenic pulmonary oedema. There may also be a role for CPAP in chest wall trauma, de-compensated or chronic obstructive sleep apnoea hypoventilation syndrome (OSAHS) and in patients developing hypoxaemia following major surgery.

CPAP in cardiogenic pulmonary oedema

Numerous studies have been performed comparing the effects of standard therapy with and without CPAP in patients with cardiogenic pulmonary oedema. One of the earlier studies assigned 39 consecutive patients to receive oxygen therapy alone or oxygen with CPAP via face mask.[7] The CPAP group showed significant improvements in a number of respiratory parameters at 30 minutes including respiratory rate, arterial pH and $PaO_2:FIO_2$ ratio.[3] The pre-defined end-point of the need for intubation also yielded a significant result, with 7 out of 20 patients requiring intubation in the standard group and 0 out of 19 patients in the CPAP group ($p = 0.005$). This study was not powered to detect a mortality effect. Subsequent studies have yielded broadly similar results with few demonstrating a statistically significant effect on mortality.

Studies have also looked at the role of bi-level NIV in cardiogenic pulmonary oedema, both in comparison with standard therapy and with CPAP. It has been argued that NIV may reduce the work of breathing more effectively than CPAP alone, and that this may confer additional benefit in cardiogenic pulmonary oedema. The studies comparing NIV with standard therapy alone have generally reported results similar to those from the CPAP studies. A reduction in the need for intubation is

---

[3] See glossary.

readily demonstrated, but effects on mortality are less clear cut. Interestingly, a study comparing CPAP with NIV reported more adverse effects in the NIV group, including a higher incidence of myocardial infarction.[8] However, it has been noted that more patients in the NIV group had chest pain at the time of randomization.

In light of these studies, the British Thoracic Society guidelines recommend the use of CPAP in acute cardiogenic pulmonary oedema and suggest that NIV be reserved for patients not responding to CPAP.[3] A recent meta-analysis has helped to clarify some of the issues.[9] Stringent quality criteria were applied to select studies for inclusion in the analysis. The mortality data comparing CPAP with standard therapy were based on 269 patients in 11 studies. A statistically significant reduction in mortality associated with CPAP was demonstrated, with a number needed to treat of 11. The mortality comparisons for NIV versus standard therapy and NIV versus CPAP were both non-significant.

In summary, the published data on the use of CPAP in acute cardiogenic pulmonary oedema show a definite reduction in the need for intubation, and when considered together suggest a worthwhile reduction in mortality. Bi-level NIV appears to offer no further advantage.

CPAP in chronic obstructive pulmonary disease

There are no randomized controlled trials comparing CPAP with standard therapy or NIV in acute exacerbations of COPD. There are theoretical reasons for believing CPAP may be beneficial in treating type II respiratory failure secondary to COPD by off-loading the inspiratory muscles and so reducing the work of breathing. Case series have been published showing improvements in oxygenation and $PaCO_2$ associated with CPAP in acute COPD. However, there is a well-established evidence base for the use of NIV in this situation (see below).

Trauma

A randomized controlled trial studied 69 patients with 3 or more fractured ribs, hypoxaemia and only mild or moderate lung injury.[10] Patients were randomized to either CPAP and regional analgesia or intubation and ventilation. Reduced ICU and hospital length of stay was demonstrated in the CPAP group. However, a higher overall injury score was noted in the intubation group despite the randomization. The British Thoracic Society recommends that CPAP be used in patients with chest wall trauma and hypoxaemia despite adequate analgesia. These patients should be monitored in a critical care environment because of the risk of pneumothorax.

Obstructive sleep apnoea

De-compensated OSAHS has been shown to respond to both CPAP and NIV. Again, no major studies comparing the two have been published. Where facilities for NIV exist, it would be logical to offer it, particularly in the presence of a respiratory acidosis. In patients with chronic stable OSAHS, long-term domiciliary CPAP plays an important role and has been shown to reduce daytime somnolence and improve symptoms of cor pulmonale.[11] A recent study looking at domiciliary nasal CPAP in patients with chronic stable OSAHS and co-existing left ventricular failure demonstrated reduced left ventricular dilatation and increased ejection fraction.[12]

Pneumonia

There are numerous reports of the beneficial effects of CPAP in acute hypoxaemic respiratory failure caused by pneumonia. In particular, CPAP has been widely used in immunosuppressed patients with pneumocystis pneumonia in an attempt to avoid the infective complications of prolonged invasive ventilation. Dalclaux and co-workers randomized 123 patients with hypoxaemic respiratory failure (of

Table 3.1 Indications and contra-indications for CPAP

Indications	Absolute contra-indications
Type I respiratory failure	• Recent trans-sphenoidal neurosurgery
• Pneumonia	Relative contra-indications
• Cardiogenic pulmonary oedema	• Surgical suture lines or anastamoses within the
• Obstructive sleep apnoea	pharynx or oesophagus.
• Chest trauma	
• Diaphragmatic splinting (obesity, ascites, bowel distension)	

which 51 had pneumonia) to either standard therapy or CPAP.[13] Improved oxygenation and dyspnoea scores were evident at one hour, but there were no detectable differences in mortality, intubation rate or hospital length of stay.

Post-operative patients

Hypoxaemia occurs in 30% to 50% of patients following major abdominal surgery. Pulmonary atelectasis occurring in the intra- and post-operative period is probably responsible for this. Although oxygen therapy and incentive spirometry are frequently effective, a recent randomized controlled trial has demonstrated a beneficial response to CPAP therapy.[14] In this study, 209 patients who developed hypoxaemia following major elective abdominal surgery were randomly assigned to receive standard therapy alone or with CPAP. The CPAP group had a statistically significant reduction in the need for intubation (1% versus 10%), pneumonia (2% versus 10%), infection, sepsis and ICU length of stay. The study was not powered to detect a difference in mortality, although a trend favouring the CPAP group was evident.

Continuous positive airway pressure summary

There are theoretical reasons for considering CPAP to be of potential benefit in a number of conditions. Good evidence exists for its efficacy in acute cardiogenic pulmonary oedema. The use of CPAP may also

be justified in other situations but the evidence is less clear-cut (Table 3.1).

Non-invasive ventilation (NIV)

It is important to acknowledge the lack of high-quality evidence for the use of invasive ventilation before reviewing the substantial evidence base for the use of NIV in acute respiratory failure associated with COPD. There are no randomized trials of conventional ventilation in COPD which have taken survival as the trial target. It is always assumed that without invasive ventilatory support, death would be inevitable. However, the variable indications for intubation in COPD coupled with reports of very different survival rates suggest that this assumption may not be correct. Invasive ventilation is associated with significant morbidity such as increased risk of hospital-acquired pneumonia, loss of respiratory muscle strength and general ICU-related problems, including those associated with the need for sedation. It therefore cannot be assumed that invasive ventilation will always improve survival.

There are also no RCTs comparing NIV alone to conventional ventilation in COPD. The majority of RCTs had protocols in which patients who 'failed' NIV were intubated and conventionally ventilated. However, the definition of failure varies from trial to trial. Also, in some studies the outcome of patients who failed NIV and were subsequently intubated was very poor. It therefore remains possible that NIV alone would result in the best outcome for severe COPD exacerbations, but it must be acknowledged that such a study would be difficult to conduct on ethical grounds.

NIV in acute exacerbations of COPD

In 1993, Dr J. Cordell Bott and co-workers at King's College Hospital, London, published a ground-breaking RCT on the use of NIV in patients with COPD.[15] They recruited 60 patients with COPD and respiratory failure ($PaO_2 > 6$ kPa) and randomized them to conventional treatment or conventional treatment with NIV. The majority of NIV was delivered on a general respiratory ward rather than a specialist area or HDU. NIV was better than conventional treatment in improving pH, reducing $PaCO_2$ and improving breathlessness. When analysed on an efficiency basis (i.e. on which patients actually received each treatment), mortality in the NIV group was significantly reduced (1/26 versus 9/30). However, on an intention-to-treat analysis, the differences were less marked and did not reach conventional significance levels. The study was criticized on a number of grounds. The mortality in the conventional group (30%) was felt to be excessive. However, subsequent comparisons with UK data from COPD patients with similar admission severity suggested that the mortality was not unrepresentative. The very low intubation rate in both groups was also controversial. This undoubtedly reflected the nihilistic view of prognosis in COPD that was current in the UK at the time of the trial. In addition, the care input received by the two groups was different. The intervention group received frequent visits from the trial physiotherapists while the control group received standard ward nursing care. Finally, it is perhaps surprising that the efficacy analysis was given preference, although the trial was clearly underpowered.

Another major RCT, reported by Brochard and his group, was based on NIV performed in critical care facilities in five university hospitals on the European mainland.[16] Entry criteria differed from those adopted in Bott's study. Eighty-five patients with known COPD and acute respiratory failure (pH < 7.35) who had been admitted to critical care were recruited and randomized to either conventional or NIV treatment. NIV significantly reduced the need for intubation (26% versus 74%), hospital length of stay (23 versus 35 days) and hospital mortality (9% versus 29%).

This important study was the first to show that NIV significantly improved outcome in COPD patients with severe exacerbations on an intention-to-treat basis. However, it should be recognized that the patients in the trial differ from the majority of those admitted with COPD. All patients entered into the study were drawn from an ICU population of 275 patients, of whom only 85 actually entered the study. Therefore patients who were not deemed 'suitable' for critical care were excluded. This contrasts with the Bott study and others that were based on patients receiving their care in a general ward. Therefore these results may not apply to patients who are not felt to benefit from conventional ventilation if they fail NIV. The location of care received should also be considered when interpreting the trial results. The critical care environment chosen for the study would give all entrants a much higher level of medical, nursing and physiotherapy care than was available on the wards. NIV is at least as time-consuming as conventional ventilation for nurses. It cannot be assumed that such good outcomes from NIV would be achieved on less well-staffed wards.

A number of these issues were subsequently addressed in an important multicentre study conducted in the Northern region of the United Kingdom in 2000.[17] This was a 'real world' study on NIV in severe COPD in 14 UK hospitals. Over a period of 22 months, 236 patients were recruited who were then randomized to either standard therapy or standard and NIV treatment. Entry criteria included evidence of respiratory failure with pH 7.25 to 7.35, despite controlled oxygen therapy. NIV was better than standard therapy in improving pH, respiratory rate and breathlessness. In-hospital mortality was also significantly better in the NIV group (10% versus 20%). The need for intubation was also reduced by NIV, although this was a post-hoc analysis based on theoretical intubation criteria. In reality, many of the patients died without intubation, presumably because the clinical teams thought that this intervention was not appropriate.

The study demonstrated that the significant benefits of NIV, observed in a critical care setting, can also be reproduced on general medical wards with less intense input (median nurse to patient ratio was 1:11) and monitoring.

The efficacy of NIV in different locations is further strengthened by the publication of an RCT conducted in 19 hospitals in mainland China in 2005.[18] Three hundred and forty-two patients with respiratory failure and COPD were recruited into standard or NIV groups. As in other trials, NIV was better at improving physiology than conventional treatment. The need for intubation was significantly reduced and there was a trend to lower mortality with NIV (5% versus 7%).

The randomized controlled trials of NIV in respiratory failure associated with COPD have been subject to a number of systematic reviews and meta-analyses. The most recent, and probably definitive, analysis was published in 2003 by the Cochrane collaboration.[19] They identified eight published studies (including the Bott, Elliott and Brochard studies) that fulfilled their criteria. Not surprisingly, they found good evidence that NIV was superior to standard care. NIV was associated with a lower mortality (relative risk 0.41), a lower need for intubation (relative risk 0.42), better improvement in physiology and reduced hospital length of stay.

The substantial evidence base for the use of NIV in severe exacerbations of COPD has led to its becoming a standard of care in several national and international guidelines. For example, in the UK, NIV is endorsed by the British Thoracic Society, Intensive Care Society and the Department of Health.[3, 20] These endorsements, which imply the availability of a continuous acute NIV service in all acute provider units, have significant resource implications. Elliott and co-workers have provided an estimate of need based on a one-year point prevalence study of COPD conducted in the North of England.[5] They concluded that a typical UK hospital (serving a population of 250 000) would expect to treat approximately 70 COPD patients per year with NIV. This figure indicates that, if properly resourced, an acute NIV service will be ventilating at least one patient at any single time and will often need to cater for two or three patients.

Despite improved hospital survival for COPD patients who receive NIV, longer term outlook remains poor. In a longer term follow up of patients who received NIV for acute exacerbation of COPD, median length of survival was only 16.8 months (mortality rate at one year was 38%) and was not significantly different from patients receiving conventional care alone.[21]

Remaining issues in COPD

The potential use of NIV in stable, severe COPD remains unresolved.[22] A number of uncontrolled trials suggest possible benefit but, as yet, no RCT has been conducted to examine the hypothesis that NIV would improve long-term outcome.

A number of issues also remain in the acute use of NIV. Many of these focus on the lack of simple, ward-based systems for monitoring ventilation. The gold standard method of assessing adequacy of ventilation remains the arterial $PaCO_2$. However, this usually requires an arterial puncture. Repeated sampling is therefore time consuming and uncomfortable for the patient. The lack of 'real time' information on $PaCO_2$ has led to little or no adjustment of ventilation in ward-based environments. It remains possible that acute outcome might be further improved if ventilation is adjusted to

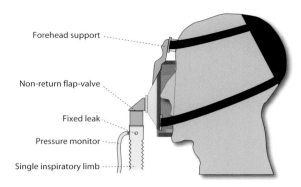

Forehead support

Non-return flap-valve

Fixed leak

Pressure monitor

Single inspiratory limb

Figure 3.10 Typical circuit and mask for non-invasive ventilation.

Unlike ventilator circuits used for anaesthesia or critical care which have two limbs, one taking fresh gas to the patient and a second returning expired gas to the ventilator, breathing circuits for non-invasive ventilation (NIV) only have one limb for taking fresh gas to the patient. The patient's inspiratory effort is detected by a fall in circuit pressure measured at the patient end of the circuit via a separate pressure monitoring line. The patient end of the circuit also has a small hole designed to provide a constant leak. At the onset of inspiration, the circuit pressure rises from the baseline pressure, called the expiratory positive airway pressure (EPAP) to the inspiratory positive airway pressure (IPAP), until the criteria for cycling into the expiratory phase have been met, which may be based on time or flow. During the expiratory phase, the circuit pressure falls to the EPAP, and expired gas escapes from the circuit through the fixed leak. Ventilators for NIV are designed to accommodate both the fixed leak at the patient end of the circuit, and a variable and almost inevitable leak between the patient's face and the mask.

individual patient need. A number of studies are currently in progress examining alternatives to arterial samples for this purpose.

The optimal level of EPAP, if any, is also unresolved. Most pressure-generating NIV machines have an obligatory low level of EPAP to promote expiratory gas flow from the circuit (Figure 3.10). Some studies reported a benefit of CPAP in COPD exacerbations. The mechanism postulated was reduced work of breathing. However, other studies have found either no benefit or a risk of inducing gas trapping and hyperinflation.

The optimal target oxygen saturation or PaO_2 is also unknown. Conventional teaching targets an SaO_2 of 90% or greater in exacerbations. However, this is not based on evidence and in one trial of ventilation in acute lung injury, patients who received low tidal volume ventilation had paradoxically poorer SaO_2 in the first 24 hours, but a better survival rate.[23] In COPD patients with chronic hypoxaemia, it is likely that a SaO_2 significantly less than 90% would be acceptable.

It is well established that conventional ventilation can cause a form of acute lung injury, identical to that reported in the acute respiratory distress syndrome.[24] It is therefore likely that NIV can also cause lung injury, although the relatively low tidal volumes and airway pressures usually generated probably minimize this risk.

Weaning and NIV

While NIV will reduce the number of patients with chronic respiratory disease who require tracheal intubation during exacerbations, a significant number will continue to require invasive support. Traditionally, these patients would mostly receive a tracheostomy followed by a conventional weaning programme of gradual reduction in support. NIV provides a possible alternative that, in selected cases, may enable a 'fast track' weaning process to be successful. Following a number of reported case series of NIV use in weaning, three RCTs of modest size have been conducted.[25, 26, 27] The first, published in 1998, recruited mechanically ventilated patients with COPD who failed a T-piece trial of weaning.[27] Patients were then randomized to receive either a conventional, pressure-supported, weaning strategy or extubation with NIV. Fifty patients were randomized in the study with 25 patients in each section.

At 60 days following study entry, 88% of the NIV group had weaned successfully compared to 68% in the conventional approach group. Mean duration of ventilation was also shorter for the NIV group. In addition, survival rates at 60 days were significantly different, with 92% of the NIV group alive while only 72% of the conventional group survived their admission.

A second study with a similar design was published in 1999.[26] From a population of 53 consecutive patients who were mechanically ventilated because of acute or chronic respiratory failure (mostly COPD), 33 who had failed a T-piece weaning trial were randomized to either conventional weaning or NIV. Unlike the first study, however, NIV did not significantly increase ultimate weaning success (NIV 76.5%; conventional approach 75%). NIV weaning also did not reduce the period of ICU or hospital stay and the three-month survival was similar in both groups. On a note of caution, patients receiving NIV had a greater total duration of respiratory support compared to those receiving a conventional approach.

More recently, a further trial involving 43 mechanically ventilated patients was reported.[25] Again, the majority had underlying COPD as the cause of their respiratory failure. These patients were selected from a large group of patients by the fact that they failed a trial of conventional weaning on three consecutive days. Despite this, weaning onto NIV reduced ventilation time, ICU and hospital length of stay, and the need for tracheostomy (5% versus 59%). Both ICU and 90-day survival were significantly increased. Using a multi-factorial model, the use of a conventional weaning strategy was associated with a 3.5-fold decrease in 90-day survival.

In otherwise stable patients who have been ventilated for exacerbations of COPD, it would therefore seem reasonable to attempt a trial of extubation onto NIV if they fail a conventional weaning attempt. However, it should be acknowledged that the numbers in the trials were relatively small and one trial did not show a significant improvement in outcome on NIV. It must also be recognized that re-intubation carries some risks (see next section, 'NIV and re-intubation') and there is a fine dividing line

between a reasonable trial of NIV and a delayed and potentially life-threatening need for re-intubation.

NIV and re-intubation

If NIV is successful in weaning patients from intubation, it would seem likely that it would also prevent the need for re-intubation. However, recent RCTs suggest that this may not be the case and even support a view that NIV may be harmful in post-extubation respiratory failure.

The first RCT comparing NIV with conventional management in post-extubation respiratory failure was published in 2002.[28] Eighty-one patients were recruited from a single tertiary care centre. These were a heterogeneous group and only a small number had COPD. Comparing NIV with conventional treatment, there was no difference in rate of re-intubation (72% versus 69%) or hospital mortality (31% in both groups). There was also no difference in length of stay.

A much larger multicentre study was subsequently published from 37 international critical care units.[29] From a group of 980 at-risk patients, 244 developed respiratory failure following extubation and 221 of these were randomized to NIV or standard treatment. The patients were heterogeneous and once again few patients with COPD were recruited. There was no difference in rate of re-intubation (48% in both groups), but the mortality rate was significantly higher in the NIV group (25% versus 14%). The cause of this is uncertain, but the authors noted that median time to re-intubation was considerably longer in the NIV group. They speculated that this delay may have resulted in the poor outcome.

The most recently conducted RCT randomized 162 ventilated patients with increased risk of post-extubation respiratory failure to immediate NIV or standard treatment.[30] This design therefore differs from the other two studies that randomized only on the development of respiratory failure. Both the development of post-extubation respiratory failure

(16% versus 27%) and ICU mortality (3% versus 12%) were less in the NIV group. A post-hoc analysis based on the presence of hypercapnia during the pre-extubation spontaneous-breathing trial found benefit from NIV only in the hypercapnic group, who predominantly had COPD.

The conclusion from both the post-extubation and weaning trials of NIV seem clear. Elective extubation of COPD patients using NIV is beneficial in terms of reduced need for re-intubation and probably overall hospital mortality. However, the use of NIV in other patient groups is without benefit and, in patients failing after extubation, may be harmful.

NIV in acute asthma

The effectiveness of NIV in acute exacerbations of COPD has led a number of groups to examine its use in acute asthma. Several case series have reported apparent success in reducing the need for conventional ventilatory support. However, a Cochrane collaboration systematic review on the topic found only one well-conducted RCT.[31] This randomized only 30 patients with acute, severe asthma to either standard treatment or standard treatment and NIV. The major benefits of NIV included reduced need for hospitalization and more rapid improvement in physiology. No patient required intubation and no patients died during their admission.

The evidence base for using NIV in severe asthma is therefore very limited. The fact that most asthmatics rapidly recover with standard treatment and the fortunate lack of 'hard' end-points of either intubation or mortality makes the conduct of NIV trials in asthma difficult. In addition, the suggestion that delayed intubation may harm patients also gives some grounds for concern in using NIV in this situation. Finally, NIV has the potential to worsen hyper-inflation and therefore increase the work of breathing.

NIV cannot therefore be recommended as a routine part of severe asthma treatment. If it is to be used, then limiting it to an HDU or ICU environment with staff with full airway skills present is recommended.

NIV in other causes of acute respiratory failure

NIV has been used in the treatment of a wide range of respiratory problems including pneumonia and acute respiratory distress syndrome. Although case reports and series tend to focus on successful use, there is little evidence in terms of RCTs to back up this view. Many RCTs that report successful results have included a significant population of patients with COPD.

One small RCT of NIV versus conventional ventilation was reported in 1995.[32] Forty-one patients with acute respiratory failure (some from cardiogenic pulmonary oedema) were randomized to either NIV or conventional ventilation. No significant difference was found in rate of intubation, length of stay or hospital mortality. NIV was associated with a trend towards a worse outcome. NIV should therefore be considered as a trial therapy in most cases of acute respiratory failure, not associated with COPD. In view of this, it should only be commenced in areas where there are the staff, equipment and monitoring available to rapidly move to intubation if NIV fails.

NIV may have an important role in the treatment of respiratory failure in the immunosuppressed patient. In one important RCT, 52 patients with immune system failure (non-HIV) who developed respiratory failure were randomized to either early NIV or standard treatment.[33] Historically, the outcome in those with immune system failure has been very poor and this was confirmed by the mortality in the standard group in which 81% died in hospital. However, NIV significantly reduced hospital mortality to 50%. It should be stressed that NIV was electively started at a relatively early stage of disease progression. This is likely to be a key to success in all forms of NIV given the need for an awake, co-operative patient.

The renewed interest in pandemic flu and the recent severe acute respiratory syndrome (SARS) outbreaks have raised issues about the possible role of NIV in highly infectious respiratory pathogens. Descriptions from the Toronto SARS outbreak suggest that SARS is a major threat to ICU workers. In particular, close contact with airway secretions appears to be a major risk factor for disease transmission in staff. This would suggest that NIV is contra-indicated in SARS-like outbreaks.[34] However, a case series drawn from the experience of hospitals in Hong Kong during their SARS outbreak concluded that NIV could be successfully used without exposing healthcare workers to increased risk.[35] The role of NIV in SARS and other highly contagious respiratory pathogens needs further research and clarification. However, current UK guidelines suggest that it should not be used.

Practical aspects of NIV delivery

A wide and increasing range of ventilations suitable for NIV delivery are available. The British Thoracic Society (BTS) standards document lists both essential and desirable features.[3] Essential features include a pressure-generating capability of at least 30 cm H_2O, the capability to support inspiratory flows of at least 60 L.min^{-1} and 40 breaths.min^{-1}, sensitive flow triggers and a disconnection alarm. Although these are fully functional ventilators, most are not suitable for intubated patients or those with tracheostomies. This is mainly because of the lack of occlusion alarms.

A wide choice of mask interfaces is also available (Figure 3.4). In the acute situation, full face masks are preferable. These need to be individually fitted and adjusted. One common problem is over-tightening of the masks (to avoid leaks), leading to pressure sores and occasional severe nasal bridge necrosis requiring skin grafting. Some alternatives to conventional masks are available, includ-

ing full head helmet-style interfaces. It should be remembered that in almost all NIV systems, expiration occurs either through a simple valve or via a small hole in the mask or tubing interface. Without this in place, the system is essentially sealed and potentially dangerous. As a safety measure, some circuits now have built-in expiratory valves that cannot be removed.

The best location for the delivery of NIV remains uncertain. It has been shown that NIV requires very significant amounts of medical and non-medical time to be successful. It is also clear that NIV should be periodically adjusted, depending on patient response and monitoring. NIV will also fail in a significant number of patients. In some of these, intubation will be appropriate. All these considerations suggest that NIV would be best carried out in an HDU type of environment. There is also some indirect evidence by comparison of outcomes in different RCTs for a benefit of NIV for patients located in HDUs and ICUs.

However, limitations on resources in many countries prevent HDU access for all potential patients and, for example, in the UK many patients are cared for on general medical wards with apparent success. One approach is to triage patients based on whether NIV is to be the limit of interventional treatment. Patients who are to be intubated if NIV fails are then placed in HDU. While pragmatic, this approach could be challenged as not providing the best care for all patients receiving NIV.

The hospital-wide organization of an NIV service is vital for success. All acute hospitals should offer a continuous NIV service. Many different models are available, including physiotherapy, nurse, technician and doctor led and delivered. Protocols are very useful for all concerned in delivery, particularly when the responsibility for immediate care is given to relatively inexperienced practitioners. Good links with critical care services need to be put in place and early decisions about treatment escalation if NIV fails need to be made. It is essential to have structured, ongoing educational packages, particularly for ward staff who are left to care for the patient once the initial setting up has been made.

NIV summary

In the last 15 years, NIV has moved from having an interesting niche role to being a standard of care in acute medicine. It is of proven benefit in COPD and can be successful in a range of other acute respiratory problems. Service provision and the interface with critical care are key determinants of the success of any programme.

REFERENCES

1. Nava S, Navalesi P, Conti G. Time of non-invasive ventilation. *Intensive Care Med.* 2006;32(3):361–70.

2. Elliott MW. Non-invasive ventilation for acute respiratory disease. *Br Med Bull.* 2004;72:83–97.

3. Non-invasive ventilation in acute respiratory failure. *Thorax.* 2002;57(3):192–211.

4. Levy MM. Pathophysiology of oxygen delivery in respiratory failure. *Chest.* 2005;128(5 Suppl 2):547S–53S.

5. Plant PK, Owen JL, Elliott MW. One year period prevalence study of respiratory acidosis in acute exacerbations of COPD: implications for the provision of non-invasive ventilation and oxygen administration. *Thorax.* 2000;55(7):550–4.

6. Jenkinson SG. Oxygen toxicity. *New Horiz.* 1993;1(4):504–11.

7. Bersten AD, Holt AW, Vedig AE *et al.* Treatment of severe cardiogenic pulmonary edema with continuous positive airway pressure delivered by face mask. *N Engl J Med.* 1991;325(26):1825–30.

8. Mehta RL. Acute renal failure and cardiac surgery: marching in place or moving ahead? *J Am Soc Nephrol.* 2005;16(1):12–14.

9. Peter JV, Moran JL, Phillips-Hughes J *et al.* Effect of non-invasive positive pressure ventilation (NIPPV) on mortality in patients with acute cardiogenic pulmonary oedema: a meta-analysis. *Lancet.* 2006;367(9517): 1155–63.

10. Bolliger CT, Van Eeden SF. Treatment of multiple rib fractures. Randomized controlled trial comparing ventilatory with nonventilatory management. *Chest.* 1990;97(4):943–8.

11. Giles TL, Lasserson TJ, Smith BJ *et al.* Continuous positive airways pressure for obstructive sleep apnoea in adults. *Cochrane Database Syst Rev.* 2006(1): CD001106.

12. Kaneko Y, Floras JS, Usui K *et al.* Cardiovascular effects of continuous positive airway pressure in patients with heart failure and obstructive sleep apnea. *N Engl J Med.* 2003;348(13):1233–41.

13. Delclaux C, L'Her E, Alberti C *et al.* Treatment of acute hypoxemic nonhypercapnic respiratory insufficiency with continuous positive airway pressure delivered by a face mask: A randomized controlled trial. *JAMA.* 2000;284(18):2352–60.

14. Squadrone V, Coha M, Cerutti E *et al.* Continuous positive airway pressure for treatment of postoperative hypoxemia: a randomized controlled trial. *JAMA.* 2005;293(5):589–95.

15. Bott J, Carroll MP, Conway JH *et al.* Randomized controlled trial of nasal ventilation in acute ventilatory failure due to chronic obstructive airways disease. *Lancet.* 1993;341(8860):1555–7.

16. Brochard L, Mancebo J, Wysocki M *et al.* Noninvasive ventilation for acute exacerbations of chronic obstructive pulmonary disease. *N Engl J Med.* 1995; 333(13):817–22.

17. Plant PK, Owen JL, Elliott MW. Early use of non-invasive ventilation for acute exacerbations of chronic obstructive pulmonary disease on general respiratory wards: a multicentre randomized controlled trial. *Lancet*. 2000;355(9219):1931–35.

18. Collaborative Research Group of Noninvasive Mechanical Ventilation for Chronic Obstructive Pulmonary Disease. Early use of non-invasive positive pressure ventilation for acute exacerbations of chronic obstructive pulmonary disease: a multicentre randomized controlled trial. *Chin Med J (Engl)*. 2005;118(24):2034–40.

19. Lightowler JV, Wedzicha JA, Elliott MW *et al*. Non-invasive positive pressure ventilation to treat respiratory failure resulting from exacerbations of chronic obstructive pulmonary disease: Cochrane systematic review and meta-analysis. *BMJ*. 2003; 326(7382):185.

20. Baudouin SV, Davidson C, Elliott MW. *National Patients Access Team Critical Care Programme: Weaning and Long Term Ventilation*. London, Department of Health, 2002.

21. Plant PK, Owen JL, Elliott MW. Non-invasive ventilation in acute exacerbations of chronic obstructive pulmonary disease: long term survival and predictors of in-hospital outcome. *Thorax*. 2001;56(9):708–12.

22. Elliott MW. Non-invasive ventilation in acute exacerbations of COPD: what happens after hospital discharge? *Thorax*. 2004;59(12): 1006–8.

23. Brower RG, Lanken PN, MacIntyre N *et al*. The Acute Respiratory Distress Syndrome Network. Ventilation with lower tidal volumes as compared with traditional tidal volumes for acute lung injury and the acute respiratory distress syndrome. *N Engl J Med*. 2000;342(18):1301–18.

24. Lionetti V, Recchia FA, Ranieri VM. Overview of ventilator-induced lung injury mechanisms. *Curr Opin Crit Care*. 2005; 11(1):82–6.

25. Ferrer M, Esquinas A, Arancibia F *et al*. Noninvasive ventilation during persistent weaning failure: a randomized controlled trial. *Am J Respir Crit Care Med*. 2003; 168(1):70–6.

26. Girault C, Daudenthun I, Chevron V *et al*. G. Noninvasive ventilation as a systematic extubation and weaning technique in acute-on-chronic respiratory failure: a prospective, randomized controlled study. *Am J Respir Crit Care Med*. 1999;160(1):86–92.

27. Nava S, Ambrosino N, Clini E *et al*. Noninvasive mechanical ventilation in the weaning of patients with respiratory failure due to chronic obstructive pulmonary disease. A randomized, controlled trial. *Ann Intern Med*. 1998;128(9):721–8.

28. Keenan SP, Powers C, McCormack DG *et al*. Noninvasive positive-pressure ventilation for postextubation respiratory distress: a randomized controlled trial. *JAMA*. 2002;287(24):3238–44.

29. Esteban A, Frutos-Vivar F, Ferguson ND *et al*. Noninvasive positive-pressure ventilation for respiratory failure after extubation. *N Engl J Med*. 2004;350(24):2452–60.

30. Ferrer M, Valencia M, Nicolas JM *et al*. Early noninvasive ventilation averts extubation failure in patients at risk: a randomized trial. *Am J Respir Crit Care Med*. 2006;173(2): 164–70.

31. Ram FS, Wellington S, Rowe B *et al*. Non-invasive positive pressure ventilation for treatment of respiratory failure due to severe acute exacerbations of asthma. *Cochrane Database Syst Rev*. 2005(3):CD004360.

32. Kramer N, Meyer TJ, Meharg J *et al*. Randomized, prospective trial of noninvasive

positive pressure ventilation in acute respiratory failure. *Am J Respir Crit Care Med.* 1995;151(6):1799–1806.

33. Hilbert G, Gruson D, Vargas F *et al.* Noninvasive ventilation in immunosuppressed patients with pulmonary infiltrates, fever, and acute respiratory failure. *N Engl J Med.* 2001;344(7): 481–7.

34. Booth CM, Stewart TE. Severe acute respiratory syndrome and critical care medicine: the Toronto experience. *Crit Care Med.* 2005;33(1 Suppl):S53–60.

35. Yam LY, Chan AY, Cheung TM *et al.* Non-invasive versus invasive mechanical ventilation for respiratory failure in severe acute respiratory syndrome. *Chin Med J (Engl).* 2005;118(17):1413–21.

Chapter 4

Management of the artificial airway

PETER YOUNG AND IAIN MACKENZIE

Introduction

In this chapter, endotracheal intubation will refer to trans-laryngeal intubation (that is oral or nasal intubation of the trachea), and tracheal intubation will refer to either endotracheal intubation or intubation via a tracheostomy (Figure 4.1). A supraglottic airway is an airway that does not pass across the vocal cords, such as an oropharyngeal airway or a laryngeal mask.

Intubation of the trachea with a cuffed tube is the only way to simultaneously provide a secure airway, repeated access to the trachea and ventilatory support. Unfortunately, the placement of an artificial airway, be it a supraglottic airway or an endotracheal or tracheostomy tube, will bypass many of the patient's natural defences and thus increase the risk of upper and lower airway colonization, aspiration and infection.[1, 2] To enable the patient to tolerate the airway, the use of sedative, analgesic or muscle relaxants may be required with the resultant risk of cardiovascular, respiratory and neuromuscular complications. Therefore, unless absolutely necessary, it is desirable to avoid the use of artificial airways, for example, by using face mask oxygen or an external airway interface to achieve non-invasive ventilation. Indeed, it has become clear that non-invasive ventilation as opposed to tracheal intubation can, in some circumstances, reduce morbidity and mortality in the critically ill (Chapter 3). When an artificial airway is required, it is the clinician's responsibility to minimize the complications consequent to its use.

The quality of care of the artificial airway is critical in preventing these complications, which are discussed in Chapter 14.

Supraglottic airways

Oropharyngeal airways

The oropharynx becomes occluded in the obtunded patient when the tongue falls posteriorly. An appropriately sized oropharyngeal airway (Figure 4.2) may be required when standard airway positioning manoeuvres (head tilt and jaw thrust) fail. The oropharyngeal airway is of the correct size when it reaches between the front incisors and the angle of the jaw when placed against the patient's cheek. The oropharyngeal airway is an anatomically contoured rigid plastic device designed to displace the tongue from the posterior pharyngeal wall. It offers no protection against pulmonary aspiration; on the contrary, it can stimulate the gag and vomiting reflexes and can only be placed and tolerated in patients with a depressed conscious level. The airway is inserted into the mouth with the concave surface towards the patient's nose and, when half-inserted, is rotated 180 degrees and gently eased into place (Figure 4.3). Normally, the oropharyngeal airway

Core Topics in Mechanical Ventilation, ed. Iain Mackenzie. Published by Cambridge University Press.
© Cambridge University Press 2008.

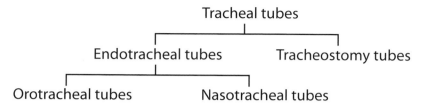

Figure 4.1 Nomenclature of tracheal tubes.

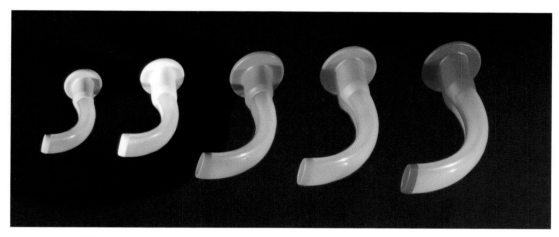

Figure 4.2 Guedel's Airways.

Sizes: Infant (size 00, light blue, 50 mm), small child (size 0, black, 55 mm), child (size 1, white, 65 mm), small adult (size 2, green, 80 mm), medium adult (size 3, orange or yellow, 90 mm) and large adult (size 4, red, 100 mm).

is used as a temporizing measure in two situations. First, it is used for patients whose conscious level is improving and an artificial airway will soon no longer be needed, such as during recovery from anaesthesia or awaiting reversal of an opiate overdose, and second for immediate assistance in ventilation and oxygenation while making preparations for a more definitive artificial airway.

Nasopharyngeal airways

Nasopharyngeal airways are commonly made of soft plastic, with a trumpeted end through which a safety pin is usually placed to prevent the airway slipping into the nose (Figure 4.4). The appropriately sized airway is lubricated with water-based gel and inserted perpendicularly to the face with a pill-rolling movement. There is a risk of trauma and bleeding, and if resistance is felt, then the other nos-

tril or a smaller diameter airway should be used. Placing the airway in hot water for one or two minutes softens it considerably, and can make it easier and less traumatic to insert. Laryngospasm and vomiting are stimulated if the nasopharyngeal airway is too long or if bleeding has been provoked. If correctly placed, nasopharyngeal airways are generally better tolerated than oropharyngeal airways in conscious patients. Although the nasopharyngeal airway will provide a temporary airway, it is also useful as an aid for secretion clearance from the hypopharynx. It is useful immediately after extubation in the critically ill when swallowing and coughing are impaired, and flexible suction catheters can be passed to the distal end to assist clearance. Nasopharyngeal airways carry the risk of erosive and infective complications.

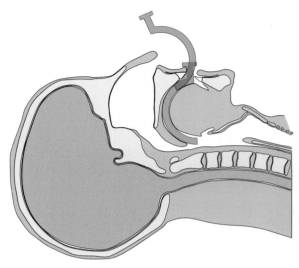

Figure 4.3 Technique for the insertion of an oropharyngeal airway.

The oropharyngeal airway is inserted upside-down with the concave surface to the patient's nose, and when half inserted, the airway is rotated 180° and gently eased home so that the straight portion of the airway lies between the patient's teeth.

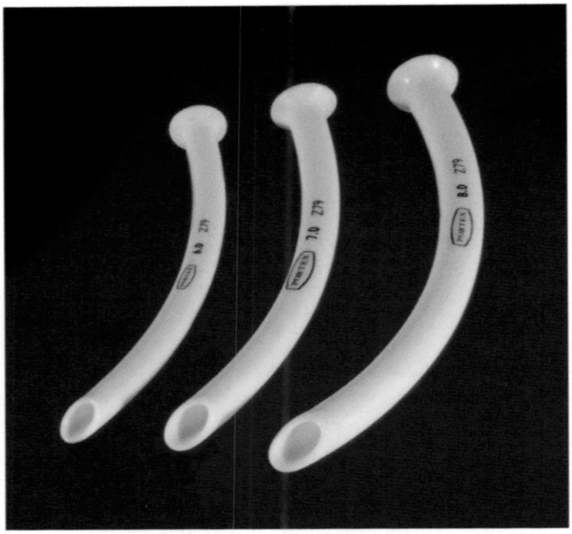

Figure 4.4 Nasopharyngeal airway.

Laryngeal mask airway

The laryngeal mask airway (LMA) is placed into the pharynx without the need for direct visualization (Figure 4.5). The insertion technique is easily mastered, and because of the rapidity of placement, it can save vital minutes. It is commonly used in the operating room for routine general anaesthesia and allows effective ventilation of the lungs to a pressure of about 20 to 30 cm H_2O. The LMA appears in the American Society of Anesthesiologists (ASA) Difficult Airway Algorithm and is a first line airway for rescue ventilation in the 'can't intubate, can't ventilate' situation. It does not, however, provide sufficient protection from aspiration in non-fasted patients and should be replaced with a definitive airway as soon as possible. The ProSeal[TM] LMA[1] and the Supreme[TM] LMA[2] are newer designs of the LMA with an oesophageal drainage tube to permit

venting of regurgitated fluid away from the laryngeal inlet. A gastric tube can be passed down the drainage tube to the stomach, if desired. The Fastrach[TM] or intubating LMA and the CTrach[TM] LMA[3] allow tracheal intubation and may be particularly useful when difficult laryngoscopy is anticipated, or if the neck needs to be immobilized in the midline position.

Combitube

The Combitube is a double lumen, double cuffed tube that may be inserted blindly through the mouth (Figure 4.6). The distal end normally passes into the oesophagus but occasionally enters the trachea. A large proximal pharyngeal balloon and a distal balloon are inflated. Depending upon the placement of the distal end, ventilation can be achieved through one or other lumen. It has been used successfully in the pre-hospital setting and in 'can't intubate, can't ventilate' situations. The Combitube is not a definitive airway and should be replaced as soon as possible.

---

[1] Laryngeal Mask Airway NV, Jersey, UK.
[2] LMA North America, Inc., San Diego, California, USA.

[3] Both made by LMA North America, Inc., San Diego, California, USA.

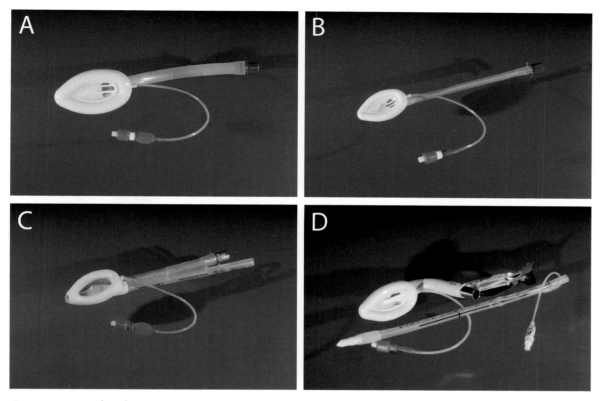

Figure 4.5 Laryngeal mask airways.

Placement of the artificial airway

In the short term, the airway can be secured in most patients with the use of simple airway adjuncts, as described above, with artificial ventilation provided manually with supplementary oxygen. For anything other than immediate life support, however, the airway needs to be secured with a cuffed endotracheal tube, or in some circumstances, a tracheostomy (Table 4.1). Endotracheal intubation in the critically ill patient carries challenges over and above those encountered during routine anaesthesia airway management because of a number of additional complicating factors (Table 4.2).

The time taken to achieve a secure airway, oxygenation and ventilation may be critical to survival, but endotracheal intubation, by whatever method,

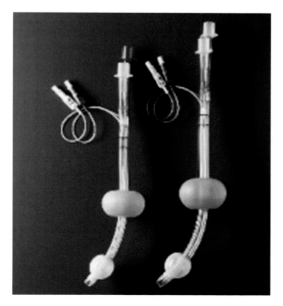

Figure 4.6 The Combitube.

Table 4.1 Indications for endotracheal intubation

- Need for assisted ventilation (failure of ventilation)
- High oxygen or positive end-expiratory pressure requirement (failure of oxygenation)
- Protection against pulmonary aspiration
- Central airway secretion clearance
- Upper airway obstruction

Table 4.2 Complicating factors in endotracheal intubation in critically ill patients

- In relation to the patient
  - Pre-existing hypoxia or hypercapnia, or both
  - Haemodynamic instability
  - Agitation or restlessness, or both
  - Potential for a full stomach
  - More likely to be elderly and edentulous, making airway control more difficult
- In relation to the environment
  - Less than ideal patient positioning (patient on the floor or in a confined space with poor access to the patient's head)
  - Reduced staff familiarity with either the equipment required (including drugs) or the procedure itself because of infrequent exposure
  - Higher risk of equipment failure (e.g. flat laryngoscope batteries, mismatch between laryngoscope blade and handle, mis-assembled bag and valve, empty oxygen cylinder)
  - Reduced availability of equipment required for difficult circumstances (e.g. a polio laryngoscope handle, a McCoy laryngoscope blade or a bougie)
  - Potential for unfamiliarity with the location and function of essential ancillary equipment (e.g. bed controls, suction, oxygen outlets)

is a skilled procedure that takes a full-time trainee in anaesthesia no less than three months to acquire in straightforward patients and no less than 12 months in more challenging ones. Complications are reduced when a junior physician is supervised by a senior colleague. The critical care team should therefore have immediate access to personnel with advanced airway skills and to appropriate monitoring and difficult-intubation equipment. When help from those with more experience is not immediately available, the non-anaesthetist is faced with a dilemma: sedate or anaesthetize the patient and risk losing the airway, or struggle on until help arrives or a cardio-respiratory arrest makes the patient easier to manage? Clearly the most appropriate course of action depends on the skill, confidence and experience of the attending clinician and the potential for someone more skilled in airway management, such as an anaesthetist, to attend. However, if the chance of experienced help arriving is low, a delay in controlling the situation merely postpones the airway management to a time when the patient is physiologically most vulnerable and least likely to do well. Details of the technique of rapid sequence induction, laryngoscopy and endotracheal intubation are beyond the scope of this chapter and readers should consult an appropriate anaesthetic text. However, familiarity with the minimum equipment requirements for acute airway management (Table 4.3) is a fundamental part of the safe and effective management of mechanical ventilation.

Oxygen supply

A primary goal of airway management is oxygenation. Many, but not all, clinical areas in an acute care setting will have a piped supply of oxygen. This is usually delivered to self-sealing wall outlets[4] at a pressure of 420 kPa (Figures 4.7, 4.8 and 4.9). The sockets for oxygen, like the sockets for other medical gases, are designed with a collar-indexing system that is gas-specific and will only accept the right probes. This means that only equipment designed for the delivery of oxygen, such as the single or double flow meters, can be plugged into these sockets. The sockets are designed to lock the probes in place

---

[4] Referred to as *Schraeder sockets*.

Table 4.3 Minimum equipment required for acute airway management

- Oxygen supply
- Physiological monitoring equipment
  - Pulse oximetry
  - Electrocardiography
  - Blood pressure
  - End-tidal carbon dioxide analysis
- Airway equipment
  - Supraglottic airways in a range of sizes
  - Two laryngoscope handles (with one set of spare batteries)
  - Standard Macintosh laryngoscope blades in sizes 3 and 4
  - McCoy laryngoscope blade
  - Gum elastic bougie
  - Malleable stylet
  - Scissors
  - 10 mL syringes
  - Endotracheal tubes in a range of sizes
- Tilting bed
- Suction apparatus
- Drugs
  - Hypnotics (propofol 1%, etomidate, midazolam)
  - Opioids (alfentanyl, fentanyl)
  - Muscle relaxants (suxamethonium, atracurium)
  - Pressors (metaraminol, ephedrine)
  - Anticholinergics (atropine)
  - Ventilation equipment

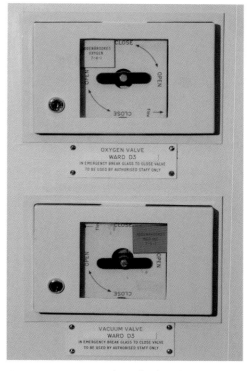

Figure 4.7 Emergency shut-off valves for piped oxygen and vacuum.

In an emergency, such as a fire, breaking the glass and turning the bar counter-clockwise will close the valves, cutting all the piped oxygen. All staff working in a clinical area should know where these valves are located.

and will only release the probe when the locking collar is depressed. In the absence of a piped supply, oxygen can be delivered in the short-term from oxygen cylinders. In the UK, these were traditionally identified by a black body with white shoulders and are available in a variety of sizes (Figure 4.10). Newer carbon fibre cylinders are designed to be lightweight for portability, have integral valves and gauges and have a higher capacity for a given size, but do not conform to the traditional colour coding, instead being white with 'Oxygen' printed on the cylinder in large black letters.[5]

[5] BOC Medical, Manchester, UK.

Monitoring

Both the ASA and the Association of Anaesthetists of Great Britain and Ireland have published minimum requirements for monitoring during anaesthesia and these should form the basic bedside monitoring in acute care areas, such as the emergency department and the intensive care unit (ICU) where the requirement for urgent airway control is likely. Of particular importance are continuous pulse oximetry and bedside capnography for rapid verification of satisfactory airway placement and both blood pressure and electrocardiogram (ECG) monitoring to recognize the instability commonly encountered during and after intubation (discussed later).

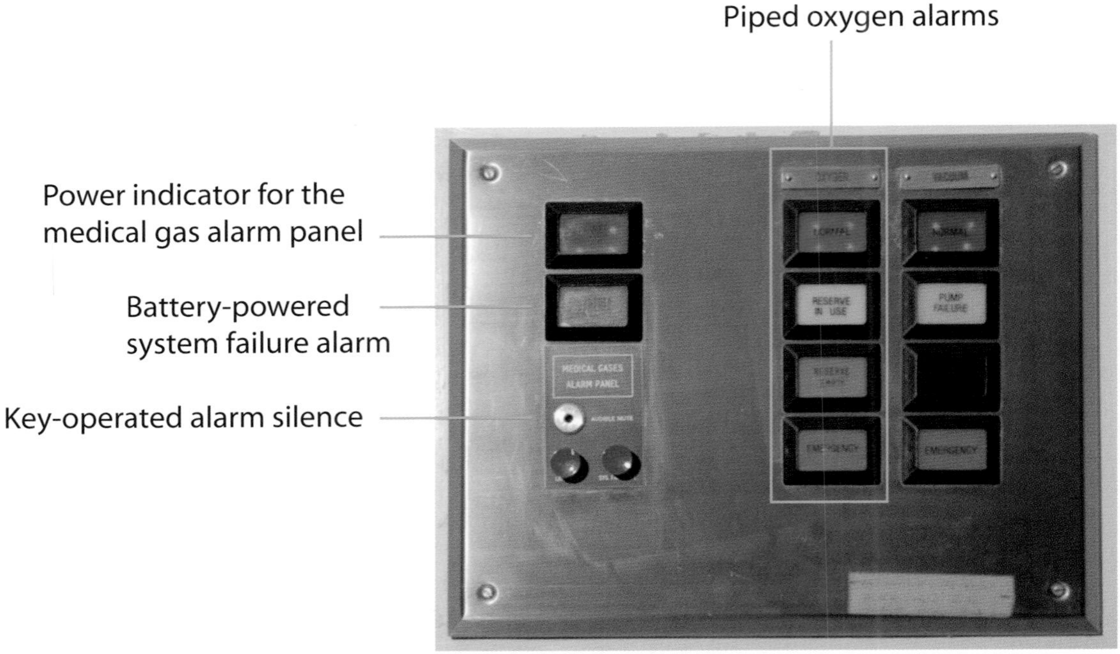

Piped oxygen alarms

Power indicator for the
medical gas alarm panel

Battery-powered
system failure alarm

Key-operated alarm silence

Figure 4.8 Medical gas alarm panel.

The alarm panel warns of a system failure, either of the panel itself or of the medical gases being monitored. This particular panel for an intensive care unit has alarms for the piped oxygen supply and the piped vacuum, with four condition indicators: 'normal', 'reserve in use', 'reserve empty' and 'emergency'. Loss of pressure in the main hospital oxygen supply, which is normally drawn from a tank of liquid oxygen, triggers a switch to a bank of back-up cylinders. Activation of the 'reserve in use' alarm should prompt senior staff to move oxygen cylinders to each bed-space where oxygen is being used in order to be prepared to switch to cylinder oxygen in the event of the piped supply failing.

Airway equipment

In addition to a range of supraglottic airways, the person performing the intubation will need access to standard equipment (Table 4.3). Vital items such as laryngoscope handles and blades should be available in duplicate in case of equipment failure. A selection of additional equipment for the management of the difficult airway should be available separately. A review of the vast array of difficult intubation techniques and associated equipment is beyond the scope of this chapter.

The importance of skilled assistance cannot be overemphasized. Correctly applied cricoid pressure reduces the risk of gastric regurgitation (Box 4.1), a likely complication in the un-fasted patient, espe-

cially when the stomach has been inflated by over-enthusiastic bag and mask ventilation. Simple aids to laryngeal visualization, such as external laryngeal manipulation and backwards upwards and right-wards pressure (the BURP manoeuvre[3]) are also useful. Intensive care nurses, however, are not only less likely to possess these skills than theatre-based staff, but are also less likely to use these skills on a regular basis. Calls for these skills to become a basic part of critical care nurse training,[4] supplemented by regular refresher training, appear to have been largely ignored.

Finally, equipment and drugs for emergency airway management should be kept in a designated location and checked regularly against an inventory to ensure that items are not missing and that all

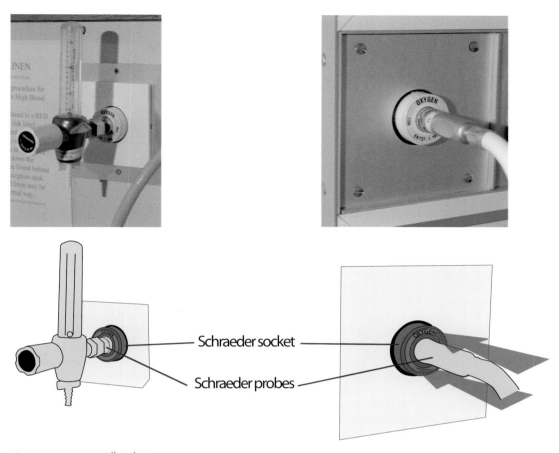

Figure 4.9 Oxygen wall sockets.

Schraeder pattern wall sockets for piped oxygen indicated in red in the diagrams below the photographs. The sockets will only accept Schraeder probes attached to equipment that uses oxygen. On the left, the Schraeder probe is attached to an oxygen flow meter and 'fir tree' connector designed to deliver oxygen through face masks. On the right, the probe is attached to oxygen hosing which in this instance provides oxygen to a mechanical ventilator. The probes can only be released from the sockets by pressing firmly against the collar, as shown by the green arrows on the right.

the equipment is clean, correctly assembled and in working order.

Tilting bed or trolley

Patients at risk of deterioration and who may need acute airway care should be nursed on beds capable of rapid positioning into the head-down position. This assists with the clearance of regurgitated fluid and also helps, in the short term, to deal with the haemodynamic consequences of mechanical ventilation.

Suction apparatus

Suction can be obtained from a wall or portable vacuum source. The apparatus should be easy to use, rugged and reliable. It should be able to both generate an appropriate maximal negative pressure (e.g. 500 mm Hg) and flow rate (e.g. 25 litres per minute). Both flexible catheters and rigid tonsillar tip (Yankaeur) catheters should be available. The rigid catheter allows the rapid removal of large volumes of fluid and particulate matter from the oropharynx. The flexible catheter can be used for

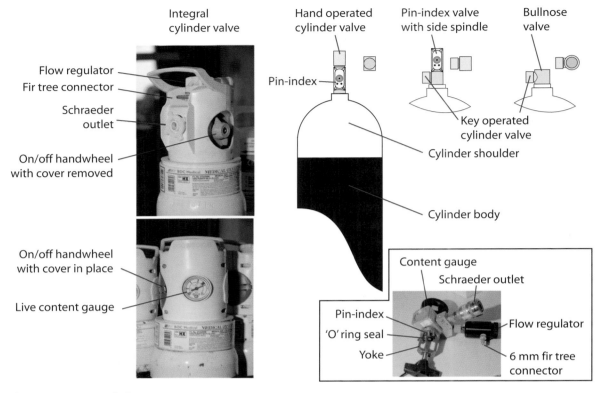

Figure 4.10 Oxygen cylinders.

Colour coding of cylinders is based on BS EN 1089–3 (for countries in the European Community) and ISO 32, but not all countries adhere to these standards. In hospitals in the UK, the commonest cylinders for ward use now have integral valves fitted with a live content gauge, an on/off handwheel, an integral flow regulator with a 6 mm fir tree connector, and in some cases (CD, HX and ZX) a Schraeder outlet. These are available as 2- or 10-litre cylinders containing, when full, 400 (AD), 460 (CD), 2300 (HX) and 3040 (ZX) litres of oxygen. Cylinders with a pin-index connector are designed to be fitted to equipment such as anaesthetic machines or resuscitation trolleys, but can be used to deliver oxygen directly to patients when fitted with an appropriate yoke and flow regulator (see inset). Cylinders with bullnose valves are now less common, and are generally found in areas where oxygen is only occasionally used. Being larger (F = 9.43 litres; G = 23.6 litres) and heavier (14.5 and 34.5 kg respectively, when empty) they are usually moved to the patient's bedside in a cylinder truck. These cylinders are often stored with the cylinder valve closed to prevent the cylinder from slowly emptying through leaky flow regulators. Unfortunately, while this often stops the cylinders from emptying, this also stops the cylinder from being used when no one can find the cylinder key.

suctioning of the tracheal tube or the pharynx, or to empty the stomach. Both types of catheter need to be used with care because they can cause mucosal damage, bradycardia, laryngospasm or de-oxygenation due to both the pause in ventilation and de-recruitment.

Drugs and venous access

The provision of intravenous fluid resuscitation and cardiovascular support is normally required during acute airway management. Haemodynamic insta-bility can be due to the pressor response of laryn-goscopy causing tachycardia and hypertension. A more common problem however is cardiovascular collapse resulting from the combination of under-lying pathophysiology, hypovolaemia, the adminis-tration of vasodilator and cardio-depressant drugs and the change from a negative to a positive intrathoracic pressure which reduces venous return. If significant hypovolaemia is likely to be present, at

Box 4.1 Correct application of cricoid pressure

Application of two-handed cricoid pressure. With one hand supporting the cervical spine behind the patient's head, the operator is applying pressure with the index finger and thumb directly over the cricoid cartilage (shown in red). The thyroid cartilage is relatively easy to locate, especially in males, as it forms the largest structure of the upper airway. Having identified the body of the thyroid cartilage, the cricoid is found immediately below, with the gap between the two being the site of the cricothyroid membrane. The cricoid is being used to occlude the oesophagus, which lies immediately behind it, in order to prevent the regurgitation of gastric contents.

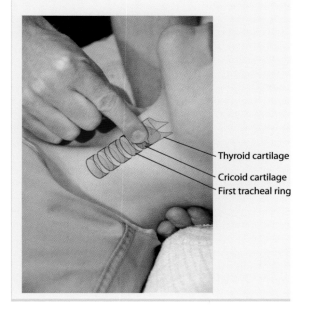

Thyroid cartilage
Cricoid cartilage
First tracheal ring

the very least aggressive fluid resuscitation should be underway before the administration of any hypnotics. Compromised patients need significantly lower doses of hypnotic drugs than one might expect for a patient of the same age and weight, and frequently respond more slowly because of a slower circulation. This can sometimes tempt the nervous or unwary into giving further doses of hypnotic before the initial dose has had an effect, with catastrophic consequences. Combinations of a short-acting benzodiazepine, such as midazolam, with a potent and rapidly acting opioid, such as fentanyl or alfentanyl, are potent, reliable and cause relatively little hypotension. This combination also has the advantage of being pharmacologically reversible. In the hands of anaesthetists propofol is a reasonably safe alternative, provided they are provided with the same concentration that they normally use in theatre (usually 1%). Etomidate, on the other hand, which is regarded as cardiovascularly 'silent', is associated with adrenal suppression but in the context of a single induction dose the relevance of this to outcome is unclear. Drug-related hypotension often responds to 0.5 or 1 mg of metaraminol and also produces a fall in heart rate. If hypotension is accompanied by bradycardia, however, 3 to 6 mg of ephedrine is preferable because this will increase both blood pressure and heart rate.

Ventilator

A minimal requirement for the critically ill patient is a mechanical ventilator capable of providing 100% oxygen, positive end-expiratory pressure (PEEP) and with appropriate monitoring and alarm functions. A simple self-inflating bag and mask system should be available in all acute areas of the hospital for temporary ventilation. The self-inflating bag should remain available in case the mechanical ventilator fails and it can be used as an aid to diagnose partial or complete airway obstruction.

Endotracheal tube

Oral or nasal

Orotracheal tubes should be used in the emergency situation as they are generally easier and more rapid to insert than nasotracheal tubes (Figure 4.11). In some units, particularly those

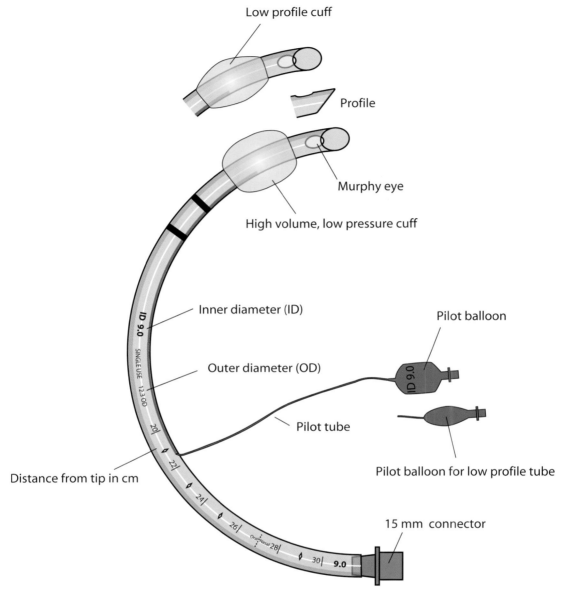

Figure 4.11 Endotracheal tubes.

Although endotracheal tubes from different manufacturers will differ in detail, they all share many of the features that are shown here. The distal end is usually bevelled, and in some brands there is an opening on the right-hand side called the Murphy eye. This is designed to prevent occlusion of the right upper lobe bronchus, which can arise directly from the trachea in some people. The distal margin of the cuff is located approximately half a centimetre above the Murphy eye, and may either be 'high-volume, low-pressure' or 'low-profile'. Proximal to the upper margin of the cuff, some brands have two black lines which indicate where the vocal cords should lie. Running up from the cuff within the anterior wall of the tube is a narrow duct that connects to the pilot tube, and pilot balloon. The pilot balloon has a Luer fitting with a spring-loaded valve that will accept a standard syringe for inflating the cuff. The proximal end of the endotracheal tube is loosely fitted with a standard 15 mm connector, which has to be seated firmly into the endotracheal tube before use.

caring for children, nasotracheal tubes are preferred because of the greater stability of fixation, protection from biting, improved comfort and swallowing and better access for oral care compared with orotracheal tubes. However, being longer and narrower than oral tubes, nasotracheal tubes result in greater airway resistance and are more difficult to pass a tracheal suction catheter through. They can kink easily and are often traumatic to insert, causing damage to the inferior turbinates and nasopharynx with associated bleeding. In patients with a haemostatic defect (therapeutic anticoagulation, thrombocytopenia, liver disease or severe sepsis) the risk of bleeding would be considered by most to be a contra-indication to the nasal route. In patients with basal skull fractures, it is even possible to intubate the cranial cavity during the insertion of the nasotracheal tube. Nasal tubes obstruct the normal drainage of mucus from the maxillary sinuses to the nasal space and significantly increase the risk of maxillary sinusitis, which in turn increases the risk of developing ventilator-associated pneumonia (see Chapter 15). Many critical care physicians avoid the use of nasal tubes because of this.

Size and length

Endotracheal tubes are available in a range of sizes given by their inner diameter (ID) measured in millimetres, with adult females normally requiring a size 7 or 8 and adult males 8 or 9 (Table 4.4). A larger ID tube provides better access for tracheal suctioning and easier passage of a fibreoptic bronchoscope. Tube blockage with secretions is common and occurs more quickly in tubes with a smaller ID (Figure 4.12). Tubes with a larger ID cause less airway resistance but are more likely to result in erosions of the laryngeal inlet. Increased airway resistance is less of a concern with more modern mechanical ventilators that can compensate for the increased work of breathing associated with the tracheal tube and breathing circuit. This compensation

Table 4.4 Typical sizes and lengths for oral and nasal endotracheal tubes in adult males and females

Inner diameter	Oral length	Female	Male	Nasal length	Female	Male
6	−			22	+	
6.5	−			23	++	+
7	21	+		24	+	++
7.5	22	++		25		+
8	23	+	+	26		
9	24		++	27		
10	25		+			
11	26					

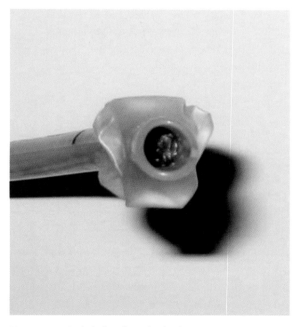

Figure 4.12 Occluded endotracheal tube.
View looking up the distal end of an endotracheal tube that is almost completely occluded by a dried mucus plug.

is less efficient if the tracheal tube becomes partially occluded with secretions, and can lead to weaning difficulties.

Endotracheal tubes are presented in sterile packaging in lengths of 31 to 33 cm. Whenever possible

Box 4.2 Technique for cutting an orotracheal tube in situ

Step 1 Remove the tapes or ties from the tube and have an assistant stabilize the tube.

Step 2 Disconnect the endotracheal tube from the ventilator circuit and remove the 15 mm connector.

Step 3 With a pair of sharp scissors, cut 2/3 across the endotracheal tube at the desired length, about 1 cm away from the patient's teeth.

Step 4 Holding the end of the tube firmly, bend it 90° at the cut so that the orifice of the distal end of the tube (which remains in the patient) is clearly visible, and then re-insert the 15 mm connector.

Step 5 Reconnect the patient to the ventilator circuit, and then cut across the remaining 1/3 of the tube to remove the unwanted section of tube.

Step 6 Re-secure the endotracheal tube with ties or tape, as before.

they should be cut to an appropriate length (Table 4.4) prior to insertion so that no more than 1 or 2 cm of tube remains outside the patient when the tip is correctly positioned mid-way between the vocal cords and the carina. Tubes cannot be cut below the point where the pilot tube joins the body of the tube, and the 15 mm connector should be replaced firmly by rotating into place *without* using lubricant. Cutting endotracheal tubes to the correct length after insertion is much more difficult, although it can be done providing the patient can tolerate loss of ventilation and positive end-expiratory pressure during the manoeuvre (see Box 4.2).

Cuff types

Since the late 1960s, the large-diameter high-volume low-pressure (HVLP) cuff has become the standard in intensive care. This type of cuff is essentially a floppy bag with a resting diameter larger than

that of the trachea. When inflated, there is no tension within the wall of the cuff and so the entire cuff pressure is transmitted to the tracheal wall. This also allows the tracheal wall pressure to be kept at a safe level by monitoring and adjusting the cuff pressure. The introduction of HVLP cuffs has led to a reduction in the incidence of tracheal injury associated with intubation. Unfortunately, HVLP cuffs allow pulmonary aspiration to occur even when correctly inflated[5] (Figure 4.13), although the rate of aspiration is reduced by preventing unintentional falls in cuff pressure.

Endotracheal tubes with low-volume cuffs remain available and are generally for use during anaesthesia. When deflated, these endotracheal tubes have a narrower outer diameter at the cuff (low-profile) that may offer some advantages when negotiating a difficult airway, for use in certain surgical procedures or during nasal intubation (with reinforced tubes, oral and nasal RAE[6] tubes, low-contour tubes, or double-lumen tubes). Therefore, a patient admitted to intensive care from the operating theatre may not have an appropriate endotracheal tube for prolonged mechanical ventilation.

Special tubes

Endotracheal tubes are available with an additional channel that opens above the cuff (to allow material lying above it to be sucked away), or with an additional channel that opens below the cuff to administer resuscitation drugs.

One lung ventilation is an established anaesthetic technique that allows surgical access to structures within the thorax, or even the lungs themselves, without the need for cardio-pulmonary bypass. The technique is made possible by the use of a double-lumen endotracheal tube that allows each lung to be ventilated (or decompressed) independently (Figure 4.14). At the end of surgery, these tubes are usually replaced by conventional endotra-

---

[6] Named after Ring, Adair and Elwin.

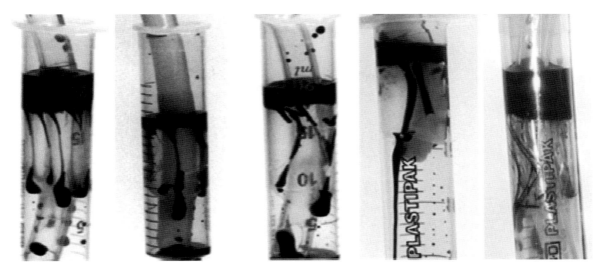

Figure 4.13 Leaks in high-volume low-pressure (HVLP) cuffs.
Five common brands of high-volume low-pressure cuff were inflated to the correct cuff pressure inside the body of a 20-mL syringe to simulate the trachea. Above each was placed a small volume of methylene blue dye, which in each case can be seen tracking down grooves formed between the cuff and the inside surface of the syringe.

cheal tubes. Occasionally double-lumen tubes are needed in intensive care, either to isolate the lungs from each other to prevent cross-contamination (for example, in focal haemorrhage), or for independent lung ventilation which may be required following single lung transplant or in the presence of a massive bronchopleural fistula. Unlike standard endotracheal tubes, the size of double-lumen tubes is given in French gauge[7].

Armoured or reinforced tubes are similar in shape to standard endotracheal tubes but are constructed of soft PVC or silicone and embedded within the wall of the tube is a spiral of wire, which makes them very resistant to kinking, although irreversible crushing can be a problem if the patient bites down onto the tube (Figure 4.15). The pilot channel exits the wall of the tube at the proximal end, rather than about 20 cm from the tip, making it impossible to reduce the length of these tubes without cutting the pilot channel and deflating the cuff. Many anaes-

thetists favour armoured tubes for neurosurgery, surgery involving the mouth, neck, jaw or face or for nasal intubation. Many of these tubes do not have HVLP cuffs and are not suitable for prolonged use.

Care of the breathing system

Securing the tube

Orotracheal tubes are commonly secured using adhesive tape or cloth ties. The type of knot used does not appear to make a difference but the method of adhesive tape fixation does. Commercial devices specifically designed to hold the tube in place allow less movement and slippage, but some are better than others. In all cases, the fixation device or material should be inelastic, and firmly attached to the endotracheal tube as near to the front teeth as possible. If the tie is attached more than one or two centimetres from the front teeth, this allows extension of the patient's head to pull the endotracheal tube down, away from the mouth and is a common cause of concealed extubation (Figure 4.16). This situation is often signalled by a 'cuff leak'

---

[7] External diameter in millimetres multiplied by three, also called *Charrier*.

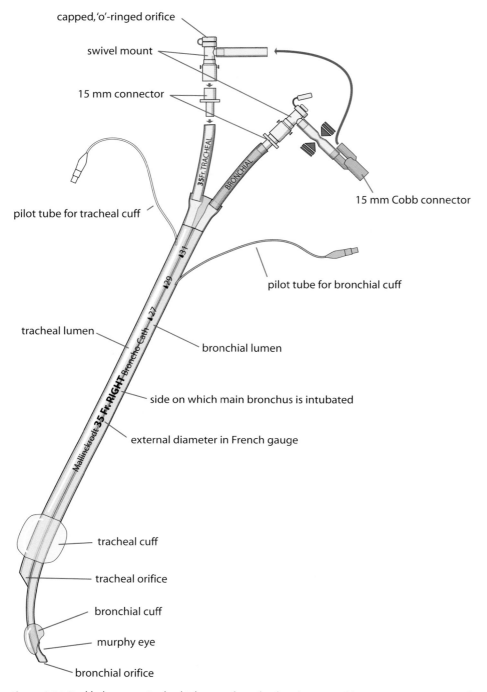

capped, 'o'-ringed orifice

swivel mount

15 mm connector

15 mm Cobb connector

pilot tube for tracheal cuff

pilot tube for bronchial cuff

tracheal lumen

bronchial lumen

side on which main bronchus is intubated

external diameter in French gauge

tracheal cuff

tracheal orifice

bronchial cuff

murphy eye

bronchial orifice

Figure 4.14 Double-lumen orotracheal tube seen from the dorsal aspect, with 15 mm connector, swivel mount and Cobb connector already attached to the bronchial lumen.

Sizes are given in French gauge, giving the external diameter of a 35Fr tube 11.6 mm, which is similar to a conventional size 8 orotracheal tube. The distal lumen intubates the main-stem bronchus either on the right or left, with the shape of the tube and distal cuff designed specifically. Right and left tubes are therefore not interchangeable. The proximal lumen opens in the trachea just distal to the tracheal cuff. The Cobb connector attaches to the swivel mounts of each lumen and allows both lungs to be ventilated simultaneously. Clamping the soft clear section of the swivel mount and uncapping the o-ring orifice allows the lung on that side to collapse, as shown here for the right lung. Attaching each 15 mm connector to a separate ventilator with conventional catheter mounts allows each lung to be ventilated independently.

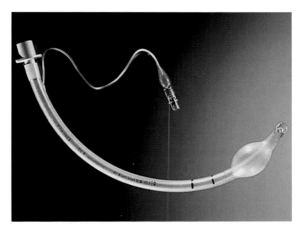

Figure 4.15 Armoured tube.

Softer and more flexible than standard tubes, the armoured tube is highly resistant to kinking because of the wire spiral within its walls. Note the low profile cuff and the position at which the pilot tube attaches to the tube wall. Armoured tubes cannot be cut, but must be used as presented.

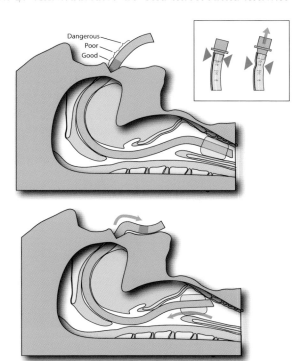

Figure 4.16 Position of tube tie and mechanism of concealed extubation.

Top: Correct tube length and tube tie position are interrelated. If the tube is cut to the correct length so that no more than 1 cm protrudes beyond the patient's front teeth, the tube tie can be secured to lie over the 15 mm connector so that the tube is clamped onto the connector (inset, left). In this position, the tube tie can be tightened very securely. If the tube is too long, the tube tie has to be secured below the 15 mm connector, and in this position will expel the connector if tied too tightly (inset, right).

Bottom: If the tube tie position is too short, the patient's trachea can become extubated by flexion at the neck or by tongue movement. This occurs relatively commonly, and often presents as a 'cuff leak'.

that cannot be eliminated by the addition of more air into the cuff. Cloth ties which pass around the back of the patient's neck should be tied with the patient's head resting on a pillow in a neutral position and slack enough to permit two fingers to slide between the tie and the patient's cheek. In patients at risk of raised intracranial pressure,[8] ties may cause cerebral venous engorgement and should not be used. Patients with significant facial or upper airway burns should also not have their orotracheal tubes tied or taped during the first two or three days. In these patients, massive facial swelling during this period can generate sufficient traction on a tied or taped tube to pull it out of the trachea. Tube fixation can be achieved by fixing the tube to healthy upper teeth, usually the front incisors, with wire. Unplanned extubation may be caused either by the patient (self-extubation) or the staff (accidental extubation), but the type of system used to secure the tube is not a factor in either.

Mechanical injury to the airway and mouth is also reduced by supporting the breathing circuit.

Cuff pressure control

Surveys have repeatedly shown that cuff pressures are not routinely monitored in the ICU, although the reasons for this are not clear. In the absence of direct monitoring, neither physicians nor nurses are

---

[8] Such as with traumatic or hypoxic head injury, fulminant hepatic failure.

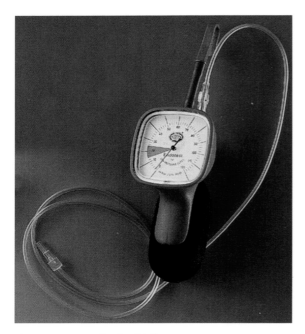

Figure 4.17 Example of cuff inflator.

able to accurately estimate the acceptable range of 20 to 30 cm H_2O, with most tending to underestimate the pressure. Both over- and under-inflation are undesirable. Over-inflation can result in tracheal injury subsequent to a restriction in capillary blood flow, and in hypotensive patients mucosal perfusion pressure is likely to be even lower. An unrecognized fall in cuff pressure is equally problematic because it causes an increased rate of aspiration,[6] and a persistent cuff pressure below 20 cm H_2O has been shown to be associated with the development of pneumonia within the first eight days of mechanical ventilation.[7]

MANUAL INFLATORS

Handheld cuff inflators with integral manometers (Figure 4.17) are convenient for intermittent measurement and adjustment and are sufficiently precise for clinical use, but can cause temporary loss of cuff pressure when measurement technique is poor. The most important problem is the compressible volume within the device that allows cuff pressure

to fall as soon as the pilot valve is connected. Unintentional depression of the deflation button on the inflator can also occur. If manual inflators are used, it is necessary for all operators to understand and be proficient in their use.

LANZ BALLOON

The Lanz inflation balloon is an integral component of a brand of tracheal tube incorporating a HVLP cuff[9] (Figure 4.18). This is an ingenious constant pressure balloon combined with a pressure-regulating valve and protected in a PVC sleeve. The device maintains the cuff pressure in the desirable range, preventing over- and under-inflation.

FOAM-FILLED CUFF

An endotracheal tube with a foam-filled HVLP cuff is also available. Air is aspirated from the cuff to collapse the foam, which remains collapsed while the spring-loaded valve in the pilot tube remains closed. Following tracheal intubation, the cap on the pilot tube is opened, allowing the cuff to expand under the force of the expanding foam. Although this method of cuff inflation avoids accidental loss of cuff pressure, aspiration can still occur by the same mechanism as with conventional cuffs[5] (Figure 4.13).

ELECTRONIC CUFF PRESSURE CONTROLLER

The Tracoe[10] cuff pressure controller is a portable electrical device with a battery back-up which is designed to be permanently attached to the pilot tube. It continuously and accurately maintains the cuff pressure at the target value set by the operator and has audible alarms for unintentional disconnections and power failure. Besides high cost, this device has two potential disadvantages. First, if the tube is unintentionally withdrawn into the larynx,

---

[9] Hi-Lo® Tracheal Tube with Lanz® Pressure Regulating Valve, Mallinckrodt

[10] See http://www.tracoe.com

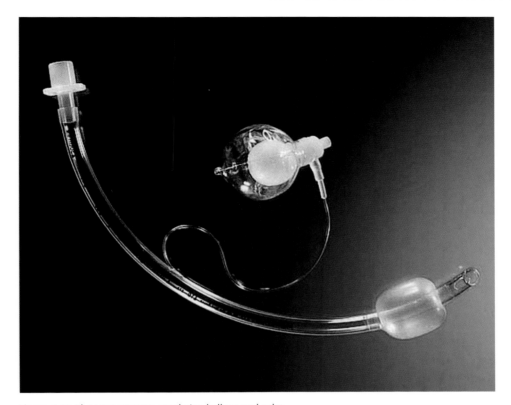

Figure 4.18 The Lanz pressure-regulating balloon and valve.

the device will further inflate the cuff, preventing re-intubation (until the situation is recognized and the cuff deflated and the tube re-positioned). Second, the inflator has a standard Luer-lock[11] connector. If this is accidentally misconnected to an intravenous line, a fatal air embolus will occur.

Failure to obtain an airtight seal immediately following intubation indicates either that the cuff has been torn during intubation, or too small a tube has been used and the tracheal diameter exceeds the diameter of the fully inflated cuff. In both situations the tube should be replaced, if possible (as will be discussed later). Cuff leaks that arise at a later date are usually caused by concealed extubation, although occasionally cuffs can become punctured

during the insertion of central venous cannulae in the neck.

Cuff deflation

Routine intermittent cuff deflation is not required if cuff pressure monitoring is used. When deflation is required both oropharyngeal and sub-glottic suctioning (if available) should be performed before-hand to prevent the airway from becoming soiled with secretions pooled above the cuff. The use of CPAP during cuff deflation may further protect against pulmonary aspiration of these secretions.

Sub-glottic secretion drainage

Radiological studies have shown that secretions pool above the cuff of an intra-tracheal tube, providing a reservoir of infected material for

---

[11] Named after the German instrument maker Hermann Wulfing Luer who made the first all-glass syringe in Paris in 1870.

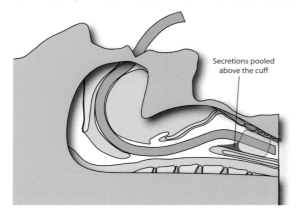

Figure 4.19 Pooling of secretions above the cuff.

micro-aspiration (Figure 4.19), leading to the development of early-onset ventilator-associated pneumonia. One type of endotracheal tube[12] includes a suction channel that runs down the dorsal aspect of the tube adjacent to the pilot channel and opens just above the cuff to allow secretions to be suctioned from the sub-glottic space (Figure 4.20). A recent meta-analysis of five randomized studies which compared normal endotracheal tubes to those with sub-glottic suction showed a 50% reduction in early-onset ventilator-associated pneumonia and significant reductions in the duration of mechanical ventilation and length of ICU stay.[8] However, the advisability of continuous suction has been questioned by animal data showing that this causes tracheal injury even at lower negative pressures,[9] and intermittent suction is likely to be less effective in reducing the incidence of pulmonary aspiration. Whether this is relevant to the clinical situation is unknown. In the absence of continuous sub-glottic suction, the sub-glottic space should be suctioned prior to tracheobronchial suctioning, adjustments of cuff pressure, extubation, or any other manoeuvre that might facilitate the movement of secretions between cuff and tracheal wall. Finally, the addition of the suction channel into the wall of the tube increases its rigidity and is prone to

blockage. This increased rigidity has been blamed for a fatal case of tracheal wall erosion[10] and a case of tube displacement,[11] although these are isolated reports.

Oral hygiene

In the critically ill, supine, ventilated patient, secretions pool in the oropharynx and sub-glottic space above the tracheal tube cuff,[1] forming a reservoir of colonized, acidic, or bilious secretions that bathe the larynx and sub-glottic space, and which is known to be damaging. Unfortunately oropharyngeal hygiene measures normally cannot hope to reach the laryngotracheal area. Good oral hygiene can reduce the volume and bacterial load of these secretions. During critical illness there is a reduction in protective secretory substances such as fibronectin, and effective oral hygiene, despite the best nursing care, will decline with a rapid shift of dental plaque colonization to pathogenic bacteria.[1] This increases the risk of ventilator-associated pneumonia[12] (VAP). Oral chlorhexidine solutions have been used successfully to reduce oral colonization and VAP. Consideration of decontamination of the digestive tract is beyond the scope of this chapter.

Management of the lower airway

In health, cilial beating on viscous mucus propels debris towards the larynx for expectoration, and inspired gases are warmed and humidified to prevent secretions from drying out. As well as providing a physical barrier to mucus clearance, tracheal intubation can reduce tracheal mucus velocity, abolish an effective cough and bypass the natural mechanisms for retaining heat and moisture. If the upper airways are bypassed by an artificial device, the inspired gases are heated and humidified by the lower rather than upper airway mucosa and this results in tracheal mucosal drying, damage to the respiratory epithelium and heat loss.[13] This then impairs the function of the mucociliary escalator,

---

[12] HiLo EVAC, Mallinckrodt, Hazelwood, Missouri, USA.

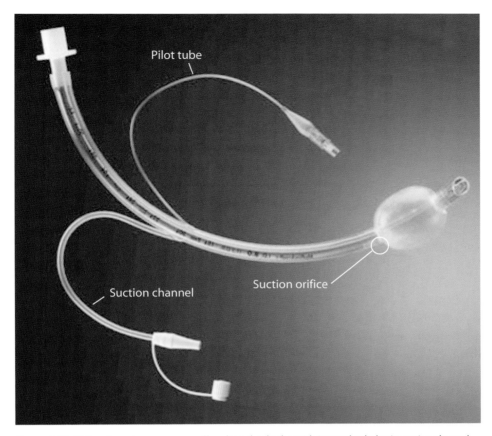

Figure 4.20 High-volume low-pressure cuff endotracheal tube with integral subglottic suction channel.

the degree of damage being proportional to the duration of ventilation with dry gases.[13]

With proper care of the ventilator circuit, the humidification device, and nebulizers, and with a sterile technique for tracheal suctioning, colonization of the lumen of the tracheal tube and breathing circuit is normally of endogenous origin. Sampling studies suggest that the oropharynx becomes colonized with pathogenic bacteria after only one to two days, followed by the stomach, the lower respiratory tract (after two to four days) and finally the inner surface of the endotracheal tube.[14] Pathogens may occasionally be inadvertently introduced if contaminated tap water is used in nebulizers, to clean respiratory equipment or to dilute enteral feed. The universal problem of aspiration past HVLP cuffs[5] leads to rapid tracheal colonization. Pneumonia develops if the pathogenicity of bacteria within the aspirated material is sufficient to overcome lung defences.[1, 2] Once a biofilm has developed on the inner lumen, the bacteria are protected from systemic antibiotics secreted in saliva and tracheal mucus, and infected material can be repeatedly propelled into the trachea and distal lung by inspiratory gas flow and tracheal suction catheters.

Effective management of the lower airway therefore involves restoring as far as possible the compromised mechanisms for maintaining optimal mucous quality and quantity and replacing the absent clearance with tracheobronchial suctioning.

Humidification

A humidifier should ideally provide inspired gas delivered into the trachea at 32 to 36 °C at 100% humidity without allowing condensate to form in the circuit, the tracheal tube, or in the tracheo-bronchial tree. This condensate may wash back into the patient, carrying biofilm with it. When an artificial airway is in place, inspiratory gases should always be heated and humidified. A number of systems are available, including heat and moisture exchange filters (HMEF), active HMEF and hot water humidifiers. Cold water humidifiers (CWH) are simple and cheap, but inefficient. Gas is delivered to the patient slightly below room temperature and they cannot provide adequate humidification for a patient whose airway is bypassed.

HEAT AND MOISTURE EXCHANGE FILTER (HMEF)

Heat and moisture exchange filters (HMEFs) have a condensation membrane and usually also a microbiological filter. During expiration, the warm moist gases condense on the membrane. The specific heat of expired gases and latent heat of water warm the membrane. During inspiration the cooler and drier inspired gas is warmed and humidified as it passes through the membrane. The expired heat and moisture is returned to the patient. HMEFs however increase both dead space and airflow resistance and should be used with caution, if at all, in weak or tired patients who are not receiving support with the work of breathing. Prolonged intubation results in progressive reduction of endotracheal tube patency to a greater extent with HMEFs than with hot water humidifiers (HWH) and this may lead to airway occlusion. Hygroscopic HMEFs are normally cheaper than HMEFs and can maintain clean ventilator circuits despite the absence of filtering media. Extended use of an HMEF is also safe and cost effective. Use for up to seven days does not increase resistance, affect circuit colonization, or increase the rate of ventilation-associated pneu-

monia. Therefore, the HMEF should not be changed unless visibly soiled or damaged.

ACTIVE HEAT AND MOISTURE EXCHANGER

In an attempt to improve the efficiency of passive HMEFs, active HMEFs have been developed recently. Water is added to an electrically heated hygroscopic–hydrophobic membrane causing evaporation and thereby increasing absolute humidity over a standard HME. There are insufficient data to recommend use of these devices at present.

HOT WATER HUMIDIFIER (HWH)

In hot water humidifiers (HWHs), inspired gas passes over or through a heated water reservoir producing gas at close to 100% humidity at higher than body temperature. The gas cools along the tubing and this results in an inspired relative humidity of 100% at 37 °C. A heated wire is normally present in the inspiratory tubing to reduce gas cooling. HWHs provide excellent humidity and heat, but they increase nursing workload and the risk of bacterial colonization of the ventilator circuit. Accumulation of condensate in the circuit due to the cooling of gases can occur (rain-out). If this is not removed regularly, it can run down the tracheal tube. Wash back of this fluid into the patient commonly occurs with changes in the tubing or patient position. The condensate may have high bacterial counts. In one study, the median level of colonization at 24 hours was 7×10^4 organisms.mL^{-1} and condensate can collect in circuits at a mean rate of 30 mL.hr^{-1}.[15] Even if the rain-out has not become heavily contaminated, it is likely to wash colonized biofilm from the inner lumen of the tracheal tube during its passage to the lungs. Other possible disadvantages include overheating malfunctions that may cause burns, a rise in core temperature and over-humidification. Patients at high risk for airway occlusion, with tenacious secretions, airway obstructive disease or hypothermia, are often considered more suitable for HWHs, although this view is not universally held.

HMEFs are passive and not capable of producing the same degree of humidification as HWHs, but they may have a protective effect through minimizing tubing condensate and colonization. Although there is disagreement among clinical studies, a meta-analysis of eight randomized controlled trials has examined the effect of the replacement of HWHs by HMEs in preventing VAP and shown a reduction in VAP in the HME group (relative risk 0.7), especially evident in ventilation for over seven days[16] (relative risk 0.57). HMEFs are convenient, reduce staff workload, reduce circuit colonization and should be used in the absence of contra-indications. A HWH should be considered in profoundly hypothermic patients in whom HMEFs may be ineffective and in patients with thick secretions.

Tracheobronchial suctioning

Airway suctioning is one of the most unpleasant experiences recalled by mechanically ventilated patients and is associated with a number of complications including hypertension, tachycardia, cough, hypoxaemia, cardiac arrhythmias, bronchospasm and both tracheal and bronchial mucosal injury. Poor aseptic technique can be a source of exogenous tracheal colonization and both movement of the tube[17] and loss of PEEP[5] may predispose to leakage of secretion past the tracheal tube cuff – all contributors to the development of VAP. However, few would dispute the value of effective suctioning in the proper management of the lower airway. In principle, the procedure is straightforward: a long flexible plastic catheter is passed aseptically through the tracheal tube into the large airways, suction is applied and the catheter slowly withdrawn. In practice, however, there is little high-quality objective evidence to guide practice in important aspects of the technique, so the following questions remain:

1. When should suctioning be performed?
2. What should be done to minimize hypoxaemia?
3. What diameter catheter should be used?
4. How far should the catheter be inserted?
5. What is a safe negative pressure to use?
6. How long should suction be applied?
7. Should suction be applied continuously or intermittently?
8. Should an 'open' or 'closed' system be used?

WHEN?

Given the potential for adverse effects, it is logical that tracheal suctioning should only be performed when indicated. Suggested criteria for identifying this include coarse or noisy breath sounds, a fall in pulmonary compliance,[13] a change in arterial blood gases, agitation, patient efforts at coughing, or if aspiration is suspected.[14] In the absence of unambiguous indications for suction, none of these have any particular value other than for a saw-tooth pattern on the flow/volume loop[18] and the presence of large airway sounds.[18] There are no absolute contra-indications to suctioning, although in some patients (with critically raised intracranial pressure, repeated suctioning-induced bradycardia or bronchospasm), consideration should be given to deepening the level of sedation beforehand.

OXYGENATION

In the vast majority of patients, the transient suction-related reduction in the arterial partial pressure of oxygen is of no consequence. This transient and modest hypoxaemia can be prevented by the administration of pure oxygen, before, during (with a closed suction system) and after, and for most, this too is harmless. This practice would be consistent with current recommendations but may, in fact, not be ideal, particularly in patients with a significant lung injury. High concentrations of oxygen are

---

13 Increased airway pressure in volume-targeted ventilation or a fall in tidal volume in pressure-targeted ventilation.
14 For example, after vomiting.

Table 4.5 Percentage of cross-sectional area of an endotracheal tube that is occupied by a suction catheter. Suction catheters and endotracheal tube combinations with a yellow background are not correct

Suction catheter Size (Fr)	Colour	Endotracheal tube size								
		6	6.5	7	7.5	8	8.5	9	9.5	10
6	Light green	11	9	8	7	6	6	5	4	4
8	Blue	20	17	15	13	11	10	9	8	7
10	Black	31	26	23	20	17	15	14	12	11
12	White	44	38	33	28	25	22	20	18	16
14	Green	60	52	44	39	34	30	27	24	22
16	Orange	79	67	58	51	44	39	35	32	28
18	Red	100	85	73	64	56	50	44	40	36
20	Yellow	123	105	91	79	69	62	55	49	44

toxic (see Chapter 14) and can promote alveolar collapse and atelectasis[19] by displacing nitrogen from lung units with modest or poor ventilation. Complete absorption of the oxygen from these lung units then causes them to collapse, worsening the ventilation/perfusion mismatch, exchanging a short-term period of hyperoxia for a long-term requirement for a higher inspired oxygen concentration. It may be preferable, therefore, to combine a modest increase in the inspired oxygen concentration (10% to 20%) with manoeuvres during or after suctioning to prevent and reverse alveolar collapse and bronchoconstriction that the procedure can cause. For example, increasing the PEEP during suctioning and performing a recruitment manoeuvre afterwards have both been shown to help. This is of particular relevance to patients whose baseline inspired oxygen concentration is 50% or more and who should also be considered for a 'closed' suctioning system (which will be discussed later).

CATHETER DIAMETER

The efficiency with which a suction catheter can aspirate secretions, particularly if they are highly viscous, is proportional to the diameter of the catheter and the suction pressure (which will be discussed later). Bigger is therefore better. On the other hand, if gas cannot enter the lungs around the suction catheter, then it will be aspirated from the lung, lead-

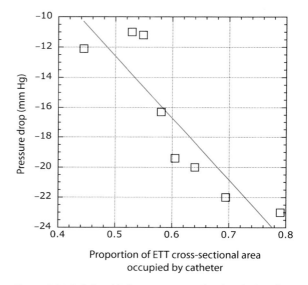

Figure 4.21 Relationship between proportional occlusion of endotracheal tube (ETT) cross-sectional area and fall in 'intrathoracic' pressure in a lung model of suctioning.

ing to lung collapse. This has been confirmed in a laboratory model in which the fall in 'intrathoracic' pressure was linearly correlated with the proportional occlusion of the tracheal tube.[20] However, providing the suction catheter occludes less than 50% of the tracheal tube, the fall in intrathoracic pressure is clinically unimportant (Figure 4.21). The proportional occlusion of adult tracheal tubes is tabulated against a range of suction catheters in Table 4.5.

HOW FAR?

Traditional teaching is that the suction catheter is introduced into the airway until it is met with resistance, and then withdrawn one or two centimetres before applying suction. This technique has been shown to cause significantly more mucosal damage than 'measured' insertion in which the catheter is introduced a predetermined distance[21] and is particularly unpleasant for the patient because it involves striking the carina each time the procedure is carried out. In relatively short-stay surgical patients an even less-invasive technique, in which the suction catheter is introduced no further than the distal end of the tracheal tube, was shown to be no less effective and caused significantly fewer suction-related adverse events.[22] While it would be premature to extrapolate this result to the wider population of patients requiring mechanical ventilation, the 'measured' technique is a sensible compromise when tailored to the needs of each patient. This is particularly easy in patients with a closed suction system in whom the correct depth can be marked by tape firmly wrapped around the outer sheath of the suction catheter.

WHICH PRESSURE?

For a given diameter of catheter (as discussed earlier), the efficacy and speed with which the procedure can be completed is proportional to the suction pressure and therefore, as with diameter, the greater, the better. However, it is commonly understood that the risk of causing mucosal damage is also related to the pressure used, leading many authorities to recommend pressures no greater than 20 kPa (150 mm Hg). However, none of the studies on which this recommendation is based consider the effect of pressure dissipation caused by the flow of material (gas, liquid or mucus) along the length of the system (Figure 4.22), and the potential harm caused by mucosal injury has to be balanced against the real harm caused by prolonged and/or ineffec-

tive suctioning. Until better information is available, a pragmatic approach would be to use no less than 20 kPa, but to use higher pressures for patients with viscous or copious secretions, or who require narrow suction catheters (<14 Fr).

HOW LONG AND CONTINUOUS OR INTERMITTENT?

The normal distance between the carina and the front teeth in adults is between 25 and 35 cm, and without making a conscious effort, it is hard to make the slow continuous withdrawal of the suction catheter last much longer than 15 or 20 seconds over this short distance. On the contrary, inexperienced caregivers tend to withdraw the suction catheter too quickly, making each pass less effective, and necessitating multiple passes to complete the task satisfactorily. The rationale behind intermittent suction is unclear and has been shown to have no advantage over continuous suction in terms of mucosal damage.[23] As continuous suction is likely to be more efficient, intermittent suction has nothing to support its use and should be abandoned.

'OPEN' OR 'CLOSED'?

In 'open' suctioning, the patient is disconnected from the ventilator by removing the catheter mount from the tracheal tube, and a sterile single-use suction catheter is introduced aseptically into the upper airway. At the end of the procedure, the patient is reconnected to the ventilator and the suction catheter discarded. With 'closed' suctioning the junction between the catheter mount and the tracheal tube is occupied by a re-usable suction catheter shrouded in a thin plastic sheath. During suctioning, the patient remains connected to the ventilator, without interruption of either ventilation or PEEP, and the catheter is simply fed into the airway without coming into contact with the caregiver's hand. Suction is applied as it is for open suctioning, but at the end of the procedure the catheter is withdrawn from the airway and 'parked' back in its sheath, ready for the next

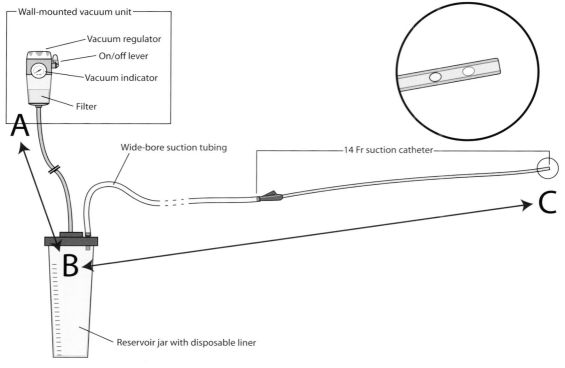

Figure 4.22 Common arrangement for endotracheal suction.

Suction pressure is regulated at the wall-mounted suction unit (A) and transferred to the wide-bore suction tubing via a reservoir with a disposable liner (B). Negative pressure is dissipated in the system between the value set at the regulator and the tip of the suction catheter at (C) depending on the total distance between (A) and (C), the internal diameter of the tubing, and the viscosity of the material being aspirated.

time it is required. Closed systems allow multiple uses of the same catheter and do not require the circuit to be opened to the environment. Closed suctioning techniques are quicker and easier than open ones, thereby reducing hypoxaemia and de-recruitment, and reducing contamination of the patient and the ICU environment. Closed suction systems are, however, more costly and can lead to circuit colonization.[24] Regular replacement is recommended by manufacturers although some studies have demonstrated that more extended use is safe.[25] The effect of closed suction systems on the risk of VAP is unclear at present and current guidance from the US Center for Disease Control does not recommend one technique over the other.[26]

SUCTION FOR AIRWAY OBSTRUCTION

An uncommon but potentially fatal problem may arise from bleeding into the airway, particularly as a complication of tracheostomy but also arising from airway trauma or pulmonary haemorrhage. Blood clots may be too large and solid to remove using suction catheters, and if they are obstructing or partially obstructing the upper airway, there may not be time to arrange for rigid bronchoscopy. In this situation, large bore suction directly in the trachea using either an endotracheal tube or the suction tubing with the end cut off may prove life-saving.

Mucoactive agents

Normal airway mucus contains viscoelastic glycoproteins that provide physical properties that are important for airway defence. Airway inflammation leads to an excessive production of this mucus and also the accumulation of products of inflammation, including neutrophil-derived DNA, filamentous actin and bacterial and cellular debris. These contribute to the purulence of sputum increasing its viscosity and adhesive properties. Tenacious mucus is not easily mobilized by cilia, cough interactions or airway suctioning. Accumulation leads to airway obstruction, bacterial colonization and infection.[27] Mucoactive agents aim to facilitate the removal of mucus by decreasing mucus viscosity (increasing mucus water content, breaking down or interfering with polymer cross-links) or by decreasing mucus production.

INCREASING MUCUS WATER CONTENT

Mucus water content is regulated by the airway epithelium which balances sodium-mediated water re-absorption,[15] chloride-mediated water secretion[16] and evaporative losses minimized by the heat and moisture preserving properties of the normal upper airway. Ineffective inspiratory gas humidification can result in mucus desiccation and the formation of mucus plugs, with dramatic consequences. Humidification of inspired gas was discussed earlier. The attempt to deliver additional moisture to the distal airway in the form of nebulized 0.9% sodium chloride is common practice in mechanically ventilated patients, but has no demonstrable effect on mucus viscosity[28] and may actually reduce bronchial mucociliary clearance.[29] In contrast, aerosolized delivery of osmotically active agents, such as hypertonic saline, powdered mannitol, or powdered dextran, increases mucus water content and enhances mucociliary clearance. In the case of hypertonic saline, regular use in patients with cystic fibrosis has been shown to slow down the deterioration in lung function.[30]

REDUCING POLYMER CROSS-LINKAGES

Mucolytics are able to break down mucus glycoprotein cross-linkages (classic mucolytics), DNA polymers (peptide mucolytics) or interfere with intermolecular ionic and hydrogen bonds (heparin), improving mobilization of secretions.

The classic mucolytics, such as N-acetylcysteine, have free thiol groups causing disulphide bond disruption to degrade mucin. In the UK, only carbocisteine[17] and mecysteine,[18] which are both oral preparations, are licensed for use as mucolytics. Parenteral N-acetylcysteine is available in the UK as Parvolex® or N-acetylcysteine injection, both with a pH of 6.5 to 7.5. Oral bioavailability of N-acetylcysteine is less than 10%, and in mechanically ventilated patients it is usually administered for mucolysis by nebulization, which should be in the air because the drug is inactivated by oxygen. In patients with chronic bronchitis, oral mucolytics, including N-acetylcysteine, significantly reduce the frequency of exacerbations and nebulized N-acetylcysteine has been shown to reduce sputum viscosity and improve both expectoration and oxygenation in post-thoracotomy patients.[28] However, no studies have been conducted on the efficacy of nebulized N-acetylcysteine in mechanically ventilated patients. Mucolytics may cause gastric irritation and should be used with caution in patients with active peptic ulceration.

Recombinant human deoxyribonuclease (rhDNase/dornase alfa) is a genetically engineered naturally occurring enzyme that degrades extracellular DNA that accumulates in sputum following infection and is responsible for increased mucus viscoelasticity and its purulent appearance. Dornase

Such agents deserve further clinical evaluation in the mechanically ventilated patient.

---

[15] Via the amiloride-sensitive apical epithelial sodium channel.
[16] Via the cystic fibrosis trans-membrane conductance regulator (CFTR).

[17] Initially, 750 mg 3 times daily, then 1.5 mg daily in divided doses.
[18] 200 mg 4 times daily for 2 days, then 200 mg 3 times daily for 6 weeks, then 200 mg twice daily.

alfa has been used extensively as a mucolytic agent in the management of cystic fibrosis, improving sputum clearance and perhaps modulating the inflammatory process in the airways. Recent reports suggest that it is safe and efficacious in mechanically ventilated children,[31] and its use has been reported in intubated patients with refractory asthma and with acute respiratory distress syndrome (ARDS). It is normally nebulized (with a dose of 2.5 mg every six hours) but has also been directly instilled into the trachea for the mobilization of impacted mucus plugs to facilitate bronchoscopic extraction. There are no large-scale studies in adult ICU patients.

There is some evidence, at least in patients with cystic fibrosis, that the combined use of classic and peptide mucolytics may be synergistic. Nebulized heparin has been advocated in patients with acute lung injury secondary to inhalation burns.

DECREASING MUCUS PRODUCTION

Basal mucus secretion is regulated by both neural and humoral control. Airway inflammation increases both the activity and number of mucus-secreting cells in the airway, while increased neural drive (induced by local inflammation and neural reflexes) only increases activity.

Anti-inflammatory drugs, particularly glucocorticoids, are effective at reducing mucus hypersecretion and have an established role in the management of chronic obstructive pulmonary disease (COPD) and asthma. Other drugs that may have useful anti-inflammatory properties include the macrolide antibiotics,[32] particularly clarithromycin and erythromycin and non-steroidal anti-inflammatory drugs, the latter delivered as an aerosol.

Neural control of mucus secretion is predominantly cholinergic acting at the M_3 muscarinic receptor. Anti-cholinergic drugs, such as ipratropium bromide, are usually used for their bronchodilating properties but some of their benefit may derive from reduced mucus production.

Fears that anti-cholinergic drugs increase mucus viscosity and lead to a reduction in bronchociliary mucus clearance are unfounded,[33] probably because mucus hydration is also under the control of other mechanisms. Anticholinergics such as hyoscine butylbromide (buscopan), hyoscine hydrobromide[19] (hyoscine injection) and glycopyrrolate are used in palliative care to control respiratory secretions. The most effective agent in this setting is hyoscine hydrobromide, but unlike the other two compounds, which are quaternary amines, the hydrobromide can cross the blood–brain barrier and may cause either sedation or agitation.

Aerosol drug delivery

In patients with pulmonary pathology, drug delivery directly to the lung through inhalation maximizes the effector-site concentration while minimizing side effects, or, in the case of some drugs, avoiding systemic absorption completely. Aerosol delivery is an appropriate method for a range of drugs (Table 4.6). Efficient drug delivery to the desired part of the airway depends on the physical properties of the particles in the aerosol, principally their diameter. Particles that are too large ($>10\,\mu$m) settle in the tubing and upper airway, while those that are too small ($<0.5\,\mu$m) do not settle at all and are exhaled. The length of time that particles in the target range (1 to 5 μm) can remain suspended, and therefore delivered, also depends on their size and the likelihood of impact against a surface. Both humidification and turbulent gas flow, for example, significantly accelerate their loss, the former by causing water adsorption, the latter by increasing surface collisions. For this reason, it is recommended that humidification be suspended before and during the delivery of drug aerosols, and that the aerosols should be delivered into spacers

---

[19] 400 to 600 micrograms by subcutaneous injection every 4 to 8 hours, or 1.5 to 2.5 μg.kg^{-1}.hr^{-1} by continuous subcutaneous or intravenous infusion.

Table 4.6 Drugs for aerosol delivery

Indication	Drug	MDI	DPI	Jet	US[a]	VM[b]	Notes
Resistant gram negative organisms	Amikacin			✓	✓	✓	
	Colistin			✓	✓	✓	
	Gentamicin			✓	✓	✓	
Pneumocystis carinii pneumonia	Pentamidine			✓	✓	✓	
Methicillin-resistant *Staphylococcus aureus*	Tobramycin			✓	✓	✓	
	Vancomycin			✓	✓	✓	
Respiratory syncytial virus (RSV) infection, SARS	Ribavirin						Delivered with small particle aerosol generator (SPAG) only. Teratogenic in animals – exposure to aerosol must be avoided by women who may become pregnant.
Bronchospasm, oedema	Adrenaline			✓	✓	✓	
Bronchospasm	Anti-muscarinics[c]	✓		✓	✓	✓	
Bronchospasm	Short-acting β2-adrenergic agonists[d]	✓	✓	✓	✓	✓	
Bronchospasm	Long-acting β2-adrenergic agonists[e]	✓	✓				
Inflammation	Corticosteroids[f]	✓	✓				
Sputum mobilization	N-acetylcysteine[g]			✓	✓	✓	Inactivated in oxygen.
Reduction of sputum viscosity in patients with cystic fibrosis	rhDNase						Deliver by jet nebulizer as temperature increase with ultrasonic device may denature the enzyme.
Inhalation burn injury	Heparin			✓		✓	
Patient–ventilator dyssynchrony	Lignocaine			✓	✓	✓	
Pulmonary hypertension	Prostacyclin			✓	✓	✓	
Acute respiratory distress syndrome, meconium aspiration	Surfactant			✓		✓	

[a] US, ultrasonic.
[b] VM, vibrating mesh.
[c] Ipratropium, oxitropium, tiotropium.
[d] Fenoterol, isoetarine, orcoprenaline, pirbuterol, reproterol, salbutamol, terbutaline.
[e] Formoterol, salmetorol.
[f] Flunisolide, becometasone, budesonide, fluticasone.
[g] Preparations outside the UK not formulated for aerosol delivery may have a low pH and cause bronchospasm.

or chambers and (in the case of jet nebulizers) in the inspiratory limb of the breathing circuit. The particles in an aerosol will have a range of sizes, with the size distribution determined by the specific device. Devices that generate a larger proportion of particles in the appropriate size range will be able to deliver a larger proportion of the prescribed dose to the patient. In mechanically ventilated patients, the efficiency of drug delivery will also depend on other factors, only some of which can be adjusted in the patient's favour. Of note is the fact that efficiency is increased by decreasing both the tidal volume and respiratory rate, increasing the inspiratory time, coordinating aerosol delivery to inspiration and suspending the bias flow. Two types of device are available for delivering drugs as aerosols – nebulizers and metered-dose inhalers.

NEBULIZERS

Nebulizers work by using a source of energy to break up a drug solution into very small droplets. Under equal conditions, solutions that are viscous and have high surface tension will produce larger droplets. Changes in the temperature of the solution also affect droplet size because of the inverse relationship between temperature and viscosity. The most widely used type, the jet nebulizer, uses a fine jet of compressed gas directed across the tip of a capillary tube. This draws the solution up into the jet by the Bernoulli effect, and breaks the liquid into droplets, the largest of which almost immediately settle following impact with internal surfaces of the device. The average size of the droplets is inversely proportional to the gas flow in the jet and the volume of solution in the device. Initially solvent is nebulized more rapidly than drugs, leading to a gradual increase in concentration and viscosity. In addition, there is a $10\,^{\circ}\mathrm{C}$ fall in the temperature of the solution, which also results in an increase in viscosity. Jet nebulizers are cheap and disposable, but are unable to deliver all

the solution placed in the delivery chamber and are slow.

Ultrasonic nebulizers use high frequency sound waves (>1 MHz) to break off small droplets from the surface of the solution. As with jet nebulizers, the larger droplets are deposited on the inner surfaces of the device, allowing the smaller ones to be released. These nebulizers have a high rate of nebulization and require a shorter operating time than jet nebulizers but they produce slightly larger droplets. In contrast to jet nebulizers these devices heat the solution being delivered by 10 to 15 $^{\circ}$C during use, and are therefore unsuitable for delivering thermolabile preparations such as enzymes and peptides. Often bulky and expensive, these devices are infrequently used with artificial airways.

Similar in principle to the ultrasonic nebulizer, the vibrating mesh nebulizer is a recent development that uses the high-frequency vibration of a mesh. Actually, the device operates at a lower frequency than the ultrasonic nebulizer and combines a number of attractive features, including quiet operation, a small dead space, a high rate of nebulization and no temperature change during operation. Of the devices available, only one is currently configured for in-line delivery to mechanically ventilated patients[20] and preliminary data are very encouraging.

With both jet and ultrasonic nebulizers, the efficiency of drug delivery to the end of the endotracheal tubes is proportional to the fill volume of the chamber. As many as 68% of in-circuit nebulizers used repeatedly in the same patient become contaminated with high levels of organisms (above $10^3.\mathrm{mL}^{-1}$). These bacteria are aerosolized to small particles capable of reaching the peripheral lung. Thorough cleaning of the nebulizers between treatments reduced this contamination to 20% and the use of modern disposable systems may reduce this further.

[20] Aeroneb Pro®, www.aeronebpro.com

METERED-DOSE INHALER (MDI)

Familiar to most as 'puffers', metered dose inhalers (MDIs) consist of a small, pressurized, canister containing a mixture of drug, surfactant, stabilizing agent, flavouring and propellant. The canister is usually presented in a colour-coded plastic inhaler which delivers a 'puff' of medication from a nozzle placed in the centre of the inhaler's mouthpiece when the device is actuated by pressing the base of the canister into the inhaler. For mechanically ventilated patients, the canister has to be removed from the inhaler and actuated through a specific in-circuit delivery device. Some ventilator circuits contain an integral MDI port in the Y-piece that connects to the catheter mount (Intersurgical, UK), but in-line adapters and adapter/chamber combinations are also available (Figure 4.23).

Which device?

Some drugs can only be delivered by one technique because of issues relating to drug stability, particle size or pharmaceutical presentation (Table 4.7), but for many drugs, a choice of delivery techniques is available. Some comparisons between jet nebulizers and MDI have either been imprecise or have used a poor MDI delivery technique. However, when optimal delivery methods are compared, the MDI is shown to be as efficient as jet nebulization, if not better, with the added advantages of a shorter delivery time. Under optimal conditions, ultrasonic nebulizers are more efficient than jet nebulizers, and on current evidence it is likely that the vibrating mesh nebulizers will be even better.

Tube exchange

The exchange of the endotracheal tube may be required urgently due to unplanned extubation or because of tube blockage. This is a clinical emergency in an often already hypoxaemic patient with an oedematous airway due to prolonged intubation. It requires a rapid response and the immediate availability of personnel with advanced airway skills. It is desirable to recognize partial endotracheal obstruction with secretions to pre-empt total obstruction. This is challenging in the clinical environment because it may be difficult to distinguish the increase in tube resistance and the artificial airway noises heard with bronchospasm. Failure to easily pass a suction catheter may alert the clinician and indicate inspection (and possibly cleaning) of the tube with a fibreoptic bronchoscope. Tube exchange may also be appropriate for patients presented to the critical care unit with low-volume high-pressure cuffs in place or if a more advanced endotracheal tube is indicated. The procedure for tube exchange is as follows:

The gel-lubricated bougie or hollow tube exchanger should be passed through a pre-cut, prepared replacement endotracheal tube to ensure adequate lubrication and easy passage, then taken off. The cuff should also be lubricated with a water soluble gel. The distance that the bougie needs to be passed to reach the tracheal tube tip should be noted. Following pre-oxygenation, upper airway secretion clearance and emptying of the stomach, the bougie or exchanger can be passed down the in-situ tracheal tube that is then removed under direct laryngoscopy. The replacement tube can be passed over the bougie and should be visualized to pass through the laryngeal inlet. An assistant should hold the bougie to stop it from slipping proximally or too far distally during the re-intubation. Position should be confirmed by auscultation and capnography, followed by radiography.

Tubing

Contamination of the ventilation circuit can occur from exogenous sources due to the breakdown of infection control measures[34] but is more commonly due to endogenous contamination from secretions returning from the patient.[14] When using active humidifiers, unless scrupulous care is used, pools of condensate can collect in the circuit

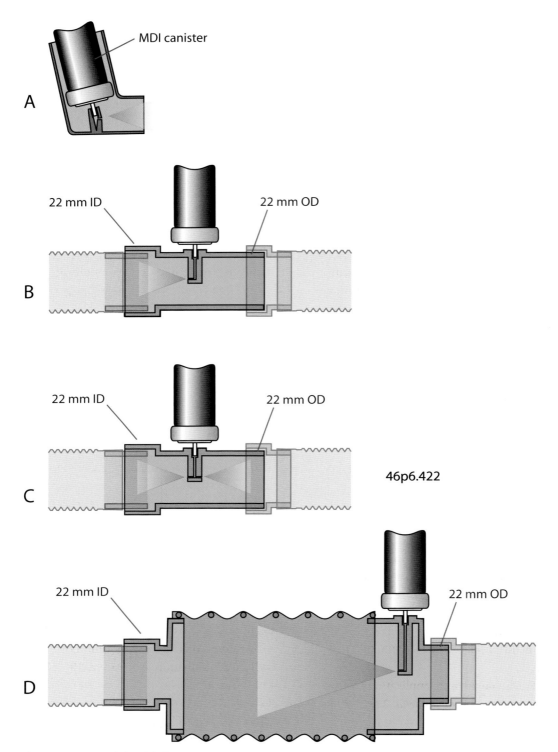

Figure 4.23 metered-dose inhalers.

A metered-dose inhaler canister presented in hand-held dispenser commonly referred to as the 'puffer'. B: In-line dispenser for MDI delivery to mechanically ventilated patients with one-way jet. C: Same as for B but with two-way jet. D: One-way in-line MDI dispenser with collapsible chamber.

Table 4.7 Factors affecting drug delivery via inhalation of aerosol		
	Fixed	Variable
Ventilator	Inspiratory flow waveform	Mode, tidal volume, respiratory rate, inspiratory time, triggering mechanism
Breathing circuit delivery system	Tracheal tube size, density of inspired gases	Humidity of inspired gases
		Type, position in circuit, presence of spacers, timing of delivery
Drug	Particle size, target site, duration of action	Formulation (for some drugs), dose, volume

and be washed back into the patient. Not only can the condensate be colonized with pathogenic bacteria,[15] but the wash back fluid can also carry biofilm from the tracheal tube lumen back into the lungs. The use of an HME reduces, but does not eliminate, the amount of condensate. Infrequent changes of the ventilator circuit tubing do not appear to be detrimental in terms of VAP acquisition[35] and circuits should only be changed for new patients or when visibly soiled.

REFERENCES

1. Estes RJ, Meduri GU. The pathogenesis of ventilator-associated pneumonia: I. Mechanisms of bacterial transcolonization and airway inoculation. *Intensive Care Med.* 1995;21(4):365–83.

2. Meduri GU, Estes RJ. The pathogenesis of ventilator-associated pneumonia: II. The lower respiratory tract. *Intensive Care Med.* 1995;21(5):452–61.

3. Knill RL. Difficult laryngoscopy made easy with a "BURP". *Can J Anaesth.* 1993;40(3): 279–82.

4. Segar EP. Cricoid pressure application by intensive care nurses. *Anaesthesia.* 2002;57 (2):184–5.

5. Young PJ, Rollinson M, Downward G *et al.* Leakage of fluid past the tracheal tube cuff in a benchtop model. *Br J Anaesth.* 1997;78(5): 557–62.

6. Young PJ, Burchett K, Harvey I *et al.* The prevention of pulmonary aspiration with control of tracheal wall pressure using a silicone cuff. *Anaesth Intensive Care.* 2000;28(6):660–5.

7. Rello J, Sonora R, Jubert P *et al.* Pneumonia in intubated patients: role of respiratory airway care. *Am J Respir Crit Care Med.* 1996;154(1): 111–15.

8. Dezfulian C, Shojania K, Collard HR *et al.* Subglottic secretion drainage for preventing ventilator-associated pneumonia: a meta-analysis. *Am J Med.* 2005;118(1): 11–18.

9. Berra L, De Marchi L, Panigada M *et al.* Evaluation of continuous aspiration of subglottic secretion in an in vivo study. *Crit Care Med.* 2004;32(10):2071– 8.

10. Siobal M, Kallet RH, Kraemer R *et al.* Tracheal-innominate artery fistula caused by the endotracheal tube tip: case report and investigation of a fatal complication of prolonged intubation. *Respir Care.* 2001;46 (10):1012–18.

11. Takara I, Fukuda A, Koja H *et al.* Unanticipated endotracheal tube displacement in a short-neck patient with a history of chronic rheumatoid arthritis: a comparison of three kinds of endotracheal tubes. *Masui.* 2004;53(10):1180–4.

12. Garrouste-Orgeas M, Chevret S, Arlet G et al. Oropharyngeal or gastric colonization and nosocomial pneumonia in adult intensive care unit patients. A prospective study based on genomic DNA analysis. *Am J Respir Crit Care Med.* 1997;156(5):1647–55.

13. Marfatia S, Donahoe PK, Hendren WH. Effect of dry and humidified gases on the respiratory epithelium in rabbits. *J Pediatr Surg.* 1975;10(5):583–92.

14. Feldman C, Kassel M, Cantrell J et al. The presence and sequence of endotracheal tube colonization in patients undergoing mechanical ventilation. *Eur Respir J.* 1999;13(3):546–51.

15. Craven DE, Goularte TA, Make BJ. Contaminated condensate in mechanical ventilator circuits. A risk factor for nosocomial pneumonia? *Am Rev Respir Dis.* 1984;129(4):625–8.

16. Kola A, Eckmanns T, Gastmeier P. Efficacy of heat and moisture exchangers in preventing ventilator-associated pneumonia: meta-analysis of randomized controlled trials. *Intensive Care Med.* 2005;31(1): 5–11.

17. Young PJ, Pakeerathan S, Blunt MC et al. A low-volume, low-pressure tracheal tube cuff reduces pulmonary aspiration. *Crit Care Med.* 2006;34(3):632–9.

18. Guglielminotti J, Alzieu M, Maury E et al. Bedside detection of retained tracheobronchial secretions in patients receiving mechanical ventilation: is it time for tracheal suctioning? *Chest.* 2000;118(4): 1095–9.

19. Santos C, Ferrer M, Roca J et al. Pulmonary gas exchange response to oxygen breathing in acute lung injury. *Am J Respir Crit Care Med.* 2000;161(1):26–31.

20. Morrow BM, Futter MJ, Argent AC. Endotracheal suctioning: from principles to practice. *Intensive Care Med.* 2004;30(6):1167–74.

21. Kleiber C, Krutzfield N, Rose EF. Acute histologic changes in the tracheobronchial tree associated with different suction catheter insertion techniques. *Heart Lung.* 1988;17(1):10–14.

22. Van de Leur JP, Zwaveling JH, Loef BG et al. Endotracheal suctioning versus minimally invasive airway suctioning in intubated patients: a prospective randomized controlled trial. *Intensive Care Med.* 2003;29(3):426–32.

23. Czarnik RE, Stone KS, Everhart CC, Jr., et al. Differential effects of continuous versus intermittent suction on tracheal tissue. *Heart Lung.* 1991;20(2):144–51.

24. Topeli A, Harmanci A, Cetinkaya Y, et al. Comparison of the effect of closed versus open endotracheal suction systems on the development of ventilator-associated pneumonia. *J Hosp Infect.* 2004;58(1):14–19.

25. Stoller JK, Orens DK, Fatica C et al. Weekly versus daily changes of in-line suction catheters: impact on rates of ventilator-associated pneumonia and associated costs. *Respir Care.* 2003;48(5):494–9.

26. Guidelines for preventing health-care-associated pneumonia, 2003 recommendations of the CDC and the Healthcare Infection Control Practices Advisory Committee. *Respir Care.* 2004; 49(8):926–39.

27. Rubin BK. The pharmacologic approach to airway clearance: mucoactive agents. *Respir Care.* 2002;47(7):818–22.

28. Gallon AM. Evaluation of nebulized acetylcysteine and normal saline in the treatment of sputum retention following thoracotomy. *Thorax.* 1996;51(4): 429–32.

29. Winters SL, Yeates DB. Roles of hydration, sodium, and chloride in regulation of canine

mucociliary transport system. *J Appl Physiol.* 1997;83(4):1360–9.

30. Elkins MR, Robinson M, Rose BR *et al.* A controlled trial of long-term inhaled hypertonic saline in patients with cystic fibrosis. *N Engl J Med.* 2006;354(3): 229–40.

31. Riethmueller J, Borth-Bruhns T, Kumpf M *et al.* Recombinant human deoxyribonuclease shortens ventilation time in young, mechanically ventilated children. *Pediatr Pulmonol.* 2006;41(1):61–6.

32. Rubin BK, Henke MO. Immunomodulatory activity and effectiveness of macrolides in chronic airway disease. *Chest.* 2004;125(2 Suppl):70S–8S.

33. Taylor RG, Pavia D, Agnew JE *et al.* Effect of four weeks' high dose ipratropium bromide treatment on lung mucociliary clearance. *Thorax.* 1986;41(4):295–300.

34. Crnich CJ, Safdar N, Maki DG. The role of the intensive care unit environment in the pathogenesis and prevention of ventilator-associated pneumonia. *Respir Care.* 2005;50(6):813–36; discussion 836–8.

35. Dodek P, Keenan S, Cook D *et al.* Evidence-based clinical practice guideline for the prevention of ventilator-associated pneumonia. *Ann Intern Med.* 2004;141(4): 305–13.

Chapter 5

Modes of mechanical ventilation

PETER MACNAUGHTON AND IAIN MACKENZIE

Introduction

Normal breathing is composed of an infinite range of breaths that vary in depth and timing to suit any and every circumstance from sleeping, yawning or coughing to singing or running. Mechanical substitution of the natural act of breathing could never hope to match what nature has achieved, but within the intensive care ventilator we do have at our disposal a range of breath types that are characterized by properties that fall into two principle domains, those of *cycling* and *inspiratory motive force*. The cycling properties of a breath describe what makes the breath start, what makes the breath end and describes the relationship the breath has with other breaths. The inspiratory motive force simply refers to the mechanism the ventilator uses to drive gas into the lungs. Mechanical breaths with specific cycling and inspiratory motive force properties are more suited to some circumstances than others. Ventilator manufacturers bring together one or more breath types, programme the rules by which the constituent breaths interact and thereby define a particular *mode of mechanical ventilation*. These modes, like the individual breaths, also may be more suited to some circumstances than others, and indeed may result in increased patient comfort, less requirement for sedatives, and even improved outcomes.[1] Understanding how a mode operates is therefore important because it allows the user to understand the physical properties of the constituent breaths, the physiological impact of the mode and allows the best mode to be chosen for the patient.

Defining features of a breath: cycling

The respiratory cycle is made up of two phases, active inspiration and passive expiration (Figure 5.1). The duration of inspiration is referred to as the *inspiratory time* (T_I, in seconds), the duration of expiration is referred to as the *expiratory time* (T_E, in seconds) and the sum of these two define the duration of the respiratory cycle, also called the *cycle time* (T_C, in seconds):

$$T_I + T_E = T_C. \tag{5.1}$$

The respiratory rate (f) is simply the number of respiratory cycles per minute, and is therefore calculated as

$$f = \frac{60}{T_C}. \tag{5.2}$$

When equations (5.1) and (5.2) are combined, it can be seen that setting two of the three variables automatically defines the third:

$$f = \frac{60}{T_I + T_E}. \tag{5.3}$$

---

[1] However, there is currently little evidence for this.

Core Topics in Mechanical Ventilation, ed. Iain Mackenzie. Published by Cambridge University Press.

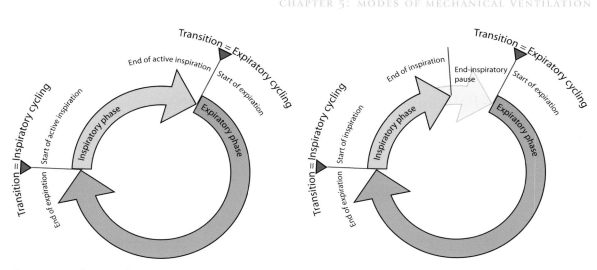

Figure 5.1 Respiratory cycle.

The inspiratory cycle is made up of two phases, the inspiratory phase and the expiratory phase, bounded by two phase transitions.

The transition from inspiration to expiration is referred to as *expiratory cycling*, while that between the expiration and inspiration is termed *inspiratory cycling*. Inspiration can itself sometimes have two phases, an active 'flow' (T_{Iflow}) phase during which gas is being delivered to the patient, and an end-inspiratory pause (T_{Ipause}), such that the total duration of inspiration is made of the sum of these two:

$$T_I = T_{Iflow} + T_{Ipause}$$

When the ventilator has complete control over the respiratory cycle in a breath, referred to as a 'mandatory' breath, two of these three variables (f, T_I or T_E) *must* be set on the ventilator, either directly or indirectly. Different ventilators use different combinations of these three as the independent timing variables. For example, on some anaesthetic ventilators[2] the independent variables are T_I and T_E, while on many intensive care ventilators the timing of the respiratory cycle is set by f and T_I, or f and the I:E ratio (Box 5.1). The duration of inspiration can also be referred to, and in some ventilators set, as the 'duty cycle', where it is expressed as a percentage of the cycle time:

$$\frac{T_I}{T_I + T_E} \times 100 = \frac{T_I}{T_C} \times 100 = \text{Duty cycle (\%)}. \quad (5.4)$$

Of mainly historical interest, the respiratory frequency can also be set *indirectly* as a derivative of

other parameters. For example, if a ventilator is supplied with a flow of gas from an anaesthetic machine ($\dot{V}$, L.min^{-1}) and the user selects a tidal volume (V_T, litres), the respiratory frequency is determined by the following:

$$f = \frac{\dot{V}}{V_T}. \quad (5.5)$$

Ventilators that worked on these principles were called *minute volume dividers* and were popular as anaesthetic ventilators because of their simplicity and reliability.[3]

Inspiratory time and inspiratory flow

In volume-controlled inflations the inspiratory time (T_I), tidal volume (V_T) and inspiratory flow ($\dot{V}_I$)

---

[2] Nuffield 200, Blease 2200, VentPac.

[3] There are still some of these ventilators in use, such as the Manley MN2, the Manley MP3, the Manley Pulmovent and the BM2 Brompton Manley, all originally manufactured by Blease. None of these ventilators is produced anymore and Blease itself has now been acquired by SpaceLabs.

Box 5.1 Calculating inspiratory and expiratory times

Many ventilators ask the user to set the I:E ratio and respiratory rate and assume that the user can calculate the duration of inspiration and expiration for themselves. This is relatively straightforward.

First, you need to calculate the respiratory cycle time in seconds. If the respiratory rate is f breaths per minute, then there are f breaths in 60 seconds, and each breath must last $60/f$ seconds.

The inspiratory time in seconds is then given by:

$$T_I = \frac{I}{I+E} \times \left(\frac{60}{f} \right)$$

and the expiratory time in seconds is given by:

$$T_E = \frac{E}{I+E} \times \left(\frac{60}{f} \right).$$

are mutually interdependent:

$$\dot{V}_I = \frac{V_T}{T_I}. \tag{5.6}$$

This is discussed in more detail in Figure 5.2.

Inspiratory cycling

The onset of inspiration marks the phase transition between expiration and inspiration, and is referred to as *inspiratory cycling*, while the phase transition between inspiration and expiration marks the onset of expiration, and is referred to as *expiratory cycling*. Exactly when a phase transition occurs can either be determined by the ventilator or by the patient.

Inspiratory cycling that is determined by the ventilator usually occurs because a certain amount of time has elapsed since the last breath (Figure 5.3, panel A), but may occur because the minute volume has fallen below a predetermined threshold. The time setting is usually obvious on intensive care ventilators because it is set directly as a respiratory rate or frequency (f).

Alternatively inspiratory cycling can be at the patient's instigation. If the ventilator does *not* contribute to the work of inspiration, the breath is referred to simply as a 'spontaneous' breath (Figure 5.3, panel B). While not supported, the patient's inspiratory effort may be *accommodated* if the patient can draw in additional gas, but in some (older) modes of ventilation, spontaneous inspiratory effort does not allow the patient to draw in more gas and is therefore *not accommodated*. If, however, the ventilator contributes partially or wholly to the work involved in the ensuing inspiration, the patient's spontaneous inspiratory effort can be said to have triggered a supported breath, referred to simply as a 'triggered' breath (Figure 5.3, panel C). The two commonest signals that are monitored by ventilators to effect triggered inspiratory cycling are changes in breathing circuit pressure or flow (Box 5.2).

Expiratory cycling

Expiratory cycling can be based on either time or flow. With time-cycled expiration, the phase transition to expiration is determined purely by the inspiratory time (T_I), which is either set as an independent parameter or is derived from the respiratory frequency and the I:E ratio, depending on the specific ventilator. Flow-dependent expiratory cycling can only operate when inspiration is pressure-controlled. In this type of breath, inspiratory flow rises rapidly to a peak and then falls exponentially. When the inspiratory flow falls below a specific threshold, measured as a percentage of the peak

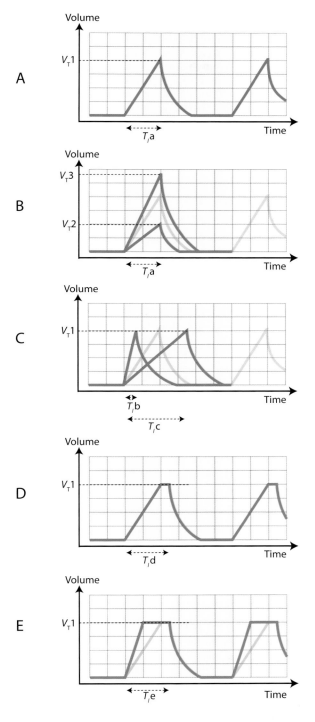

inspiratory flow, the ventilator cycles into expiration (Figure 5.4).

All modern ventilators will also cycle immediately into expiration if the airway pressure exceeds the upper pressure alarm limit, as well as activate both visual and auditory alarms. This is to prevent dangerously high airway pressures from developing in the event of the patient resisting inspiration, coughing, or should the airway become occluded.

Figure 5.2 Relationship between tidal volume, inspiratory time and flow in a volume-controlled inspiration.

A: Volume/time curve for a volume-controlled inspiration with a tidal volume of V_T1 litres and an inspiratory time of T_Ia seconds. The inspiratory flow ($\dot{V}_I$) is the slope of the volume/time profile between the beginning and end of inspiration, and because flow is constant, this line is straight:

$$\dot{V}_I = \frac{V_T1}{T_I a}.$$

B: Volume/time curve for a volume-controlled inspiration with the same inspiratory time as in A, but now with either a larger (V_T3) or smaller (V_T2) inspiratory volume. As can be seen, inspiratory flow is increased (steeper) if the delivered tidal volume is increased and, conversely, inspiratory flow is decreased (flatter) if inspiratory tidal volume is decreased.

C: Volume/time curve for a volume-controlled inspiration with the same tidal volume as in A, but now with either a shorter (T_Ib) or longer (T_Ic) inspiratory time. Inspiratory flow is increased (steeper) if inspiratory time is shortened, and conversely inspiratory flow is decreased (flatter) if inspiratory time is increased. Note also that changing the inspiratory time while keeping the cycle time and respiratory rate the same necessarily means changing the I:E ratio.

D: In some ventilators, it is possible to programme an end-inspiratory pause that divides the inspiratory time into an initial flow phase (T_{Iflow}), and an end-inspiratory pause (T_{Ipause}). The total inspiratory time is now composed of the sum of these two components:

$$T_I = T_{Iflow} + T_{Ipause}.$$

E: With an end-inspiratory pause, it is now possible to change the inspiratory flow rate by increasing or decreasing the duration of the end-inspiratory pause without changing the total duration of inspiration. If the total inspiratory time remains constant, an increase in the end-inspiratory pause causes inspiratory flow to increase, and conversely decreasing the end-inspiratory pause decreases the inspiratory flow rate.

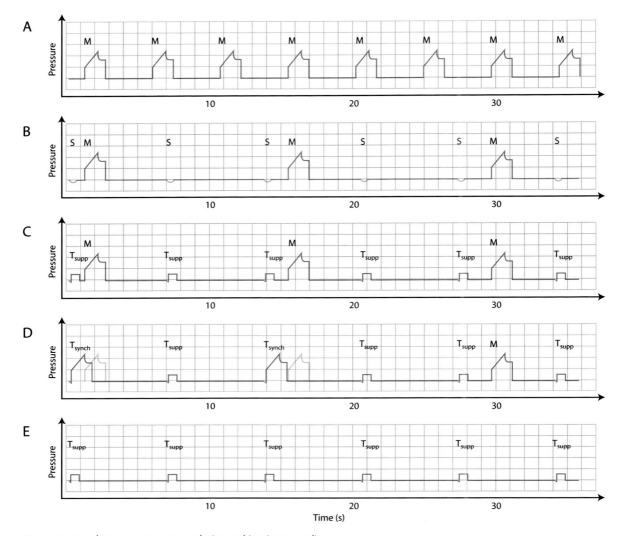

Figure 5.3 Mandatory, spontaneous and triggered inspiratory cycling.

These graphs show the pressure/time profile for different patterns of inspiratory cycling, where M indicates mandatory inspiratory cycling, S indicates spontaneous inspiratory cycling and T indicates triggered inspiratory cycling.

A: In this tracing, the ventilator is delivering all the breaths with mandatory inspiratory cycling. The pressure profile indicates that these breaths are volume-controlled and are being delivered at approximately 12 breaths per minute.

B: In this tracing, the mandatory inspiratory cycling rate has been reduced to about 6 breaths per minute, and now we can see evidence of spontaneous inspiratory cycling at a rate of about 8.5 breaths per minute. We can tell that these are unsupported breaths because during inspiration the airway pressure falls. The proximity of the spontaneous breath and mandatory breath at 0.5 and 1.5 seconds and again at 14 and 15.5 seconds suggests that the mandatory breaths are neither suppressed by, nor synchronized to, spontaneous inspiratory cycling.

C: This tracing is very similar to B, but now the patient's inspiratory effort is clearly triggering inspiratory pressure-controlled support. Note the difference in the pressure profile between the volume-controlled breaths (M) and the pressure-controlled breaths (T).

D: This tracing is very similar to C, but we can see an interaction between spontaneous and mandatory inspiratory cycling at 0 seconds and 14 seconds. In both of these instances, a spontaneous inspiratory effort occurred sufficiently close to the time that a mandatory breath was due to be delivered that the ventilator synchronized the delivery of these volume-targeted breaths to the patients inspiratory effort. Note that this tracing now has triggered breaths that are volume-controlled (Tsynch), triggered breaths that are pressure-controlled (Tsupp), and one volume-controlled mandatory breath (M).

E: In this tracing, there is no evidence of mandatory inspiratory cycling and all the breaths are pressure-targeted and trigger inspiratory-cycled.

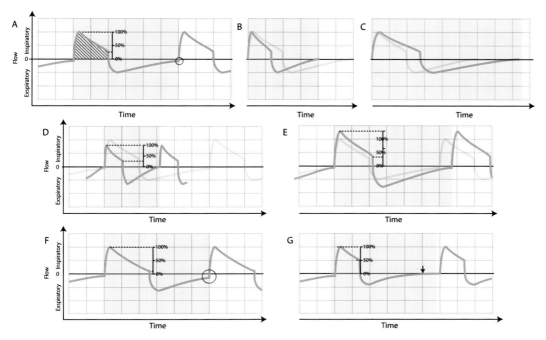

Figure 5.4 Flow-dependent expiratory cycling.

A: When inflation is driven by pressure, inspiratory flow rises rapidly to a peak, and then falls exponentially. With flow-dependent expiratory cycling, the ventilator monitors inspiratory gas flow as a proportion of the peak inspiratory flow. When inspiratory flow has fallen to a preset proportion of the peak inspiratory flow, the ventilator cycles into expiration. On many ventilators, this flow threshold for expiratory cycling is 25% of peak inspiratory flow, as illustrated here. The tidal volume is determined by the area under the flow/time profile and is indicated here by the dark blue hatch.

The duration of the inspiratory phase is proportional to both the resistance and compliance of the respiratory system.

B: The inflating pressure is the same as in A, but the respiratory resistance and compliance are both lower. Therefore, with the same expiratory flow threshold of 25%, the duration of inspiration is shorter.

C: in contrast, both the resistance and compliance of the respiratory system are higher, and so the duration of inspiration is prolonged.

D: If the patient resists inspiration by contracting their expiratory muscles, the criteria for cycling into expiration are met very quickly, resulting in a very short inspiratory phase and a small tidal volume. This situation most commonly arises if the patient is converted from a mandatory mode to pressure support when the respiratory system compliance is still very low. The small tidal volumes and rapid respiratory rate commonly lead to arterial haemoglobin desaturation. Occasionally, this situation can be managed by increasing the inspiratory pressure support and decreasing pulmonary sensitivity to the high inspiratory flow rates with nebulized local anaesthetic. Alternatively, the benefit of inspiratory triggering can be maintained by converting to assist/control in which expiratory cycling is determined by the ventilator and not the patient.

E: If the patient is making a significant contribution to inspiration, the augmentation of the peak inspiratory flow can result in a prolonged inspiratory phase and large tidal volumes. This situation can be improved by increasing the expiratory cycling threshold if the ventilator allows this to be set.

F: If there is significant airflow obstruction (high resistance), the inspiratory flow rate falls relatively slowly, leading to a relatively prolonged inspiration and a large tidal volume. This, in turn, prolongs the duration of expiratory flow to the point where the next inspiratory phase starts before expiratory gas flow has reached zero, indicated in A by the black circle. If the threshold for expiratory flow-cycling is reduced from 25% to 10%, which is only possible on some ventilators (F), the situation described above is exacerbated. Increasing the expiratory flow-cycling threshold to 50% (G) now limits the duration of inspiration allowing expiratory flow to reach zero (arrow) well before the start of the next inspiration.

Box 5.2 Inspiratory triggering

Pressure triggering. In this type of triggering, the patient's inspiratory effort causes the breathing circuit pressure to drop, which the ventilator detects and cycles to inspiration. The sensitivity of the trigger can be adjusted by changing the pressure drop required for inspiratory cycling to be triggered, and this can be set to a value between -1 cm H_2O (very sensitive) and -20 cm H_2O (very insensitive). If the setting is too sensitive, minor fluctuations in breathing circuit pressure (e.g. from cardiac pulsations) can trigger the ventilator inappropriately. This is most likely to occur in young patients with a hyperdynamic circulation.

Flow triggering.[a] With flow triggering, the ventilator delivers a constant background flow of gas into the breathing circuit called the 'bias flow'. If the patient starts to breath in, the flow in the return limb of the ventilator circuit[b] immediately falls below the flow being delivered to the patient in the other limb of the circuit,[c] and this flow difference causes the ventilator to cycle into inspiration. The reduction in return flow that has to be detected for triggering to occur can be adjusted between 1 (very sensitive) and 10 (insensitive) litres/minute. Flow triggering is considered to require less work from the patient to initiate a breath and therefore may enhance patient comfort and reduce the work of breathing.

Other techniques. Neurally Adjusted Ventilatory Assist (NAVA) is a recently introduced method of improving synchronization between the patient's respiratory efforts and the ventilator. A modified nasogastric tube that contains two electrodes to record the diaphragmatic electrical activity is used to sense the patient's respiratory efforts. As soon as the diaphragmatic electrical activity exceeds a threshold level, a ventilator breath is triggered, resulting in no delay between the patient's inspiratory effort and the increase in airway pressure. Furthermore, the reduction in electrical activity signifying the end of inspiration can be used for expiratory cycling. Theoretically this method of triggering should improve coordination of patient and ventilator during support modes. Preliminary clinical experience is encouraging.

[a] Also called 'flow-by' (Puritan-Bennett).
[b] The efferent limb.
[c] The afferent limb.

Breath types and ventilation modes

The following classification system has been created by the authors to bring some order into what can otherwise seem a confusing subject.

When inspiratory cycling is determined by the *ventilator*, which is almost always on the basis of time, the breath is referred to as a 'mandatory' breath (Table 5.2). If all the breaths supplied to the patient are controlled in this way, then the mode of ventilation is also referred to as being mandatory (Table 5.3).

When inspiratory cycling is determined by the *patient*, and the ventilator provides assistance with the work of inspiration, expiratory cycling, by definition, is determined by the ventilator.[4] These

Table 5.1 Comparison of 'volume-controlled' and 'pressure-controlled' breaths		
	Volume	Pressure
Tidal volume	Fixed	Variable
Airway pressure	Variable	Fixed
Minute volume	Set	Measured
Inspiratory flow	Constant	Decelerating

[4] Expiratory cycling in pressure support may *seem* to be 'patient cycled' because the resistance and compliance of the patient's respiratory system determine when the flow threshold has been reached. As respiratory system compliance can be increased by the use of inspiratory muscles and decreased by the use of expiratory muscles, the patient has some influence over expiratory cycling. Ultimately, however, the precise time

Table 5.2 Classification of breath types based on the control of inspiratory and expiratory cycling

Inspiratory cycling	Expiratory cycling	Inspiratory support	Breath type	Example
Ventilator	Ventilator	Yes	Mandatory	IPPV breath
Patient	Ventilator	Yes	Triggered	Pressure support
Patient	Patient	No	Spontaneous	CPAP breath

Table 5.3 Classification of mode types based on the type of breaths available within the mode

Breath types	Mode	Examples
Mandatory only or mandatory + spontaneous	Mandatory	IPPV
Triggered only	Triggered	Pressure support
Spontaneous only	Spontaneous	CPAP
Mandatory + triggered	Hybrid	SIMV, Assist/control

breaths are referred to as *triggered*.[5] If *all* the breaths are triggered, the mode is also referred to as triggered.

When both inspiratory *and* expiratory cycling are determined by the patient, the breath is referred to as *spontaneous* and, by definition, is unsupported. Obviously, patients who have the capacity and the desire to make an inspiratory effort, may do so at any time. The important point is whether the patient's inspiratory effort allows gas to be inspired, in which case the spontaneous respiratory effort is *accommodated*. Alternatively, the ventilator may not allow additional gas to be inspired, and the patient's inspiratory effort results in a fall in circuit pressure. This spontaneous breath is *not accommodated*. Spontaneous breaths are accommodated in some mandatory and hybrid modes.

If a mode allows a mixture of mandatory and triggered breaths, it is referred to as a 'hybrid' mode. At its most basic, two types of breath can operate together but without any interaction between triggered and mandatory breaths (Figure 5.3, panel C). More sophisticated hybrid modes have been made possible by the development of microprocessor-

based ventilators that have allowed manufacturers to design and implement complex algorithms to control the interaction between breath types in a single mode. Nowadays a more common interaction is to allow the triggered breaths to take precedence over the mandatory breaths, either by *suppressing* them (Figure 5.5) or by *synchronizing* with them (Figure 5.6). Some ventilators will automatically switch between a triggered and mandatory mode depending on the patient's activity (see automated modes below).

Triggered breaths in a hybrid mode may be of two types. Where the triggered breaths have exactly the same control parameters as the mandatory ones, these breaths are referred to as being of *mandatory-pattern*.[6] In some hybrid modes, such as in assist-control, all the triggered breaths are mandatory-pattern, and when the patient's spontaneous respiratory rate exceeds the set rate, the mandatory breaths are effectively suppressed. In other modes, such as synchronized intermittent mandatory ventilation (SIMV), mandatory-pattern triggered breaths are only delivered when the patient's inspiratory effort occurs within a 'trigger window' that opens

at which expiratory cycling occurs is determined by the flow threshold set on the ventilator.

[5] Referred to as 'demand' breaths by Viasys.

[6] These breaths are referred to by Puritan-Bennett as *Patient Initiated Mandatory*.

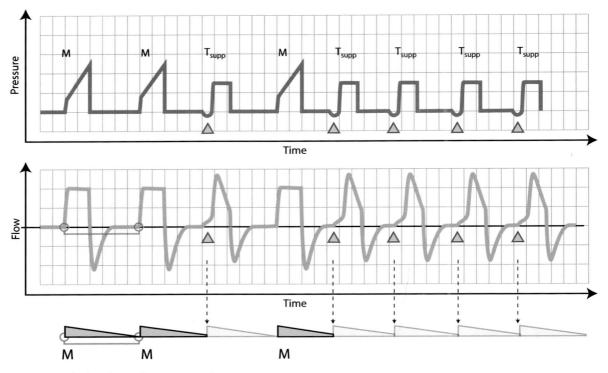

Figure 5.5 Hybrid mode ventilation: suppression.

This is a relatively simple algorithm in which the mandatory cycle time is determined by the mandatory respiratory frequency. In the example above, the mandatory frequency for volume-controlled breaths is 10 breaths.min^{-1}, which gives a mandatory cycle time of six seconds from the start of one breath to the start of the next. The first breath shown here is a mandatory breath, and six seconds later a second mandatory breath is delivered. Before another six seconds have elapsed from the start of the second mandatory breath, the patient makes an inspiratory effort and triggers a pressure-supported breath. At the onset of this triggered breath, the internal clock is reset and six seconds later the fourth breath is delivered as a mandatory volume-controlled breath. The last four breaths all occur with a cycle time that is less than six seconds, suppressing the underlying mandatory breaths.

for a set time prior to the next mandatory breath. If a breath is triggered in this period, it replaces the mandatory breath that would otherwise have been delivered at the end of the 'trigger window'. If the patient makes an inspiratory effort outside the trigger window, then the breath is 'supported' using a different set of control parameters.

When inspiratory cycling is entirely dependent on being triggered by the patient, the majority of intensive care ventilators will operate a back-up system. The operator sets the apnoea interval in seconds and if the delay between triggered breaths exceeds the apnoea interval the ventilator automat-ically switches to a mode with mandatory inspiratory cycling and sounds an alarm. The ventilator continues with mandatory inspiratory cycling until the alarm is acknowledged and re-set.

Defining features of a breath: inspiratory motive force

During inflation, a mechanical ventilator causes gas to flow into a patient's lungs and it can only do so by creating a pressure gradient between the upper airway and the alveoli. However, there are two ways of generating this pressure gradient. Either the ven-tilator can cause the pressure at the alveoli to fall

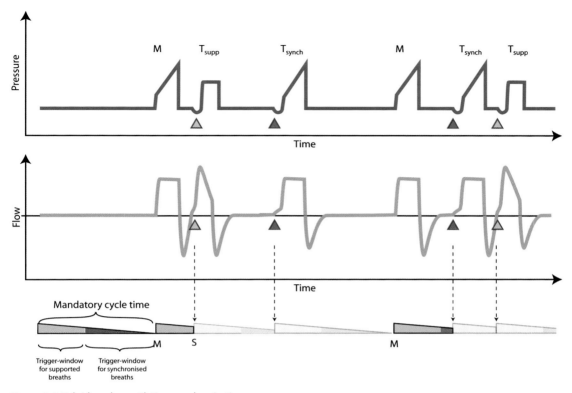

Figure 5.6 Hybrid mode ventilation: synchronization.

This algorithm is slightly more complex and may differ in detail between ventilators. In the example illustrated, the mandatory frequency (SIMV rate) is 6 breaths.min^{-1}, with volume-controlled mandatory breaths and pressure support for triggered breaths.

The mandatory cycle time is divided into two phases. The first phase, which in the Puritan-Bennett SIMV algorithm is 60% of the mandatory cycle time,[7] is the trigger window for mandatory breaths. If no breath is triggered during this period, the patient receives a ventilator-initiated mandatory breath, and for the remaining 40% of the cycle time, the patient may trigger supported breaths. In the sequence illustrated here, the first breath is a ventilator-initiated mandatory breath (M), and the second is a pressure-supported breath triggered by the patient. The third breath is also a ventilator-initiated mandatory breath because no inspiratory activity was detected during the trigger-window for mandatory breaths. The fourth breath, however, is a patient-triggered mandatory breath (TM) that was initiated early in the trigger-window for mandatory breaths, and the remainder of the mandatory cycle time now becomes a trigger-window for supported breaths.

Breath synchronization ensures that a mandatory breath, either ventilator-initiated or patient-initiated, occurs once during every mandatory cycle time.

by creating a negative pressure around the chest wall, which is called negative pressure ventilation, or the ventilator can increase the pressure at the upper airway, which is called positive pressure ventilation. Negative pressure ventilators, such as tank or cuirass ventilators, are rarely used in general intensive care practice and are discussed in Chapter 19.

As the respiratory system is elastic, it exhibits the property of compliance,[8] which means that the volume and pressure of the system are interdependent.

---

[7] Or 10 seconds, whichever is shorter.

[8] Compliance = change in volume (ΔV)/change in pressure (ΔP).

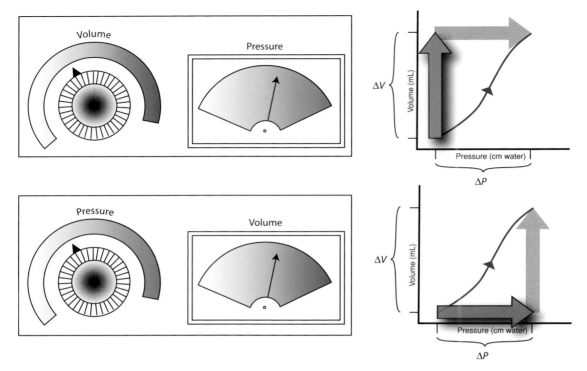

Figure 5.7 Volume-driven or pressure-driven inflation.

Top: The desired tidal volume is set on the ventilator, and the resulting airway pressure excursion is merely observed. Inspiratory volume is thus the primary, or independent, variable (ΔV) and the change in airway pressure (ΔP) resulting from this is the secondary, or dependent, variable. The value of ΔP is determined by the compliance of the respiratory system, which is given by $\Delta V/\Delta P$. If the compliance of the respiratory system falls, ΔV remains constant but ΔP increases.

Bottom: The desired inflating pressure is set on the ventilator, and the tidal volume that this delivers is merely observed. The change in airway pressure is thus the primary, or independent, variable (ΔP) and the volume change (ΔV) resulting from this is the secondary, or dependent, variable. The value of ΔV is determined by the compliance of the respiratory system, which is given by ($\Delta V/\Delta P$). If the compliance of the respiratory system falls, ΔP remains constant but ΔV falls.

Changing the gas volume in the respiratory system will result in a pressure change that depends on the compliance. Conversely, changing the pressure in the respiratory system will result in a volume change that similarly depends on the compliance. In each case, one variable is the primary, independent variable whose change in value is predetermined, and the other is the secondary, dependent variable whose change in value can only be measured. In other words, to effect positive pressure ventilation, we can either choose to deliver a predetermined volume and accept the pressure change that this causes, or effect a predetermined

pressure change and accept the volume that this delivers (Figure 5.7). Originally, positive pressure ventilators were designed with one or more driving mechanism. Those in which the tidal volume was the set variable became known as 'volume-controlled' machines, and were preferred in Europe, while those in which the inflating pressure was the set variable became known as 'pressure-controlled' machines and for historical reasons were more popular in North America. Subsequent generations of ventilator designs combined the capacity to deliver volume-controlled or pressure-controlled breaths in the same machine, and the terms retained

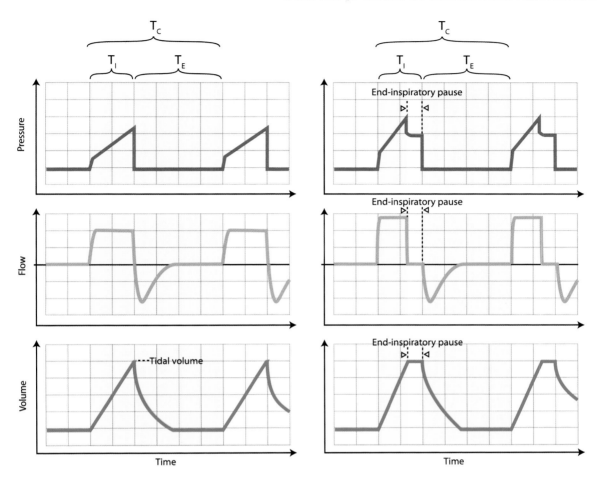

Figure 5.8 Volume-controlled inflation.

Pressure/time (red), flow/time (yellow) and volume/time (green) curves for volume-controlled breaths with an inspiratory time of 2 seconds, an expiratory time of 4 seconds, and a respiratory rate of 10 breaths.min^{-1} respectively.

On the left, there is no end-inspiratory pause and inspiratory flow continues right up to the time of expiratory cycling.

On the right, although the inspiratory tidal volume is the same, inspiratory flow terminates after 1.3 seconds, leaving an end-inspiratory pause of 0.7 seconds. Note the differences in the profiles for pressure, flow and volume compared to their profiles when there is no end-inspiratory pause. In particular, note that the peak airway pressure is higher, and during the pause drops to a shoulder value. Also, the peak inspiratory flow is higher.

value because they specified certain characteristics of the inflation phase (Table 5.1).

Volume as the drive to inspiration

With a volume-controlled inflation, the tidal volume is preset and the ventilator generates the flow required to deliver this volume in the available inspiratory time, with the airway pressure being entirely dependent on the resistance and compliance of the respiratory system. In its classical form, this is achieved by delivering a constant inspiratory flow for a fixed period of time (square wave profile, Figure 5.8), but some ventilators now

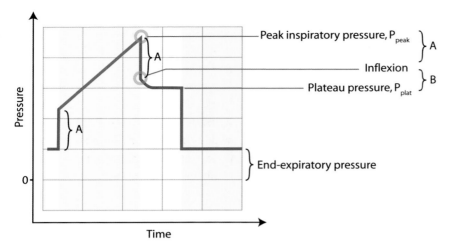

Figure 5.9 Pressure profile of a volume-controlled breath with an end-inspiratory pause.

In this illustration, the pressure baseline is above zero (atmospheric pressure) because the patient is receiving a positive end-expiratory pressure (PEEP). At the start of inflation, the airway pressure immediately rises because of the resistance to gas flow (A), and at the end of inspiratory gas flow the airway pressure immediately falls by the same pressure (A) to an inflexion point. Thereafter, the airway pressure more gradually declines to the plateau pressure. The loss of airway pressure after the inflexion (B) is due to gas redistribution and tissue deformation.

have the option of delivering the inflation with decelerating inspiratory flow. After an initial sudden rise in pressure, caused by resistance to gas flow, pressure increases gradually throughout the inspiratory phase to reach a peak at the end of inspiration (Figure 5.9). Lung volume increases progressively and uniformly.

Volume-controlled inflation has the advantage of a predictable tidal volume that remains constant with varying respiratory system compliance and resistance, thereby ensuring a stable arterial partial pressure of carbon dioxide ($PaCO_2$) and pH. The disadvantage is that maximum airway pressure is not directly controlled and the lungs may be exposed to excessive and potentially damaging pressures. The airway pressure alarm cannot be used to limit pressures on a breath-by-breath basis because whenever the high airway pressure alarm is activated, the ventilator immediately cycles to expiration. To address this problem, some ventilators now allow an inspiratory pressure limit to

be set for volume-controlled breaths,[9] which prevents the inspiratory pressure from exceeding the set limit without cycling into expiration and terminating inspiration prematurely.

The constant inspiratory flow rate that is associated with most volume modes may be a cause of patient discomfort and what is termed *patient–ventilator asynchrony*.[10] In patients who are making spontaneous breathing efforts that trigger the ventilator, the inspiratory flow rate in a volume mode needs to be set to match the patient's desired flow rate. If the flow rate is set too low, the patient will

---

[9] This is done either *overtly* as an upper pressure limit that is set separately from the peak pressure limit, or *covertly* by never allowing ventilator-generated pressures to come within 5 cm H_2O of the upper pressure limit. Unless the user is very familiar with a ventilator that operates in this way, the latter can cause consternation because when the airway pressure reaches this unapparent ceiling, the ventilator issues an advisory warning that the pre-set tidal volume could not be delivered. However, inspection of the pressure/time profile shows that the airway pressure never exceeds the pressure alarm limit.

[10] This is also referred to as 'fighting the ventilator'.

experience discomfort because of flow restriction. The patient will respond by trying to increase inspiratory flow rate by generating a greater spontaneous effort, but as the flow rate is constant, the result is that a large negative pressure is generated in the airway without any increase in inspiratory flow.

Pressure as the drive to inspiration

In pressure-controlled inflation, the airway pressure generated during inspiration is set with the resulting tidal volume depending upon the respiratory system compliance and resistance. Airway pressure rapidly increases to a maximum and is then held at this pressure for the duration of the inspiratory phase. The initial rate of rise of the airway pressure to the maximum pressure is termed the *rise time* and can be adjusted on most ventilators. The inspiratory flow that results from the increase in airway pressure also rises very rapidly to a peak and declines in an exponential manner (decelerating inspiratory flow) as lung volume increases. The lung volume increases rapidly in the early part of inspiration when flow is high (Figure 5.10).

The advantages of pressure modes include that the airway pressure is limited because it will not exceed the set value. This may improve safety in terms of the risk of barotrauma. In addition, the flow profile of pressure modes is associated with enhanced patient comfort. Flow is not preset the way it is in the volume modes but depends upon the set inspiratory pressure, respiratory system resistance, respiratory system compliance and patient effort. If the patient makes a greater effort during inspiration, there will be a corresponding increase in flow rate. There is no restriction of inspiratory flow in pressure modes, which is in contrast to volume modes. Pressure control may be associated with improved gas exchange compared to volume control because there is more rapid filling of the lungs in the early part of inspiration.

The main disadvantage of pressure modes is that tidal volume, and therefore minute volume,

are not controlled and will vary according to respiratory compliance and resistance. Tight control of $PaCO_2$ and pH may be difficult without a high degree of vigilance and frequent adjustment of the ventilator. In addition, it may be difficult to ensure maintenance of tidal volume within appropriate limits, particularly if the respiratory system compliance and resistance change rapidly. Thus a sudden improvement in compliance may result in the delivery of excessive tidal volumes.

Pressure modes of ventilation have become increasingly popular over the last decade although there is little evidence that the choice of ventilator mode has a significant impact upon patient outcome.

Control, target and limit: multi-parameter breaths

Modern microprocessor-based ventilators equipped with rapidly responding valves and sensors can not only mimic the characteristics of the original volume-controlled or pressure-controlled breaths, but can now use secondary parameters to limit or augment gas delivery either during a breath or in subsequent breaths. Most intensive care ventilators now offer dual parameter modes that combine the volume guarantees of volume-controlled ventilation with the pressure and flow characteristics of pressure-controlled ventilation. This additional sophistication means that to adequately describe the parameters that contribute to tidal volume and airway pressure in some types of breath, the original terminology is no longer sufficient. These more complex breaths are in fact best characterized by describing the parameter that is manipulated to drive inflation as the 'control' parameter, while the parameter that is measured to provide feedback to limit or augment the control parameter is described as the 'target' or 'limit' parameter, depending on whether the breath is pressure-controlled

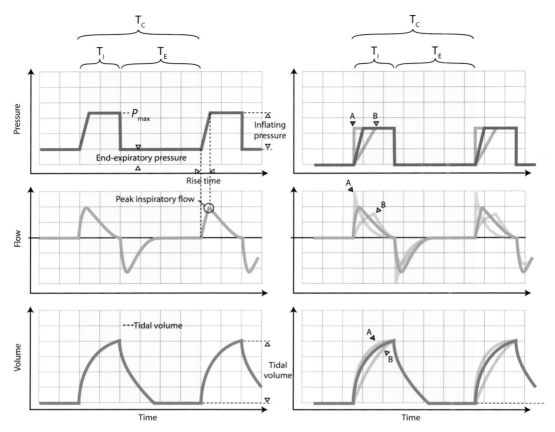

Figure 5.10 Pressure-controlled inflation.

Left: Pressure/time (red), flow/time (yellow) and volume/time (green) curves for pressure-controlled inspiration. The breath is targeted to a pressure that is set on the ventilator either as the inflating pressure[11] (P_{inf}) or maximum airway pressure[12] (P_{max}). The former is more useful because (1) it allows the user to set the pressure that determines the tidal volume as a primary variable, and (2) it allows changes to be made to the end-expiratory pressure (P_{EE}) without affecting the inflating pressure. The inflating pressure, maximum airway pressure (P_{max}) and the end-inspiratory pressure are inter-dependent as follows:

$$P_{max} = P_{inf} + P_{EE}.$$

Users must be aware that some manufacturers do not allow the same parameters to be set between mandatory and triggered pressure-controlled breaths. For example, one manufacturer sets mandatory breaths as P_{max} and P_{EE}, but triggered breaths as P_{inf} and P_{EE}.

Right: In pressure-controlled breaths, the user often has control of the time taken for the airway pressure to rise from the baseline to the maximum, known as the *rise time*. With a very short rise time (A), the peak inspiratory flow is very high, while with a much slower rise time (B), the peak inspiratory flow is much lower.

or volume-controlled, respectively. For example, a breath where the inspiration is driven by pressure but where this pressure is increased or

decreased based on the volume of gas delivered would be called a 'pressure-controlled, volume-targeted' breath. This feedback can either be used

---

[11] Also called inspiratory pressure (P_I, Puritan-Bennett), support pressure (P_{supp}, Puritan-Bennett), ΔP (Draeger) and pressure support above PEEP (PSAP, Draeger).

[12] Also, rather confusingly, called inspiratory pressure (P_{insp}, Draeger).

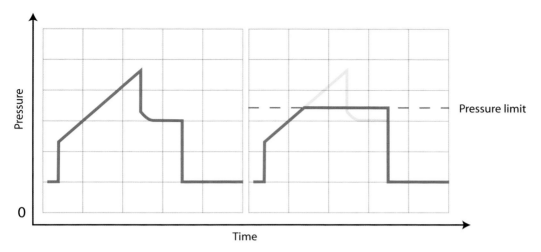

Figure 5.11 Effect of a pressure-limit on a volume-controlled breath.

The figure shows the pressure/time profile for two volume-controlled breaths. On the left, the breath is not pressure-limited, and shows the expected profile. On the right is the same breath in terms of tidal volume and inspiratory flow, but now the activation of a pressure-limit has prevented the airway pressure reaching the previous peak value. This pressure limitation means that flow has needed to continue until the end of the inspiratory time, and it may not have been possible for the ventilator to deliver the desired tidal volume.

instantaneously to influence gas delivery within the same breath (intra-breath), or can be used to influence gas delivery in the following breath (inter-breath). In the case of volume-controlled breaths, in which pressure is expected to vary during inspiration (Figure 5.11), the addition of a 'pressure limit' provides a means of limiting the peak pressures, while *trying* to maintain a constant inspiratory volume.

Classification of modes

Ventilation modes do not conform to any internationally agreed terminology, allowing ventilator manufacturers to use the same or similar names for modes that operate in quite different ways, or, in deference to trademark laws, to use completely different names for modes that operate in very similar ways (Box 5.3). Broadly speaking, modes fall into four categories, as described above: mandatory, triggered, spontaneous and hybrid modes (Table 5.3).

Within these categories the wide and often confusing range of positive pressure ventilation modes offered by the modern intensive care ventilator can be understood by considering the following key elements:

- In mandatory breaths (if present)
  - What determines inspiratory cycling?
  - What drives inflation (control parameter) and what is the breath targeted to or limited by?
  - Is feedback intra-breath or inter-breath?
  - What determines expiratory cycling?
- In triggered breaths (if present)
  - What breath types are present? Mandatory-pattern, supported or both?
  - In supported breaths (if present), what drives inflation (control parameter) and what is the breath targeted to or limited by?
  - Is feedback intra-breath or inter-breath?
  - What determines expiratory cycling?
- Are spontaneous breaths accommodated and if so, when?

Box 5.3 What in a name?

Example 1: Pressure-targeted breaths with trigger inspiratory cycling are called ressure supportby most ventilator manufacturers except one, which uses the term ssisted spontaneous breathingfor its ventilators marketed in Europe.

Example 2: ynchronised intermittent mandatory ventilationis now a dual-control inspiratory cycling mode in which the breaths with mandatory inspiratory cycling are either volume- or pressure-targeted.

- The classic description of SIMV in the literature describes a mode in which volume-targeted breaths are delivered either with mandatory inspiratory cycling, or synchronised with the patient inspiratory effort providing this occurred within a rigger window Unlike modern implementations of SIMV, however, respiratory activity that occurred outside the trigger window was not supported.
- In one version of SIMV currently on the market breaths that occur with triggered inspiratory cycling, which are pressure-targeted, can completely suppress mandatory inspiratory cycling which generates volume-targeted breaths.

Example 3: One manufacturer uses the term BiPAP and another uses the term BIPAP and these are substantially different modes of ventilation.

Mandatory modes

Continuous Mandatory Ventilation (CMV) is the simplest mode of ventilatory support (Table 5.4). The tidal volume and frequency are fixed and there is no synchronization with the patient's respiratory efforts. No additional breaths can be triggered. It is the mode of ventilatory support typically used during general anaesthesia when the patient has received a muscle relaxant. Intensive care ventilators can be made to function in CMV mode by disabling the trigger, although this would cause significant discomfort if the patient made an inspiratory effort. This mode is now rarely used in modern intensive care practice.

Intermittent mandatory ventilation is now of historical interest only and was developed from CMV to allow patients to breath spontaneously in between the mandatory breaths. Initially, this was achieved by inserting a one-way valve connected to a simple breathing circuit with a reservoir bag to the inspiratory limb of the ventilator breathing circuit. IMV was developed as a method of weaning patients from the ventilator,[1] which would be achieved by progressively reducing the preset frequency while the patient increased the number of spontaneous breaths.

Pressure control is analogous to CMV, but an inspiratory pressure rather than tidal volume is pre-set (Table 5.4). Cycling is always by time, which may be directly set or derived from the set frequency and I:E ratio. Respiratory rate is set and there is no ability to trigger additional breaths.

Volume-targeted pressure control combines the benefits of volume and pressure control (Table 5.4). The volume is set, but rather than being delivered as a constant flow rate for a set period of time, it is delivered as a pressure-controlled breath with a square wave of pressure and a decelerating flow rate. Tidal volume is guaranteed with minimum airway pressure. The algorithm used varies according to the individual ventilator but typically the ventilator delivers an initial volume-controlled breath to assess the lung mechanics. The next breath is then delivered as a pressure-controlled breath to achieve the set tidal volume. The tidal volume is monitored on a breath-by-breath basis and the airway pressure constantly adjusted to ensure that the desired volume is delivered. If the compliance

Table 5.4 Mandatory modes of ventilation

Mandatory breaths				
Inspiratory cycling	Time	Time	Time	Time
Control	Volume[a]	Volume	Volume	(Pressure)
Target/Limit	–	–	Pressure-limited	Volume-targeted
Feedback	–	–	Intra-breath	Inter-breath
Expiratory cycling	Time	Time	Time	Time[b]
Triggered breaths				
Types	None	None	None	None
Supported breaths				
Control	–	–	–	–
Target	–	–	–	–
Feedback	–	–	–	–
Expiratory cycling	–	–	–	–
Spontaneous breaths				
During mandatory inspiration	Not accommodated[c]	Not accommodated	Not accommodated	Accommodated
Otherwise	Not accommodated	Accommodated	Not accommodated	Accommodated
Synonyms	IPPV (Draeger[d]), Controlled Mandatory Ventilation or (historically) Control Mode Ventilation	Intermittent Mandatory Ventilation	IPPV (Draeger[e])	IPPV (Draeger[f])

Notes

a: Viasys default is for decelerating flow, but constant flow is an option.

b: Viasys offers an option for flow cycling (called *Flow Cycle*) with an adjustable expiratory cycling threshold of 0% to 45% peak inspiratory flow. The default setting is for this to be set to 0% (off) and for expiratory cycling to be time-based.

c: Accommodated with Viasys' Intra-Breath Demand System that supports inspiratory effort from the patient and even provides inspiratory support.

d: With Flowtrigger OFF, AutoFlow OFF and pressure-limited Ventilation OFF. If Flowtrigger is ON, mode behaves as assist-control. If AutoFlow is ON, mode behaves as pressure-controlled, volume-targeted.

e: With Flowtrigger OFF, AutoFlow OFF and pressure-limited Ventilation ON. If Flowtrigger is ON, mode behaves like assist-control. If AutoFlow is ON, mode behaves as pressure-controlled, volume-targeted. If inspiratory pressure is limited, the set tidal volume may not be delivered, generating a 'volume not constant' alarm.

f: With Flowtrigger OFF and AutoFlow ON (pressure-limited Ventilation N/A). If Flowtrigger is ON, mode behaves like assist-control. If inspiratory pressure is limited, the set tidal volume may not be delivered, generating a 'volume not constant' alarm. Accommodated with Draeger's AutoFlow that supports inspiratory effort from the patient.

changes, the pressure will progressively increase or decrease (usually in 2 to 3 cm H_2O increments) in order to maintain the tidal volume. With dual parameter breaths, there is a limit to which the airway pressure can be increased, which is typically 5 to 10 cm H_2O below the peak airway pressure alarm setting, but it varies according to the ventilator. Dual parameter breaths function well for most patients, although some may not cope well when there are marked changes in compliance between breaths. This may occur in the patient who makes occasional large respiratory efforts due to the respiratory depressant effects of opiates.

Triggered modes

In pressure support, spontaneous breathing is assisted with an increase in airway pressure following each inspiratory effort (Table 5.5). The difference between the expiratory pressure and inspiratory pressure is the level of pressure support. The patient's spontaneous efforts set the respiratory rate so pressure support can only be used in patients with an adequate respiratory drive. Pressure support may be combined with a back-up controlled mode (either pressure or volume), termed *apnoea ventilation*, which will be activated if the patient makes no respiratory effort for a preset time (e.g. 15–30 seconds). Pressure support was introduced as a method of partial ventilatory support to assist with weaning but is increasingly used as a method of full support in patients with a normal respiratory drive.

In pressure support, expiratory cycling is primarily determined by the change in inspiratory flow. The pressure support is maintained until the inspiratory flow rate falls to a predetermined level. For most ventilators cycling occurs when the inspiratory flow rate falls to 25% of the peak inspiratory flow rate. Some ventilators allow the flow threshold for expiratory cycling to be adjusted between 10% and 90% of the peak flow rate rather than default to a value of 25%. Increasing the threshold may be appropriate in patients with high airway resistance such as COPD while a lower threshold may be indicated in patients with poor lung compliance. In COPD, the associated high airways resistance is associated with a low peak inspiratory flow rate that falls only slowly and is still above 25% of peak inspiratory flow when the patient starts to exhale. The patient therefore has to actively exhale against the pressure support to reduce inspiratory flow rate and cause the ventilator to cycle to expiration. Active exhalation may be detected by observing the patient during expiration or from noting an increase in airway pressure above the set pressure support level towards the end of the inspiratory phase. This is associated with an increase in the expiratory work of breathing and significant patient discomfort. Increasing the threshold flow rate for cycling allows expiration to occur at an earlier stage and avoids the patient having to actively exhale.

Expiratory cycling is impaired if there is a significant leak in the circuit as the inspiratory flow rate may not fall to the trigger level, with the result that the inspiratory phase could be extremely prolonged. For this reason, pressure support will also cycle to expiration after a default time that is usually between 2 and 3 seconds. Pressure support may be used as the sole method of ventilatory support or combined with SIMV to support additional spontaneous breaths. Inspiratory time is not set in pressure support, and when patients are changed from pressure control to pressure support ventilation there may be a deterioration in gas exchange due to a significant fall in inspiratory time.

Volume-targeted pressure support (volume support) is a modification of pressure support and can be considered a dual parameter mode applied to a support mode (Table 5.5). This is a triggered mode and the patient needs to have an adequate respiratory drive and be able to trigger ventilator breaths. Rather than set an inspiratory pressure as in pressure support, the minimum tidal volume is set. Whenever the patient makes an inspiratory effort, the ventilator will deliver a pressure-supported breath with an appropriate airway pressure to achieve the desired tidal volume. If in subsequent breaths the tidal volume is excessive, the level of pressure support will be automatically adjusted. Theoretically, this mode should automatically reduce the level of pressure support as the patient becomes more active resulting in automated weaning. However, there is limited experience in clinical trials to assess if this mode is effective in shortening the process of weaning.

Table 5.5 Triggered modes of ventilation

Mandatory breaths			
Inspiratory cycling	–	–	–
Control	–	–	–
Target	–	–	–
Feedback	–	–	–
Expiratory cycling	–	–	–
Triggered breaths			
Types	Supported breaths only	Supported breaths only	Supported breaths only
Supported breaths			
Control	Pressure[a]	(Pressure[b])	(Pressure[b])
Target/Limit	–	Volume-targeted	Flow and volume
Feedback	–	Inter-breath	Intra-breath
Expiratory cycling	Flow[c]	Flow[c]	Flow[c]
Spontaneous breaths			
During mandatory inspiration	–	–	–
Otherwise	–	–	–
Synonyms	Assisted Spontaneous Breathing (Draeger), Spontaneous mode (Hamilton, Puritan-Bennett), Pressure support (Maquet), CPAP (Respironic), Pressure Support Ventilation (Viasys)	Volume Support (Maquet, Puritan-Bennett)	Proportional assist ventilation, Proportional Pressure Support (Draeger), Proportional Assist Ventilation Plus (Puritan-Bennet)

Notes

a: Set as P_{ASB} (Draeger), $P_{support}$ (Hamilton), PS (Maquet), P_{supp} (Puritan-Bennett) or PSV (Respironics, Viasys) relative to PEEP.

b: Pressure not set by user.

c: Threshold fixed (Draeger) or variable (Hamilton, Maquet, Puritan-Bennett, Respironics, Viasys). May also have secondary (pressure) and tertiary (time) expiratory cycling criteria.

Proportional assist[13] ventilation[2] is a triggered mode which is similar to pressure support in that each inspiratory effort is supported by an increase in airway pressure (Table 5.5). However, the degree of support varies according to patient effort such that with increasing patient effort more support is provided. It has been described as the ventilator equivalent of power steering. By contrast, pressure support is an all-or-nothing mode; whatever the patient effort, the amount of support in terms of airway pressure generated is identical.

For a given inspiratory airway pressure, the flow rate will increase if the patient's inspiratory effort increases. During PAV, the inspiratory support that is delivered is in proportion to the inspiratory flow rate and therefore patient effort. There are two main forces to overcome when breathing in: the resistance of the airways and breathing circuit and the elasticity of the chest wall and lung. In PAV, the support that is applied at any time point during inspiration is

[13] Proportional Assist Ventilation® and PAV® are registered trademarks owned by the University of Manitoba.

in proportion to the work required to overcome the individual resistive and elastic forces. To offload the resistive work, pressure is applied in proportion to the flow rate ($cm.L^{-1}s^{-1}$), and to offload the elastic work, pressure is applied in proportion to the volume inhaled ($cm.L^{-1}$). To apply PAV correctly, the resistance and elastance need to be known. The degree of support applied is then set as a percentage between 0% and 90%. Levels of support above 90% are not applied due to the risk of amplification or 'runaway'. This describes the circumstances when the support applied is greater than that needed to offload the work of breathing such that lung volume continues to increase uncontrollably even when inspiratory effort has stopped.

PAV has been associated with improved patient comfort when compared to pressure support. The main limitation has been the requirement to have an accurate estimate of resistance and compliance to ensure correct application.

Spontaneous modes

The only spontaneous mode that can be delivered from a ventilator is continuous positive airway pressure (CPAP) which is discussed in more detail in Chapter 3.

Hybrid modes

In assist volume control the patient is able to trigger ventilator breaths (Table 5.6). Tidal volume and frequency are set as in CMV. However, the set frequency should be considered as the minimum or back-up rate that the ventilator will deliver if the patient makes no respiratory efforts when the mode is effectively identical to CMV. However, if the patient makes an inspiratory effort, the ventilator delivers a breath of the set tidal volume. The frequency is therefore dictated by the patient's efforts as long as it is above the preset value. Assist control can therefore act as a fully controlled mode if the patient makes no efforts or a support mode if the patient has a normal respiratory drive. Assist volume control

is the most common mode of ventilatory support used worldwide. When appropriately set, it will significantly reduce the patient's work of breathing. In order to ensure patient comfort, the inspiratory flow rate needs to be carefully set to match the patient's demands. The main disadvantage of assist volume control is that inappropriate hyperventilation may occur in patients with a high respiratory drive.

Assist Pressure Control is the pressure-targeted version of assist (volume) control. The rate, inspiratory pressure and inspiratory time are set as in pressure control. As in assist volume control, the set respiratory rate acts as a minimum or back-up rate. Whenever the patient makes an inspiratory effort, the ventilator will deliver a pressure breath, and if the patient's own respiratory rate is greater than the set rate, all breaths will be patient-triggered. The duration of inspiration is dictated by the set inspiratory time.

Synchronized intermittent mandatory ventilation (Table 5.7) was the natural development of IMV and was designed to synchronize the mandatory breaths with the patient's inspiratory effort, when this occurred within a trigger window immediately prior to the time the mandatory breath was due to be given. In the absence of an inspiratory effort from the patient, the mandatory breath is delivered to ensure the set frequency is achieved.

As originally described, SIMV was volume-controlled and inspiratory efforts that did not occur within the trigger window were unsupported. This is an important distinction to the modern implementation of SIMV, which is almost always used in conjunction with pressure support for inspiratory efforts outside the trigger window (SIMV + PS), which may have a significant bearing on the assessment of SIMV as a weaning mode.[3] More recently manufacturers have implemented a pressure-targeted version of SIMV.

The difference between assist control and SIMV is that in assist control there is only one type of breath delivered by the ventilator while in SIMV

Table 5.6 Hybrid mode: Assist control

Mandatory breaths			
Inspiratory cycling	Time or trigger	Time or trigger	Time or trigger
Control	Volume	Pressure[a]	(Pressure[b])
Target	–	–	Volume-targeted
Feedback	–	–	Inter-breath
Expiratory cycling	Time	Time	Time
Triggered breaths			
Types	Mandatory-pattern only	Mandatory-pattern only	Mandatory-pattern only
Supported breaths			
Control	–	–	–
Target	–	–	–
Feedback	–	–	–
Expiratory cycling	–	–	–
Spontaneous breaths			
During mandatory inspiration: Otherwise	Not accommodated[c]	Accommodated	Accommodated
Synonyms	IPPV$_{Assist}$ (Draeger[d]), Synchronized Controlled Mandatory Ventilation (Hamilton), Volume Control (Maquet), VCV-A/C (Puritan-Bennett, Respironics), Volume A/C (Viasys)	BIPAP$_{Assist}$ (Draeger), P-CMV (Hamilton), Pressure Control (Maquet), PCV-A/C (Puritan-Bennett, Respironics), Pressure A/C (Viasys)	Adaptive Pressure Ventilation CMV (Hamilton), Pressure Regulated Volume Control (Maquet), VC+ A/C (Puritan-Bennett), Pressure Regulated Volume Control A/C (Viasys), IPPV Assist Autoflow (Draeger)

Notes

a: Set as P$_{insp}$ (Draeger) or PRESSURE (Respironics) relative to atmospheric pressure. Set as P$_{control}$ (Hamilton), PC (Maquet), P$_I$ (Puritan-Bennett), Insp Pres (Viasys) relative to *PEEP*.

b: Not set by user.

c: Accommodated in the Maquet implementation by switching to pressure support while the patient demand exceeds that predicted for the volume-control breath.

d: With Flowtrigger ON. With Flowtrigger OFF, mode becomes IPPV.

there are two types of breath administered: mandatory breaths (volume or pressure) according to the set frequency, and additional triggered breaths are either unsupported or supported with pressure support.

In its simplest form, bi-level ventilation can be likened to a form of CPAP in which the level of CPAP cycles between two different pressures with the phase transitions synchronized to the patient's inspiration and expiration (Table 5.8). The patient's spontaneous breathing activity is unsupported and the user simply sets the duration (T$_{high}$) and pressure (P$_{high}$) for the high-pressure phase as well as the duration (T$_{low}$) and pressure (PEEP) for the low-pressure phase. More recent implementations of the bi-level concept have added pressure support

Table 5.7 Hybrid mode: Synchronized intermittent mandatory ventilation (SIMV)

Mandatory breaths			
Inspiratory cycling	Time or trigger	Time or trigger	Time or trigger
Control	Volume	Pressure[a]	(Pressure[b])
Target/Limit	–	–	Volume-targeted
Feedback	–	–	Inter-breath
Expiratory cycling	Time	Time	Time
Triggered breaths			
Types	Mandatory-pattern[c] and supported	Mandatory-pattern and supported	Mandatory-pattern and supported
Supported breaths			
Control	Pressure[d]	Pressure[d]	Pressure[d]
Target	–	–	–
Feedback	–	–	–
Expiratory cycling	Flow[e]	Flow[e]	Flow[e]
Spontaneous breaths			
During mandatory inspiration	Not accommodated	Accommodated	Accommodated
Otherwise	Only if support is OFF.	Only if support is OFF.	Only if support is OFF.
Synonyms	SIMV (Draeger, Hamilton), SIMV (VC) + PS (Maquet), VCV-SIMV (Puritan-Bennett, Respironics), Volume SIMV (Viasys)	P-SIMV (Hamilton), SIMV(PC) + PS (Maquet), PCV-SIMV (Puritan-Bennett, Respironics), Pressure SIMV (Viasys)	SIMV + Autoflow (Draeger), Adaptive Pressure Ventilation SIMV (Hamilton), SIMV (PRVC) + PS (Maquet), VC+ SIMV (Puritan-Bennett), PRVC SIMV (Viasys)

Notes

a: Set as PRESSURE (Respironics) relative to atmospheric pressure. Set as $P_{control}$ (Hamilton), PC (Maquet), P_I (Puritan-Bennett), Insp Pres (Viasys) relative to PEEP.

b: Not set by user.

c: Triggered mandatory-pattern breaths do not increase the set frequency of mandatory breaths.

d: Set relative to PEEP (Maquet, Respironics, Viasys).

e: Threshold fixed (Draeger) or variable (Hamilton, Maquet, Puritan-Bennett, Respironics, Viasys). May also have secondary (pressure) and tertiary (time) expiratory cycling criteria.

to breaths triggered during the low-pressure phase or during both low and high phases (Figure 5.12). The ability to maintain spontaneous ventilation throughout all phases of ventilation is claimed to improve comfort as it prevents the patient 'fighting the ventilator'. Maintaining spontaneous ventilation is also associated with improved matching of ventilation and perfusion, particularly in the basal segments of the lung and has been associated with improved gas exchange compared to

pressure control without any superimposed spontaneous breathing.

Airway pressure release ventilation is a variant of bi-level ventilation where a relatively high airway pressure is maintained for a prolonged period with brief episodes when the airway pressure falls to a lower value (Figure 5.13). Spontaneous ventilation is maintained throughout. APRV maintains a high mean airway pressure promoting lung recruitment and is an effective method of improving

Table 5.8 Hybrid mode: Bi-level ventilation

Mandatory breaths

Inspiratory cycling	Time or trigger	Time or trigger	Time or trigger	Time or trigger
Control	Pressure[a]	Pressure[b]	Pressure[c]	Pressure[d]
Target	–	–	–	–
Feedback	–	–	–	–
Expiratory cycling	Time or trigger	Time or trigger	Time or trigger	Time or trigger

Triggered breaths

Interaction	Mandatory-pattern and supported	Mandatory-pattern and supported	Mandatory-pattern[e] and supported	Mandatory-pattern and supported

Supported breaths

Control	Pressure[f]	Pressure[g]	Pressure[h]	Pressure[i]
Target	–	–	–	–
Feedback	–	–	–	–
Expiratory cycling	Flow[j]	Flow[j]	Flow[j]	Flow[j]

Spontaneous breaths

During mandatory inspiration	Accommodated	Triggers support to $PEEP + P_{support}$ if this is > P_{high} (Hamilton DuoPAP), $P_{low} + P_{support}$ if this is > P_{high} (Hamilton APRV), or $PEEP_L + P_{supp}$ if this is > $PEEP_H$ (Puritan-Bennett)	Triggers support to PRES HIGH + PSV if T_{high} PSV is activated	Triggers support to PSV above P_{High}
Otherwise	Triggers support	Triggers support to $PEEP + P_{support}$ (Hamilton DuoPAP), $P_{low} + P_{support}$ (Hamilton APRV), or $PEEPL + P_{supp}$ (Puritan-Bennett)	Triggers support to PRES LOW + PSV	Triggers support to PSV above PEEP
Synonyms	BIPAP (Draeger)	DuoPAP/APRV (Hamilton), Bi-level (Puritan-Bennett)	APRV/Bi-phasic (Viasys)	Bi-vent (Maquet)

Notes
a: Set as P_{insp} (Draeger) relative to atmospheric pressure.
b: Set as P_{High} (Hamilton) or $PEEP_H$ (Puritan-Bennett) relative to atmospheric pressure.
c: Set as PRES HIGH (Viasys) relative to atmospheric pressure.
d: Set as P_{High} (Maquet) relative to atmospheric pressure.
e: The trigger window is adjustable in steps of 5% from 0% to 50% of T_{high} (expiratory cycling) and T_{low} (inspiratory cycling). If the window is adjusted to 0% mandatory breath cycling is not synchronized to spontaneous respiratory activity but occurs at interval set by T_{high} and T_{low}.
f: Set as P_{ASB} (Draeger) relative to PEEP.
g: Set as $P_{support}$ (Hamilton) or P_{supp} (Puritan-Bennett) relative to PEEP.
h: Set as PSV (Viasys) relative to PRES LOW.
i: Set as PSV above P_{High} and PSV above PEEP (Maquet).
j: Threshold fixed (Draeger) or variable (Hamilton, Maquet, Puritan-Bennett, Respironics, Viasys). May also have secondary (pressure) and tertiary (time) expiratory cycling criteria.

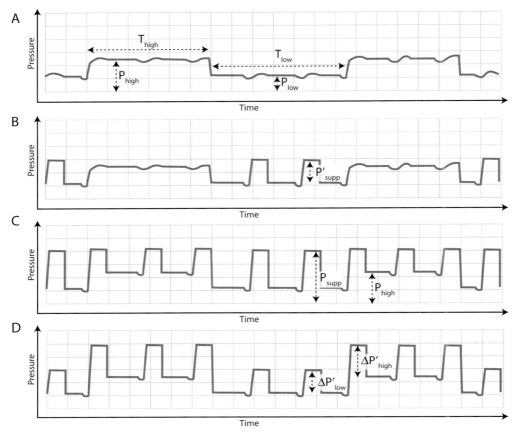

Figure 5.12 Bi-level ventilation.

A: Baseline pressure cycles between P_{low} and P_{high} with spontaneous, unsupported, patient breaths during high and low phases. Transition from low to high phase is synchronized to the patient's inspiration, and transition from high to low phase is synchronized to patient's expiration.

B: As in A, but now inspiratory efforts during the P_{low} phase trigger support (P_{supp}).

C: As in A, but now inspiratory effort during both P_{low} and P_{high} phase trigger support which is targeted to the same absolute support pressure (P_{supp}). If P_{high} is greater than P_{supp}, patient effort during P_{high} becomes unsupported.

D: As in A, but now inspiratory effort during both P_{low} and P_{high} phase trigger support which is set specifically for each phase, relative to the baseline pressure of the phase.

oxygenation in patients with severe acute respiratory distress syndrome (ARDS). Alveolar ventilation and carbon dioxide clearance occur from the unassisted spontaneous respiratory efforts augmented by the transient change in lung volume which occurs following the intermittent fall in airway pressure to the lower level, which increases minute ventilation. Theoretically, APRV should be a lung protective strategy as maximum airway pressure is limited by the upper pressure level and there are no superimposed large tidal volumes.

Automation

The sophisticated processing power within a modern intensive care ventilator has allowed the development of modes that automatically adjust a

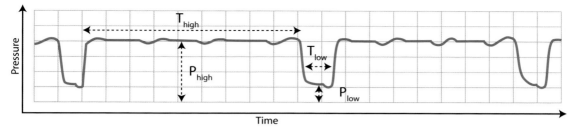

Figure 5.13 Airway pressure-release ventilation (APRV).

The ventilator settings for APRV do not usually include the respiratory frequency but instead the duration of P_{high}, T_{high} in seconds; the duration of P_{low}, T_{low} in seconds; as well as the absolute value of P_{high} and P_{low}. As with bi-level ventilation, different ventilators offer different options for supporting inspiratory efforts during the high and low phases.

number of ventilatory parameters to ensure optimal support to the patient. These modes tend to be specific to a particular manufacturer.

Automode®

Automode[14] allows the ventilator to switch automatically between a mandatory mode (volume control, pressure control and pressure-regulated volume control) and a triggered mode (pressure support or volume support). If the patient starts to make respiratory efforts the ventilator will change to the support mode as long as there is an adequate respiratory drive. If the respiratory effort subsequently becomes inadequate the controlled mode will be reactivated. When combined with volume support, the pressure support will be automatically adjusted to maintain desired tidal volume. Thus one setting can be used throughout, and the patient will theoretically be automatically weaned as they improve and their respiratory function returns. There is some preliminary evidence that this mode can reduce duration of ventilatory support post-operatively, but clinical trials are limited.

Adaptive support ventilation® [15]

This is a single automated mode that theoretically offers optimal ventilatory support throughout the patient's stay.[4] The target minute ventilation is

set as a percentage of resting minute ventilation corrected for body weight. The ventilator is able to switch between a controlled mode and pressure support. The target tidal volume and respiratory rate is based on the Otis equation that predicts the optimal combination which should be associated with minimal mechanical work of breathing.[5] As the lung mechanics are continuously monitored, the optimal tidal volume and frequency can vary as mechanics change. The applied inspiratory pressure is automatically adjusted to achieve the desired tidal volume (either in controlled mode or pressure support mode). The ventilator will change between controlled and support mode depending on the patient's respiratory rate compared to the optimal respiratory rate. The mode functions within some preset safety limits for frequency (high and low) and tidal volume (high and low). Again, clinical evidence of benefit compared to conventional modes is lacking although there are some data to suggest that weaning may be more rapid following cardiac surgery than with the more conventional mode of SIMV.[6]

SmartCare® [16]

This is a closed-loop, knowledge-based weaning system that automatically adjusts the level of pressure support. From continuous monitoring of respiratory rate, tidal volume and end-tidal carbon

---

14 Maquet.
15 Hamilton Medical.

16 Draeger.

dioxide concentration, the pressure support is automatically adjusted to ensure the patient remains within a comfort zone. This is defined as a respiratory rate between 15 and 30, a tidal volume above a minimum threshold and an end-tidal carbon dioxide concentration below a maximum threshold. As long as the patient remains in the comfort zone, the algorithm will continually try to wean the patient by assessing the response to an incremental reduction in pressure support (usually by 2 to 3 cm H_2O). If the patient has signs of respiratory distress, the pressure support level will be increased. The aim of the system is to automatically reduce pressure support to a minimum level that is dictated by the method of humidification, type, diameter and length of artificial airway. If a spontaneous breathing trial at the minimal level of pressure support is tolerated, the ventilator will display a message informing that the patient is ready for separation from the ventilator. In a recently published multi-centre randomized controlled trial comparing this system to a nurse-directed protocol, the automated knowledge-based weaning system was associated with quicker weaning.[7] Applying guidelines to clinical practice is often difficult to implement and this knowledge-based weaning system effectively ensures compliance with a weaning protocol by making it integral to the functioning of the ventilator.

Compensation for resistance from the tracheal tube

The endotracheal or tracheostomy tube applies an imposed work to spontaneously breathing patients. This work is reflected by the pressure gradient across the tracheal tube which can be calculated from the airway flow at any time point together with knowledge of the resistance of the tube. If details of the diameter and length of the tracheal tube are entered into the ventilator, the pressure gradient across the tracheal tube, both during inspiration and expiration, can be estimated as flow within the airway is measured continuously. The ventilator can use the estimated pressure drop to adjust the inspiratory and expiratory pressures to minimize the work of breathing imposed by the tracheal tube. It is the equivalent to the patient breathing without the resistance of the tracheal tube and can be used during spontaneous breathing trials to assess readiness for extubation. This type of compensation is referred to as *Automatic Tube Compensation* (ATC, Draeger), *Artificial Airway Compensation* (AAC, Viasys), *Tube Resistance Compensation* (TRC, Hamilton), or *Tube Compensation* (Puritan-Bennett).

REFERENCES

1. Downs JB, Klein EF, Jr., Desautels D *et al.* Intermittent mandatory ventilation: a new approach to weaning patients from mechanical ventilators. *Chest.* 1973;64(3):331–5.

2. Younes M. Proportional assist ventilation, a new approach to ventilatory support. Theory. *Am Rev Respir Dis.* 1992;145(1):114–20.

3. Brochard L, Rauss A, Benito S *et al.* Comparison of three methods of gradual withdrawal from ventilatory support during weaning from mechanical ventilation. *Amer J Respir Crit Care Med.* 1994;150(4):896–903.

4. Linton DM, Potgieter PD, Davis S *et al.* Automatic weaning from mechanical ventilation using an adaptive lung ventilation controller. *Chest.* 1994;106(6):1843–50.

5. Otis AB, Fenn WO, Rahn H. Mechanics of breathing in man. *J Appl Physiol.* 1950; 2(11):592–607.

6. Sulzer CF, Chiolero R, Chassot PG *et al.* Adaptive support ventilation for fast tracheal extubation after cardiac surgery: a randomized controlled study. *Anesthesiology.* 2001; 95(6):1339–45.

7. Lellouche F, Mancebo J, Jolliet P *et al.* A multicenter randomized trial of computer-driven protocolized weaning from mechanical ventilation. *Am J Respir Crit Care Med.* 2006;174(8):894–900.

Chapter 6

Oxygenation

BILL TUNNICLIFFE AND SANJOY SHAH

Introduction

Oxygenation is one of the primary gas exchange functions of the lung. Acute hypoxaemic respiratory failure is defined as an arterial partial pressure of oxygen (PaO_2) of less than 8 kPa. This specific value is to a degree arbitrary, but reflects the beginning of the relatively steep portion of the oxy-haemoglobin dissociation curve (Figure 6.1).

This chapter will briefly review how to assess the adequacy of oxygen uptake and, in the context of each of the mechanisms of arterial hypoxaemia, examine how this can be improved in the mechanically ventilated patient.

Is the patient adequately oxygenated?

The assessment of oxygenation has two facets, one pulmonary, and one extra-pulmonary. The pulmonary facet is asking the question 'how well are this patient's lungs able to take up the oxygen I am supplying?' This is an important question to answer because it provides information on how sick the patient is, and provides an impetus for further action to improve pulmonary function. The extra-pulmonary facet is asking the question 'is enough oxygen being supplied to the patient's vital organs?' This too is an important question, because inadequate oxygen delivery will lead to organ failure, but in the absence of arterial hypoxaemia the man-

agement of this problem cannot be addressed by ventilatory strategies.

From the pulmonary perspective the clinical assessment of the adequacy of oxygenation is deceptively difficult and most clinical signs attributable to hypoxaemia have many other causes. Mental status, pulse rate and breathing pattern are notoriously unreliable clinical indicators of hypoxaemia. Also the detection of cyanosis suffers from significant inter-observer variation, has other causes (methaemoglobinaemia, sulphaemoglobginaemia), and may not be present in patients with anaemia despite life-threatening hypoxaemia. As a consequence, if hypoxaemia is suspected, some measure of oxygenation is mandatory. In clinical practice, this usually equates to the measurement of the PaO_2 or the percentage saturation of arterial haemoglobin with oxygen (SaO_2), or both. It is important to appreciate that the PaO_2 and SaO_2 are not equivalent and provide different information.

Most oxygen carried in the blood is bound reversibly to haemoglobin, with only a small quantity dissolved in plasma (Figure 6.1). As each molecule of haemoglobin can only carry four molecules of oxygen, the *maximum* amount of oxygen that can be bound is determined by the haemoglobin concentration, not the PaO_2. Nevertheless, the extent to which the available binding

Core Topics in Mechanical Ventilation, ed. Iain Mackenzie. Published by Cambridge University Press.
© Cambridge University Press 2008.

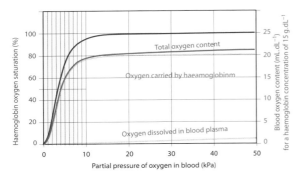

Figure 6.1 The haemoglobin/oxygen saturation curve (blue) and the oxygen content of blood (red).

The blue curve represents the relationship between the partial pressure of oxygen in blood (x-axis) and the associated haemoglobin oxygen saturation (left y-axis). A partial pressure of 8 kPa in arterial blood is usually regarded as the threshold for hypoxaemic respiratory failure. Values below this are shaded in grey. The oxy-haemoglobin saturation curve is not completely fixed, but shifts to the left and right depending on certain factors. A shift to the left means that haemoglobin's affinity for oxygen has *increased*, and is caused by alkalosis, temperature less than 36.8 °C and reduced red blood cell concentration of 2,3-diphosphoglycerate (2,3-DPG). It is worth noting that stored blood often has reduced 2,3-DPG because of reduced red blood cell glycolysis. Conversely, a shift to the right means that haemoglobin's affinity for oxygen has *decreased*, and is caused by acidosis, temperature above 36.8 °C and increased 2,3-DPG. The precise position of the oxy-haemoglobin saturation curve can be referred to by the partial pressure of oxygen at which 50% of the haemoglobin is saturated, and it is referred to as the P_{50}. A normal P_{50} is 3.53 kPa, as indicated above, and varies between 3.33 and 3.86 kPa.

The red curves represent the relationship between the partial pressure of oxygen in blood (x-axis) and the blood oxygen content (right y-axis). This is composed of the oxygen dissolved in the blood plasma (lower interrupted pink line) and the oxygen bound to haemoglobin (upper interrupted pink line) which together form the total blood oxygen content (red line) in the relationship described by Equation 6.5. The curve shown here is based on a haemoglobin of 15 gm.dL^{-1}.

sites on haemoglobin are occupied by oxygen, in other words haemoglobin's *oxygen saturation* which is expressed as a percentage, depends on three things. First, and principally, it depends on the partial pressure of oxygen around the haemoglobin. Second, it depends on haemoglobin's *affinity* for oxygen. Finally, it depends on the concentration

of other molecules that can preferentially occupy oxygen's binding site, such as carbon monoxide and nitric oxide (Figure 6.2). Once bound to haemoglobin, the oxygen molecules do not contribute to the partial pressure of oxygen within the red cell. Therefore, during the process of oxygen uptake within the pulmonary capillaries, oxygen diffuses down a partial pressure gradient from alveolar gas (P_AO_2) to capillary blood plasma to the inside of the red blood cell.

However, neither the PaO_2 nor the SaO_2 *alone* provide any information on how well the lungs are functioning in taking up alveolar oxygen. Thus a PaO_2 of 5.5 kPa might indicate mildly impaired lung function in a subject breathing air at an altitude of 3500 metres, but severely impaired lung function if they were breathing 100% oxygen at sea level. In order to incorporate the fractional inspired oxygen concentration (FiO_2) into a single measure of oxygenation, clinicians frequently refer to the 'PF ratio'. Rather confusingly, this is not a ratio at all,[1] but refers to the PaO_2 divided by the FiO_2, and has the units in which the oxygen pressure is measured – in this case, kPa. The PF ratio can take any value between 0 and 65 kPa. Thus, for the examples given earlier, the subject breathing air at altitude has a PF ratio of 26 kPa, while the individual breathing pure oxygen at sea level has a PF ratio of 5.5 kPa. The PF ratio is in fact the index of oxygenation incorporated in the definitions of acute lung injury (ALI) and the acute respiratory distress syndrome[1] (ARDS), and by these criteria, our subject at altitude fulfils the *oxygenation* criteria for ARDS. This demonstrates the weakness of the PF ratio: it fails to account for either the barometric pressure or the alveolar partial pressure of carbon dioxide. A more sophisticated but laborious index of oxygenation is to calculate the difference between the partial pressure of oxygen in the alveoli (P_AO_2) and arterial blood (PaO_2), known as the *alveolar–arterial difference* or the Aa

---

[1] A true ratio is dimensionless; in other words it has no units.

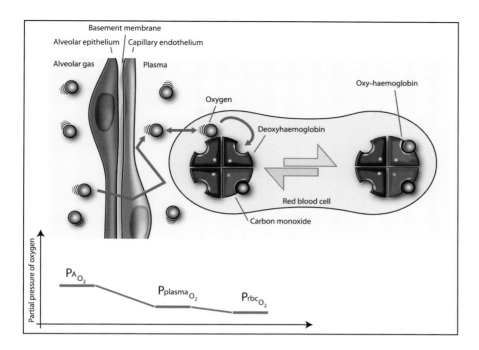

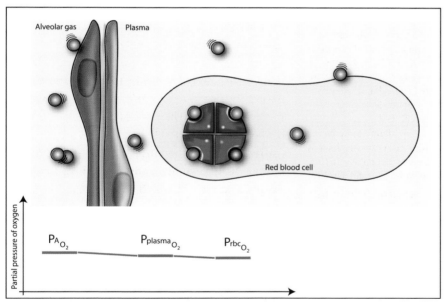

Figure 6.2 Diffusion of oxygen across the alveolar–capillary interface and uptake by haemoglobin.

The upper panel of this diagram represents a red cell that has just come into contact with a ventilated alveolus. At this point, there is quite a steep oxygen partial pressure gradient between the alveolar gas, capillary plasma and red blood cell cytoplasm. Oxygen molecules (green) diffuse down this partial pressure gradient but once bound to haemoglobin the oxygen *no longer exerts a partial pressure*. Haemoglobin's *affinity* for oxygen varies according to local conditions (see Figure 6.1). Each haemoglobin molecule can bind four molecules of oxygen, and as each binding site becomes occupied, the oxygen affinity of the remaining sites *increases*, a phenomenon known as co-operative binding. The saturation of any one haemoglobin molecule can only be 0, 25, 50, 75 and 100% as each of the four binding sites become occupied by oxygen. The molecule illustrated here already has one of the binding sites occupied by carbon monoxide.

The bottom panel illustrates the situation just before the red blood cell loses contact with the alveolus. At this stage, there is almost no partial pressure gradient between the alveolus and the interior of the red cell, and the illustrated haemoglobin molecule is 75% saturated with oxygen and 25% saturated with carbon monoxide.

difference:

Alveolar–arterial (Aa) difference $= P_{A_{O_2}} - Pa_{O_2}$.

$$(6.1)$$

The $P_{A}O_2$ can be calculated using the following approximation:

$$P_{A_{O_2}} = \left[F_{I_{O_2}} \times (Pb - 6.3) \right] - \frac{Pa_{CO_2}}{0.8}, \qquad (6.2)$$

where P_b is the barometric pressure and 6.3 is the partial pressure of saturated water vapour. The Aa difference can take any value between 0 and 100 kPa. Using Equations (6.1) and (6.2), a normal subject breathing air at sea level with a $PaCO_2$ of 5 kPa and a PaO_2 of 13 kPa would have an Aa difference of only 0.6 kPa. The subject at altitude with the same $PaCO_2$ has an Aa difference of 5.6 kPa, which is only very marginally increased. By the same token the subject breathing 100% oxygen with a $PaCO_2$ of 5 kPa has an Aa difference of 88.4 kPa, which is significantly elevated. The Aa difference can also be adapted to account for the use of positive end-expiratory pressure (PEEP), as follows:

$$P_{A_{O_2}} = \left[F_{I_{O_2}} \times \left(Pb + \frac{PEEP}{10.197} - 6.3 \right) \right] - \frac{Pa_{CO_2}}{0.8}.$$

$$(6.3^2)$$

Unfortunately, better oxygen uptake is indicated by a *smaller* Aa difference, while the opposite is true for both the $PaCO_2$ and PF ratio. This problem can be corrected by simply subtracting the calculated Aa difference from 100, as shown in Figure 6.3. In paediatric practice, an alternative oxygenation index that is sometimes used incorporates mean airway pressure ($P\overline{aw}$). This is simply referred to as the *oxygenation index* (OI):

$$OI = \frac{100 \times F_{I_{O_2}} \times P\overline{aw}}{Pa_{O_2}}. \qquad (6.4)$$

From the *extra-pulmonary* perspective, neither the PaO_2 nor the SaO_2 tells us whether vital organs

[2] PEEP has to be divided by 10.197 to convert cm H_2O into kPa.

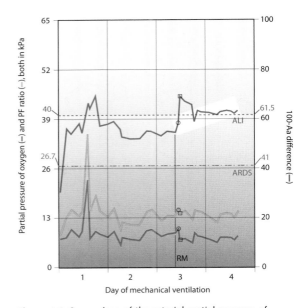

Figure 6.3 Comparison of the arterial partial pressure of oxygen (PaO_2), the PF ratio and 100-Aa difference as indices of oxygenation.

Because the Aa difference can theoretically take values between 0 (perfect oxygen transfer) to 100 (no oxygen transfer), comparison with the PF ratio is made easier by subtracting the Aa difference from 100. This value will be referred to as the *–Aa difference*.

Values for the PF ratio and –Aa difference are shown falling into three zones, based on consensus criteria for acute lung injury (ALI) and the acute respiratory distress syndrome (ARDS). A PF ratio of 26.7 kPa or less meets the oxygenation criteria for ARDS and is proportionally equivalent to an –Aa difference of less than 41 kPa. This zone is coloured pink with an upper boundary indicated by the purple interrupted line. A PF ratio of 40 kPa or less meets the oxygenation criteria for ALI and is proportionally equivalent to an –Aa difference of less than 61.5 kPa. This zone is coloured amber with an upper boundary indicated by the blue interrupted line.

This patient, whose data is illustrated, was intubated following two days of continuous positive airway pressure for respiratory failure as a result of bleomycin-induced lung fibrosis. Both the PaO_2 and the PF ratio show some improvement in oxygenation following intubation, but the latter remains within the oxygenation criteria for ARDS. In contrast, the –Aa difference shows a marked improvement, with the second blood gas showing a transition from the oxygenation criteria for ARDS to those of ALI. Mid-day on day one, the patient's positive end-expiratory pressure was increased, resulting in marked improvements in PaO_2 and PF ratio, but only a modest improvement in –Aa difference. On day three the patient was

Figure 6.3 (continued) subjected to a recruitment manoeuvre (RM). By the criteria of the PaO_2 and PF ratio, this resulted in a very small improvement in oxygenation (black circles), followed by a deterioration (black square). In marked contrast, by the criterion of the –Aa difference, the RM resulted in a proportionally larger improvement in oxygenation (black circle), followed by a *further* improvement which was even greater (black square). Moreover, neither the PaO_2 nor the PF ratio demonstrate the trend for improvement in gas exchange during days three and four, which is demonstrated by the –Aa difference.

are receiving enough oxygen to meet metabolic demand. In terms of systemic oxygen delivery, knowledge of the arterial oxygen content is usually sufficient in patients with normal cerebral function and normal, or near normal, cardiac output. Both PaO_2 and SaO_2 are frequently used as clinical surrogates for the arterial oxygen content. The total oxygen content of arterial blood is composed of oxygen bound to haemoglobin and oxygen dissolved in plasma. When the blood haemoglobin concentration is known, total arterial oxygen content can be calculated as follows:

$$Ca_{O_2} = \left(Hb \times 1.34 \times \frac{Sa_{O_2}}{100}\right) + (0.0225 \times Pa_{O_2}),$$

$$(6.5)$$

where the blood haemoglobin concentration (Hb) is measured in g.dL^{-1} and the PaO_2 is in kPa.

The arterial oxygen content alone may be insufficient in circumstances where cardiac output is reduced, and in these circumstances, oxygen delivery should be calculated. The quantity of oxygen delivered by global arterial blood flow per unit time[3] is the product of total cardiac output[4] and the oxygen content of arterial blood:

$$\dot{D}_{O_2} = \dot{Q}_t \times \frac{Ca_{O_2}}{100}.$$

$$(6.6)$$

Deficiency in oxygen content may be offset, to a degree, by a compensatory increase in the cardiac

output and vice-versa. This compensatory mechanism may operate globally or within a regional blood supply.

In addition to oxygen delivery, we can also calculate how much oxygen is being consumed,[5] which is simply the product of total cardiac output and the difference in the oxygen content between arterial and mixed venous blood:[6]

$$\dot{V}_{O_2} = \dot{Q}_t \times \left(\frac{Ca_{O_2} - C\bar{v}_{O_2}}{100}\right).$$

$$(6.7)$$

However, to do this we also need to calculate the oxygen content of mixed venous blood. This can be done using a similar equation to that used to calculate the arterial oxygen content (Equation 6.5), but using the mixed venous oxygen saturation[7] and the mixed venous partial pressure of oxygen:

$$C\bar{v}_{O_2} = \left(Hb \times 1.34 \times \frac{S\bar{v}_{O_2}}{100}\right) + (0.0225 \times P\bar{v}_{O_2}).$$

$$(6.8)$$

This calculation allows us to assess the global oxygen consumption but does not reflect the oxygen consumption of individual organs. Specific organ hypoxia is usually recognized only after damage has occurred. This limitation is important, as some clinical conditions (e.g. septic shock) may result in selective organ hypoxia even though global oxygen supply is adequate.

Probably the single best measure of oxygenation in patients with impaired cardiac function or

---

[3] Oxygen delivery, $\dot{D}O_2$, in mL.min^{-1}.
[4] Total cardiac output, $\dot{Q}t$, in mL.min^{-1}.
[5] Oxygen consumption, $\dot{V}O_2$, in mL.min^{-1}.
[6] Oxygen content of mixed venous blood, $C\bar{v}O_2$, in ml.dL^{-1}; but what is *mixed* venous blood? Venous return flows into the right atrium from the superior vena cava, which drains the head and upper limbs; from the inferior vena, which drains blood from most of the rest of the body; and from the coronary sinus, which drains the heart itself. Each of these venous returns has a different venous oxygen content because of the difference in the metabolic activities of the organs that they drain. To get a proper estimate of *global* oxygen consumption, the venous blood sampled must be a thorough mixture of these three venous returns, which requires sampling blood from the pulmonary outflow tract using a pulmonary artery catheter. This sample is called mixed venous blood.
[7] Mixed venous oxygen saturation, $S\bar{v}O_2$, in %.

haemodynamic instability is the mixed venous oxygen saturation. When cardiac output falls, or is unable to compensate for a decrease in arterial oxygen content, the mixed venous oxygen content and mixed venous oxygen saturation will fall. Normally, both cardiac output and the arterio-venous content difference can each increase up to three-fold (15 L.min^{-1} for cardiac output, and 15 ml.dL^{-1} for the arterio-venous oxygen content difference). Increasing the arterio-venous oxygen content difference is almost always at the expense of lowering the mixed venous oxygen content, thus mixed venous oxygen saturation generally reflects adequacy of oxygen delivery for the body's needs. When mixed venous oxygen saturation falls below 40%, which is equivalent to a mixed venous oxygen partial pressure of ~3.6 kPa at a pH of 7.36, the limits of compensation are such that any further fall is likely to result in lactic acidosis; this should be considered a pre-terminal event unless it is corrected rapidly.

While mixed venous oxygen saturation is a useful measure of oxygenation, it is not without its problems. First, its measurement requires a sample of blood from the pulmonary artery. Second, the interpretation of the resultant value needs careful consideration. Thus a low mixed venous oxygen saturation indicates inadequate oxygen delivery for the body's metabolic needs, and the lower the value, the more severe the derangement. However, and herein lies the problem, a *normal* mixed venous oxygen saturation does not necessarily mean that oxygen delivery is adequate. This may be encountered in several different circumstances; for example, regional hypoperfusion may be masked by an adequate blood flow to the rest of the body resulting in an organ being oxygen deficient with its oxygen-poor venous blood flow being insufficient to cause a significant reduction in the mixed venous oxygen saturation. Similarly, peripheral arterio-venous shunts may have the same effect; such shunts have been described in septic and cardiogenic shock. Finally, consumption may be inadequate in some

conditions despite an acceptable oxygen delivery because of the inhibition of mitochondrial oxidative phosphorylation, a condition termed *cytopathic hypoxia*.[2] Classically, this is recognized as the mechanism of cyanide poisoning, but may be an important contributor to the organ dysfunction seen in sepsis.

Mechanisms of hypoxaemia and their management

Oxygen moves from the alveolar gas to the pulmonary capillary blood by diffusion. The rate at which diffusion occurs, and therefore the maximum rate at which oxygen can be taken up by the lungs, is dictated by the physical characteristics of the alveolar–capillary interface, and is described by Fick's Law:

$$\text{Diffusion flux} = \text{surface area for diffusion} \times \text{speed of diffusion} \quad (6.9)$$

and

$$\text{Speed of diffusion} = K \times \frac{\left(P_{A_{O_2}} - Pa_{O_2}\right)}{d}, \quad (6.10)$$

where K is the gas-specific diffusion coefficient[8] and d is the distance that the gas needs to diffuse. In the context of oxygen diffusing across the alveolar–capillary interface, d comprises the thickness of the alveolar epithelium, the thickness of the basement membrane, and the thickness of the capillary endothelium. Substituting the speed of diffusion defined in Equation 6.10 into Equation 6.9 gives the following equation:

$$\text{Rate of diffusion} = \text{surface area for diffusion} \times K \times \frac{\left(P_{A_{O_2}} - Pa_{O_2}\right)}{d}. \quad (6.11)$$

However, Equation 6.11 assumes an alveolus with two essential components: tidal ventilation and perfusion with blood. The ideal situation is where ventilation ($\dot{V}$) and perfusion ($\dot{Q}$) are perfectly matched;

---

[8] For an explanation of the diffusion coefficient see 'Diffusion Coefficient' later in the chapter.

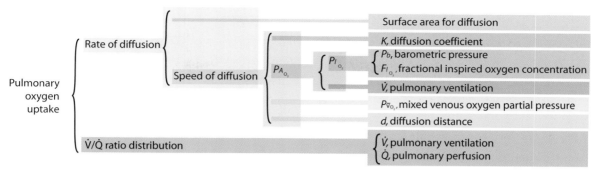

Figure 6.4 Determinants of pulmonary oxygen uptake.
The rate of diffusion depends on the surface area for diffusion and the speed of diffusion.

in other words, a nominal $\dot{V}/\dot{Q}$ ratio of 1. In alveoli where ventilation exceeds perfusion and the $\dot{V}/\dot{Q}$ ratio is greater than 1, the rate of oxygen uptake will be limited by *perfusion*. Conversely, in alveoli where perfusion exceeds ventilation and the $\dot{V}/\dot{Q}$ ratio is less than 1, the rate of oxygen uptake will be limited by *diffusion*. At one end of the spectrum of $\dot{V}/\dot{Q}$ ratios are alveoli with no ventilation at all, and these constitute a true pulmonary shunt. These two key components provide all the variables that contribute to pulmonary oxygen uptake (Figure 6.4), which not only lead to arterial hypoxaemia, but also provide means by which oxygen uptake can be improved.

Surface area

If one assumes, for simplicity, that the lungs are equivalent to a large spherical balloon, the relationship between the volume of the balloon and its surface area is obvious. The larger the volume of gas in the balloon, the larger the surface area. Measuring absolute lung volumes in a clinical setting is not practical, but because lung volume and airway pressure are related by the pulmonary compliance, we can use pressure as an index of volume. Of course, the volume of the lungs during normal tidal ventilation does not remain static, but alternates between the end-expiratory and end-inspiratory volumes. Thus the end-expiratory and end-inspiratory pressures may be used to mark the lower and upper lim-

its of the pulmonary surface area, and the mean airway pressure is a useful proxy for the average pulmonary surface area.

It is now evident that any manoeuvre that increases the mean airway pressure will result in an increase in the surface area available for gas diffusion. However, in an alveolus in which the capillary blood haemoglobin is not diffusion-limited and *already* fully saturated with oxygen, this increase in surface area *cannot* increase oxygen uptake.[9] Of course, the lung is not as simple as a single balloon, but actually consists of approximately 300 million alveoli. Again, for the sake of simplicity, we can assume that these alveoli fall into one of two groups: alveoli that are open and ventilated, and alveoli that are not ventilated (Figure 6.5).

With this slightly more sophisticated view of the lung, it is now apparent that increasing the volume of intra-pulmonary gas can have one of two effects (Figure 6.6). As before, the additional volume can cause the open alveolus to increase its surface area, or the additional volume can convert the previously closed alveolus into an open one. If it is assumed that alveoli are spherical, the difference between these two situations is quite striking. In the first instance, doubling the volume of

---

[9] In fact, in some circumstances, the increased intra-alveolar pressure may actually cause the oxygen uptake to *fall*. See Figure 6.11, Panel B.

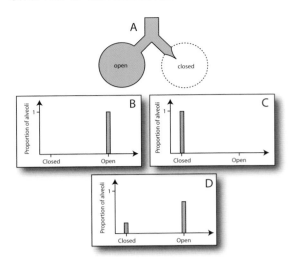

Figure 6.5 Lung model in which alveoli are either open or closed.

In the lung model shown in A, it is assumed, for simplicity, that each of the lung's 300 million alveoli is either open and ventilated, or closed and non-ventilated, as in A. For the lung as a whole, the alveoli can therefore be all open (B), all closed (C) or somewhere in-between. D shows the frequency histogram for a lung in which 25% of the alveoli are closed.

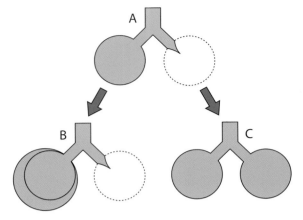

Figure 6.6 Possible outcomes from increasing intra-pulmonary gas volume.

The top diagram represents two alveoli, one of which is not available for ventilation. Doubling the volume can have two outcomes. In B, the volume of the open alveolus has doubled, and the surface area has increased by $\sqrt[3]{2}$, or approximately 1.26 times. In C, the extra volume has 'recruited' a previously closed alveolus, and in this instance the surface area for diffusion *has also doubled*.

the open alveolus results in a surface area increase of $\sqrt[3]{2}$, or approximately 1.26 times. In the second instance, converting a previously closed alveolus into an open one *doubles* the surface area. Moreover, the opening, or 'recruiting', of a previously closed alveolus has a big impact on oxygen uptake because the capillary blood to this previously closed alveolus can now be oxygenated. Alveolar recruitment also has an impact on the lung's physical characteristics because the intra-pulmonary volume is now distributed across twice the surface area, meaning that the wall stresses are reduced. For the lung as a whole, this is reflected as an increase in pulmonary compliance. So far, only two alveoli have been considered in the argument: an open one and a closed one. The overall effect of increasing intra-pulmonary volume for all 300 million alveoli will depend on the proportion of these alveoli that are closed at baseline, and the proportion of the *closed* alveoli that are recruited. At present, it

is clinically impractical to measure either of these things.

In practical terms, there are a number of ways of increasing the mean airway pressure, which is represented graphically by the area under the pressure/time profile (Figure 6.7). The most obvious way is to use a larger inflating pressure, but this inevitably increases the minute volume and without changing the ventilatory rate would result in a fall in the $PaCO_2$, which may not be desired. Alternatively, and much more effectively, mean airway pressure can be increased by adding PEEP. Finally, prolongation of inspiration at the expense of expiration increases mean airway pressure. This mechanism is used by two forms of mechanical ventilation, inverse-ratio ventilation and airway pressure release ventilation (APRV). Ultimately mean airway pressure, and therefore surface area, can be maximized by dispensing completely with a traditionally expiratory phase by using high-frequency oscillatory ventilation (HFOV).

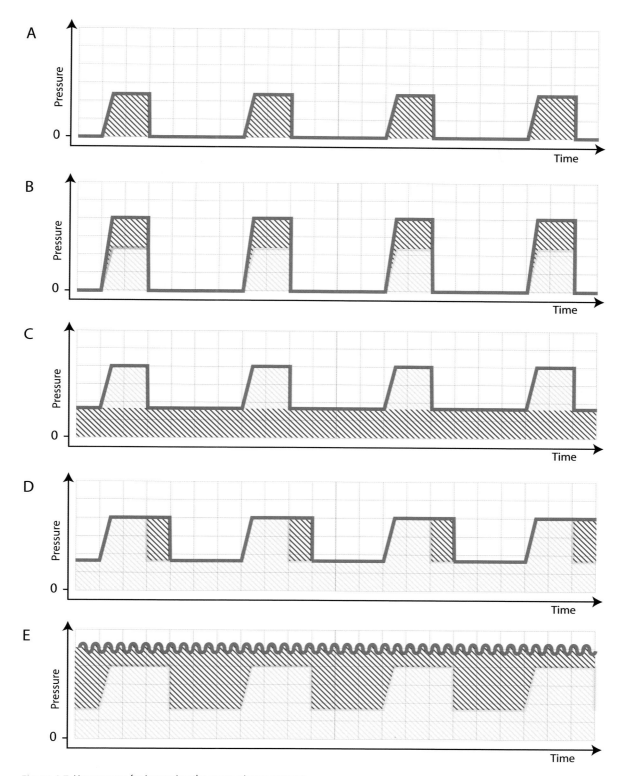

Figure 6.7 Manoeuvres for increasing the mean airway pressure.

The mean airway pressure is given by the area under the pressure/time profile, as indicated by the blue hatch in panel A. This area, and therefore the mean airway pressure, can be increased by using a larger inflating pressure (panel B), by adding positive end-expiratory pressure (PEEP, panel C), or by increasing the duration of inspiration at the expense of expiration (panel D). Ultimately, mean airway pressure can be maximized by dispensing completely with an expiratory pressure drop by using high-frequency oscillatory ventilation (HFOV, panel E).

Positive end-expiratory pressure (PEEP)

In the critical care setting, PEEP is almost universally applied, although in general, increases in PEEP in response to worsening hypoxaemia tend to occur long after the fractional inspired oxygen concentration has been increased above 60%. While an increase in the fractional inspired oxygen concentration improves the PaO_2, this does not address the most likely cause for the deterioration in gas exchange and risks oxygen toxicity.

PHYSIOLOGICAL PEEP

Small amounts of PEEP (3 to 5 cm H_2O) are commonly applied to intubated patients to overcome the decrease in functional residual capacity that results from the bypassing of the glottic apparatus by the endotracheal intubation.

PEEP FOR HYPOXAEMIA

There is now some evidence supporting the use of a limited tidal volume, limited airway pressure 'open lung' strategy in the mechanical ventilation of patients with ALI or ARDS[3] (ALI/ARDS). As part of this strategy, the relative safety of permissive hypercapnia has been recognized, as have the benefits of incorporating spontaneous breathing efforts, where possible. From its introduction to clinical practice more than 40 years ago, the use of PEEP has been a cornerstone of ventilator management for this challenging group of patients. The rationale for its use in patients with ALI/ARDS is primarily to increase the aerated lung volume (i.e. 'to open the lungs and keep them open').[4] In addition, its appropriate use is thought to be able to improve respiratory mechanics, reduce intrapulmonary shunt, stabilize unstable lung units and reduce the risks of ventilator-induced lung injury (VILI).

While the application of PEEP can undoubtedly increase end-expiratory lung volumes and produce varying lung recruitment, there are very large differences in its effects between individuals. This would

suggest that in some subjects, PEEP can increase lung volumes without achieving recruitment (Figure 6.6), which can only occur by increasing the distension of previously normally aerated lung units. Such PEEP-induced distension has been shown in several studies, most of which show recruitment and distension occuring simultaneously rather than sequentially in different lung regions, challenging the view that a single value of PEEP might be 'optimal' for the lung as a whole.[5] This phenomenon has been shown to be dependent on several factors including ARDS aetiology, lung and chest wall mechanics, stage of disease and lung morphology.

Despite the clarity of the aims of applying PEEP in ARDS and its widespread clinical use, no single method for determining the 'optimal' PEEP in patients with ALI/ARDS has proved to enhance any clinical outcome. The range of targets proposed to select optimal PEEP is extensive and includes achieving maximal oxygen delivery, achieving intrapulmonary shunt <15%, achieving a drop in mixed venous oxygen tensions, achieving adequate PaO_2 with minimal FiO_2, achieving the minimal end-tidal carbon dioxide gradient, linear airway pressure/time profiles, using 'lower inflection point plus 2 cm H_2O pressure' on the inspiratory pressure/volume curve, achieving maximal static compliance, among others. A more pragmatic approach to selecting PEEP was used in the ARDSnet trial, which was set empirically on the basis of a predefined table and PEEP being determined by the FiO_2 required to achieve an adequate PaO_2 (Table 6.1).

The second ARDSnet trial (ALVEOLI) attempted to compare the impact of 'high' and 'low' levels of PEEP on clinical endpoints;[6] the low PEEP values were those used in the first ARDS network study. Subjects were randomized to high or low PEEP levels, while undergoing IMV with a tidal volume of 6 mL.kg^{-1} (predicted body weight) and a plateau pressure of <30 cm H_2O. PEEP was titrated on the

Table 6.1 Selection of positive end-expiratory pressure according to the inspired oxygen concentration; based on the 2001 ARDSnet study

Inspired oxygen concentration (%)	PEEP (cm H$_2$O)
30	5
40	5
40	8
50	8
50	10
60	10
70	10
70	12
70	14
80	14
90	14
90	16
90	18
100	18 to 24

values selected on the basis of the ARDSnet trial table will sustain significant regional alveolar over-distension.[7]

Where does this leave us when faced with a patient with ARDS requiring ventilation? Pragmatically, we would advocate the use of a low tidal volume strategy and the lowest PEEP–FiO$_2$ combination (based on the ARDSnet trial) that produces acceptable oxygenation as a starting point, particularly where an FiO$_2$ < 0.6 can be achieved. Beyond this, subsequent optimal PEEP might currently best be determined by a combination of clinical judgement (e.g. whether there is likely still to be recruitable lung) and a trial of higher and lower PEEP values; therefore, achieving an adequate mixed venous oxygen saturation would seem to be a reasonable goal. Volumetric CT scanning of the thorax would currently seem to offer an objective way to select optimal PEEP, but its limited practicality means this technique is unlikely to be adopted widely. The additional role of recruitment manoeuvres remains to be established (and will be discussed later).

COMPLICATIONS OF AND CONTRA-INDICATIONS TO THE USE OF PEEP

The application of PEEP may have potential drawbacks; these need to be carefully considered within the clinical context. Complications are directly related to the level of PEEP applied (Table 6.2), and the contra-indications to PEEP are listed in Table 6.3.

Prolongation of inspiratory time
INVERSE RATIO VENTILATION

Inverse ratio ventilation (IRV) is the use of extended inspiratory times during mechanical ventilation so that the inspiratory period extends beyond 50% of the total cycle time. It was first described in the early 1970s in infants with ARDS[8] and was soon being reported in many, predominantly uncontrolled, trials in adults with ARDS, producing improved indices of oxygenation.[9, 10] IRV can be applied in either volume- (VC) or pressure-controlled (PC)

basis of two pre-defined tables (high and low) of combinations of PEEP and FiO$_2$ to achieve identical goals. The trial was interrupted after an interim analysis showed no difference in any of the pre-defined clinical outcomes. This apparent null effect has been subject to considerable scrutiny, and post hoc analysis restricted to a subset of patients enrolled after a protocol amendment, that produced greater separation in the levels of PEEP used in each group, demonstrated a survival advantage in the high PEEP group. This probably means that the trial was interrupted prematurely rather than confirming that the high PEEP strategy was superior. It would also suggest that higher PEEP values are relatively safe.

The application of a pre-defined PEEP on the basis of the FiO$_2$ required to achieve adequate oxygenation has been investigated with volumetric CT scanning in ventilated patients with ARDS. These studies have confirmed that, in general, measured physiological variables (including oxygenation) are poor predictors of an individual's response to a particular level of PEEP. They also suggest that again, in general, around one third of subjects with PEEP

Table 6.2 Complications of positive end-expiratory pressure (PEEP)

- Pulmonary over-distension
- Barotrauma
- Ventilator-induced lung injury (VILI)
- Increased dead space
- Impaired carbon dioxide elimination
- Reduced diaphragmatic force-generating capacity
- Reduced cardiac output and oxygen delivery
- Impaired renal perfusion
- Reduced splanchnic blood flow
- Hepatic congestion
- Reduced lymphatic drainage

Table 6.3 Contra-indications to positive end-expiratory pressure (PEEP)

Absolute	Relative
Hypovolaemic shock	Bronchopleural fistula
Undrained tension pneumothorax	↑ ICP with reduced cerebral compliance
	Chronic restrictive chest wall disorders
	Hyperinflation with exp flow limitation

ventilatory modes, though more commonly referred to now as PC-IRV.

The rationale for the use of IRV again centres on achieving and maintaining an open lung in ALI/ARDS. The concept is that in the injured lung the spectrum of alveolar time constants (slower and faster alveolar compartments) is increased. Intrinsic PEEP is generated by deliberately shortening expiratory times, thereby preventing collapse of the slower alveolar compartments and improving oxygenation. This implies using regional gas-trapping to prevent alveolar collapse, with an inevitable increased risk of biotrauma. The delivery of IRV requires profound sedation and frequently the use of neuromuscular blockade. In addition, the technique inevitably raises mean intrathoracic pressures with potentially adverse consequences to cardiac output; any perceived benefits to oxygenation may well be offset by consequent reductions in oxygen delivery.

Overall, clinical studies have failed to demonstrate any benefit in outcomes associated with IRV. In addition, most of the claimed benefits of IRV can generally be achieved more safely with controlled mechanical ventilation and adequate levels of externally applied PEEP. Given this, whether there is any role for IRV in the mechanical ventilation of patients with ALI/ARDS is uncertain. In our own experience, alternative strategies, including the use of recruitment manoeuvres or the use of HFOV (where available), should probably be considered in preference to IRV as rescue therapy in such patients with persistently inadequate oxygenation.

AIRWAY PRESSURE RELEASE VENTILATION

APRV was first described in 1987[11] and is a form of bi-level assisted ventilation utilizing continuous positive airway pressure (CPAP) with periodic pressure releases, either to a lower CPAP pressure or to atmospheric pressure. These periodic releases provide a background tidal volume and respiratory rate enabling carbon dioxide clearance, while the periods of sustained CPAP produce a high mean airway pressure resulting in lung recruitment and effective oxygenation. Unrestricted spontaneous breathing throughout the ventilator cycle also enables carbon dioxide clearance. Advantages claimed over conventional ventilation include superior lung recruitment, higher mean airway pressure but lower peak airway pressure, superior haemodynamic and renal/splanchnic perfusion, and the patient's ability to breath spontaneously from the time of intubation to the point of separation from the ventilator. Protagonists suggest a theoretically lower risk of biotrauma and accelerated weaning, but these claims remain unproven.

In contrast to conventional ventilation, where short sharp breaths are delivered to cyclically inflate the lung from a low resting volume to a higher volume with PEEP used to prevent de-recruitment and inspiratory pressures limited to prevent excessive tidal volumes, the sustained periods of CPAP maintain a high resting lung volume. The CPAP pressures delivered are dominant in determining mean airway pressure (determined by the CPAP value and the $T_{high}:T_{low}$ ratio), which in turn essentially determines the lung volume and therefore governs oxygenation. Intermittent low frequency (<16 minute^{-1}) pressure releases produce an exhaled tidal volume resulting in carbon dioxide clearance; the fall in lung volume resulting from the pressure releases is controlled by the pressure gradient and the release time. Tidal volumes are limited by raising the lower pressure level or alternatively by reducing the release time, prematurely terminating expiratory airflow and producing intrinsic PEEP; in essence, excessive tidal volumes signify de-recruitment and small tidal volumes imply gas trapping.

When APRV is classically applied, P_{low} is typically fixed at 0, P_{high} at 25 to 30 cm H_2O with T_{high} being determined by the respiratory rate, typically 16 breaths.min^{-1}. The $T_{high}:T_{low}$ ratio is adjusted to achieve tidal volumes of 6 to 8 mL.kg^{-1} and a mean airway pressure of less than 5 cm H_2O below P_{high}. With successful recruitment over time, P_{high} should be reduced with improving PF ratios. Changes in $PaCO_2$ should prompt review of T_{high} (respiratory rate). Typically, no pressure support would be offered to spontaneous breathing efforts, although this is an option with some ventilators.[10]

When then should APRV be used? One of its key theoretical advantages over conventional ventilation is that it allows spontaneous breathing efforts and as a consequence does not impose the need for deep sedation and the use of muscle relaxants.

Also APRV can be delivered by most conventional intensive care unit ventilators and does not require the use of special circuits or equipment. Given this, protagonists suggest that it should be seen as a ventilatory technique that should be considered early in the course of ARDS rather than as a method of rescue for those failing conventional techniques. They argue that its early institution will limit the possibility of ventilator-associated lung injury adding to the inflammatory cascade sustaining the pathogenesis of ALI/ARDS. As yet, this view is not supported by trial data.

Currently in the UK, as with HFOV (discussed later), APRV is typically used as a rescue technique for those failing to achieve adequate oxygenation with conventional ventilation. Its safe application requires considerable knowledge as ventilator adjustments may seem counter-intuitive. Familiarity with the technique is obviously important, and it seems that this is one of the determinants as to where and when it is used. There are currently no data available comparing the use of APRV and HFOV in this setting.

High-frequency oscillatory ventilation (HFOV)

HFOV is an unconventional mode of ventilation, but conceptually is seen as an extension of the open lung approach to mechanical ventilation. By eliminating the need for the bulk gas flow of tidal ventilation, it tends to avoid the potential problems of cyclical over-inflation and collapse in differing lung zones that may accompany conventional ventilatory methods.

In adult practice in the UK, HFOV is generally used as a rescue method for patients with ARDS failing conventional ventilation, principally because of poor oxygenation. Clinical trial data are accumulating supporting the contention that in ARDS, HFOV appears to be as safe and effective as conventional ventilation.[12] To date, no adequately powered trial has been undertaken

---

[10] Supported spontaneous breathing during APRV may result in volutrauma, whereas unsupported spontaneous effort tends to improve the intrathoracic blood pump mechanism and limit the risk of volutrauma.

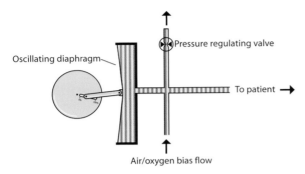

Oscillating diaphragm

Pressure regulating valve

To patient →

Air/oxygen bias flow

Figure 6.8 Diagram illustrating the principles of high-frequency oscillatory ventilation (HFOV).

The mean airway pressure is determined by both the bias flow, set in L.min^{-1}, and the resistance to outflow generated by the pressure regulating valve, which on the SensorMedics 3100B is adjusted using the 'mean pressure' dial (see Figure 6.10). The FIO_2 of the source gas for the bias flow is set on a separate mixer unit.

to explore whether HFOV, if applied as the primary ventilatory strategy in ARDS, might improve outcomes.

The principles of the technique are relatively simple. Oxygenation and carbon dioxide clearance are in essence disconnected, being controlled through generally independent mechanisms. Oxygenation is determined by the delivered FIO_2 and the degree of alveolar recruitment that is achieved, and maintained, by means of the mean airway pressure. This acts like 'super CPAP' with pressures of up to 55 cm H_2O and is controlled by the fresh gas flow into the circuit, the bias flow, and a variable resistance to outflow from the circuit (Figure 6.8).

Carbon dioxide clearance is managed principally through an oscillating diaphragm that has both active inspiratory and expiratory travel. The cycle volume delivered by the piston is referred to in the SensorMedics 3100B as the 'power' and can be varied from 0 to 10, representing displacements of approximately 40 to 300 mL. These cause symmetric oscillations of intrapulmonary pressure around the mean airway pressure (Figure 6.9) at a fre-

quency of 3 to 9 Hz[11] which equates to 180 to 540 breaths.minute^{-1}. The amplitude of the pressure excursions generated is proportional to both the cycle volume, or 'power', and the inspiratory time – but *inversely* proportional to the frequency. This process, when applied at the airway opening, induces rapid gas mixing within the lungs with net gas transport occurring along the partial pressure gradients for oxygen and carbon dioxide.

At initiation, an FIO_2 of 1 is selected and the starting mean airway pressure determined by adding 5 cm H_2O pressure to the plateau pressures being generated with conventional ventilation. Sequential increases in the mean airway pressure, in 5-cm H_2O increments up to a maximum of 55 cm H_2O, are then applied to achieve alveolar recruitment. Successful recruitment is demonstrated by improved oxygenation and confirmed where necessary by chest radiography. Over-distension is usually accompanied by reductions in indices of oxygenation. If and when alveolar recruitment is achieved, the FIO_2 is sequentially reduced to achieve the target PaO_2, with the goal of achieving adequate oxygenation with an FIO_2 below 0.6. The time course of recruitment varies between patients, but in general occurs more rapidly when HFOV is initiated early.

Sequential reductions in the mean airway pressure, in 2-cm H_2O decrements, are then attempted to exploit the hysteresis of the lungs, with the aim of maintaining alveolar recruitment but at lower distending pressures. De-recruitment will occur if pressures are reduced too much (conceptually to a value beyond that on the deflation limb of the pressure/volume curve) and is generally evidenced by a fall in PaO_2. In this case, pressures tend to be increased transiently by 8 to 10 cm H_2O to achieve

[11] Because HFOV uses such high ventilatory frequencies, these are measured in cycles/breaths per second (Herz, Hz) rather than cycles/breaths per minute as in conventional ventilation.

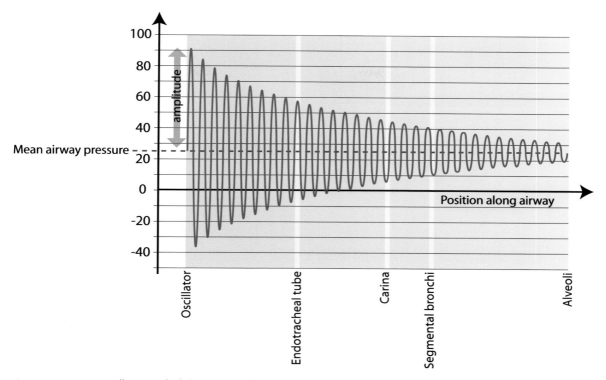

Pressure oscillations in high frequency oscillatory ventilation.

re-recruitment, and then lowered again to an intermediate value.

The ventilatory costs of inadequate recruitment are reflected in atelectrauma, with pressure transmission (hence energy transfer) to the lung being sharply increased at low lung volumes; in contrast, volutrauma results from excessive recruitment. In general, investigation into the use of HFOV supports the use of a vigorous lung recruitment strategy, as accepting ongoing atelectasis tends to carry disproportionate risk.[13]

Arbitrary starting settings for the oscillating piston are usually selected at the initiation of HFOV. These values reflect the physical properties and dimensions of the piston and diaphragm used on the HFOV ventilator currently available in the UK (SensorMedics 3100B, see Figure 6.10), and may not be applicable to machines likely to become available in the future with differing characteristics. The

frequency is usually initially set to 6 Hz and the 'power' to 6.

Unless hypercarbia and the resultant respiratory acidosis are extreme, adjustments to these controls are delayed until adequate recruitment is achieved; in general, if adequate recruitment is achieved, managing carbon dioxide clearance is relatively straightforward. To increase carbon dioxide clearance, power tends to be increased initially in steps that produce an increase in amplitude (ΔP) of 5 cm H_2O. Power increments are generally halted when amplitude exceeds 100 to 120 cm H_2O or the power adjustment reaches 10. If these adjustments fail to produce adequate carbon dioxide clearance, then sequential reductions in frequency are generally undertaken, in 0.5-Hz steps down to a minimum of 4 Hz. For optimal lung protection, one should use the lowest power (equating to smallest tidal volume) and highest frequency that achieve

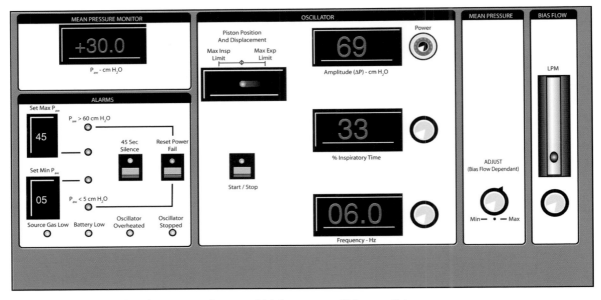

Figure 6.10 Control panel for the SensorMedics 3100B high frequency oscillatory ventilator.

$PaCO_2$ elimination targets. The ventilatory costs of frequency reduction are generally disproportionately higher than increments in power, hence the hierarchy of adjustment recommended previously. In addition to these adjustments, carbon dioxide elimination can be enhanced by deliberately causing a cuff leak, exploiting the resultant bulk gas flow out of the lungs that will result. In terms of the position of this technique in the risk hierarchy, this is generally very safe and can effectively reduce the stroke volume needed to achieve relative normocapnia by up to 50%. As a consequence, the instigation of a cuff leak is now often undertaken at initiation of HFOV and certainly should be considered before reductions in frequency below 6 Hz are undertaken.

HFOV tends to be a sensitive detector of hypovolaemia; volume resuscitation and increased vasopressor support are often required at the time of initiation of HFOV. Concerns about an increased risk of air leaks with HFOV have, in general, been discounted; in experienced hands, the incidence of pneumothorax tends to be no higher than that encountered with conventional ventilation.

Most of the perceived limitations of HFOV currently reflect limitations of the machines available to provide HFOV rather than the technique itself. Such limitations include the lack of demand flow to augment spontaneous breaths, meaning that adults tend to have to be converted back to APRV or conventional ventilation for final weaning. Limited alarms and feedback from the ventilator, and its tendency to be noisy during use, also tend to put off novice users. Indeed, a major limitation to the use of HFOV is the need to develop and maintain HFOV skills in medical and nursing staff and allied health professionals; most encounter HFOV only rarely, and then only when it is being used as a late intervention or as a measure of last resort.

We tend to use HFOV when it is agreed by two independent critical care consultants that adequate oxygenation cannot be maintained in a patient with ARDS undergoing conventional ventilation at an inspired oxygen concentration of less than 60%, despite being appropriately resuscitated, sedated and expertly ventilated. Our own experience is that in the majority of cases striking improvements in gas exchange are achieved as well as, in some, considerable reductions in vasopressor support, and that these improvements are often sustained. Whether these apparent benefits are reflected in improved survival in this group is uncertain.

As experience with the technique develops, the need grows for an adequately powered clinical trial examining the efficacy of HFOV relative to conventional ventilation as the primary mode of ventilatory support for patients with ARDS.

Recruitment manoeuvres

Recruitment manoeuvres (RMs) are techniques devised to improve the volumes of aerated lung and consequently hypoxaemia, principally in patients receiving invasive mechanical ventilation for ALI/ARDS. RMs generally involve the application of a static pressure to the lung that would generally be considered hazardous during tidal ventilation. Both the magnitude of the pressure and the duration of its application seem to be important in determining their effects.

RMs are seen by many as complementary to the process of optimal PEEP selection. Leading on from the discussion regarding the appropriate selection of PEEP in patients with ALI/ARDS, they argue that applied PEEP will be unable to 'keep open' any lung units that were not open at an earlier point in the respiratory cycle. They suggest that these refractory units of the acutely injured lung may require pressures considerably higher than $25 \, cm \, H_2O$ to achieve patency. Once opened, however, these lung units are believed to close at lower pressures, allowing ventilation to be achieved with the same tidal volume and PEEP, though in the context of a more open lung. Proponents argue that to consolidate the benefit of a successful RM, PEEP will generally need to be increased following a manoeuvre and otherwise potential benefits of an RM will tend to be short-lived if PEEP is returned to its original value.

Various techniques for RM have been described; one of the simplest is the static application of 40 cm H_2O pressure to the airway for 40 seconds which, if tolerated, is followed by the re-instatement of PEEP 2 to 5 cm H_2O higher than the initial value.

When sustained pressure is applied to the airway, mean and peak airway pressures are identical; this occurs through its effects principally on right ventricular after-load (and to a lesser degree its preload) which may produce significant falls in cardiac output and result in hypotension. In addition, barotrauma may be sustained. Clinicians performing an RM should remain vigilant to these effects and be prepared to both rapidly re-instate typical mechanical ventilation and perform resuscitation. Currently, no data exist to demonstrate clinical benefit from the application of RMs or to support the use of one manoeuvre over another. Similarly, no prescription for suggested timing and frequency of RMs is supported by outcome data.

So, should we be performing RMs? This remains highly controversial. Given the current state of knowledge, we believe the role for RMs should generally be limited to those patients with ALI/ARDS who require high inspired concentrations of oxygen ($FiO_2 > 0.6$) despite an apparently adequate level of applied PEEP (following a trial of various PEEP levels). It is probably prudent to attempt recruitment earlier in the course of these patients rather than later, and carefully monitor the ability of the patient to tolerate attempts at recruitment. Again, in general we suggest that if benefits accrued through recruitment are maintained, further attempts at recruitment should not be attempted. If initial benefits are lost (despite an increase in PEEP), then we would generally attempt further recruitment at that point, with further increases in PEEP, if successful. In our hands, failure to re-recruit or repeated de-recruitment, and the requirement for an $FiO_2 > 0.6$ to achieve adequate oxygenation would prompt us to consider alternative forms of ventilatory support, e.g. HFOV (as discussed earlier).

Sigh

Sigh is a ventilatory technique where 'larger than normal' tidal volumes/inspiratory pressures are delivered, usually in a predetermined sequence, interspersed with routine tidal breaths. A typical example would be the delivery of three consecutive sigh breaths, with inspiratory pressures of 45 cm H_2O, each minute superimposed on the regular pattern of delivered breaths.

The proposed rationale for the use of sigh is to try to achieve further recruitment of lung segments with unresolved atelectasis, similar in concept to the use of recruitment manoeuvres discussed previously, and then to 'keep them open'. While conceptually this seems attractive, and clinical data reflecting respiratory parameters during the use of sigh tend to be improved, there is no clinical evidence available to demonstrate any benefit with sigh in terms of clinical outcome.

Whether sigh can in fact maintain recruitment in patients with unstable lung segments undergoing low tidal volume ventilation is not clear. Much as with recruitment manoeuvres, how sigh might best be used is unknown; also its relative benefit when adequate PEEP or manual recruitment manoeuvres are employed is uncertain. Given this, many clinicians have abandoned sigh in the management of patients with ALI/ARDS.

Diffusion coefficient

The diffusion coefficient for a gas is proportional to the gas's solubility in the medium through which the gas has to diffuse, and is inversely proportional to the square root of the gas's relative molecular mass. As these are fixed physical properties of a gas, they cannot be manipulated.

Alveolar partial pressure of oxygen

The factors that contribute to the alveolar partial pressure of oxygen are shown in Equation 6.1 and consist of factors that affect the *inspired* partial pressure of oxygen on the one hand, and the alveolar partial pressure of carbon dioxide, which contributes to the alveolar gas composition, on the other.

Low inspired partial pressure of oxygen

The partial pressure of inspired oxygen[12] is determined by the barometric pressure[13] and the fractional inspired oxygen concentration:

$$P_{I_{O_2}} = Pb \times F_{I_{O_2}}. \tag{6.12}$$

At sea level, the barometric pressure is approximately 101 kPa, and the inspired fractional oxygen concentration is 0.21, giving an inspired partial pressure of oxygen of 21.2 kPa. With modern ventilators and anaesthetic machines that prevent the administration of hypoxic gas mixtures, low inspired oxygen concentrations should not account for hypoxaemia in ventilated patients or the critically ill. Prior to hospital admission, patients may be exposed to hypoxic atmospheres either where a fire in a confined space has consumed the oxygen or where oxygen has been displaced by other gases such as methane.

Low barometric pressure as a cause of arterial hypoxaemia is only a problem at altitudes of around 2500 metres[14] or greater and is therefore unlikely in a European clinical environment. This is not the case in other parts of the world where there are very significant populations living at these high altitudes.[15]

OXYGEN THERAPY

Oxygen is the commonest and one of the most important drugs used in the clinical setting. It is unfortunately poorly prescribed and considerable misconceptions about its use remain. Oxygen should be administered to all patients who are

[12] Inspired partial pressure of oxygen, $P_{I_{O_2}}$, in kPa.
[13] Barometric pressure, Pb, in kPa.
[14] 2500 m = 8200 feet.
[15] La Paz, Bolivia (population 1 million, altitude 3600 m); Mexico City (population 8.7 million, altitude 2240 m); Lhasa, Tibet (population 0.25 million, altitude 3650 m).

suspected to be, or who have been confirmed to be, hypoxaemic, with the goal of restoring normoxia. The inspired oxygen concentration should be titrated to response, in general 'starting high and titrating down' as the situation allows. In circumstances where hypoxaemia does not respond to an increased FIO_2, (as described earlier), the FIO_2 should be limited to protect the lung from potential oxygen toxicity. It is worth emphasizing that oxygen delivery relies, in all patients, on the maintenance of a patent airway. The administration of oxygen and the use of continuous positive airway pressure (CPAP) in a self-ventilating patient is discussed in Chapter 3.

At the time of the initiation of ventilation, high concentrations of inspired oxygen are usually employed, and these are subsequently titrated downwards, based on the results of arterial blood gas analysis or SaO_2 measurements, or both, so that adequate oxygen delivery can be achieved with relatively modest inspired concentrations of oxygen. High inspired concentrations of oxygen have been shown to damage cells and may induce alveolar injury. The precise mechanism of injury is unknown, but oxygen is a free radical with the propensity to react with metals to form superoxide, which may attack double bonds in many organic molecules including the unsaturated fatty acids in cells. Under normal circumstances, the body has many defences against such damage (glutathione, catalase, superoxide dismutase), but with a high enough inspired oxygen concentration these defences are rapidly overwhelmed. Patients ventilated in intensive care units are *traditionally* considered to be safe from pulmonary oxygen toxicity if their inspired oxygen concentrations remain below 60%, although this assumption is open to question (see Chapter 14).

Hypoventilation

Hypoventilation alters the alveolar oxygen tension in proportion to the rise of $PaCO_2$. This may be an important cause of hypoxaemia, particularly when breathing room air.

Reduced mixed venous partial pressure of oxygen

Although a reduction in the mixed venous oxygen partial pressure *increases* the oxygen partial pressure gradient between alveolus and the pulmonary capillary, and would therefore *increase* the speed of diffusion (see Equation 6.11), this would only improve oxygenation in alveoli in which oxygenation was limited by the speed of diffusion. This improved oxygenation would be more than offset by the deterioration in PaO_2 that this low PO_2 blood would have from passing through alveolar units with a low $\dot{V}/\dot{Q}$ ratio (Figure 6.11).

Diffusion distance

Diffusion

The importance of impaired pulmonary diffusion capacity for oxygen as a significant cause of hypoxaemia is disputed. Nevertheless, there are many clinical circumstances in which transpulmonary blood flow is accelerated[16] and diffusion distances lengthened[17] in which it is likely to contribute to hypoxaemia. In each of these situations, the relationship between PaO_2 and FIO_2 will be linear; that is, they will tend to be responsive to increased FIO_2.

Ventilation/perfusion mismatch

Imbalance between pulmonary ventilation and pulmonary perfusion ($\dot{V}/\dot{Q}$) is the most common cause of hypoxaemia and is discussed in Chapter 1. Its responsiveness to increments in FIO_2 is variable and depends on the distribution of

---

[16] Any condition, for example, that causes an increased cardiac output, such as anaemia or sepsis.
[17] By material (1) lying between the capillary endothelium and the alveolar epithelium, such as fibrotic tissue, malignant cells, interstitial pulmonary oedema, or (2) lining the alveolar epithelium, such as inflammatory exudate, alveolar fluid, necrotic cells or proteinaceous material.

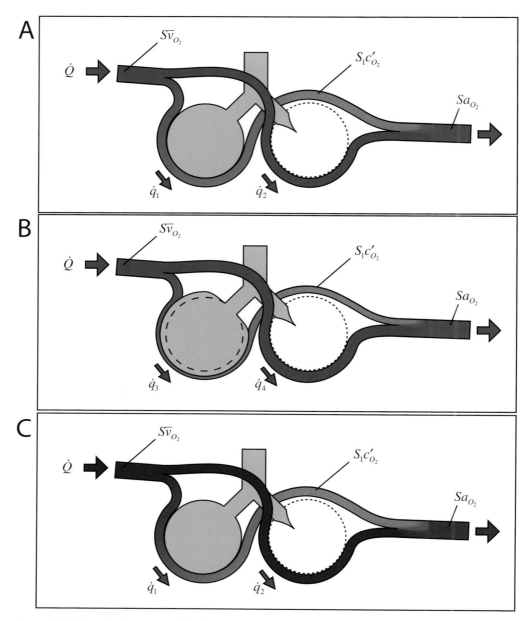

Figure 6.11 Effect of pulmonary venous admixture on oxygen content. Panel A: Pulmonary venous blood flow ($\dot{Q}$ mL.min^{-1}) is divided equally between two alveoli: a ventilated alveolus with a flow of $\dot{q}_1$ mL.min^{-1}, and a non-ventilated alveolus with a blood flow of $\dot{q}_2$ mL.min^{-1} such that

$$\dot{Q} = \dot{q}_1 + \dot{q}_2.$$

To a very reasonable approximation, the saturation of the 'arterial' blood draining these two alveoli is given by the 'flow-average' from these two alveoli as follows:

$$Sa_{O_2} = \frac{\left(\dot{q}_1 \times S_1c'_{O_2}\right) + (\dot{q}_2 \times Sv_{O_2})}{\dot{q}_1 + \dot{q}_2}.$$

Figure 6.11 (continued) If $\dot{q}_1$ is 0.8 and $\dot{q}_2$ is 0.2, $S_1c'_{O_2}$, the end-capillary saturation of blood draining the ventilated alveolus is 99% and $S\bar{v}_{O_2}$, the mixed venous saturation is 75% (i.e. normal), the saturation of the arterial blood would be

$$Sa_{O_2} = \frac{(0.8 \times 99) + (0.2 \times 75)}{1} = 94.2\%.$$

Panel B: If the intra-alveolar pressure in the ventilated alveolus rises sufficiently, blood flow will be diverted to the unventilated alveolus which is not exposed to the increased intra-alveolar pressure. In this situation, the total flow would remain the same:

$$\dot{Q} = \dot{q}_3 + \dot{q}_4$$

but $\dot{q}_3$ might fall to 0.7, and $\dot{q}_4$ might increase to 0.3. Under these conditions, and with the same end-capillary and mixed venous saturation, the arterial saturation would become

$$Sa_{O_2} = \frac{(0.7 \times 99) + (0.3 \times 75)}{1} = 91.8\%.$$

Panel C: Alternatively, the mixed venous saturation might be reduced to only 50% but with the same distribution of flow:

$$Sa_{O_2} = \frac{(0.8 \times 99) + (0.2 \times 50)}{1} = 89.2\%.$$

abnormal $\dot{V}/\dot{Q}$ units contributing to the problem. Shunting is an extreme form of $\dot{V}/\dot{Q}$ imbalance in which blood passes from the right to the left side of the heart without coming into contact with a ventilated alveolus. Under normal circumstances, a small amount of venous blood draining the pulmonary parenchyma (bronchial veins) and left ventricle (Thebesian veins) enters the left ventricle directly and constitutes what is referred to as the 'anatomical' shunt. Pathological right-to-left shunts usually arise in the context of congenital cardiac malformations which have been present for long enough to cause pulmonary hypertension and are very unlikely to be a cause of *unexplained* hypoxaemia. However, right-to-left intra-cardiac shunting *can* occur in the absence of longstanding pulmonary hypertension, or in patients whose pulmonary hypertension is acute.[18] In these circumstances, care providers may not know about a septal lesion, which may be a simple patent foramen ovale or an atrial septal defect. These lesions can be very difficult to detect by trans-thoracic echocardiography in ventilated patients and where suspicions are strong should be sought using bubble-contrast echocar-

diography.[14] True *intra-pulmonary* shunts are even more uncommon. These pulmonary arterio-venous malformations may arise in patients with severe liver disease,[15] in patients with hereditary haemorrhagic telangiectasia,[16] or occasionally as a complication of pulmonary artery catheterization. The hepatopulmonary syndrome is not amenable to any intervention other than liver transplantation, whereas other symptomatic pulmonary arteriovenous malformations can be closed by coiling. Hypoxaemia caused by shunting is unresponsive to increased F_{IO_2}.

A low $\dot{V}/\dot{Q}$ ratio is much more common than any form of shunt. The obstruction to alveolar ventilation can occur at the alveolar level or more proximally. Proximal obstruction in the mechanically ventilated patient is usually accompanied by a sudden deterioration in gas exchange and rise in airway pressures, most commonly by mucus plugging of a bronchus (Figure 6.12), or inadvertent intubation of the right main bronchus. Occasionally, significant obstruction can be caused by blood from the upper airway which rapidly coagulates into bronchial casts. The absence of breath sounds over one side of the chest and a failure to respond to withdrawing the endotracheal tube 1 or 2 cm

---

[18] Pulmonary thromboembolism, ARDS/ALI.

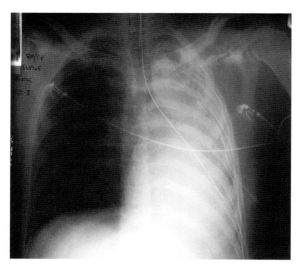

Figure 6.12 Collapse of left lung.

Table 6.4 Causes of reduced focal alveolar ventilation contributing to a low ventilation:perfusion ratio

- Proximal obstruction
  - Mucus plug
  - Blood clot
  - Aspirated foreign body
- Distal obstruction
  - Alveolar collapse
  - Alveolar plugging
    * Foam
  - Alveolar occupation
    * Fluid (exudate or transudate)
    * Inflammatory infiltrate and cellular debris
    * Blood

is strongly suggestive of bronchial plugging, which may require bronchoscopy.

Distal obstruction to alveolar ventilation may arise in a number of ways (Table 6.4). The most widely accepted cause in patients with ALI/ARDS is alveolar collapse,[17] which is managed by alveolar recruitment using PEEP and the techniques described earlier. The role of alveolar collapse has recently been challenged on the basis of animal data[18] that suggests that alveolar flooding and plugging with foam are responsible. In humans, it is likely that both mechanisms operate.[19]

Alveolar flooding may respond to a variety of therapeutic manoeuvres. The passage of fluid from capillary to interstitium and then from the interstitium to alveolar lumen is determined by the balance between the hydrostatic and colloid osmotic pressures in the three compartments (capillary, interstitium and alveolus), the reflection co-efficients of the interceding endothelium (capillary/interstitium interface) or epithelium (interstitial/alveolar interface), and the function of the drainage mechanisms.[19] Currently, nothing can be done to alter

the pulmonary capillary endothelial reflection co-efficient which falls as a result of the relaxation of inter-endothelial tight junctions precipitated by inflammatory mediators. The alveolar epithelial reflection co-efficient has two components: the first is the inter-epithelial tight junctions (similar to the pulmonary capillary endothelium), the second arises from the effect of alveolar surfactant. As with the capillary endothelium, relaxation of inter-epithelial tight junctions is currently not amenable to intervention. Loss of alveolar surfactant occurs by a number of mechanisms which include the degradation of alveolar surfactant by plasma proteins that have leaked into the alveolar lumen, loss by alveolar surfactant 'milking' consequent upon large volume changes[4] and the loss of alveolar type II pneumocytes which synthesize surfactant. The administration of surfactant has been shown to improve lung mechanics, oxygenation and outcome in neonates with hyaline membrane disease,[20] but has yet to be shown to be of benefit in adults. Capillary fluid efflux may be reduced, or even reversed, by minimizing the pulmonary capillary filtration pressure, which in disease may not equate to the pulmonary artery occlusion pressure because of the presence of significant pulmonary venous

[19] Pneumocyte abluminal Na^+/K^+-ATPase and pulmonary lymphatics.

flow restriction; in patients with ARDS, the resultant reduction of extra-vascular lung water has been shown to be associated with a better outcome.[21] Alveolar fluid reabsorption (but not interstitial fluid absorption)[22] may be promoted by positive end-expiratory pressure and results in improved oxygenation. Alveolar fluid reabsorption is promoted in animal models of pulmonary oedema by activation of the abluminal pneumocyte Na^+/K^+-ATPase by β-adrenoreceptor agonists,[23] suggesting that these agents may be helpful in promoting the resolution of pulmonary oedema in patients.[24] A preliminary study in patients with ARDS has confirmed that intravenous β-adrenoreceptor agonists reduce extra-vascular lung water,[25] but in this small study, this did not translate into a significant improvement in oxygenation. In contrast, a similarly small study investigating the effect of diuretic combined with albumin supplementation compared to diuretic alone did have a significant effect in improving oxygenation.[26] Interstitial fluid drainage through the pulmonary lymphatics may be encouraged by minimizing central venous pressures.

Loss of alveolar airspace by the influx of inflammatory cells, fibrin and cellular debris, resulting in pulmonary consolidation, is not amenable to any form of physical intervention and depends on the resolution of the underlying condition. Hypoxic pulmonary vasoconstriction, which normally operates to minimize blood flow to poorly ventilated alveolar units,[27] is attenuated by pneumonia[28] and systemic endotoxaemia. There is evidence that hypoxic pulmonary vasoconstriction may be compromised in *some* patients with ARDS.[29] Almitrine bismesylate, a piperazine respiratory stimulant, enhances hypoxic pulmonary vasoconstriction and has been shown to significantly improve $\dot{V}/\dot{Q}$ matching and oxygenation in patients with ARDS.[30] Unfortunately, almitrine is not licensed for use in the UK.

Diffuse alveolar haemorrhage is a feature of a number of conditions (Table 6.5), and presents

Table 6.5 Causes of diffuse alveolar haemorrhage

- Vasculitis (Wegener's granulomatosis, systemic lupus erythematosus, microscopic polyarteritis, Goodpasture's syndrome, Henoch-Schönlein purpura, antiphospholipid syndrome, IgA nephropathy, Behcet's, essential mixed cryoglobulinaemia)
- Coagulopathy (disseminated intravascular coagulation, thrombolytic therapy, therapeutic anticoagulation)
- Infections (leptospirosis, scrub typhus, Hanta virus, dengue fever)
- Bone marrow transplantation
- Drugs (propylthiouracil, diphenylhydantoin, penicillamine, platelet glycoprotein IIb/IIIa receptor inhibitors, infliximab)
- Envenomation (snake, jelly fish, bee)
- Malignancies (lymphangioleiomyomatosis, leukaemia, Langerhans cell histiocytosis)

with severe hypoxaemia and bilateral alveolar infiltrates. The presence of blood in the lower respiratory tract may not be immediately apparent. Unlike focal pulmonary haemorrhage, physical isolation of the bleeding site with a bronchial blocker or double-lumen tube is of no help because of the diffuse nature of the bleeding. Management therefore relies on treatment of any underlying condition[20] and aggressive correction of any coagulopathy. Control of bleeding may require the use of anti-fibrinolytics such as tranexamic acid or aprotinin or, in refractory cases, recombinant activated human factor seven. Recruitment manoeuvres, not surprisingly, yield little improvement by way of pulmonary mechanics (Figure 6.13), but may yield surprising benefit in terms of oxygenation.

Under normal circumstances, variations in mixed venous oxygen content should not influence the arterial oxygen content. In the presence of a significant shunt or severe $\dot{V}/\dot{Q}$ mismatch, venous

---

20 For example, steroids, cyclophosphamide, azothioprine, and in some cases, plasma exchange in patients with vasculitis.

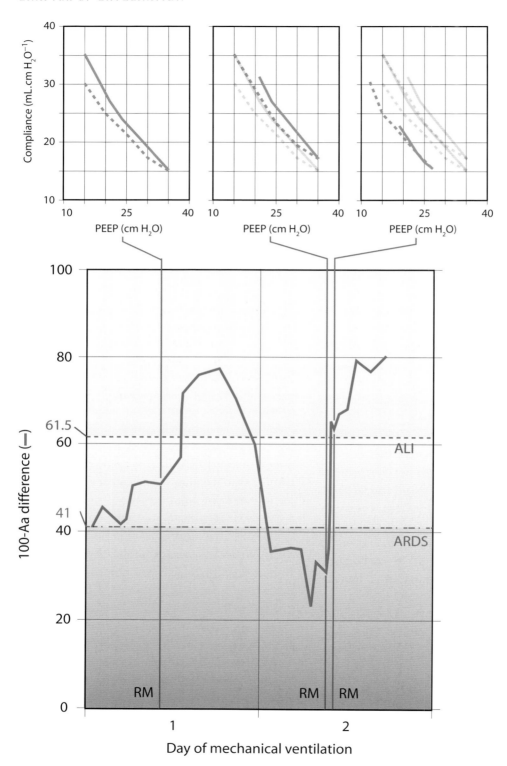

oxygen content influence might become important. Because mixed venous oxygen saturation is influenced primarily by the ratio of oxygen consumption to oxygen delivery, hypoxaemia may be responsive to improving oxygen delivery or reducing oxygen demand.

PRONE POSITION

The goal of the prone position is to improve oxygenation in patients with ARDS principally by reordering $\dot{V}/\dot{Q}$ relationships in previously dependent lung units. Improvements in gas exchange are observed in around two thirds of patients with refractory hypoxaemia when they are placed in the face-down position. While these improvements have been impressive, clinical trials have to date failed to demonstrate a survival benefit from this technique when it is used routinely, typically for a minimum of six hours daily.

Potential complications of the prone position include, among others, inadvertent extubation, loss of central venous access and chest drains, delayed cardiopulmonary resuscitation and blindness.

Given these potential complications and the lack of an evidence base supporting its use, we no longer use this technique routinely. We do occasionally resort to the prone position in patients undergoing HFOV when adequate oxygenation at an FiO_2 of <0.6 cannot be achieved or maintained, or when bronchorrhoea makes supine HFOV challenging. Our experience with this combination is limited, but unexpected survival of a number of patients has been observed.

NITRIC OXIDE

Inhaled nitric oxide (NO) is a selective pulmonary vasodilator that improves blood flow to ventilated lung units. When administered to patients undergoing conventional ventilation for ARDS, acute improvements in oxygenation are observed in around two thirds of patients. Unfortunately, despite considerable early enthusiasm for the routine use of NO, clinical trials have failed to demonstrate any survival benefit from NO; on the contrary, three trials showed a trend towards increased mortality in patient groups receiving NO.

Our own practice is now to not use NO as routine or rescue therapy in patients with ARDS and refractory hypoxaemia. Currently, we tend to rely on HFOV, initiated relatively early where possible (plus the prone position in a very limited number of cases) in this group of patients.

REFERENCES

1. Bernard GR, Artigas A, Brigham KL *et al.* The American-European consensus conference on ARDS: definitions, mechanisms, relevant outcomes, and clinical trial coordination. *Am J Respir Crit Care Med.* 1994;149:818–24.
2. Fink MP. Bench-to-bedside review: cytopathic hypoxia. *Crit Care.* 2002;6(6):491–9.

Figure 6.13 Effect of a recruitment manoeuvre (RM) in a patient with diffuse alveolar haemorrhage.

Recruitment manoeuvres were performed by ventilating in pressure-controlled mode with an inflating pressure of 15 cm H_2O at 12 breaths.min^{-1} and an I:E ratio of 1:1 using 5-cm H_2O increments of PEEP, starting at the baseline PEEP and increasing to a maximum PEEP of 35 cm H_2O. Each level of PEEP was maintained for up to 60 seconds. At the end of the recruitment phase, PEEP was reduced to 24 cm H_2O and withdrawn in decrements of 3 cm H_2O. The top panels show respiratory system compliance (y-axis) against PEEP (x-axis) for each of the recruitment manoeuvres with the recruitment phase indicated with a dotted orange line and the down-titration phase with a solid orange line. These show sharp reductions in compliance with increasing PEEP and little gain in respiratory system compliance following the manoeuvre, suggesting little benefit from the manoeuvre. However, the –Aa difference, which is plotted in the bottom panel against time, shows that each of the recruitment manoeuvres was followed by significant improvements in oxygenation. The deterioration in oxygenation that occurred during the first night was caused by premature reduction of PEEP.

3. The Acute Respiratory Distress Syndrome Network. Ventilation with lower tidal volumes as compared with traditional tidal volumes for acute lung injury and the acute respiratory distress syndrome. *N Engl J Med*. 2000;342(18):1301–8.

4. Lachmann B. Open up the lung and keep it open. *Intensive Care Med*. 1992;18:319–21.

5. Puybasset L, Gusman P, Muller JC *et al*. Regional distribution of gas and tissue in acute respiratory distress syndrome. III. Consequences for the effects of positive end-expiratory pressure. CT Scan ARDS Study Group. Adult Respiratory Distress Syndrome. *Intensive Care Med*. 2000;26(9):1215–27.

6. Brower RG, Lanken PN, MacIntyre N *et al*. Higher versus lower positive end-expiratory pressures in patients with the acute respiratory distress syndrome. *N Engl J Med*. 2004;351(4):327–36.

7. Nieszkowska A, Lu Q, Vieira S *et al*. Incidence and regional distribution of lung overinflation during mechanical ventilation with positive end-expiratory pressure. *Crit Care Med*. 2004;32(7):1496–1503.

8. Reynolds EO. Effect of alterations in mechanical ventilator settings on pulmonary gas exchange in hyaline membrane disease. *Arch Dis Child*. 1971;46(246):152–9.

9. Cole AG, Weller SF, Sykes MK. Inverse ratio ventilation compared with PEEP in adult respiratory failure. *Intensive Care Med*. 1984;10(5):227–32.

10. Gurevitch MJ, Van Dyke J, Young ES *et al*. Improved oxygenation and lower peak airway pressure in severe adult respiratory distress syndrome. Treatment with inverse ratio ventilation. *Chest*. 1986;89(2):211–13.

11. Stock MC, Downs JB, Frolicher DA. Airway pressure release ventilation. *Crit Care Med*. 1987;15(5):462–6.

12. Mehta S, Lapinsky SE, Hallett DC *et al*. Prospective trial of high-frequency oscillation in adults with acute respiratory distress syndrome. *Crit Care Med*. 2001;29(7):1360–9.

13. Pillow JJ, Sly PD, Hantos Z. Monitoring of lung volume recruitment and derecruitment using oscillatory mechanics during high-frequency oscillatory ventilation in the preterm lamb. *Pediatr Crit Care Med*. 2004;5(2):172–80.

14. Mackenzie IM, Banning A, Dyar O. Pharmacologic exposure of an occult atrial septal defect. *Crit Care Med*. 2001;29:1832–4.

15. Naeije R. Hepatopulmonary syndrome and portopulmonary hypertension. *Swiss Med Wkly*. 2003;133(11–12):163–9.

16. Morrell NW. Screening for pulmonary arteriovenous malformations. *Am J Respir Crit Care Med*. 2004;169(9):978–9.

17. Gattinoni L, Caironi P, Pelosi P *et al*. What has computed tomography taught us about the acute respiratory distress syndrome? *Am J Respir Crit Care Med*. 2001;164(9):1701–11.

18. Hubmayr RD. Perspective on lung injury and recruitment: a skeptical look at the opening and collapse story. *Am J Respir Crit Care Med*. 2002;165(12):1647–53.

19. Rouby JJ, Puybasset L, Nieszkowska A *et al*. Acute respiratory distress syndrome: lessons from computed tomography of the whole lung. *Crit Care Med*. 2003;31(4 Suppl):S285–95.

20. Jobe AH. Pulmonary surfactant therapy. *N Engl J Med*. 1993;328(12):861–8.

21. Humphrey H, Hall J, Sznajder I *et al*. Improved survival in ARDS patients associated with a reduction in pulmonary capillary wedge pressure. *Chest*. 1990;97(5):1176–80.

22. Hopewell PC, Murray JF. Effects of continuous positive-pressure ventilation in experimental pulmonary edema. *J Appl Physiol*. 1976;40(4):568–74.

23. Charron PD, Fawley JP, Maron MB. Effect of epinephrine on alveolar liquid clearance in the rat. *J Appl Physiol*. 1999;87(2):611–18.

24. Barker PM. Transalveolar Na$^+$ absorption. A strategy to counter alveolar flooding? *Am J Respir Crit Care Med*. 1994;152:302–3.

25. Perkins GD, McAuley DF, Thickett DR *et al.* The beta-agonist lung injury trial (BALTI): a randomized placebo-controlled clinical trial. *Am J Respir Crit Care Med*. 2006;173(3): 281–7.

26. Martin GS, Moss M, Wheeler AP *et al.* A randomized, controlled trial of furosemide with or without albumin in hypoproteinemic patients with acute lung injury. *Crit Care Med*. 2005;33(8):1681–7.

27. Brimioulle S, Julien V, Gust R *et al.* Importance of hypoxic vasoconstriction in maintaining oxygenation during acute lung injury. *Crit Care Med*. 2002;30(4):874–80.

28. Yaghi A, Mehta S, McCormack DG. Delayed rectifier potassium channels contribute to the depressed pulmonary artery contractility in pneumonia. *J Appl Physiol*. 2002;93(3): 957–65.

29. Benzing A, Mols G, Brieschal T *et al.* Hypoxic pulmonary vasoconstriction in nonventilated lung areas contributes to differences in hemodynamic and gas exchange responses to inhalation of nitric oxide. *Anesthesiology*. 1997;86(6):1254–61.

30. Reyes A, Roca J, Rodriguez-Roisin R *et al.* Effect of almitrine on ventilation-perfusion distribution in adult respiratory distress syndrome. *Am Rev Respir Dis*. 1988;137(5): 1062–7.

Chapter 7

Carbon dioxide balance

BRIAN KEOGH AND SIMON FINNEY

Carbon dioxide is produced as a by-product of the Kreb's cycle[1] that links the metabolism of glucose, lipids and amino acids to oxidative phosphorylation and the aerobic generation of energy within cells. Carbon dioxide is excreted by the lungs. The partial pressure of carbon dioxide (PCO_2) in arterial blood ($PaCO_2$) can be viewed in reasonably simple mathematical terms as the equilibrium between its production and elimination, modified by the balance between arterial and venous carbon dioxide content (Figure 7.1). It is less subject to the confounding elements seen in oxygen physiology, namely the effects of shunt and the oxy-haemoglobin dissociation curve.

The basic physiology of carbon dioxide elimination has been considered in Chapter 1. In essence, since inspired carbon dioxide concentration is minimal and carbon dioxide production relatively constant over short periods of time, the $PaCO_2$ depends on alveolar ventilation, regulated largely via central chemoreceptors sensitive to $PaCO_2$ and pH that influence both respiratory frequency and tidal volume. This usually results in normocapnia and a $PaCO_2$ between 4.5 and 6.0 kPa. Nevertheless, this balance may be stressed, and even overwhelmed, in unusual physiological states such as extreme exercise, although this is often limited by the onset of fatigue. In pathophysiological states, carbon dioxide production may be increased, elimination may be impaired, or frequently both aberrations may co-exist. Acute compensatory mechanisms, aimed at increasing alveolar ventilation, may be impaired centrally by sedatives or neurological abnormalities or may prove inefficient as a consequence of pulmonary or chest wall disease.

Irrespective of the aetiology, hypercapnic respiratory failure ensues. Hypercapnic respiratory failure, defined as a $PaCO_2$ in excess of 6.7 kPa, is also referred to as *Type 2 respiratory failure*. It may occur in isolation, with normal oxygenation, or may co-exist with *Type 1 respiratory failure* in which arterial oxygen tension is less than 8.0 kPa. The more common conditions that may give rise to hypercapnic respiratory failure are listed in Table 7.1. The threshold 'failure' values for $PaCO_2$ and PaO_2 broadly indicate the need for medical therapy in acute respiratory failure but do not, per se, mandate the institution of either non-invasive or invasive mechanical ventilation. Other key clinical factors that influence the decision to initiate such therapy are listed in Table 7.2. This sometimes difficult clinical judgment is considered in Chapter 2.

[1] Also known as the tricarboxylic acid cycle.

Core Topics in Mechanical Ventilation, ed. Iain Mackenzie. Published by Cambridge University Press.
© Cambridge University Press 2008.

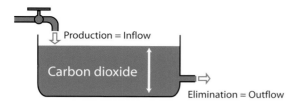

Figure 7.1 Effect of carbon dioxide production and carbon dioxide elimination on blood carbon dioxide tension.

Carbon dioxide production

Carbon dioxide production is based on metabolic rate and the substrates that are being utilized to drive the Kreb's cycle. Typically, an adult male at rest produces around 200 mL.min^{-1} of carbon dioxide. Many factors common to critically ill patients can influence this value (Table 7.3). The therapeutic administration of bicarbonate ions, in particular, may considerably increase carbon dioxide production in the short term.

Pulmonary elimination of carbon dioxide

Carbon dioxide is carried to the lungs in pulmonary arterial blood that in health has a mixed venous PCO_2 of approximately 6.1 kPa. Since alveolar PCO_2 is 5.3 kPa, the partial pressure gradient is only 0.8 kPa across the alveolar–capillary membrane, compared to approximately 8 kPa for oxygen. Despite this low gradient, the favourable diffusion constant for carbon dioxide allows 200 mL.min^{-1} of carbon dioxide to be cleared via the lungs. Typically, this equates to approximately 15% of the pulmonary arterial carbon dioxide content. The high solubility and diffusion constants of carbon dioxide mean that its clearance is rarely limited by diffusion and considerably more than 15% of arterial carbon dioxide content can be cleared, if required.

Factors that influence pulmonary elimination of carbon dioxide include the volume of dead space, tidal volume, respiratory frequency and positive end-expiratory pressure (PEEP).

Table 7.1 Aetiology of hypercapnic respiratory failure
• Increased airways resistance – Chronic obstructive pulmonary disease – Asthma
• Upper airway obstruction – Airway tumours – *Foreign body inhalation (uncommon in adults)* – *Airway infection (epiglottitis, paratonsillar abscess)*
• Pulmonary parenchymal disease – Pneumonia – Acute respiratory distress syndrome – Pulmonary oedema – Emphysema – Non-traumatic pneumothorax – Fibrotic pulmonary conditions – Cystic fibrosis
• Abnormal chest wall mechanics – Kyphoscoliosis – Obesity – Abdominal distension
• Trauma – Flail chest – Pneumothorax – Haemothorax
• Altered pulmonary blood flow – Pulmonary embolism – Hypovolaemia
• Depressed central respiratory drive – Central nervous system depressants – Brain stem disease
• Respiratory muscle impairment – *Guillain–Barré syndrome* – *Spinal cord lesions* – *Myasthenia gravis* – *Muscular dystrophies*

Dead space

A major influence on the efficiency of carbon dioxide clearance is the dead space. This refers to those compartments of the respiratory system which receive part of the tidal volume but do not contribute to gas exchange. The dead space is composed of the *anatomical dead space*, which includes the airways from nose and mouth down to the

Table 7.2 Clinical factors that influence the decision to initiate respiratory support

- Clinical history
  - Aetiology of the acute disease
  - Natural history of any underlying chronic respiratory disease
  - Assessment of respiratory and cardiovascular reserve
- Physiological assessment
- Mental state and degree of distress
  - Respiratory rate and pattern
  - Effectiveness of cough
  - Metabolic and acid-base status
  - Degree of compensation for respiratory acidosis
- Therapeutic response
  - Response to immediate therapy
  - Direction of clinical vectors

Table 7.3 Influences on the production of carbon dioxide

- Factors associated with increased carbon dioxide production
  - Systemic inflammation
  - Sepsis
  - Burnt patients
  - Hyperpyrexia
  - Thyrotoxic crisis
  - Muscular activity (seizures, excessive respiratory work)
  - Predominance of glucose as metabolic substrate
  - Administration of exogenous bicarbonate
- Factors associated with reduced carbon dioxide production
  - Hypothermia
  - Hypothyroidism
  - Sedation and neuromuscular blockade
  - Predominance of fatty acids as metabolic substrate

terminal bronchioles (airway generation 16), and the *alveolar dead space*, which refers to that volume of alveoli that are ventilated but not perfused. The sum of these two dead spaces is usually referred to as the *physiological dead space*:

$$\text{Alveolar } (V_{D_A}) + \text{Anatomical } (V_{D_{anat}})$$
$$= \text{Physiological dead space } (V_D). \qquad (7.1)$$

An additional dead space element must be considered in patients who are mechanically ventilated. The *equipment dead space* represents an extension of the anatomical dead space and represents the circuit sections which have bi-directional flow and from which re-breathing of end-expired gas from the last exhalation will occur at the commencement of the next inspiration. This equipment dead space extends from the point of fresh gas renewal, which is usually the Y-piece of a standard circuit, to the tip of the endotracheal or tracheostomy tube. Inappropriately sized catheter mounts or particularly large heat and moisture exchangers can adversely impact small patients with existing carbon dioxide clearance difficulties. The equipment dead space replaces some of the anatomical dead space of the upper airway in the intubated patient. The total dead space volume is thus composed of the sum of the alveolar, anatomical and equipment dead spaces:

$$\text{Alveolar } (V_{D_A}) + \text{Anatomical } (V_{D_{anat}})$$
$$+ \text{Equipment } (V_{D_{equip}}) = V_D. \qquad (7.2)$$

The total physiological dead space can be estimated using the Bohr equation if the carbon dioxide in mixed expiratory gases is measured (Box 7.1).

Dead space ventilation is effectively wasted ventilation that still requires its associated muscular effort. In health, anatomical dead space is approximately 150 mL, alveolar dead space is negligible, and the V_D/V_T ratio is roughly 0.3. As V_D/V_T increases, minute ventilation and hence the work of breathing must increase to maintain carbon dioxide clearance. When V_D/V_T exceeds 0.7 to 0.8, spontaneous breathing is usually no longer able to maintain carbon dioxide homeostasis.

Changes in physiological dead space that occur in disease are usually due to variations in alveolar dead space. Notable exceptions include the variation of anatomical dead space that occurs with varying air

Box 7.1 Estimation of total physiological dead space using the Bohr equation

The Bohr equation for estimating physiological dead space is

$$\frac{V_D}{V_T} = \frac{Pa_{CO_2} - P\bar{E}_{CO_2}}{Pa_{CO_2}},$$

where V_D is the physiological dead space (anatomical + alveolar + equipment), V_T is the tidal volume, Pa_{CO_2} is the partial pressure of carbon dioxide in arterial blood (used to estimate the partial pressure of carbon dioxide in alveolar gas), and $P\bar{E}_{CO_2}$ is the partial pressure of carbon dioxide in mixed expiratory gases.

flows through chest drains in pulmonary leaks and in equipment dead space when errors in recent circuit changes have been made. The gravitational distribution of pulmonary blood flow has been discussed in Chapter 1. The least dependent parts of the lung, which are apical in the erect patient, and anterior in the supine patient, are often referred to as *West's Zone 1*. The alveoli in this zone exhibit end-inspiratory alveolar pressures greater than pulmonary capillary inflow pressures. Thus, these alveoli are ventilated but unperfused and represent alveolar dead space. If the volume of Zone 1 increases, as may occur with higher PEEP or lower cardiac output, then physiological dead space will increase, and carbon dioxide clearance will be impaired in the absence of compensatory measures.

Tidal volume and frequency

When ventilating healthy lungs, normocapnia is often achieved with a tidal volume of 6 to 8 mL.kg^{-1} and a frequency of 10 to 12 breaths.min^{-1}. Hypercapnia can often be reduced by a simple increase in respiratory rate. This holds true while the V_D/V_T ratio is not excessively high. When the ratio exceeds 0.6, a simple increase in frequency will have mini-

mal effects on carbon dioxide clearance. The V_D/V_T ratio may be high if either the dead space volume is high or the tidal volume is low. Low tidal volumes are frequently employed in the critically ill, since there is good evidence that they prevent ventilator-induced lung injury. Thus, it is important to recognize that the increase in ventilatory frequency that corrects hypercapnia when ventilating normal lungs is not always the answer to carbon dioxide clearance problems in pulmonary disease. A recent study investigating the effect of increased ventilatory frequency in acute respiratory failure showed that while $PaCO_2$ did not change, adverse changes were observed in the V_D/V_T ratio and haemodynamics, consistent with the development of end-expiratory gas trapping.[1] Unfortunately, the alternative approach of increasing tidal volume may risk further lung trauma and exacerbate ventilation perfusion matching.

Positive end-expiratory pressure (PEEP)

Positive end-expiratory pressure (PEEP) maintains alveolar stability at end expiration, enhances lung volume recruitment in lung injury and pulmonary oedema, reduces intra-pulmonary shunt and improves oxygenation (see Chapter 6). However, the application of PEEP may also affect carbon dioxide clearance.

Low levels of PEEP (3 to 5 cm H$_2$O) have little effect on carbon dioxide clearance in normal lungs. Higher levels of PEEP (8 to 15 cm H$_2$O) applied to diseased lungs may increase the V_D/V_T ratio by increasing West's Zone 1 volume and reduce the efficiency of carbon dioxide clearance. This is particularly evident if low tidal volumes are used. By contrast, in patients who display recruitable lung volume, PEEP may enhance carbon dioxide clearance by improving pulmonary compliance and alveolar ventilation. Patients who show limited or no lung recruitment potential are more likely to display reduced carbon dioxide clearance with high PEEP levels. PEEP may also increase

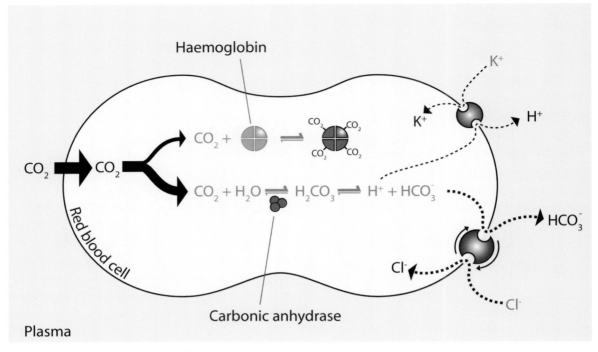

Figure 7.2 Carbon dioxide transport in blood.

Carbon dioxide diffuses into the red blood cell where the majority is converted to bicarbonate by the enzyme carbonic anhydrase, which is then exchanged for plasma chloride. A small fraction (5% to 10%) binds to uncharged amino groups (-NH$_2$) on the globin chains in haemoglobin, with a similarly small fraction (5% to 10%) remaining as dissolved carbon dioxide.

the VD/VT ratio by its effects on cardiac output, since PEEP-induced increased intrathoracic pressures may impair right ventricular function and retard venous return, resulting in a net reduction in pulmonary blood flow.

Ventilatory protocols that employ short expiratory times, whether by inverse ratio ventilation or high respiratory rates, may result in the generation of intrinsic PEEP or may limit delivered tidal volume in pressure-limited modes. These effects will also limit carbon dioxide clearance. Nevertheless, intrinsic PEEP may be beneficial,[2] and indeed, intrinsic PEEP may have averaged around 6 cm H$_2$O in the ARDSNet study of lower tidal volumes.[3,4] Intrinsic PEEP is likely to be less beneficial in conditions such as chronic obstructive pulmonary disease when it is the result of airway collapse. In this scenario, application of extrinsic PEEP that closely approximates

the level of intrinsic PEEP may splint the airway open, favourably influencing expiratory mechanics, and enhancing carbon dioxide clearance.

Arterio-venous carbon dioxide balance

Carbon dioxide is transported in arterial and venous blood predominantly (80% to 90%) as bicarbonate ions, produced by the action of carbonic anhydrase on carbon dioxide and water in erythrocytes (Figure 7.2). A further 5% to 10% is dissolved in plasma, and 5% to 10% is bound to haemoglobin. Haemoglobin has a lower affinity for carbon dioxide at high oxygen tensions (the Haldane effect) promoting its unloading from blood as it passes through the lungs. By contrast, the affinity for oxygen falls when carbon dioxide tensions increase (the

Bohr effect) promoting unloading of oxygen in the tissues.

The balance between arterial and venous carbon dioxide is based in part upon cardiac output. While low perfusion states are associated with higher veno-arterial PCO_2 differences,[5] this is primarily due to venous hypercapnia.[6] In the setting of severe lung disease limiting carbon dioxide elimination or causing significant intra-pulmonary shunt, then low cardiac output states may exacerbate arterial hypercapnia.

Effects of altered arterial carbon dioxide

A $PaCO_2$ below 3.7 kPa is referred to as hypocapnia, whereas a $PaCO_2$ in excess of 6.7 kPa is termed *hypercapnia*.

Hypocapnia

Hypocapnia results in systemic vasoconstriction and thus may be associated with reduced organ blood flow, notably in the brain and placenta.[7] By contrast, in the pulmonary circulation, hypocapnia attenuates hypoxic pulmonary vasoconstriction and increases intrapulmonary shunting.[8] Hypocapnia also produces an increase in blood pH (alkalosis) and leads to hypokalaemia, ionized hypocalcaemia, neuronal excitability and leftward shift of the oxy-haemoglobin dissociation curve. The latter effect reduces unloading of oxygen in peripheral tissues. Ionized hypocalcaemia results in the classic symptoms of acute hypocapnia that include perioral tingling and paraesthesia of the hands and feet. Finally, it is important to note the susceptibility of the brain to ischaemia in the setting of hypocapnia with its reduced cerebral blood flow, poor unloading of oxygen, and increased neuronal activity. This is particularly true in the setting of neurological injuries and explains the detrimental effects of prolonged hypocapnia on outcome in these patients.

Hypercapnia

Hypercapnia typically causes systemic vasodilatation, notably of the skin and cerebral circulation. Increased cerebral blood flow increases intracranial and intraocular pressures. Once more, the effect of hypercapnia differs in the pulmonary circulation which is characterized by vasoconstriction and increased pulmonary arterial pressures.[9] Hypercapnia results in an acidosis and thus impaired myocardial contractility and rightward shift of the oxy-haemoglobin dissociation curve. Stimulation of central chemoreceptors in the brain stem by carbon dioxide increases ventilatory drive and sympathetic outflow resulting in sweating, mydriasis, tachycardia, hypertension and arrhythmias. Finally, marked hypercapnia results in neurological depression, somnolence and coma, an effect often termed *CO_2 narcosis*.

Manipulation of arterial carbon dioxide

Typically, mechanical ventilation is applied to maintain the $PaCO_2$ between 4.5 and 6.0 kPa.

Hypocapnia can be controlled relatively easily through adjustment of ventilator settings to reduce minute ventilation in the sedated patient. In the non-sedated patient with high respiratory drive, such as those with a metabolic acidosis or following some brain injuries, sedation may be needed to normalize the $PaCO_2$. This is unlikely to be appropriate in the setting of a metabolic acidosis since it will exacerbate arterial acidaemia.

Hypercapnia may be difficult to manage, and this clinical challenge forms the basis of much of the discussion that follows. Techniques include general measures to reduce carbon dioxide production, manipulation of mechanical ventilation, adjunctive pulmonary therapies and extracorporeal removal of carbon dioxide. Alternatively, it may be appropriate to allow a degree of hypercapnia (permissive hypercapnia), cogniscent that it may be beneficial per se, or at least that therapies aimed to reduce it have significant adverse effects. Finally, the effects of hypercapnia and the associated acidaemia may be mitigated through the use of buffering agents.

General techniques to lower carbon dioxide production

The causes of altered carbon dioxide production presented in Table 7.3 suggest some techniques that could be used to reduce carbon dioxide production and thereby reduce $PaCO_2$.

Increasing body temperatures are associated with greater resting energy expenditure, oxygen consumption and carbon dioxide production,[10] although this is not universal.[11] Thus, avoidance of pyrexia is a simple strategy that may limit carbon dioxide production. Techniques include the control of sepsis, anti-pyretics such as paracetamol, and external cooling. By extrapolation it may be possible to reduce carbon dioxide production further by inducing hypothermia. Indeed, in a study of fifteen brain-injured patients, induced hypothermia to $32\,°C$ was associated with resting energy expenditures of around 85% of that predicted by the Harris-Benedict equation.[12] Interestingly, most of the benefit was accrued by about 34 to 35 °C, suggesting that moderate hypothermia is sufficient. Such levels of hypothermia are easily induced during extracorporeal haemofiltration and are well tolerated in patients with multi-organ failure. There are no data to support profound hypothermia as a method of carbon dioxide control. Alternative cooling techniques include the use of intravascular cooling catheters, cooling blankets, cooling mattresses and the application of ice packs.

Lowering the respiratory quotient (see Chapter 1) will result in less carbon dioxide production for a similar rate of oxygen utilization, which is a surrogate for the metabolic rate. The respiratory quotient can be lowered by encouraging the use of fatty acids as metabolic substrate through the use of enteral feeds that are low in carbohydrates and high in lipids. Indeed, studies have demonstrated that this approach does lower total body carbon dioxide production in both ambulatory patients with respiratory disease and the critically ill.[13] Interestingly, this reduced carbon dioxide production does not always translate to lower $PaCO_2$ levels when compared to standard enteral feeds.[13] To date, two studies have examined the effects of a commercial low-carbohydrate, high-lipid enteral feed (Pulmocare: Ross Products, Abbott Laboratories) in 20 and 32 mechanically ventilated patients.[13,14] These studies provide contrasting results with one study demonstrating accelerated weaning from mechanical ventilation and no change in minute ventilation, while the other study demonstrated reduced minute ventilation but no reduction in the time taken to wean. While the studies were too small to come to any conclusions about the effects of low-carbohydrate, high-lipid feeds, they do suggest some moderate effect that may merit further investigation. Undoubtedly, the total amount of energy supplied in a feeding regimen as well as its composition will influence carbon dioxide production. This is of particular relevance if nutrition is supplied parenterally since this route of administration is predictable by comparison to enteral feeding, which is often limited by gastrointestinal function (see Chapter 9).

Sedation and neuromuscular blockade reduce metabolic rate by around 9%[15] and can result in a moderate reduction in carbon dioxide production. Although minimization of sedation and paralysis has been associated with improved outcome,[16] these agents are often necessary in patients with severe hypercapnia in order to facilitate mechanical ventilation.

Conventional mechanical ventilation

The basic ventilatory modes in modern ventilators have been discussed in detail in Chapter 5. With respect to carbon dioxide clearance, alveolar ventilation is the key variable. It may be increased by increased respiratory frequency, tidal volume, or endeavouring to lower physiological dead space (as discussed earlier).

There are no data to suggest that one mode of mechanical ventilation has a more favourable outcome than any other. However, the decelerating inspiratory flow pattern typical of pressure control ventilation may increase carbon dioxide clearance due to the longer inspiratory dwell time[2] allowing greater cross ventilation among alveoli and better mixing of expiratory gases. This mode is favoured often in hypercapnia complicating pulmonary air leaks. The theoretical advantages of constant flow patterns are fewer than the decelerating inspiratory flow pattern. Nevertheless, the choice of ventilator mode is based frequently on available hardware and individual or unit preference.

Adjunctive pulmonary therapies

Nebulized bronchodilators such as β_2-agonists are often used to treat bronchoconstriction in mechanically ventilated patients. In patients with severe acute asthma, effective bronchodilator therapy allows greater tidal volumes for similar peak airway pressures, and hence increased clearance of carbon dioxide. Beta-agonists also stimulate apical sodium chloride channels in the alveolar epithelial cells and appear to reduce extravascular lung water.[17] There are no data regarding how this influences carbon dioxide clearance (personal communication, Dr DF McAuley).

Physiotherapy is also seen as an essential component of the care of mechanically ventilated patients. Techniques undertaken include positioning, manual hyperinflation, percussion and vibration and suctioning. The rationales for these techniques are outlined in Table 7.4. Physiotherapy may cause

[2] In pressure-controlled breaths a much larger proportion of the tidal volume is delivered in the first half of the inspiratory time than in the second half. This is not the case with volume-controlled breaths which have a constant flow. To get around this, some ventilators offer volume-controlled breaths with a decelerating flow-time profile.

Table 7.4 Rationales for use of physiotherapy techniques in the care of mechanically ventilated patients

Technique	Rationale
Positioning	Improve ventilation perfusion matching
	Enhance mucus clearance
	Increase functional residual capacity
	Reduce work of breathing
Manual hyper-inflation	Recruitment of collapsed lung
	Enhance mucus clearance
Percussion and vibration	Enhance mucus clearance
Suction	Enhance mucus clearance

a transient rise in oxygen consumption and carbon dioxide production[18] which may result in increased arterial carbon dioxide tensions in the most severely hypercapnic. However, this occurs rarely and hypercapnia is often seen as a trigger for physiotherapy if it is due to conditions such as pulmonary collapse or sputum retention.

High frequency ventilation

High frequency ventilation (HFV) refers to the use of ventilatory frequencies above the physiological range (i.e. over 60 breaths.min^{-1} in adults) with small tidal volumes near or below the volume of the anatomical dead space. High frequency techniques are commonplace in neonatal critical care but have not been widely adopted in adult critical care. HFV is particularly appealing because smaller tidal volumes and lower peak airway pressures may limit lung injury while maintaining end-expiratory volumes and preventing cyclical collapse of alveoli. As such, it represents a potentially lung-protective ventilator strategy. High frequency oscillatory ventilation (HFOV), a form of HFV that employs even higher respiratory frequencies and lower tidal volumes, utilizes an oscillating diaphragm to rovide active inspiration and expiration, as opposed to older HFV versions with passive expiratory phase. HFOV is now available for adults (Sensor Medics 3100B, Viasys Healthcare, USA) operating at a frequency of 5 to 20 Hz. It has been the subject of several small studies which have demonstrated its efficacy at maintaining oxygenation in severe lung injury.[19,20] The bulk flow of expiratory gases containing carbon dioxide does not occur during HFV. Indeed, the physiology of carbon dioxide clearance during HFV is far from fully understood. Additional clearance mechanisms include bulk convection, asymmetric velocity profiles, pendelluft, Taylor dispersion, cardiogenic oscillation and molecular diffusion.

A striking observation in the use of HFV in patients with lung injury is that lung volume and thereby oxygenation can usually be maintained with normal or even low carbon dioxide levels. This suggests that HFOV, the currently favoured version, may find its niche where permissive hypercapnia is contraindicated such as in severe pulmonary hypertension. This theoretical advantage has not yet, to the authors' knowledge, led to widespread application of HFOV in such conditions.

Caution should always be applied when considering HFV in patients with obstructive lung disease or increased airways resistance. HFV can be considered analogous to pressure-limited inverse ratio ventilation extended along the frequency spectrum. Both techniques maintain lung volume by generating significant levels of intrinsic PEEP, although in HFV, carbon dioxide clearance is almost always superior. In chronic obstructive pulmonary disease and asthma, active expiration during HFO may be less effective and substantial gas trapping may occur. It is very difficult to accurately measure distal airway pressures with HFV, and indirect and reasonably unsatisfactory measures such as changes in thoracic circumference or haemodynamic indices have to suffice. HFV has been reported in paediatric acute severe asthma with a favourable outcome,[21] but the risks of occult gas trapping with HFV render it a considerably more dangerous option in this condition than controlled, low-frequency ventilation combined with haemodynamic support and patience.

Tracheal gas insufflation

On each inspiration, end-expiratory gases from the previous breath that are present in the anatomical and equipment dead spaces form a significant portion of the alveolar ventilation. The carbon dioxide present in these gases reduces the diffusion gradient between blood and alveolar gas thereby reducing carbon dioxide clearance. Tracheal gas insufflation (TGI) reduces this effect by flushing the expiratory gases from the dead space with fresh gas delivered proximally into a central airway.

leaflong14pt Gas can be delivered close to the carina using dedicated apparatus such as special endotracheal tubes with separate channels or (deflated) bronchial blockers. Alternatively, and using more readily available equipment, oxygen can be delivered continuously (1 to 5 $L.min^{-1}$) down the catheter of a closed endotracheal suction system. The catheter is advanced to the region of the carina and the valve taped open to allow gas to flow. Gas may be delivered throughout the respiratory cycle or timed to occur only during expiration. Optimal gas flow is determined by capnography, which demonstrates progressive dilution of expiratory carbon dioxide to near zero (Figure 7.3).

There are several drawbacks to TGI. First, insufflated gas is typically cold and dry and may result in inspissated secretions and mucosal damage: the bubble-through humidifiers often used only generate, at best, a relative humidity of 40% at body temperature. Second, the additional gas flow and physical size of the catheter can generate resistance to flow during expiration and inadvertently generate intrinsic PEEP. This may be lessened with bidirectional catheters which deliver the majority of flow in a retrograde manner. Finally, delivering

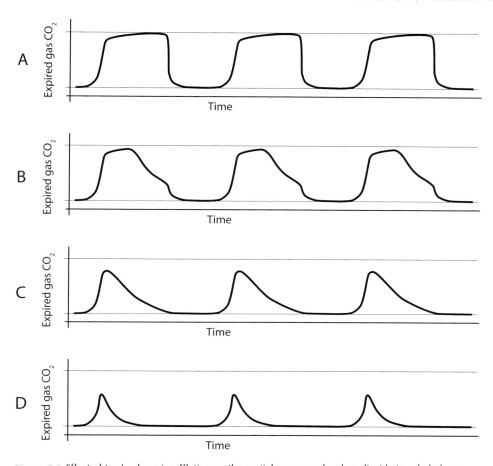

Figure 7.3 Effect of tracheal gas insufflation on the partial pressure of carbon dioxide in exhaled gas.

A: Normal exhaled carbon dioxide trace.

B: Low-flow tracheal gas insufflation.

C: Optimum flow tracheal gas insufflation.

D: High-flow tracheal gas insufflation.

additional gas into a ventilator circuit may alter performance of the ventilator particularly with respect to flow triggering, the measurement of inspiratory and expiratory volumes and the measurement of intrinsic PEEP. Typically, alarm conditions are generated unless pressure-based modes are selected. TGI integrated into ventilators could minimize this problem but none are presently available.

The reduction in arterial PCO$_2$ depends on the catheter flow rate, expiratory time and underlying disease process. TGI is most efficacious in the setting

of hypercapnia and a high anatomical and equipment dead space. By contrast, it is less efficacious when anatomical and equipment dead spaces are relatively small or there is substantial alveolar dead space. This is borne out in studies that demonstrated that a continuous 5 L.min^{-1} reduced the arterial PCO$_2$ by 1.0 to 1.5 kPa in acute lung injury,[22] and that this increased to 2.5 to 3.5 kPa in patients with significant hypercapnia.[23] TGI has little efficacy in hypercapnic tracheostomied patients with chronic obstructive pulmonary disease,[24] presumably at least in part due to their substantial alveolar dead space.

Extracorporeal gas exchange

Traditionally, extracorporeal gas exchange (ECGE) has been utilized in patients only as a rescue therapy. Extracorporeal support can range from a pumped veno-arterial device which supports and oxygenates the entire cardiac output to lung assist devices that are veno-venous or arterio-venous and which process only a limited proportion of the cardiac output. Lung assist devices provide partial oxygenation and carbon dioxide removal, augmenting what can be achieved by mechanical ventilation.

Cannulae for blood flow to and from such devices are now almost always inserted percutaneously. Cannulae for veno-venous systems are usually anatomically distant from each other due to the cannula dimensions and in order to minimize recirculation. Recirculation refers to the scenario where a proportion of oxygenated and carbon dioxide depleted blood from the outflow cannul immediately returns to the device and not the patient since the inflow and outflow are so close to one another. In the setting of haemodialysis, this can account for up to 20% of flow in the extracorporeal circuit. Arterio-venous devices are usually pumpless with the flow dependent upon systemic arterial pressure; such devices require the patient to have sufficient cardiac reserve to provide the flow through the device.

Extracorporeal gas exchange devices that return blood to the venous system are limited in their ability to increase the content of oxygen in arterial blood because they usually do not support a major proportion of the cardiac output. Although the outflow cannula from the device contains fully oxygenated blood, this is immediately mixed with other systemic venous blood creating an effective right-to-left shunt. The characteristics of the oxy-haemoglobin dissociation curve and the shunt effect seen in mixing a higher proportion of de-oxygenated venous blood with a low volume of device-oxygenated blood renders such a system poorly effective in improving venous oxygenation. In addition, an inherent mechanical inefficiency exists in that any proportion of the resultant, mixed device-oxygenated and venous blood that passes through a normally functioning alveolus will be fully saturated in the pulmonary vein regardless of the mixed venous or pre-pulmonary saturation. Thus, a considerable volume of any calculated oxygen transfer from the device will be rendered irrelevant by pulmonary physiology. Systems designed to support arterial oxygenation by delivering oxygenated blood to the venous system need to have the capacity to increase the mixed venous oxygen saturation to a level that will substantially reverse the adverse effect of intra-pulmonary shunt on arterial oxygenation. This mandates that they achieve mixed venous oxygen saturations preferably in the high eighties and this usually requires a flow in excess of two thirds of cardiac output. This limited oxygenation capacity is the main reason for the failure of innovative devices such as the intracorporeal IVOX miniaturized multifibre oxygenator which was the subject of multicentre investigations in the 1990s.[25]

This physiological inefficiency is not seen in relation to carbon dioxide clearance in the performance of extracorporeal gas exchange devices. Carbon dioxide clearance is a net effect and indeed can be reasonably measured by measuring gas flows and exhaust gas content from the device. Thus, recently developed, simply inserted lung assist devices are more effective at carbon dioxide removal than oxygenation and these systems are often designated as providing extracorporeal CO_2 removal (ECCOR). Pure oxygen is still employed as the sweep gas to enhance carbon dioxide removal by the Haldane effect and for its moderate effects on oxygenation.

Currently only two, relatively old, randomized studies of ECGE have been undertaken.[26,27] Neither demonstrated any mortality benefit.

Haemorrhage and coagulopathies are the most significant complications of ECGE, occurring in up to two thirds of adult patients.[28] By contrast, in uncontrolled studies greater success has been reported.[28,29] While the lack of control groups prevents critical evaluation of the data, it is possible that newer extracorporeal circuits that do not stimulate the coagulation and complement cascades as much, together with improved anticoagulation, non-occlusive roller pumps, and better mechanical ventilation explain this difference. This hypothesis formed the basis of the UK CESAR trial which compared pumped veno-venous or veno-arterial extracorporeal oxygenation to conventional therapy in patients with severe acute respiratory failure. This study has recently completed recruitment and is presently in its follow-up phase.[30] Success has been reported also with the pumpless arterio-venous Novalung (Novalung GmbH, Hechingen, Germany) lung assist device.[31] The Novalung has been described in the settings of bridge-to-recovery, bridge-to-transplant and facilitation of inter-hospital patient transport. The device is licensed for 28 days of use and is reported to be able to eliminate up to 200 mL.min^{-1} carbon dioxide with a blood flow of 1.5 L.min^{-1} through 15 Fr (~5 mm diameter) cannulae. Heparin-bonding on the cannulae and membrane aim to improve biocompatibility.

Permissive hypercapnia

Traditionally, mechanical ventilation was applied with the aim of normalizing blood gas values, particularly $PaCO_2$. However, it is now appreciated that hypercapnia is often well tolerated and possibly advantageous in patients with pulmonary disease. Indeed, survival following arterial PCO_2 tensions as high as 30 kPa has been reported.[32]

A potential advantage of permissive hypercapnia is that it allows deliberate hypoventilation and a reduction in tidal volumes and transpulmonary pressures. Indeed, application of mechanical ventilation with high tidal volumes increases mortality in patients with the acute respiratory distress syndrome,[4] and is associated with elevated levels of circulating cytokines that may propagate both pulmonary and systemic inflammation. It is this theory that underpinned the original clinical study that suggested that permissive hypercapnia may be beneficial.[33] It is also possible that hypercapnia, per se, may limit pulmonary injury. *In vitro*, hypercapnia reduces the activation of NF-κB, intercellular adhesion molecule-1 (ICAM-1) and interleukin-8 (IL-8) in human pulmonary endothelial cells.[34] NF-κB is a key regulatory molecule in the activation of many pro-inflammatory genes, including those that produce ICAM-1 and IL-8, molecules that trigger the movement of leukocytes into the inflamed lung. *In vivo*, studies have demonstrated that hypercapnia may reduce inflammation in experimental lung injury.[35] Finally, hypercapnia may improve ventilation perfusion matching[36] and intestinal and subcutaneous tissue oxygenation.[37]

Hypercapnia is associated with a respiratory acidosis. The resulting acidaemia and associated cardiovascular instability are the limiting factors on ever-increasing elevations in $PaCO_2$. Therefore, permissive hypercapnia is often titrated to a target pH rather than a specific $PaCO_2$ threshold. A commonly selected target is pH 7.20,[38] above which cardiovascular disturbance is minimal. The threshold of 7.20 is at least in part based on data from animal experiments which demonstrate profound myocardial dysfunction below this level.[39] The target has never been subjected to formal study[4] in humans and specifically not in the ARDSNet study[4] of low tidal volume ventilation in ARDS. The acidifying effects of carbon dioxide can be mitigated by the use of buffers, or by inducing a metabolic alkalosis. Such a metabolic alkalosis can be a welcome side effect of furosemide administered to counter fluid overload, a frequent intercurrent pathophysiological entity. Other adverse effects of hypercapnia include impaired neuromuscular transmission, impaired diaphragmatic function and an increased need for sedation and pharmacological paralysis. All these factors may prolong weaning from mechanical ventilation.

Hypercapnia is poorly tolerated in the settings of a concomitant metabolic acidosis, pulmonary hypertension, or intracranial hypertension. A mixed metabolic and respiratory acidosis often results in severe acidaemia and cardiovascular instability. Hypercapnia results in elevated pulmonary pressures and can exacerbate right ventricular dysfunction. Indeed, in the setting of lung injury, right ventricular failure is associated with a particularly poor outcome. Finally, hypercapnia is associated with cerebral vasodilatation and increased intracranial pressure. In patients with significant neurological injuries, the rises in intracranial pressure are associated often with a prohibitive reduction in cerebral perfusion pressure, thereby preventing the use of even moderate permissive hypercapnia in these patients. Indeed, intraventricular haemorrhages have been associated with hypercapnia in neonates.

Permissive hypercapnia has been the subject of several clinical investigations in adults with ARDS. In the original study by Hickling *et al.*, 50 patients treated with lower peak inspiratory pressures and permissive hypercapnia had reduced mortality with respect to an historical cohort.[33] In randomized studies, hypercapnia was part of a lower tidal volume strategy in three studies.[38,40,41] Only in one study was mortality reduced and the interpretation of that study was complicated by an unusually high mortality and significant incidence of barotrauma in the control group.[38] Hypercapnic acidosis was limited in the ARDSNet study[4] of lower tidal volume through the use of increased respiratory frequency or the use of sodium bicarbonate (discussed later). Nevertheless in a *post hoc* analysis of that study, hypercapnic acidosis was associated with a lower mortality in those ventilated with larger tidal volumes[42] (10 to 12 mL.kg^{-1}). It had no additional benefit in patients ventilated with lower tidal volumes (4 to 6 mL.kg^{-1}). In patients with acute severe asthma, hypercapnia was associated with increased mortality, although the confounding effects of more severe disease may contribute to this observation.[43] Thus, although the evidence for permissive hypercapnia is limited, its use is common because it allows easier application of lower tidal volume and lower pressure mechanical ventilation with only minor disadvantages.

Buffering agents

SODIUM BICARBONATE THERAPY

Intravenous sodium bicarbonate is the most commonly employed buffering agent used to counteract acidaemia. It is usually administered in a millimolar 8.4% w/v solution via a central vein. Enteral bicarbonate has high bioavailability but is generally not used outside the setting of chronic renal impairment due to the unreliability of this route in critically ill patients.

The administration of sodium bicarbonate generates large volumes of carbon dioxide (see Figure 7.2), which must be cleared. If they are not cleared then intracellular carbon dioxide levels will increase and there will be a paradoxical exacerbation of intracellular acidosis. The acute effect and time scale of a bolus of sodium bicarbonate can be observed during cardiopulmonary bypass. A bolus of 1 mmol.kg^{-1} sodium bicarbonate results in an immediate doubling of carbon dioxide concentration in the oxygenator exhaust, reflecting the marked rise in carbon dioxide production. This persists for 10 or more minutes. An analogous situation can be inferred in a patient not on bypass, when the extra carbon dioxide must be cleared via the lungs. In patients with impaired carbon dioxide clearance, the time scale of clearance may be considerably prolonged. Large rises in myocardial and vascular smooth muscle carbon dioxide production can result in a paradoxical intracellular acidosis and thus have negative inotropic and vasodilatory effects respectively. Other adverse effects of sodium bicarbonate administration are the associated sodium load (1 mmol.mL^{-1}) and volume of fluid required for its administration.

The administration of sodium bicarbonate in a pure metabolic acidosis is controversial, though only really in terms of degree and threshold for treatment. In the presence of a metabolic acidosis, it is essential to correct causative factors such as hypovolaemia and address the need for inotropic support. If metabolic acidosis persists and is associated with haemodynamic compromise, many physicians would consider administration of bicarbonate if the pH < 7.20 and the base excess lower than −10 mEq.L^{-1}. Individual treatment thresholds vary considerably between clinicians since there are no data that demonstrate improved outcome with the administration of bicarbonate in this setting. If it is decided to administer sodium bicarbonate, then a typical dose aims to half correct the metabolic acidosis and can be estimated using the following formula:

$$NaHCO_3 \text{(mL of 8.4\%)}$$
$$= 0.3 \times \text{lean body weight (kg)}$$
$$\times \text{base deficit (mEq.L}^{-1}\text{).} \quad (7.3)$$

The dose is administered over 30 to 60 minutes with appropriate adjustments of ventilator settings (within safe limits) to allow for the increased need for carbon dioxide clearance.

The administration of sodium bicarbonate to counteract a pure respiratory acidosis is the subject of considerable debate. The therapeutic generation of the resultant rise in carbon dioxide production appears counterintuitive in a situation when intracellular and extracellular carbon dioxide levels are already high. Many clinicians regard the effects of sodium bicarbonate as undesirable and inappropriate in this context, although others consider it as part of their therapeutic approach to respiratory acidosis. Proponents of sodium bicarbonate therapy in

respiratory acidosis tend to regard a pH < 7.20 from whatever cause as undesirable and are prepared to accept the risk of a transient increase in intracellular carbon dioxide production in order to achieve an eventual increase in total body bicarbonate. Indeed, such an approach was adopted in the ARDSNet study of lower tidal volumes.[4] Slow administration[44] or manipulation of ventilator settings in the short term to deal with the obligatory excess carbon production may overcome the perceived disadvantages. In acute severe asthma, however, manipulation of ventilation may not be possible. Those who do not support the use of sodium bicarbonate in this context note that permissive hypercapnia and respiratory acidosis are usually well tolerated (as discussed earlier) and that the paradoxical intracellular acidosis is undesirable. This approach advocates that if renal compensation mechanisms are intact, bicarbonate ions will be retained by the kidney over a period of a few days resulting in a more balanced acidosis. Sometimes this group of clinicians may administer bicarbonate if the pH falls below threshold levels, for example, 7.1 or 7.0, in the belief that the benefits may outweigh the risks as acidaemia becomes more extreme. Ironically, the potential adverse effects of a paradoxical intracellular acidosis inevitably increase as pH falls. While there are no studies that provide definitive evidence supporting either approach, the authors do not generally administer sodium bicarbonate in this setting.

Mixed metabolic and respiratory acidosis are more common in the acute setting, and modest derangements of both components can profoundly affect the resultant pH. Again, there is limited evidence to guide decision making. Hypercapnia is less well tolerated in the setting of a metabolic acidosis. This is typically the case in patients with severe acute asthma. These patients often present with respiratory exhaustion, profound hypercapnia and carbon dioxide narcosis, and a severe metabolic acidosis. The latter is typically the product of prehospital hypoxia, metabolic demands of respiratory muscles creating lactic acidosis and severe hypo-volaemia due to fluid losses associated with tachyp-noea and adrenergic stimulation. Typically, $PaCO_2$ levels may be as high as 15 to 25 kPa and a base deficit more negative than -10 mEq.L^{-1}, result-ing in a pH of 6.8 or less. In these patients, pri-mary emergency treatment entails ensuring effec-tive oxygenation and circulatory resuscitation with fluids and inotropes. Mechanical ventilation can be extremely difficult in this situation and a substantial degree of hypercapnia must be tolerated (see Chap-ter 10). Indeed, carbon dioxide clearance is so lim-ited that the administration of sodium bicarbonate could not be justified during acute resuscitation.

In acute renal failure, it is not possible for the kidney to retain bicarbonate ions and a metabolic acidosis may ensue. If renal replacement therapy is instituted, bicarbonate is often administered sepa-rately or in the diafiltrate solution. Lactate-buffered solutions indirectly administer bicarbonate since the generation of glucose in liver from lactate con-sumes energy and hydrogen ions. Haemofiltration itself alleviates some of the difficulties encountered with bicarbonate therapy as the excess sodium load and potential fluid overload can be regulated by filtration settings. In the presence of a respiratory acidosis, doses of sodium bicarbonate, however administered, may need to be adjusted to create an artificial form of metabolic compensation for respi-ratory acidosis. An initial target approach might be to achieve a pH > 7.25, but in more chronic situa-tions, and particularly during respiratory weaning, it may be appropriate to ensure that titrated bicar-bonate therapy during renal support achieves a near normal pH.

Alternative buffering agents

An alternative buffer is tromethamine or THAM. THAM is a biologically inert amino-alcohol that is a more effective buffer than sodium bicarbonate at physiological pH. Moreover, THAM is particularly appealing since its administration does not increase

carbon dioxide production and is not associated with a large sodium load. Following its adminis-tration, THAM distributes primarily to the extracel-lular compartment, but also intracellularly in ery-throcytes and hepatocytes. It is eliminated by the kidney in its acidified form and should be used with caution in those with renal insufficiency. Negative aspects of THAM include the large volume of fluid within which it is administered and the induction of hypoglycaemia. Small studies have demonstrated benefits in physiological indices following THAM administration to adults with permissive hypercap-nia.[45] However, no study has investigated the mer-its of this buffer rigorously. In general, it is more often used in the paediatric arena.

Finally, Carbicarb, an equimolar mixture of sodium carbonate and sodium bicarbonate, is theo-retically advantageous to sodium bicarbonate since it is a better buffer at physiological pH and does not result in the production of carbon dioxide. Despite experimental data confirming these characteristics in animal models,[39] only a single small study has examined its use in humans.[46]

SUMMARY

The clearance of carbon dioxide is a vital function of the lungs. While in health, the lungs achieve this role with considerable reserve, clearance is often impaired in diseased lungs. In mechanical ventila-tion of patients with severe pulmonary disease, nor-mocapnia may not be achievable simply by alter-ations in respiratory frequency. Alternative interven-tions include induced-hypothermia, manipulation of the cardiovascular system, optimization of PEEP and tidal volume, high frequency ventilation, tra-cheal gas insufflation, extracorporeal gas exchange and buffering agents. None of these therapies have proven benefits. Although the evidence is not clear, it may be appropriate to accept a degree of permis-sive hypercapnia in the knowledge that techniques to lower the $PaCO_2$ further may be detrimental. In practice, clinicians adopt a technique somewhere between optimal carbon dioxide clearance and more liberal clearance targets, based on assessment of the severity of lung disease and the risks and benefits of ventilatory manipulations or associated interventions.

REFERENCES

1. Vieillard-Baron A, Prin S, Augarde R et al. Increasing respiratory rate to improve CO_2 clearance during mechanical ventilation is not a panacea in acute respiratory failure. Crit Care Med. 2002;30(7):1407–12.

2. Patroniti N, Pesenti A. Low tidal volume, high respiratory rate and auto-PEEP: the importance of the basics. Crit Care. 2003; 7(2):105–6.

3. de Durante G, del Turco M, Rustichini L et al. ARDSNet lower tidal volume ventilatory strategy may generate intrinsic positive end-expiratory pressure in patients with acute respiratory distress syndrome. Am J Respir Crit Care Med. 2002;165(9):1271–4.

4. Ventilation with lower tidal volumes as compared with traditional tidal volumes for acute lung injury and the acute respiratory distress syndrome. The Acute Respiratory Distress Syndrome Network. N Engl J Med. 2000;342(18):1301–8.

5. Inoue T, Sakai Y, Morooka S et al. Venoarterial carbon dioxide tension gradient in acute heart failure. Cardiology. 1993;82(6):383–7.

6. Zhang H, Vincent JL. Arteriovenous differences in PCO_2 and pH are good indicators of critical hypoperfusion. Am Rev Respir Dis. 1993;148(4 Pt 1):867–71.

7. Laffey JG, Kavanagh BP. Hypocapnia. N Engl J Med. 2002;347(1):43–53.

8. Domino KB, Lu Y, Eisenstein BL et al. Hypocapnia worsens arterial blood oxygenation and increases VA/Q heterogeneity in canine pulmonary edema. Anesthesiology. 1993;78(1):91–9.

9. Balanos GM, Talbot NP, Dorrington KL et al. Human pulmonary vascular response to 4 h of hypercapnia and hypocapnia measured using Doppler echocardiography. J Appl Physiol. 2003;94(4):1543–51.

10. Chapot G, Muller M, Barrault N et al. A correlation between $PaCO_2$ and body temperature in febrile patients. Thorax. 1974; 29(1):104–5.

11. McIntyre J, Hull D. Metabolic rate in febrile infants. Arch Dis Child. 1996;74(3):206–9.

12. Tokutomi T, Morimoto K, Miyagi T et al. Optimal temperature for the management of severe traumatic brain injury: effect of hypothermia on intracranial pressure, systemic and intracranial hemodynamics, and metabolism. Neurosurgery. 2003;52(1): 102–11.

13. van den Berg B, Bogaard JM, Hop WC. High fat, low carbohydrate, enteral feeding in patients weaning from the ventilator. Intensive Care Med. 1994;20(7):470–5.

14. al-Saady NM, Blackmore CM, Bennett ED. High fat, low carbohydrate, enteral feeding lowers PaCO2 and reduces the period of ventilation in artificially ventilated patients. Intensive Care Med. 1989;15(5):290–5.

15. Vernon DD, Witte MK. Effect of neuromuscular blockade on oxygen consumption and energy expenditure in sedated, mechanically ventilated children. Crit Care Med. 2000;28(5):1569–71.

16. Kress JP, Pohlman AS, O'Connor MF et al. Daily interruption of sedative infusions in critically ill patients undergoing mechanical ventilation. N Engl J Med. 2000;342(20): 1471–7.

17. Perkins GD, McAuley DF, Thickett DR et al. The beta-agonist lung injury trial (BALTI): a randomized placebo-controlled clinical trial. Am J Respir Crit Care Med. 2006;173(3): 281–7.

18. Horiuchi K, Jordan D, Cohen D *et al.* Insights into the increased oxygen demand during chest physiotherapy. *Crit Care Med.* 1997; 25(8):1347–51.

19. Mehta S, Granton J, MacDonald RJ *et al.* High-frequency oscillatory ventilation in adults: the Toronto experience. *Chest.* 2004; 126(2):518–27.

20. Bollen CW, van Well GT, Sherry T *et al.* High frequency oscillatory ventilation compared with conventional mechanical ventilation in adult respiratory distress syndrome: a randomized controlled trial [ISRCTN24242669]. *Crit Care.* 2005;9(4): R430–9.

21. Duval EL, van Vught AJ. Status asthmaticus treated by high-frequency oscillatory ventilation. *Pediatr Pulmonol.* 2000;30(4): 350–3.

22. Ravenscraft SA, Burke WC, Nahum A *et al.* Tracheal gas insufflation augments CO_2 clearance during mechanical ventilation. *Am Rev Respir Dis.* 1993;148(2):345–51.

23. Kalfon P, Rao GS, Gallart L *et al.* Permissive hypercapnia with and without expiratory washout in patients with severe acute respiratory distress syndrome. *Anesthesiology.* 1997;87(1):6–17; discussion 25A–26A.

24. Nakos G, Lachana A, Prekates A *et al.* Respiratory effects of tracheal gas insufflation in spontaneously breathing COPD patients. *Intensive Care Med.* 1995;21(11):904–12.

25. Sim KM, Evans TW, Keogh BF. Clinical strategies in intravascular gas exchange. *Artif Organs.* 1996;20(7):807–10.

26. Zapol WM, Snider MT, Hill JD *et al.* Extracorporeal membrane oxygenation in severe acute respiratory failure. A randomized prospective study. *JAMA.* 1979;242(20): 2193–6.

27. Morris AH, Wallace CJ, Menlove RL *et al.* Randomized clinical trial of pressure-controlled inverse ratio ventilation

and extracorporeal CO_2 removal for adult respiratory distress syndrome. *Am J Respir Crit Care Med.* 1994;149(2 Pt 1):295–305.

28. Bartlett RH, Roloff DW, Custer JR *et al.* Extracorporeal life support: the University of Michigan experience. *JAMA.* 2000;283(7): 904–8.

29. Ullrich R, Lorber C, Roder G *et al.* Controlled airway pressure therapy, nitric oxide inhalation, prone position, and extracorporeal membrane oxygenation (ECMO) as components of an integrated approach to ARDS. *Anesthesiology.* 1999; 91(6):1577–86.

30. Peek GJ, Clemens F, Elbourne D *et al.* CESAR: conventional ventilatory support vs extracorporeal membrane oxygenation for severe adult respiratory failure. *BMC Health Service Res.* 2006;6:163.

31. Elliot SC, Paramasivam K, Oram J *et al.* Pumpless extracorporeal carbon dioxide removal for life-threatening asthma. *Crit Care Med.* 2007;35(3):945–8.

32. Urwin L, Murphy R, Robertson C *et al.* A case of extreme hypercapnia: implications for the prehospital and accident and emergency department management of acutely dyspnoeic patients. *Emerg Med J.* 2004;21(1): 119–20.

33. Hickling KG, Henderson SJ, Jackson R. Low mortality associated with low volume pressure limited ventilation with permissive hypercapnia in severe adult respiratory distress syndrome. *Intensive Care Med.* 1990; 16(6):372–7.

34. Takeshita K, Suzuki Y, Nishio K *et al.* Hypercapnic acidosis attenuates endotoxin-induced nuclear factor-[kappa]B activation. *Am J Respir Cell Mol Biol.* 2003;29(1):124–32.

35. Laffey JG, Tanaka M, Engelberts D *et al.* Therapeutic hypercapnia reduces pulmonary and systemic injury following in vivo lung

reperfusion. *Am J Respir Crit Care Med.* 2000;162(6):2287–94.

36. Brogan TV, Robertson HT, Lamm WJ *et al.* Carbon dioxide added late in inspiration reduces ventilation-perfusion heterogeneity without causing respiratory acidosis. *J Appl Physiol.* 2004;96(5):1894–8.

37. Ratnaraj J, Kabon B, Talcott MR *et al.* Supplemental oxygen and carbon dioxide each increase subcutaneous and intestinal intramural oxygenation. *Anesth Analg.* 2004; 99(1):207–11.

38. Amato MB, Barbas CS, Medeiros DM *et al.* Effect of a protective-ventilation strategy on mortality in the acute respiratory distress syndrome. *N Engl J Med.* 1998;338(6): 347–54.

39. Kraut JA, Kurtz I. Use of base in the treatment of severe acidemic states. *Am J Kidney Dis.* 2001;38(4):703–27.

40. Stewart TE, Meade MO, Cook DJ *et al.* Evaluation of a ventilation strategy to prevent barotrauma in patients at high risk for acute respiratory distress syndrome. Pressure- and Volume-Limited Ventilation Strategy Group. *N Engl J Med.* 1998;338(6):355–61.

41. Brochard L, Roudot-Thoraval F, Roupie E *et al.* Tidal volume reduction for prevention of ventilator-induced lung injury in acute respiratory distress syndrome. The Multicenter Trail Group on Tidal Volume reduction in ARDS. *Am J Respir Crit Care Med.* 1998;158(6):1831–8.

42. Kregenow DA, Rubenfeld GD, Hudson LD *et al.* Hypercapnic acidosis and mortality in acute lung injury. *Crit Care Med.* 2006;34(1): 1–7.

43. Gupta D, Keogh B, Chung KF *et al.* Characteristics and outcome for admissions to adult, general critical care units with acute severe asthma: a secondary analysis of the ICNARC Case Mix Programme Database. *Crit Care.* 2004;8(2):R112–21.

44. Landow L, Visner MS. Does NaHCO₃ exacerbate myocardial acidosis? *J Cardiothorac Vasc Anesth.* 1993;7(3):340–51.

45. Kallet RH, Jasmer RM, Luce JM *et al.* The treatment of acidosis in acute lung injury with tris-hydroxymethyl aminomethane (THAM). *Am J Respir Crit Care Med.* 2000;161(4 Pt 1):1149– 53.

46. Leung JM, Landow L, Franks M *et al.* Safety and efficacy of intravenous Carbicarb in patients undergoing surgery: comparison with sodium bicarbonate in the treatment of mild metabolic acidosis. SPI Research Group. Study of Perioperative Ischemia. *Crit Care Med.* 1994;22(10):1540–9.

Chapter 8

Sedation, paralysis and analgesia

RUSSELL R. MILLER III AND E. WESLEY ELY

Introduction

The benefits of therapeutic interventions among critically ill, mechanically ventilated, intensive care unit (ICU) patients must outweigh the risk of adverse consequences. The art and science of medicine converge when selecting medications to bring comfort to, and ensure the safety of, mechanically ventilated, critically ill patients. Evidence for improved care of ICU patients has expanded significantly in the last twenty years in this regard. For instance, new data favouring low tidal volume ventilation in acute respiratory distress syndrome (ARDS), recombinant human activated protein C (drotrecogin alfa) for severe sepsis, and conservative fluid management in ARDS have all been proclaimed, if not widely adopted, for their ability to impact both morbidity and mortality. New agents to ensure adequate sedation, paralysis and analgesia of ICU patients are being investigated. The Society of Critical Care Medicine's (SCCM) 2002 guidelines for the use of sedatives and analgesics[1] and for the use of neuromuscular blocking agents (NMBAs)[2] are the most recent consensus recommendations. In weaving art and science together, critical care practitioners constantly seek to improve the quality of life for patients who are frequently unable to relate their anxiety and pain.

Because of the ubiquity of discomfort or pain among mechanically ventilated patients, sustained analgesia is the foundation of therapy. Oftentimes, two or more sedatives (as opposed to analgesics) are used concurrently to diminish anxiety and facilitate positive pressure ventilation. Unfortunately, the additive or synergistic effect of multiple sedatives applies not only to therapeutic benefit but also to adverse effects. Occasionally, though perhaps less frequently than necessary, has enough attention been paid to adequate sedation, analgesia and paralysis as is required.

This chapter will include a discussion of sedation, analgesia and paralysis for mechanically ventilated, adult ICU patients and attempt to highlight the central role of analgesia. Each of these three topics will be formatted as follows: overview and general discussion, monitoring and medications used (including mechanism of action, adverse effects and common adverse effects for each). Also, because of the likely aetiologic connection, the related topic of delirium will be included. This chapter is not intended as a summary of guidelines for clinical practice because the SCCM task forces serve that function; nor will we discuss costs of medications because these are fluid in today's ICU practice and often vary by institution.

Core Topics in Mechanical Ventilation, ed. Iain Mackenzie. Published by Cambridge University Press.
© Cambridge University Press 2008.

Sedation

Overview

In addition to pain, critically ill patients constantly and uniformly are exposed to other noxious environmental, human and emotional stimuli while in the ICU. Unpleasant experiences such as pain, sensory overload or sensory deprivation, tracheal suctioning, isolation, immobilization, physical restraint, noise and sleep deprivation provoke anxiety, fear, anger and agitation. The resultant stress response leads to increased myocardial oxygen consumption, dys-synchronous mechanical ventilation, accidental removal of either endotracheal tubes or large intravenous lines and immunosuppression. Sedation is primarily intended to prevent and treat unpleasant experiences, provide comfort and ameliorate the stress response; in so doing, it also facilitates treatment of critically ill patients. Yet anxiety in the ICU is complex, and sedation also serves other functions. For instance, acidosis, hyperventilation and institution of mechanical ventilation may cause patients post-operatively or with sepsis, stroke and cardiogenic shock to become more tachypnoeic, tachycardic and diaphoretic. Such autonomic hyperactivity is the hallmark of both anxiety and critical illness. Sedation helps to reduce complications generated by both anxiety as well as the underlying medical condition.

Sedatives are therefore used nearly ubiquitously in mechanically ventilated patients to lessen the unpleasant experiences of the ICU stay, the underlying medical or surgical condition and the complications of critical illness. Among the forms of sedation used in critically ill patients, benzodiazepines have been studied most extensively. Newer agents may prove safer and more effective in preventing long-term complications of critical illness.

Monitoring

Sedation in the ICU involves selecting appropriate agents and giving them to a patient in the right amount. Early incorporation of spontaneous breathing trials into management of ventilated, critically ill patients reduces the duration of ventilation[3] and attendant risks and consequences. Preparation for a spontaneous breathing trial in patients frequently receiving continuous sedative infusions requires appropriate tools for monitoring the effect of sedatives in the form of sedation scales and guidelines.

Subjective sedation scales provide standardized methods for the assessment of a patient's level of arousal or consciousness. Use of such validated sedation scales allows the multidisciplinary ICU team to use a succinct, common language when discussing goals and treatments for patients. Examples of adult sedation scales include the Riker Sedation-Agitation Scale, Motor Activity Assessment Scale and the Ramsay scale. Each has been validated in ICU patients with good, and sometimes excellent, inter-rater reliability and has been tested to identify sedation endpoints. A sedation goal is established by the multidisciplinary medical team and regularly refined according to changes in a patient's course of illness.[1] Although the Ramsay scale has been criticized for lack of clear differentiation among the various sedation levels, it has been shown in a randomized, controlled trial to shorten the duration of mechanical ventilation as well as ICU and hospital lengths of stay.[4]

More recently, the Richmond Agitation Sedation Scale (RASS)[5] (Table 8.1), has been validated to detect changes in sedation level over consecutive ICU days and correlates with doses of sedatives and analgesics. Validated use in medical, surgical, cardiac surgery, coronary and neuroscience patients and excellent reliability among physicians, nurses and a pharmacist enhance its value. It is equally valid among verbal and non-verbal patients, highlighting its utility among ventilated ICU patients. Two unique features of the tool serve to objectify the level of sedation: (1) verbal and physical stimuli are separated so that the patient's arousal may

Table 8.1 The Richmond agitation and sedation scale (RASS)

+4	**Combative**	Combative, violent, immediate danger to staff
+3	**Very agitated**	Pulls or removes tube(s) or catheter(s); aggressive
+2	**Agitated**	Frequent non-purposeful movement, fights ventilator
+1	**Restless**	Anxious, apprehensive, but movements not aggressive or vigorous
0	**Alert and calm**	
−1	**Drowsy**	Not fully alert, but has sustained awakening to voice (eye opening and contact > 10 sec)
−2	**Light sedation**	Briefly awakens to voice (eye opening and contact < 10 sec)
−3	**Moderate sedation**	Movement or eye opening to voice (but no eye contact)
−4	**Deep sedation**	No response to voice, but movement or eye opening to physical stimulation
−5	**Unarousable**	No response to voice or physical stimulation

be graded according to stimulus potency and (2) the duration of eye contact serves as the principal means of quantifying arousal.

The bispectral index (BIS) monitor, potentially an even more objective tool for monitoring wakefulness, mathematically analyses the electroencephalogram and provides a discrete number corresponding to the level of consciousness. Worn on the patient's forehead, the BIS monitor has historically been used in the operating room to ensure adequate suppression of consciousness. While a number from 0 (deep sedation) to 100 (awake) is reported as a marker of consciousness among anaesthetized patients, distinctions between wakefulness and sedation are not as clear as one might hope in the ICU. The confounding impact on BIS of metabolic brain abnormalities and muscle activity makes determinations of level of consciousness less clear. It is not known whether the BIS can perform better than sedation scales, and determination of its validity in the ICU is needed.

The value of guidelines for sedative use in the ICU cannot be overstated. A protocolized approach to the management of sedation in preparation for weaning from mechanical ventilation improves patient outcomes. As such, multidisciplinary 'buy-in' of sedation scales enhances the compliance with and success of guidelines while minimizing adverse consequences of sedative use.

Sedative medications

Sedatives are generally thought to be helpful in prevention and treatment of anxiety. Yet absolute indications for their use are not evidenced-based, except in specific circumstances such as alcohol or other drug withdrawal syndromes and in the event of neuromuscular blockade, when amnesia is essential. Frequently reported indications include a desire to potentiate analgesia, anxiety, patient–ventilator dys-synchrony, or poor oxygenation, or the need to perform a procedure. In some cases, treatment of the underlying condition may suffice. Sometimes an assumption, such as one that sedatives improve sleep quantity or quality, is unclear or probably wrong. In addition, overuse of sedatives can lead to prolonged ventilation and its attendant consequences (e.g. ventilator-associated pneumonia, delirium, increased length of ICU stay, increased cost and even death). Clinicians also cannot prevent some patients from developing increasingly apparent long-term neurocognitive impairment. For all these reasons, appropriate selection of sedative is important.

Three categories of intravenous sedative (benzodiazepines, propofol, and central α_2-agonists) will be discussed and are compared pharmacologically in Table 8.2. Currently, etomidate is used for rapid sequence intubation rather than sustained sedation and so will not be discussed. Likewise, diazepam

Table 8.2 Pharmacologic properties of sedatives commonly used for continuous sedation in mechanically ventilated ICU patients

	Midazolam	Lorazepam	Propofol	Dexmedetomidine
Bolus dose (70-kg man)	1–5 mg	1–5 mg	2 mg.kg^{-1}	0.2–1.0 µg.kg^{-1}.hr^{-1}*
Intermittent dosing	Yes	Yes	No	No
Onset	2–5 min	2–20 min	1–2 min	1–2 min
Elimination half-life	1–5 h	10–40 h	30–60 min	2 h
Metabolism	Hepatic	Hepatic	Hepatic	Hepatic
Excretion	Renal	Renal	Renal	Renal
Lipophilic	High	Moderate	High	Minimal
Complications	Respiratory suppression	Respiratory suppression	Respiratory suppression	Hypotension
	Long elimination	Longer elimination	Hypotension ±	Bradycardia
	Withdrawal	Withdrawal	Withdrawal	
Active metabolites	Yes	No	No	No

* Dexmedetomidine may be initiated either without a bolus (maintenance dose 0.2 to 0.7 µg.kg^{-1}.hr$^{-1)}$) or with a small bolus (1.0 µg.kg^{-1}.hr$^{-1)}$) and careful haemodynamic monitoring. See text for further details.

is not routinely employed in ICUs for general sedation and will not be included. Ideal sedatives in the ICU would have rapid onset, predictable duration of action, minimal adverse effects on cardiovascular stability and respiratory function, easy administration, available reversing agents, no active metabolites, a favourable therapeutic index, minimal or no withdrawal syndrome, and favourable cost.

Benzodiazepines

By binding to a specific, high-affinity receptor in the brain that facilitates γ-aminobutyric acid (GABA) neurotransmitter activity, benzodiazepines hyperpolarize (and so prevent depolarization of) central neurons, resulting in non-specific central nervous system depression. In addition to sedation-hypnosis and anxiolysis, benzodiazepines cause varying degrees of anticonvulsant effects, antegrade amnesia, muscle relaxation and potentiation of analgesic effects. Furthermore, they are central to treatment of alcohol and certain other drug withdrawal states. Benzodiazepines commonly used in ventilated patients include midazolam and

lorazepam. Their use should be guided, as discussed previously, by frequent monitoring of the patient's sedation level and by titration based upon clinical parameters (e.g. ability to ventilate or oxygenate for a given level of sedation) rather than in an undirected manner or based on ease of patient care.

Popular because of their familiarity, benzodiazepines are widely used for sedation in ventilated ICU patients. In 1998, 39% of American critical care physicians interviewed used lorazepam, while 25% used midazolam at least 70% of the time in their critically ill patients.[6] Less than one third of hospitals (including academic hospitals) had sedation protocols in place by that time. In a multicentre survey published in 2005 of 5183 adult patients that were ventilated for >12 hours, 68% received sedatives for a median of three days (interquartile range, two to six days).

Midazolam, a short-acting benzodiazepine, has a rapid onset of action, owed in part to its high lipid solubility, and is useful for short-term sedation, amnesia and as an anticonvulsant. Midazolam should be used short term (up to 72 hours), titrated to a defined end-point according to sedation guidelines or for rapid sedation of an acutely agitated patient[1] (although antipsychotics may prove more helpful in that circumstance). The declining use of midazolam among some ICUs is undoubtedly multifactorial. However, biologically plausible explanations suggest that midazolam results in proportionally greater adverse effects because as fat becomes fully saturated with the drug, the sedative properties are exaggerated, leading to less predictable extubation times and higher cost than lorazepam. Central nervous system depressants, ethanol and barbiturates potentiate the sedative effects of benzodiazepines.

For years, lorazepam has been the sedative drug of choice in ventilated ICU patients in North America. As an intermediate-acting benzodiazepine, lorazepam requires several hours to reach maximal effect. Intermittent bolus dosing is generally preferred over continuous infusion to minimize over-sedation. Lorazepam is the least costly of intravenous sedatives, and its safe extensive use suggests its effectiveness.

The benzodiazepines are theoretically reversible. Flumazenil is approved for reversal of benzodiazepine-induced sedation in the ICU to enable neurologic evaluation, hasten preparedness for extubation or treat overdose. However, routine use of the competitive GABA-receptor antagonist can increase myocardial oxygen consumption or induce withdrawal symptoms after administration of only 0.5 mg.[7] It is not indicated for routine use in ICU patients who have been on continuous benzodiazepine infusion.

Propofol

A general anaesthetic with sedative and hypnotic properties at lower doses, the isopropylphenol, propofol, causes GABA-ergic central nervous system depression. Like benzodiazepines, propofol has additional properties, including anxiolysis, anticonvulsion, antiemesis, reduction of intracranial pressure and potentially dose-dependent antegrade

amnesia. Its rapid onset and offset[1] are particularly important qualities during endotracheal intubation and occasionally other bedside procedures such as bronchoscopy. Length of recovery on discontinuation of infusions appears to be dose- and time-related, where higher or longer dosing predict longer recovery (as with lorazepam).

Parameters for cost-effective and reliable use of propofol are being evaluated. Historically, short-term use of sedation (under 72 hours) most frequently prompts consideration of propofol. For use under 24 hours, propofol may offer cost savings over benzodiazepines. Also, propofol allows more rapid and more predictable recovery than lorazepam (or midazolam) *beyond 72 hours* (provided that sedation is targeted to a specified goal) among ICU patients.[8] When used for more than 48 hours, propofol appears to result in fewer ventilator days when compared with intermittent lorazepam.[9] Finally, although benzodiazepines largely remain the historical standard of care for alcohol withdrawal, propofol may treat delirium tremens equally safely and equally well.

Dexmedetomidine

A combined sedative-analgesic with properties of anxiolysis and sympatholysis, dexmedetomidine is a highly selective α_2-agonist.[2] Sedation appears to be by α_2-adrenergic receptor-mediated inhibition of noradrenaline release in the locus coeruleus of the brainstem. The inhibition of noradrenaline release subsequently decreases concentrations of GABA, serotonin, histamine, and orexin, resulting in its sedative properties. Concomitant analgesia may occur via spinal cord nociceptors.

Dexmedetomidine is approved for use in North America for up to 24 hours in ventilated patients, although data on use of the drug beyond 24 hours has been equally encouraging when administered

---

[1] Offset following a bolus dose occurs because of drug redistribution rather than metabolism and elimination, so does not depend on hepatic or renal function.

[2] This drug is not licensed for use in Europe.

without a loading dose. Additional randomized, controlled trials of the proposed safety and efficacy of dexmedetomidine beyond 24 hours have recently been completed.

Where the benefits of dexmedetomidine have been studied, most are in post-surgical patients. In post-surgical patients, where the goal is sedation and analgesia that does not interfere with respiration, dexmedetomidine has been shown to enable both easy arousability and sleep. Importantly, dexmedetomidine has not yet been shown to enable better sleep quality or pain relief compared with propofol. Another potential benefit of dexmedetomidine is a decreased incidence of postoperative delirium, but here, too, the evidence to date is mixed; additional study is warranted. Dexmedetomidine has been confirmed as needing less supplemental propofol, midazolam or morphine when used alone or with these agents, thereby exposing patients to fewer adverse effects.[10] The drug appears relatively safe and may have a better safety profile than once feared when routinely administering loading boluses. As such, its incorporation into the sedative armamentarium of intensivists awaits further study.

Adverse effects

Sedative medications have been demonstrated to result in prolonged ventilation, longer lengths of ICU and hospital stay, longer exposure to ICU complications (e.g. nosocomial pneumonia or deep venous thrombosis) and sometimes death. How these adverse events come about is less clear, although oversedation can attend all sedative medications. Acutely or chronically, oversedation is associated with hypotension, arrhythmia, gastrointestinal hypomotility, inhibition of cough, excessive loss of spontaneous ventilation and risk of withdrawal. Other adverse effects of sedatives by drug class are discussed later. Unknown risks assuredly exist.

Benzodiazepines are frequently the cause of haemodynamic and/or respiratory suppression.

Acutely, venodilatation and impaired myocardial contractility can result in hypotension, especially in hypovolaemic patients. Benzodiazepines are distributed into fat, but once fat stores are saturated, sedative effects are enhanced. Delayed awakening, particularly with midazolam and its metabolites when compared with lorazepam, leads to prolonged ventilation. Also, paradoxical excitation and tachyphylaxis can occur, prompting additional benzodiazepine use. A unique adverse effect of lorazepam is propylene glycol (or polyethylene glycol) toxicity associated with serum propylene glycol concentrations >18 mg.dL^{-1}. This toxic level can be achieved either by prolonged use (perhaps for weeks), high doses (>25 mg.hr^{-1}) or both, and appears to predict a syndrome of metabolic acidosis, lactic acidaemia, acute tubular necrosis and hyperosmolarity. Finally, exposure to benzodiazepines for as little as one week at high doses can cause physiologic dependence and thus precipitate withdrawal if discontinued abruptly. Characterized by tremor, nausea, diaphoresis, anxiety, agitation, muscle cramps, sleep disturbance, delirium, seizure, headache and dysphoria, benzodiazepine withdrawal results in reinstitution of therapy (not necessarily as an infusion), longer ICU stay, longer duration of mechanical ventilation and higher total doses of drug. Liver failure inhibits the metabolism of midazolam but not lorazepam, because the glucuronidation process for lorazepam is commonly spared in liver failure. Finally, in addition to neuroexcitation, benzodiazepines may be causative in agitation and delirium (which will be discussed later).

Propofol, as with the benzodiazepines, is associated with myocardial suppression, tachyphylaxis and paradoxical neurological excitation (as myoclonus). Many of these effects can be averted by using small boluses and either intermittent administration or low-dose continuous infusion. With prolonged use at high doses, physiologic dependence may cause a withdrawal syndrome similar to that seen with benzodiazepines. Other adverse effects, especially related to use over 72 hours, include hypertriglyceridaemia, nosocomial infection (perhaps due to contamination of the lipid diluent) and the propofol infusion syndrome. Hypertriglyceridaemia occurs in up to 10% of patients and may prompt discontinuation, in part because the phospholipid emulsion provides 1.1 kcal.mL^{-1} from fat. Adjustment of caloric intake (including parenteral intake) should be made for the emulsion. Nosocomial infection, presumably due to contamination of the lipid emulsion, has been reported although not proven, and is retarded by additives in the preparation. The propofol infusion syndrome is characterized by hypertriglyceridaemia, rhabdomyolysis with metabolic acidosis, hypotension, and bradycardia leading to fatal arrhythmia. Precipitating factors are unclear, but use of >65 mcg.kg^{-1}.min^{-1} for $\geq$ 48 hours is likely to be harmful.

Dexmedetomidine, the newest of the sedative agents, appears to cause bradycardia and hypotension. When used with a loading dose, bradycardia occurs in a small minority of patients and hypotension in nearly one third. However, the haemodynamic effects of dexmedetomidine are complex. Initially, the drug can cause transient hypertension when given as a bolus. Bradycardia and hypotension can occur during the first four hours after administration and then stabilize. Use in hypovolaemic patients, or those with known bradycardia or low cardiac output, may exaggerate these effects. The bradycardia, while potentially life-threatening, may also be cardioprotective – for example, in post-operative patients. Moreover, using a low-dose bolus ($\sim$0.4 μg.kg^{-1}.hr^{-1}), or none at all, may avert adverse haemodynamic effects. The impact of adverse effects when using dexmedetomidine for more than 24 hours requires additional study.

Management of sedation

The balance between art and science is perfectly exemplified by the desire to sedate but not oversedate critically ill patients in the ICU. In fact, as compelling as avoidance of undersedation may be in preventing unpleasant experiences that might lead to post-ICU emotional distress in some and post-traumatic stress symptoms in others, avoidance of oversedation has proven beneficial in enabling earlier liberation from ventilation. Two principles of sedation in the ICU aim to tip favourably the balance of risk and benefits, namely intermittent administration and daily interruption of sedation. Intermittent dosing of sedatives prevents exposing patients to risk unnecessarily, as is the case of continuous infusion. Continuous sedative infusions prolong mechanical ventilation and length of stay in the ICU, prompting recommendations for intermittent use, whenever possible.[11]

Daily discontinuation of sedatives has proven effective in improving clinical outcomes among medical ICU patients. In a seminal paper by Kress et al.,[12] daily interruption of sedative infusions (so-called 'spontaneous awakening') reduced duration of mechanical ventilation by 2.4 days (p = 0.004) and ICU length of stay by 3.5 days (p = 0.02). Follow-up analysis confirmed decreased incidence of complications of prolonged intubation and mechanical ventilation in the intervention group.[13] The authors concluded that a 'strategy of daily sedative interruption allowed a focused downward titration of sedative infusion rates over time, streamlining administration of these drugs and minimizing the tendency for accumulation.'[12] In fact, protocolization of sedation in the ICU may alone be partially responsible for beneficial outcomes. For example, compared with standard care, a nurse-implemented sedation protocol conveys a nearly 50% reduction in duration of ventilation and about a 25% reduction in duration of ICU and hospital lengths of stay.[4] Regardless of whether the effect is mediated by protocolization alone or by spontaneous awakening, the new standard of care for ICU patients is protocolized sedation with spontaneous awakening. A forthcoming trial will investigate the impact of combining daily spontaneous awakening and spontaneous breathing trials on clinical outcomes among a cohort of medical and surgical ICU patients.

After ensuring adequate analgesia, choosing the 'best' sedative agent ultimately depends on balancing the risks and benefits. Pharmacologic properties of sedative drugs, intended duration of use and clinical factors, such as presence of renal or hepatic dysfunction, are all important. One adverse event associated with sedative use, delirium, deserves further consideration.

Delirium

Definition

A form of acute organ dysfunction much like acute renal failure or acute respiratory failure, delirium originates from the Latin word, *delirus*, meaning 'to be crazy, deranged, or silly.' Although the medical community has historically reserved 'delirium' to describe agitated, confused patients and has used 'encephalopathy' to describe lethargic, confused patients, the *Diagnostic and Statistical Manual of Mental Disorders*, Fourth Edition (DSM-IV) does not make this distinction. It defines delirium as a confusional state characterized by acute onset, fluctuating level of consciousness, inattention and disorganized thinking. Disruption of the sleep–wake cycle and psychomotor or perceptual disturbances (e.g. hallucinations) are associated features of delirium but are not required for its diagnosis.

Attempts to characterize delirium according to motor subtype have led to characterization of hyperactive versus hypoactive subtypes, with the distinguishing feature being the level of activity observed. Patients with hyperactive delirium demonstrate psychomotor agitation, semi-purposeful activity and emotional lability, while those with hypoactive delirium demonstrate decreased responsiveness, inactivity and lethargy. Although certain aetiologies are commonly associated with a particular sub-

type of delirium (e.g. alcohol withdrawal and anti-cholinergic toxicity tend to cause hyperactive delirium, whereas hepatic insufficiency and traumatic brain injury tend to cause hypoactive delirium), patients frequently develop mixed delirium, exhibiting features of both hyperactive and hypoactive subtypes during the course of their illness. Hypoactive and mixed delirium are more common than isolated hyperactive delirium, as determined by the Confusion Assessment Method for the ICU (CAM-ICU). In a study of 307 medical ICU patients, persistently hyperactive delirium is uncommon in both mechanically ventilated and non-ventilated patients (<2%), and most ventilated patients have either mixed or hypoactive delirium. Regardless of subtype, delirium is clearly much more than psychomotor agitation and confusion, as has been historically assumed.

Diagnosis

Routine assessment for delirium in all ICU patients is warranted. A well-validated, reliable, brief assessment tool to easily equip critical care practitioners in monitoring both level of arousal and *content* of consciousness is ideal. Such an instrument would allow for goal-directed titration of sedatives and analgesics as well as rapid recognition of delirium. Two tools for monitoring delirium in ICU patients include the Intensive Care Delirium Screening Checklist[14] and the CAM-ICU.[15] The Intensive Care Delirium Screening Checklist is an eight-item checklist with a reported sensitivity of 99% and specificity of 64% and excellent inter-rater reliability ($\kappa = 0.94$).[14] Each of the eight items is scored as absent or present (0 or 1, respectively), and the item scores are summed for a total, in which patients with a score ≥ 4 are considered delirious. The CAM-ICU was adapted for use in non-verbal ICU patients from the original Confusion Assessment Method[16] and includes a four-feature assessment (Figure 8.1), the results of which yield a dichotomous result for delirium: present or absent. The presence of

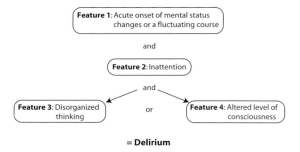

Figure 8.1 Diagnosis of delirium with the Confusion Assessment Method for the Intensive Care Unit (CAM-ICU).

Used with permission, copyright © 2002, E. Wesley Ely, MD, MPH and Vanderbilt University, all rights reserved.

Table 8.3 Risk factors for delirium		
Baseline characteristics	Iatrogenic/ environmental factors	Disease factors
Age	Sedative medications	Sepsis
Cognitive impairment	Analgesic medications	Hypoxaemia
Co-morbidities	Use of bladder catheter	Metabolic derangements
	Anticholinergic medications	Severity of illness score
	Sleep quality or quantity	

feature 1 *and* feature 2 *and either* feature 3 *or* feature 4 indicates delirium. The CAM-ICU[3] is a well-validated, bedside evaluation instrument (i.e. sensitivity and specificity values both >90%) that is easy to administer, takes on average less than a minute to complete, is widely used, requires minimal training, and is highly reliable. Using the CAM-ICU, delirium occurs in as many as three of every four mechanically ventilated patients and one of every two non-ventilated patients.

Risk factors

Proven or potential risk factors for delirium include: (1) host characteristics, (2) features of the acute illness and (3) environmental or iatrogenic factors (Table 8.3). The accumulation of risk factors appears to portend the development of delirium, and the cumulative prevalence of myriad risk factors in ICU patients relates to the high occurrence of delirium in the ICU. Probably the most universal and potentially modifiable risk factor among critically ill patients is exposure to sedatives and analgesics. Pethidine[4] and morphine have separately been shown to predict delirium occurrence.

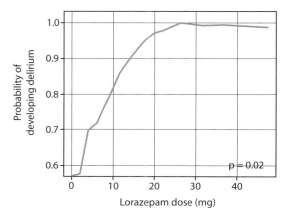

Figure 8.2 Lorazepam is an independent risk factor for transitioning to delirium in ICU patients.

Used with permission from Marinelli WA, Leatherman JW, Neuromuscular disorders in the intensive care unit. *Crit Care Clin*. 2002.

Additionally, in a cohort of 198 mechanically ventilated medical and cardiac ICU patients, Pandharipande *et al.*[17] found that lorazepam had an independent and dose-related temporal association with delirium with the adjusted odds for daily transition to delirium increasing by 20% *per milligram* of lorazepam (p = 0.003) in a multivariable model (Figure 8.2). Delirium may represent an idiosyncratic reaction to psychoactive medications, and it is not clear that all psychoactive medications present an equal risk. Novel sedative agents

---

[3] A complete description of the CAM-ICU and training materials including several language translations can be found at www.icudelirium.org.

[4] Called *meperidine* in North America.

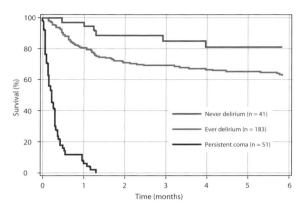

Figure 8.3 Delirium predicts six-month mortality among ICU patients.

Kaplan-Meier curves of survival to six months among ICU patients. Patients with delirium in the ICU had significantly higher mortality than patients without delirium (p = 0.008). Used with permission from Hund E., *Curr Opin Neurol.* 2001.

which spare GABA receptors, such as dexmedetomidine, may diminish the cognitive dysfunction seen in ICU patients. For now, the detrimental impact of sedatives on ICU outcomes must be recognized.

Outcomes

Delirium is associated with numerous, independent adverse outcomes. An altered level of consciousness complicates bedside monitoring, drug delivery and life-supporting therapies, raising the risk of aspiration, nosocomial infection, self-extubation and air embolism. Using the CAM-ICU for diagnosing delirium in ICU patients, additional untoward outcomes independently associated with delirium in multivariable models include increased mortality at six months (p = 0.008, Figure 8.3),[18] longer duration of hospital stay, failure of extubation and probably long-term cognitive impairment. In a multivariate model intended to evaluate the relationship of delirium to hospital length of stay, each of delirium, severity of illness, age, gender, race and duration of sedative and analgesic drug administration were found to be related, with delirium as the

strongest predictor (p = 0.006).[19] The increased risk has been subsequently confirmed using multivariate analyses among large cohorts. Extubation failure (i.e. the need for re-intubation within 48 hours) exposes patients to risk of prolonged ventilation or of re-intubation, such as nosocomial pneumonia and death. Delirium specifically (and abnormal mental status more generally) may increase the need for re-intubation within 48 hours of extubation three-fold. Chronic complications may be as consequential to ICU survivors as acute events, even if less well-described in the literature. Nearly 50% of all acute respiratory distress syndrome (ARDS) survivors, for example, exhibit neuropsychological impairment up to two years following their ICU stay.[20] Given the high importance many place on cognitive abilities and the independence derived from them, the presence of long-term cognitive impairment among critically ill patients represents a potentially devastating, lasting burden for patients, their families and society. Future study of long-term cognitive outcomes in survivors of critical illness is warranted.

Prevention and treatment

Ultimately, prevention of adverse events requires careful consideration of how resources in the ICU are used. The pharmacology of sedative agents combined with medical co-morbidities of an ICU patient may direct, for instance, the selection of a narcotic alone over a benzodiazepine. Likewise, prevention of delirium requires contemplation of both pharmacologic and non-pharmacologic options for addressing potentially reversible risks. Employment of standardized intervention protocols for delirious patients outside the ICU has resulted in significant reductions in the incidence and the duration of delirium. Although unproven to date, such strategies may portend improvements in ICU delirium as well. Early treatment of hypercapnia, hypoglycaemia, hypoxia, shock and other metabolic derangements may prevent the occurrence of delirium altogether. Also, careful selection of sedative and analgesic agents may prevent delirium. For example, while benzodiazepines are the drugs of choice for the treatment of alcohol withdrawal, this class of drugs is not recommended for the routine treatment of delirium because of the likelihood of promoting confusion, oversedation and respiratory depression. For the prevention of delirium, as well as beneficial clinical outcomes mentioned earlier, goal-directed sedation protocols are crucial.

A general lack of awareness of hypoactive delirium and its risks, as well as the absence of clinical trial data, have resulted in medical indifference regarding ICU delirium and wide variation in pharmacologic treatment strategies. Antipsychotics such as haloperidol and the 'atypicals' (e.g. olanzapine, risperidone, ziprasidone, aripiprazole and quetiapine) are thought to exert an anti-delirium effect by 'normalizing' cerebral function via disinhibition of acetylcholine, blockade of dopamine receptors and activation of serotonin receptors and, for haloperidol, by antagonizing the production of pro-inflammatory cytokines. Unfortunately, atypical antipsychotics do not have intravenous formulations. Therefore, despite the absence of randomized, placebo-controlled clinical trials or FDA approval, haloperidol has been recommended for treatment of ICU delirium.

Haloperidol is a butyrophenone with neuroleptic and purported anti-inflammatory properties that may work by stabilizing cerebral function via dopamine blockade and acetylcholine disinhibition. Data supporting the use of haloperidol either alone or versus other medications for the treatment and prevention of delirium are limited. Among elderly, non-ICU hip surgery patients, prophylactic treatment with low-dose haloperidol reduced the duration, but not the incidence, of delirium.[21] Retrospectively, critically ill patients who received haloperidol within two days of initiation of mechanical ventilation had a significantly lower hospital mortality when compared with patients

who did not receive haloperidol.[22] How haloperidol works in this regard is unknown.

The pharmacokinetics of haloperidol, as with sedatives, reflects its risk. With a half-life of about 21 hours, haloperidol reaches peak plasma concentrations within 2 to 6 hours of enteral administration, or under 20 minutes of intramuscular or intravenous administration. Most commonly, the drug is administered intravenously in the ICU to patients with hyperactive delirium at a dose of 2 to 10 mg followed by higher doses as needed and then switched to dosing every 6 hours once stable.

Haloperidol use in critically ill patients appears safe, although adverse effects do occur. These can include hypotension (antagonization of adrenaline when given intravenously), dose-dependent QTc prolongation (possibly resulting in tachyarrhythmias such as torsades de pointes in those with pre-existing cardiac disease or those receiving cumulative daily doses >35 to 40 mg), extrapyramidal symptoms (e.g. rigidity), neuroleptic malignant syndrome and akathisia. Patients should be monitored for these signs and symptoms while receiving haloperidol. Importantly, haloperidol is not sedating, does not suppress respiratory drive and has, not surprisingly, been shown as superior to lorazepam for treatment of delirium. It is recommended for treatment of delirium in the ICU, although the optimal dose, formulation, and timing of administration as well, as any difference between hyperactive and hypoactive delirium, are all unknown.

The atypical antipsychotics may also be helpful in treating delirium. With half-lives typically of at least 20 or more hours (ziprasidone is approximately seven hours), the atypical antipsychotics usually reach peak plasma concentration within 5 to 8 hours following enteral administration (shorter for risperidone) or within one hour for drugs administered intramuscularly. Their mechanisms of action are similar to haloperidol, but instead of blocking primarily dopamine, they affect a variety of other neurotransmitters including noradrenaline, serotonin, histamine and acetyl-choline. In contrast to haloperidol, the atypical antipsychotics usually cause few side effects. Although weight gain, hypotension and dysglycaemia are not uncommon, the risks of extrapyramidal symptoms or neuroleptic malignant syndrome are lower. The drugs variably contribute to sedation and suppression of the respiratory drive. In early 2005, the U.S. Food and Drug Administration issued an alert that atypical antipsychotic medications are associated with a mortality risk among elderly patients. However, no such generalization to patients treated with antipsychotics for delirium is warranted in 2008.

Paralysis

Overview

Prolonged paralysis of patients in the ICU has come under increased scrutiny in the last decade. Historically, the most common reported indication for prolonged use of neuromuscular blockade agents (NMBAs) in ICU patients has been facilitation of complex mechanical ventilation (e.g. pressure control or inverse ratio ventilation, permissive hypercapnia, or high levels of positive end-expiratory pressure), where muscle paralysis is intended to minimize lung injury and optimize ventilation and oxygenation. It is known, for example, that patients may actively contract expiratory muscles to oppose the volume-recruiting effects of positive end-expiratory pressure, so it makes logical sense that preventing the active contraction could improve clinical outcome. Expressed reasons for using paralytic agents are listed in Table 8.4.

While frequency of paralytic use prior to the early 1990s is unknown, in 1991 most U.S. academic critical care practitioners routinely used NMBAs in up to 20% of ventilated patients.[23] Following the 1995 publication of the SCCM guidelines, use of NMBAs declined. However, at enrolment into the ARDS Network trial of low versus high tidal volume ventila-

Table 8.4 Indications for therapeutic paralysis among ventilated ICU patients
• Facilitation of complex mechanical ventilation
• Intra-operative muscle relaxation
• Reduction of oxygen consumption
• Prevention of physical injury and preserving adequate ventilation and haemodynamic stability in patients with status epilepticus
• Minimization of shivering during post-operative rewarming
• Prevention of muscle spasm and rigidity in those with neuromuscular agent poisoning, tetanus or neuroleptic malignant syndrome
• Minimization of transient increases in intracranial pressure because of coughing or agitation

tion during the late 1990s, 1 in 4 patients received NMBAs[24] and 1 in 7 were still receiving NMBAs after as many as 14 days of mechanical ventilation for ARDS. Overuse of paralytic agents persists among ventilated ICU patients.

Three problems associated with the routine use of NMBAs are well known: lack of demonstrable efficacy, difficulty in monitoring level of sedation and degree of paralysis and poor risk:benefit ratio because of adverse effects. Much attention will be given in this chapter to the myriad adverse effects of NMBAs. Most adverse effects are avoidable, given that appropriate attention is paid to sedation and analgesia in mechanically ventilated patients and that paralytic agents are only used in short-term rescue, when necessary. For those patients in whom paralysis is necessary, determination of safest practice based on patient and pharmacologic factors, using the lowest possible dose and establishing local practice guidelines on monitoring is paramount.

Monitoring

Monitoring paralysis is necessary to minimize the potential for adverse events. Careful adherence to a protocol for monitoring sedation and analgesia (see the appropriate sections of this chapter for monitoring in sedation and analgesia) is of fore-most importance. Patients interviewed after their ICU stays who remember being ventilated fre-quently describe it as stressful or unpleasant. Mean-while, attention must be paid to the host of poten-tial adverse effects of NMBA use. These are dis-cussed in further detail below and include appro-priate eye care and deep venous thrombosis pro-phylaxis. A combined approach of objective bed-side assessment along with tests such as peripheral nerve stimulation has been recommended as central to monitoring paralysis.[25]

Bedside assessment by a critical care practitioner is important partly because of the uniqueness of paralytic agents and partly because of the imperfec-tion of presumably more objective tests to deter-mine the level of paralysis. The diaphragm, lar-ynx and laryngeal adductor muscles require higher concentrations of NMBA at the neuromuscular junction to prevent neuromuscular transmission than other skeletal muscles. Patient–ventilator asyn-chrony, tachypnea, diaphoresis, lacrimation, hyper-tension, tachycardia and occasionally overt agita-tion with facial or eye movements indicate incom-plete, or awake, paralysis. Bedside evaluation of skeletal muscle and respiratory effort for any of these findings in a patient receiving a NMBA is essential. However, because the diaphragm tends to be paralysed only at high levels of paraly-sis, reliance upon simple observation (such as of spontaneous ventilatory effort) to titrate NMBAs is unreliable.

Increasingly in the last few years, peripheral nerve stimulation, particularly train-of-four (TOF) test-ing, has been recommended to estimate the extent of paralysis. TOF is a painless technique where four bursts of electrical current are administered in 0.5 seconds from a handheld device, then the mag-nitude of contraction of the adductor pollicis or orbicularis oculi muscle is assessed for each of the electrical bursts. No response elicited is thought to correspond to >90% blockade of receptors, while

response to all four bursts indicates <50 to 75% blockade of receptors. Although recommended by the SCCM for monitoring of all patients receiv-ing paralytic agents, the TOF is imperfect and, sometimes, clinically confusing. Moreover, it does not predict the development of adverse effects of NMBAs such as myopathy.

Clinical assessment on withholding paralysis not infrequently demonstrates that continued paraly-sis is unnecessary. Therefore, the most practical method of monitoring paralysis, when required, is to allow the patient to move prior to administer-ing additional, intermittent doses of NMBA. This approach permits assessment of undiscovered med-ical conditions (including lack of adequate sedation or analgesia) and does not require special training or equipment.

Neuromuscular blocking agents (NMBAs)

Neuromuscular blocking agents (NMBAs) have his-torically been administered by continuous infusion. However, intermittent dosing of paralytic agents might result in a lower occurrence of perhaps the most common adverse effect of NMBA use: acute myopathy and/or neuropathy. De Lemos et al.[26] prospectively assigned 30 patients to receive either continuous or intermittent pancuronium in order to assess the incidence of neurologist-proven resid-ual muscle weakness. The investigators noted a 30% absolute risk reduction during their study in inci-dence of severe muscle weakness favouring the inter-mittent paralysis group, yet the small sample size did not permit statistical significance to be achieved. Although lacking in statistical and methodologi-cal rigor, the study is analogous to the random-ized daily interruption of sedation and spontaneous awakening trials performed by Kress et al.,[12] and as with interrupted use of sedatives, intermittent use of paralytic agents appears superior to contin-uous infusion in the incidence of acute myopathy. Due to the difficulty of monitoring paralysis, the true effect is likely to be larger than that which is measured. Also, intermediate-acting agents such as cisatracurium or vecuronium might demonstrate an even greater degree of difference in the incidence of myopathy.

Another concern with use of paralytic agents has to do not so much with the difficulty in monitoring but in determining the effectiveness of paralysis in obtaining the stated goal of NMBA use. The level of evidence among patients in whom the goal of NMBA use was treatment of muscle spasms or reduction of intracranial pressure does not rise above that of retrospective case reports. At a meeting of representatives from 11 international medical organizations, the summary statement reads, in part, 'When appropriately utilized, NMBAs may improve chest wall compliance, prevent respiratory dyssynchrony, and reduce peak airway pressures. Muscle paralysis may also decrease the work of breathing.'[27] Yet, paralysis has not been shown as effective in achieving two of the purported goals for the use of paralytic agents; decreasing oxygen consumption or improving oxygen delivery in severe sepsis.[23] Instead, despite achieving adequate sedation and paralysis and improving lung compliance among 18 ventilated patients with severe sepsis in a randomized, placebo-controlled trial, Freebairn et al. in 1991 demonstrated that vecuronium was not associated with reduction of oxygen consumption or improvement in oxygen delivery.[28] The authors concluded that routine use of NMBAs for the purpose of reducing oxygen consumption 'should be abandoned'. There have been no placebo-controlled trials of NMBAs for the express purpose of facilitating mechanical ventilation (e.g. permissive hypercapnia, inverse ratio ventilation, etc.) to date, and despite frequent use of paralytic agents in patients who receive newer modes of ventilation such as high-frequency oscillatory ventilation, the superiority of that mode of ventilation, let alone the need for paralysis as opposed to adequate sedation and analgesia, has not been established.

While the absence of data need not 'paralyse' critical care practitioners, a thoughtful consideration of the risk:benefit ratio has come to suggest a new guideline for use of NMBAs. Regardless of the paucity of data supporting efficacy of paralysis, and irrespective of the inability to unequivocally monitor when a patient is paralysed, the use of paralytic agents has deservedly come under scrutiny in recent years. Evidence of a mounting number of adverse effects, from awake paralysis to sustained paralysis or critical illness myopathy after discontinuation of paralysis, are the most concerning aspects of NMBA use, even if paralysis proves to be manageable and worthwhile.

Mechanism of action

Normal physiology involves conduction of neural impulses to the neuromuscular junction, provoking the release of acetylcholine from pre-synaptic vesicles into the junctional space. From there, acetylcholine binds to specific receptors on the post-synaptic membrane (e.g. on the skeletal muscle), causing sodium–potassium flux and depolarization. The ability of muscle to contract repeatedly is achieved by a combination of acetylcholine reuptake and degradation by acetylcholinesterase, both 'true' acetylcholinesterase and pseudocholinesterase which has the additional capability of metabolizing acetylcholine-like molecules. Depolarizing NMBAs stereochemically resemble acetylcholine and so bind and activate acetylcholine receptors; however, they are not degraded by acetylcholinesterase and so cause persistent depolarization (preventing repolarization of the motor endplate) until the agent diffuses out of the synaptic cleft. Non-depolarizing NMBAs block acetylcholine receptors without activating them. Because a sustained decrease in acetylcholine binding results in a compensatory increase in the number of acetylcholine receptors, only depolarizing NMBAs will have increased responsiveness to this up-regulation of receptors. The muscle will, in fact, become relatively resistant to non-depolarizing NMBAs as a consequence of this same up-regulation. This difference in mechanism of action has important consequences not only for pharmacologic and pharmacokinetic properties of the medications but also for potential adverse effects. Most importantly, the mechanism of action of NMBAs confirms their paralytic properties as well as their lack of sedative or analgesic properties.

Depolarizing agents

The only depolarizing agent in current use is succinylcholine, and it is no longer used to maintain continuous paralysis. The agent has a rapid onset of action (in seconds) and brief duration of action (<10 min) as a result of rapid degradation by pseudocholinesterase. In fact, so rapid is this degradation that only a minority of the administered dose (typically 1 mg.kg^{-1}) reaches the neuromuscular junction, where it results in skeletal muscle depolarization and fasciculation. With this, potassium is released from muscles. Plasma concentrations can rise as much as 1 mmol.L^{-1} in patients with rhabdomyolysis, multiple trauma, burns, neuromuscular disease or peritonitis and thus represent a life-threatening complication. Hypothermia is particularly well-known to decrease metabolism of succinylcholine, resulting in sustained paralysis. Frequently, the administration of succinylcholine results in a sympathomimetic response; subsequent histamine release and hypotension are particularly common in combination with barbiturates. Because of its rapid onset, succinylcholine is a useful agent for rapid sequence intubation. However, prolonged use results in vagal stimulation and bradycardia. Malignant hyperthermia is a rare but potentially lethal and adverse effect of use, especially in genetically susceptible individuals. It is characterized by intractable jaw muscle spasm, hyperventilation, tachycardia, labile blood pressure, fever, severe acidosis, hyperkalaemia and rhabdomyolysis. While the paralytic effects of succinylcholine are pharmacologically irreversible, dantrolene may be used to treat malignant hyperthermia.

Non-depolarizing agents

Non-depolarizing NMBAs are most conveniently grouped according to pharmacologic properties (Table 8.5), including duration of action, route of metabolism and excretion, propensity to release histamine (resulting in hypotension and bronchospasm) and propensity of vagolysis (resulting in tachycardia). Classically, the benzylisoquinolinium agents are associated with histamine release but not vagolytic properties, while aminosteroid agents are more commonly associated with vagolysis rather than histamine release. The following brief review of common non-depolarizing NMBAs focuses on newer agents, which typically have fewer of the deleterious properties than did the original drug identified in each class. They also are less commonly reversible than depolarizing agents. The ideal agent would have a rapid onset of action, fairly short recovery period, no dependence upon renal or liver clearance or metabolism, no associated hypotension or tachycardia and would be inexpensive.

Benzylisoquinolinium NMBAs

Cisatracurium is an intermediate-acting benzylisoquinolinium NMBA that causes few cardiovascular effects, in part because it does not cause significant histamine release. Because it is degraded in the blood by Hoffman elimination independent of organ function, it does not need to be adjusted for renal or hepatic dysfunction. It has been compared to vecuronium and atracurium in non-randomized, prospective trials of a broad spectrum of ICU patients. Each trial utilized either clinical endpoints or TOF. Similar clinical effects to vecuronium and atracurium were demonstrated,[29,30] although recovery of TOF >0.7 may occur more quickly with cisatracurium than with vecuronium.

Like cisatracurium, atracurium is an intermediate-acting agent with minimal cardiovascular adverse

Table 8.5 Selected neuromuscular blocking agents used for continuous paralysis of mechanically ventilated patients in the ICU

	Cisatracurium	Atracurium	Doxacurium	Pancuronium	Vecuronium	Rocuronium
Initial dose (mg.kg^{-1})	0.1 to 0.2	0.4 to 0.5	0.025 to 0.05	0.06 to 0.1	0.08 to 0.1	0.6 to 1.0
ED95^a dose (mg.kg^{-1})	0.05	0.25	0.025 to 0.03	0.05	0.05	0.3
Onset of action (min)	2 to 3	2 to 3	5 to 11	2 to 3	2 to 5	1 to 4
Duration (min)	45–60	25–35	120–150	90–100	35–45	30
Infusion dose (µg.kg^{-1}.min^{-1})	2.5 to 3.0	4.0 to 12.0	0.3 to 0.5	1.0 to 2.0	0.8 to 1.2	10.0 to 12.0
Recovery (min)	90	40 to 60	120 to 180	120 to 180	45 to 60	20 to 30
Duration in renal failure	No change	No change	Increased	Increased	Increased	Minimal
Duration in hepatic failure	Minimal/none	Minimal/none	N/A	Mild increase	Mild, variable	Moderate increase
Active metabolites	No	No	N/A	Yes	Yes	No
Vagolysis	No	No	No	Yes	No	Yes (high doses)

^{a} ED95 = effective dose for 95% of patients.

effects and is degraded in the bloodstream. Unlike cisatracurium, atracurium is associated with dose-dependent histamine release. In patients with multi-organ system failure, liver failure and brain injury, atracurium has proven safe for use for more than one week. It may have several niches: (1) patients with renal failure because the drug is not cleared by the kidney, (2) older patients because its termination is not impaired by advanced age or (3) patients with cardiovascular or haemodynamic instability. However, tachyphylaxis may occur with long-term use, and the drug has a metabolite, laudanosine, that is thought to lower the seizure threshold or directly excite the brain in patients who have liver failure or who have received high NMBA doses. Also, although a class effect is thought to exist, atracurium has specifically been associated with protracted paralysis after discontinuation.[31]

Doxacurium[5] is a potent, long-acting NMBA not associated with cardiovascular effects. Its use in elderly patients and those with renal failure may

result in significantly prolonged duration of paralysis. In a randomized, double-blind controlled trial with pancuronium intended to facilitate mechanical ventilation or to lower intracranial pressure, patients receiving doxacurium had significantly shorter and more reliable length of recovery time on discontinuation of the NMBA.[32] The drug's long duration of action, longer time to onset and excretion by the kidney, however, limit its clinical utility.

Aminosteroidal NMBAs

Introduced in 1972, pancuronium is one of the oldest NMBAs. It is a long-acting agent. As one of the least expensive NMBAs, its widespread use in ventilated patients is appealing. However, it is almost uniformly vagolytic (>90% of ventilated patients are reported to have a rise in their pulse by ≥ 10 beats.min^{-1}),[32] may cause histamine release and has been associated with prolonged effects in patients with either renal or liver dysfunction due to production of active metabolites. The increased heart rate frequently results in avoidance of use in cardiovascular ICUs.

---

[5] Only available in North America.

Vecuronium, an intermediate-acting aminos-teroid NMBA, is an analogue of pancuronium devoid of its vagolytic properties. Together with a brief onset of action and relatively short duration, the absence of vagolytic properties makes vecuronium useful for rapid sequence intubation in the ICU. However, metabolism of the parent drug by the liver results in prolonged duration of action in patients with liver dysfunction. Owing to the accumulation of a toxic metabolite that is 50% as active as the parent drug, vecuronium use in patients with renal failure may be detrimental because of prolonged duration of action. The longer duration of recovery using TOF compared with cisatracurium, accumulation by the liver and poor clearance in renal failure suggest the reasons for its occasional replacement with pancuronium, cisatracurium or rocuronium in ICU practice.

The newest agent reviewed, rocuronium, was first introduced in 1994 as an intermediate-acting agent (similar to vecuronium) with more rapid onset and shorter duration of recovery than vecuronium. Its use is similarly limited in patients with liver but not always renal failure.

Adverse effects from non-depolarizing NMBAs are common and require careful monitoring. All nondepolarizing NMBAs are capable of being reversed, although careful cardiac and haemodynamic monitoring is warranted when using edrophonium, neostigmine or pyridostigmine for this purpose.

Adverse effects

Clinical outcomes related to use of NMBAs have recently been elucidated among an international cohort of 5183 adult patients from 361 ICUs in 20 countries who received mechanical ventilation for more than 12 hours.[33] Paralysis was employed in 13% of patients for a median of 2 days.[34] Use of NMBAs was associated with prolonged durations of mechanical ventilation, weaning, and ICU stay (all $p < 0.001$). Their use independently increased the

odds of mortality by nearly 40% ($p < 0.001$),[34] at least partly reflecting the fact that NMBAs were used (in accordance with SCCM guidelines) as a final option in severely ill ventilated patients.

Many dangers of paralysis, ranging from cough suppression to awake paralysis to life-threatening weakness and, rarely, to malignant hyperthermia, have been identified. Difficulty in recognizing inadequate sedation makes awake paralysis a feared complication of paralysis. The detrimental effects of inadequate sedation with paralysis were documented again in 2006 in a descriptive case series of 11 patients who vividly recalled fear, loss of control, and a sense of 'almost dying'.[35] Unrecognized ventilator malfunction, arterial line dysfunction, or even extubation can be fatal in paralyzed patients regardless of sedation level. Corneal erosions or ulcerations may result from the absence of diligent eye care and hydration. Nerve compression syndromes leading to contractures or paresis are possible without careful attention to frequent repositioning and padding, although these are now standard care in most ICUs. Not surprisingly, NMBAs predispose patients to formation of deep venous thrombi and to muscle atrophy. While standard ICU care currently prevents many complications, other serious adverse effects continue to occur. For instance, paralytic agents prevent patient communication and conceal such time-sensitive physical signs of distress as intra-abdominal catastrophe from lack of abdominal rigidity, hypoglycaemia, seizures, angina and stroke.

Numerous medications and medical conditions can impact the effect of NMBAs as a result of impaired ability to assess the patient, complications of prolonged immobility, reduction in protective reflexes and respiration, and consequences from adverse effects of NMBAs (e.g. protracted neuromuscular weakness, neuroleptic malignant syndrome and neuropsychiatric distress). A special clinical situation is that of oedema, whereby an increased volume of distribution may initially make paralysis more difficult to achieve. Eventually the large reservoir of accumulated drug in oedema fluid prolongs recovery. Prolonged paralysis may be related to genetic or acquired (e.g. through advanced age or pregnancy) cholinesterase deficiency, varying pharmacologic properties of NMBAs, metabolic conditions or drugs that potentiate drug effects, or accumulation of metabolites due to failed excretion. Up to 5% of patients are heterozygous for plasma cholinesterase deficiency while <0.04% of patients are homozygotes. Avoidance in patients at known risk is prudent. Myopathy was once thought to be more common in NMBAs with a steroid base (e.g. vecuronium, pancuronium) because of their extensive hepatic metabolism and creation of active metabolites; however, this conventional wisdom is no longer thought to be unique to the aminosteroids. Tachyphylaxis to both classes of NMBAs has been reported and may reflect saturation of neuromuscular junctions and compensatory increase in acetylcholine receptor expression. Increasing the dose of a given NMBA subjects patients to increased risk of adverse effects, and guidelines recommend that patients should receive a different drug if paralysis is still required.[2]

Acute quadriplegic myopathy syndrome

A syndrome of often profound quadriplegic muscle weakness, acute quadriplegic myopathy syndrome (AQMS), is characterized by symmetric weakness of extremities and trunk muscles while sparing facial muscles and cranial nerves.[36] Often obscured early in the course of recovery from paralysis and then requiring differentiation from prolonged paralysis, AQMS becomes apparent as weakness once paralytic agents are weaned. In most cases, AQMS occurs in patients who have received mechanical ventilation for severe airflow obstruction and who have usually been treated with corticosteroids and NMBAs concomitantly. However, AQMS can occur in the absence of either or both agents,[37]

and the effect of an interaction between corticosteroids and NMBAs remains unproven. Although prolonged neuromuscular paralysis may not be the sine qua non for development of AQMS in patients who receive steroids while undergoing mechanical ventilation, it seems reasonable to conclude that NMBAs markedly increase the risk of myopathy.

AQMS likely encompasses a collection of syndromes, including critical illness myopathy associated with sepsis, thick filament myopathy related to use of corticosteroids and NMBAs, and necrotizing myopathy. A series of 107 mechanically ventilated asthmatic patients demonstrated similar prevalence of AQMS for patients treated with atracurium (35%) and vecuronium (31%).[36] The exact incidence is not known, partly because of overlap of the syndromes clinically, electrophysiologically and pathologically. A recent suggestion to use the term 'critical illness myopathy'[38] might avoid confusion. Diagnostic findings on examination include diminished deep tendon reflexes, preserved sensation and muscle atrophy. Frequently, but not always, creatine kinase levels are elevated. Diagnosis is confirmed electromyelographically in most cases.

When it occurs, critical illness myopathy is a serious complication of NMBA use resulting in prolonged ventilation, ICU stay, and hospital stay, prolonged rehabilitation (up to four months), potentially diminished quality of life (especially in those with permanent deficits), and increased costs.[39] Avoidance of critical illness myopathy should be a priority for all critical care practitioners because no specific treatment exists. Unfortunately, as stated by Marinelli and Leatherman, 'it may not be possible to prevent this complication in patients with severe sepsis and multiorgan failure or with severe, protracted status asthmaticus that requires use of corticosteroids and either prolonged deep sedation or neuromuscular paralysis'.[37] As such, avoidance of paralytic agents may be the best preventive strategy available.

Analgesia

Overview

Prompt, initial attention to analgesia when considering how best to 'sedate' a mechanically ventilated patient is prudent. Narcotic-based sedation has been proposed as an alternative to or replacement for traditional benzodiazepine-based sedation strategies among the ventilated critically ill. In fact, despite widespread use of benzodiazepines for sedation and exposure to adverse cardiopulmonary, neurologic and other effects, analgesia is underutilized. Reasons for the under use of analgesics are likely to be multifactorial. First, relief of pain has been traditionally minimized, perhaps because of fear that the history or examination might not reveal new symptoms or signs. Second, decreased bowel motility, cardiopulmonary instability (at least when combined use of narcotics and NMBAs was more commonplace) and other adverse effects have discouraged their use. Finally, over-reliance on benzodiazepines and other sedatives, where monitoring with sedation scales is more widely accepted, has tilted the scales toward a focus on anxiolysis rather than analgesia. Unfortunately, unrelieved pain creates numerous complications in its own right. Basal pulmonary atelectasis from abdominal splinting may impair oxygenation and pain discourages activity, thereby promoting deconditioning and deep venous thrombosis formation. Indeed, as more cumulative adverse effects of benzodiazepines become known, the risk to benefit balance favours more liberal use of analgesia.

Monitoring

To date, relatively little work has been done to identify appropriate analgesia scales. In a 2006 prospective cohort study measuring the impact of systematically evaluating pain and agitation along with sedation (using the RASS) in 230 patients in a medical–surgical ICU, incorporation of the protocol resulted in significantly decreased incidences of both pain (and severe pain) and agitation (p = 0.002 for both).[40] Fewer nosocomial infections were noted among the intervention group, probably due to decreased duration of mechanical ventilation. The authors concluded that systematic evaluation of pain and agitation was beneficial. Further study, particularly with appropriate randomization of patients, is warranted.

Many patients monitored with sedation scales concomitantly receive both benzodiazepines and narcotics. As such, studies of valid, reliable sedation protocols have included patients receiving narcotics for analgesia, and narcotics are often used with the express purpose of sedation or treating agitation at times when benzodiazepines are avoided. Yet pain among hospitalized and ICU patients is prevalent, and its long-term effects to date not well characterized. Six months after experiencing severe pain while hospitalized, patients are more than four times as likely to report continued pain than patients who had the least pain.[41] Establishing an analgesic scale akin to the RASS that is appropriate for use among frequently non-verbal ICU patients is appropriate for future investigation. Such scales will hopefully be validated in the near future among the critically ill.

Analgesic medications

OPIOID AGONISTS

Acting centrally at stereospecific opioid receptors, opioid agonists result in predictable dose-related sedation in addition to blocking pain nociception. Titration to patient response is advisable, as it is essential to maintain a balance between the patient's comfort and level of awareness. Minimizing opioid complications involves using the lowest effective dose (as with sedatives), using slow administration rates, and adequately repleting intravascular volume prior to administration. Commonly used opioids and their properties are outlined in Table 8.6.

Morphine is the best-recognized opioid. A pure opioid receptor agonist, morphine induces both

Table 8.6 Pharmacologic properties of selected opioids used for analgesia in mechanically ventilated ICU patients

	Morphine	Fentanyl	Pethidine	Remifentanil
Intermittent dosing	Yes	Yes	Yes	No
Onset	1–3 min	< 30 sec	5–15 min	1–3 min
Elimination half-life	2–3 h	3–4 h	3–4 h	10–20 min
Metabolism	Hepatic	Hepatic	Hepatic	Plasma/tissue esterase
Excretion	Renal	Renal	Renal	Renal
Active metabolites	Yes	No	Yes	No
Reversible	Yes	Yes	Yes	Yes
Serious complications	Hypotension ± Bradycardia	Hypotension Muscle rigidity	Hypotension Tachycardia Cardiac arrest Seizures	Bradycardia Muscle rigidity Cost

sedation and euphoria within minutes that lasts for two to three hours. It may be administered by the oral, intramuscular, subcutaneous, intrathecal, epidural, or intravenous routes. Of these, the intravenous route is unaffected in cases of impaired absorption and is most commonly employed in ventilated ICU patients. Analgesia is associated with dose-dependent respiratory depression. In large doses, or when administered as a large (>10 mg) intravenous bolus, analgesia may cause cardiopulmonary complications to occur. Otherwise, constipation, urinary retention, nausea, vomiting and bronchial constriction may complicate therapy. Histamine release seems causative in some of these adverse effects. A reduction in dose at less frequent intervals is prudent in patients with renal, hepatic or cardiac failure.

Fentanyl, a lipophilic synthetic opioid receptor agonist, is a more potent analgesic than morphine. Its extremely rapid onset of action when administered intravenously is mitigated somewhat by initial redistribution to inactive tissue sites such as muscle and fat. Transient profound chest wall rigidity has been noted anecdotally, particularly in elderly patients administered large intravenous doses. Administered either by intravenous or transcutaneous route (a patch), fentanyl avoids

histamine release and is thus thought to be associated with less hypotension or myocardial depression than morphine. The drug accumulates with repeated administration. As with morphine, a reduction in dose and increase in dosing interval is prudent in patients with liver or kidney disease.

Pethidine[6] is a phenylpiperidine opioid agonist with minimal potency relative to morphine and fentanyl and numerous adverse effects. Historically used to induce sedation and for short procedures, pethidine causes histamine release (i.e. hypotension, nausea and vomiting), myocardial depression, delirium and tachycardia. The active metabolite, norpethidine, is epileptogenic, and seizures in patients with impaired excretion of norpethidine are not uncommon. Pethidine use should generally be avoided in ICU patients.

A newer synthetic opioid agonist, remifentanil, may prove useful as a continuous infusion sedative and analgesic. It reportedly does not require adjustment in patients with liver or renal failure because it is metabolized in the plasma by non-specific esterases. Remifentanil also avoids histamine release and only causes hypotension via

[6] Called *meperidine* in North America.

bradycardia. The drug does not appear to accumulate over time, minimizing the duration of 'off time' upon discontinuation that might otherwise prolong mechanical ventilation. It also lacks anxiolytic or amnestic properties and enables rapid neurologic assessment. Preliminary investigation suggests it may not cause as much delirium as other medications, at least in part because of its short 'off' time. Because of favourable pharmacodynamic and pharmacokinetic properties, remifentanil may prove to be a key component of sedation and analgesia regimens in coming years pending controlled trials.

Reversal of opioids is achieved using the antagonist naloxone. In intravenous doses of 0.4 to 2.0 mg, naloxone reverses respiratory suppression and, if administered in repeated low doses or a slow infusion, can do so without reversing analgesia. This property suggests that naloxone may be most useful in chronic narcotic users thought to have unintentionally oversedated themselves. A single dose is likely to be insufficient in reversing respiratory suppression in patients who accumulate drug in tissues during long-term narcotic infusions. Conversely, use of naloxone in remifentanil may be unnecessary given the rapidity of reversal of respiratory suppression with remifentanil.

ACETAMINOPHEN
Combining oral acetaminophen with opioids has been shown to exert analgesic synergism.

NON-STEROIDAL ANTI-INFLAMMATORY DRUGS (NSAIDS)
Combining NSAIDs with opioids may result in decreased opioid requirements. Oral ibuprofen, in particular, is thought to exert synergistic analgesia when used with opioids, though this effect likely extends to aspirin and COX-2 inhibitors also. All NSAIDs are given orally with the exception of rectal liquid ibuprofen (limited use due to perceived risk) and intravenous ketorolac (expensive).

As noted below, concern about adverse effects may be exaggerated among ICU patients.

Adverse effects
OPIOID AGONISTS
Long-term infusion of narcotics may result in an accumulation of drug and thus an accumulation of adverse events. These effects vary by drug and according to the amount of histamine release (vasodilatation), but they do include suppression of spontaneous ventilation, decreased gastrointestinal motility, cardiopulmonary compromise, peripheral vasodilatation and cognitive abnormalities (including delirium). Cardiopulmonary compromise is exacerbated when large doses are administered in the context of hypovolaemia. Impaired gastrointestinal mobility, while often multifactorial, is frequently exacerbated by opioids and may result in decreased or impaired absorption of enteral nutrition or medications. Concern about rare biliary spasm with opioid use (less so with pethidine) is generally unwarranted. Also, while addiction is conceivable, fear of narcotic addiction among ventilated ICU patients with real pain and no history of substance dependence is unjustified. However, there is a clear risk of narcotic withdrawal in patients who receive large doses of narcotics over long periods of time when their infusion is abruptly discontinued. Narcotic withdrawal frequently mimics infection or systemic inflammation in ICU patients and may require weaning.

ACETAMINOPHEN
There is real risk of hepatotoxicity associated with acetaminophen, particularly in those with pre-existing hepatic dysfunction or those inadvertently receiving multiple sources of acetaminophen simultaneously. While the effectiveness of acetaminophen to diminish hyperthermia is exaggerated in the ICU, its pain-relieving properties support its use in selected patients able to tolerate oral or rectal medication.

NSAIDS

Well-known complications of NSAIDs, such as gastrointestinal bleeding, renal impairment, and platelet inhibition, have historically resulted in preferential use of opioids and their attendant risks. COX-2 inhibitors are purported to cause less gastrointestinal irritation, yet the severity and frequency of adverse events associated with NSAIDs are emerging. Renal dysfunction is frequently multifactorial, and attributing the cause to NSAIDs may be challenged and perhaps incorrect. Platelet inhibition, moreover, is not uniformly detrimental. More frequently, the use of NSAIDs, if selective, may be appropriate.

REFERENCES

1. Jacobi J, Fraser GL, Coursin DB *et al.* Clinical practice guidelines for the sustained use of sedatives and analgesics in the critically ill adult. *Crit Care Med.* 2002;30(1): 119–41.

2. Murray MJ, Cowen J, DeBlock H *et al.* Clinical practice guidelines for sustained neuromuscular blockade in the adult critically ill patient. *Crit Care Med.* 2002; 30(1):142–56.

3. Ely EW, Baker AM, Evans GW *et al.* The prognostic significance of passing a daily screen of weaning parameters. *Intensive Care Med.* 1999;25(6):581–7.

4. Brook AD, Ahrens TS, Schaiff R *et al.* Effect of a nursing-implemented sedation protocol on the duration of mechanical ventilation. *Crit Care Med.* 1999;27(12):2609–15.

5. Sessler CN, Gosnell MS, Grap MJ *et al.* The Richmond Agitation-Sedation Scale: validity and reliability in adult intensive care unit patients. *Am J Respir Crit Care Med.* 2002; 166(10):1338–44.

6. Rhoney DH, Murry KR. National survey of the use of sedating drugs, neuromuscular blocking agents, and reversal agents in the intensive care unit. *J Intensive Care Med.* 2003;18(3):139–45.

7. Kamijo Y, Masuda T, Nishikawa T *et al.* Cardiovascular response and stress reaction to flumazenil injection in patients under infusion with midazolam. *Crit Care Med.* 2000;28(2):318–23.

8. Kress JP, O'Connor MF, Pohlman AS *et al.* Sedation of critically ill patients during mechanical ventilation. A comparison of propofol and midazolam. *Am J Respir Crit Care Med.* 1996;153(3):1012–18.

9. Carson SS, Kress JP, Rodgers JE *et al.* A randomized trial of intermittent lorazepam versus propofol with daily interruption in mechanically ventilated patients. *Crit Care Med.* 2006;34(5):1326–32.

10. Dasta JF, Jacobi J, Sesti AM *et al.* Addition of dexmedetomidine to standard sedation regimens after cardiac surgery: an outcomes analysis. *Pharmacotherapy.* 2006;26(6): 798–805.

11. Kollef MH, Levy NT, Ahrens TS *et al.* The use of continuous i.v. sedation is associated with prolongation of mechanical ventilation. *Chest.* 1998;114(2):541–8.

12. Kress JP, Pohlman AS, O'Connor MF *et al.* Daily interruption of sedative infusions in critically ill patients undergoing mechanical ventilation. *N Engl J Med.* 2000;342(20): 1471–7.

13. Schweickert WD, Gehlbach BK, Pohlman AS *et al.* Daily interruption of sedative infusions and complications of critical illness in mechanically ventilated patients. *Crit Care Med.* 2004;32(6):1272–6.

14. Bergeron N, Dubois MJ, Dumont M *et al.* Intensive Care Delirium Screening Checklist: evaluation of a new screening tool. *Intensive Care Med.* 2001;27(5):859–64.

15. Ely EW, Inouye SK, Bernard GR *et al.* Delirium in mechanically ventilated patients:

validity and reliability of the confusion assessment method for the intensive care unit (CAM-ICU). *JAMA*. 2001;286(21):2703–10.

16. Inouye SK, van Dyck CH, Alessi CA *et al.* Clarifying confusion: the confusion assessment method. A new method for detection of delirium. *Ann Intern Med*. 1990; 113(12):941–8.

17. Pandharipande P, Shintani A, Peterson J *et al.* Lorazepam is an independent risk factor for transitioning to delirium in intensive care unit patients. *Anesthesiology*. 2006;104(1):21–6.

18. Ely EW, Shintani A, Truman B *et al.* Delirium as a predictor of mortality in mechanically ventilated patients in the intensive care unit. *JAMA*. 2004;291(14):1753–62.

19. Ely EW, Gautam S, Margolin R *et al.* The impact of delirium in the intensive care unit on hospital length of stay. *Intensive Care Med*. 2001;27(12):1892–1900.

20. Hopkins RO, Weaver LK, Collingridge D *et al.* Two-year cognitive, emotional, and quality-of-life outcomes in acute respiratory distress syndrome. *Am J Respir Crit Care Med*. 2005;171(4):340–7.

21. Kalisvaart KJ, de Jonghe JF, Bogaards MJ *et al.* Haloperidol prophylaxis for elderly hip-surgery patients at risk for delirium: a randomized placebo-controlled study. *J Am Geriatr Soc*. 2005;53(10):1658–66.

22. Milbrandt EB, Kersten A, Kong L *et al.* Haloperidol use is associated with lower hospital mortality in mechanically ventilated patients. *Crit Care Med*. 2005;33(1):226–9; discussion 263.

23. Hansen-Flaschen JH, Brazinsky S, Basile C *et al.* Use of sedating drugs and neuromuscular blocking agents in patients requiring mechanical ventilation for respiratory failure. A national survey. *JAMA*. 1991;266(20):2870–5.

24. Ventilation with lower tidal volumes as compared with traditional tidal volumes for acute lung injury and the acute respiratory distress syndrome. The Acute Respiratory Distress Syndrome Network. *N Engl J Med*. 2000;342(18):1301–8.

25. Gehr LC, Sessler CN. Neuromuscular blockade in the intensive care unit. *Semin Respir Crit Care Med*. 2001;22(2):175–88.

26. de Lemos JM, Carr RR, Shalansky KF *et al.* Paralysis in the critically ill: intermittent bolus pancuronium compared with continuous infusion. *Crit Care Med*. 1999; 27(12):2648–55.

27. Vender JS, Szokol JW, Murphy GS *et al.* Sedation, analgesia, and neuromuscular blockade in sepsis: an evidence-based review. *Crit Care Med*. 2004;32(11 Suppl):S554–61.

28. Freebairn RC, Derrick J, Gomersall CD *et al.* Oxygen delivery, oxygen consumption, and gastric intramucosal pH are not improved by a computer-controlled, closed-loop, vecuronium infusion in severe sepsis and septic shock. *Crit Care Med*. 1997;25(1):72–7.

29. Pearson AJ, Harper NJ, Pollard BJ. The infusion requirements and recovery characteristics of cisatracurium or atracurium in intensive care patients. *Intensive Care Med*. 1996;22(7):694–8.

30. Newman PJ, Quinn AC, Grounds RM *et al.* A comparison of cisatracurium (51W89) and atracurium by infusion in critically ill patients. *Crit Care Med*. 1997;25(7):1139–42.

31. Meyer KC, Prielipp RC, Grossman JE *et al.* Prolonged weakness after infusion of atracurium in two intensive care unit patients. *Anesth Analg*. 1994;78(4):772–4.

32. Murray MJ, Coursin DB, Scuderi PE *et al.* Double-blind, randomized, multicenter study of doxacurium vs. pancuronium in intensive care unit patients who require

neuromuscular-blocking agents. *Crit Care Med.* 1995;23(3):450–8.

33. Esteban A, Anzueto A, Frutos F *et al.* Characteristics and outcomes in adult patients receiving mechanical ventilation: a 28-day international study. *JAMA.* 2002; 287(3):345–55.

34. Arroliga A, Frutos-Vivar F, Hall J *et al.* Use of sedatives and neuromuscular blockers in a cohort of patients receiving mechanical ventilation. *Chest.* 2005;128(2):496–506.

35. Ballard N, Robley L, Barrett D *et al.* Patients' recollections of therapeutic paralysis in the intensive care unit. *Am J Crit Care.* 2006; 15(1):86–94; quiz 95.

36. Fischer JR, Baer RK. Acute myopathy associated with combined use of corticosteroids and neuromuscular blocking agents. *Ann Pharmacother.* 1996;30(12): 1437–45.

37. Marinelli WA, Leatherman JW. Neuromuscular disorders in the intensive care unit. *Crit Care Clin.* 2002;18(4):915–29.

38. Hund E. Critical illness polyneuropathy. *Curr Opin Neurol.* 2001;14(5):649–53.

39. Fletcher SN, Kennedy DD, Ghosh IR *et al.* Persistent neuromuscular and neurophysiologic abnormalities in long-term survivors of prolonged critical illness. *Crit Care Med.* 2003;31(4):1012–16.

40. Chanques G, Jaber S, Barbotte E *et al.* Impact of systematic evaluation of pain and agitation in an intensive care unit. *Crit Care Med.* 2006; 34(6):1691–9.

41. Desbiens NA, Wu AW, Alzola C *et al.* Pain during hospitalization is associated with continued pain six months later in survivors of serious illness. The SUPPORT Investigators. Study to Understand Prognoses and Preferences for Outcomes and Risks of Treatments. *Am J Med.* 1997;102(3):269–76.

Chapter 9

Nutrition in the mechanically ventilated patient

CLARE REID

Introduction

Respiratory failure and the need for mechanical ventilation brought about by a variety of medical, surgical and traumatic events makes the optimum nutritional requirements of this group of patients difficult to determine. Nonetheless, nutritional support is an important adjunct to the management of patients in the intensive care unit, mechanically ventilated patients being especially vulnerable to complications of under- or over-feeding. This chapter will consider the nutritional requirements, route and timing of nutritional support, and complications associated with feeding mechanically ventilated, critically ill patients.

Nutritional status and outcome

The metabolic response to critical illness, which features a rise in circulating levels of the counter-regulatory hormones and pro-inflammatory cytokines, is characterized by insulin resistance, increased metabolic rate and marked protein catabolism. The loss of lean body mass impairs function, delays recovery and rehabilitation and, at its most extreme, may delay weaning from artificial ventilation. The degree of catabolism and its impact on outcome depends on the duration and severity of the inflammatory response.

Anthropometric techniques routinely used to measure changes in body mass and composition are inaccurate in the presence of excess fluid retention and therefore the assessment and monitoring of the nutritional status in critically ill patients is difficult. A pre-illness weight and weight history may provide useful information on pre-existing malnutrition, but once admitted to the intensive care unit (ICU), acute changes in body weight largely reflect changes in fluid balance. Assessment of nutritional status should in such cases be based on clinical and biochemical parameters.

Malnourished critically ill patients are consistently found to have poorer clinical outcomes than their well-nourished counterparts,[1] and up to 80% of ICU patients are malnourished.[1] Complications occur more frequently in these patients resulting in prolonged ICU and hospital length of stay and a greater risk of death.[1]

Nutritional requirements

Despite the negative impact of malnutrition on outcome, evidence that nutritional support actually influences *clinically* important outcomes is difficult to obtain. Therefore, the optimum nutritional requirements of critically ill patients remain unknown.

Energy requirements

Resting energy expenditure of the ICU patient is variable, influenced by the impact of the illness and its treatment, but requirements rarely exceed

Core Topics in Mechanical Ventilation, ed. Iain Mackenzie. Published by Cambridge University Press.
© Cambridge University Press 2008.

2000 kcal per day.[2] Indirect calorimetry is considered the gold standard method for determining energy expenditure despite having several limitations in the ICU setting.[3] Routine use of indirect calorimetry can be impractical due to the cost of the device and time taken to calibrate equipment and perform measurements. Therefore, most institutions lack this methodology and must estimate nutritional goals based on predictive equations, of which there are more than 200. There are essentially two types of predictive equation. The first involves calculating basal metabolic rate, using equations previously derived from healthy subjects (e.g. Harris Benedict), then adding a stress or correction factor to account for the illness or injury.[4] The addition of stress factors is very subjective and may introduce substantial error into estimates of energy expenditure. Typically, stress factors between 1.2 and 1.6 have been used for mechanically ventilated ICU populations. The second type of predictive formula is multivariate regression equations. These include an estimate of healthy resting energy expenditure or parameters associated with resting energy expenditure plus clinical variables that relate to the degree of hyper-metabolism. The Ireton–Jones equations are perhaps best known in the ICU and use categorical stress modifiers which take into account diagnosis, obesity and ventilator status.[5] Some studies have shown that these equations correlate well with measured energy expenditure.[6] An alternative and simpler method for estimating energy expenditure is to use a 'calorie per kilogram' approach. The American College of Chest Physicians recommend using 25 kcal.kg^{-1} to estimate the energy requirements of ICU patients.[2] Since all of these equations use body weight, fluid retention during critical illness may make it difficult to assess true body weight and thus increase the inaccuracy of these equations. Ideally, a pre-morbid weight should be used when calculating energy needs.

Comparison of these different approaches with indirect calorimetry show that no single prediction equation is suitable in all patients and may be dependent on age, adiposity and type of illness.[4,6] There is no evidence that achieving a positive energy balance in critically ill patients can prevent the loss of lean body mass or consistently improve clinical outcome; therefore, the level of accuracy provided by prediction equations in estimating energy expenditure may be sufficient to guide short-term nutritional support strategies. In the long term, however, more precision may be required if the complications associated with prolonged under- and over-feeding are to be prevented.

Over-feeding

Over-feeding critically ill patients can negatively affect respiratory function. Any excessive intake, particularly excessive carbohydrate load, results in a significant increase in carbon dioxide production.[7] In order to expel excess carbon dioxide and to maintain normal blood gas concentrations, the body increases alveolar ventilation (i.e. minute ventilation). This compensatory mechanism is limited in patients whose ventilatory response is impaired and is further restricted in those whose response is controlled with mechanical ventilation. These patients are therefore at risk of hypercapnia from over-feeding. This can result in prolonged requirement for mechanical ventilation or even precipitate respiratory failure in the marginally compensated patient.

Enteral formulations have been marketed with reduced carbohydrate and increased lipid contents, specifically for patients with respiratory compromise, but their use is rarely indicated provided that over-feeding is avoided.

Hypocaloric feeding

Weight-based predictive equations, used to estimate energy expenditure, increase the risk of over-feeding in overweight and obese patients.[6] With increasing evidence that a positive energy balance will not improve outcome from critical illness, hypocaloric feeding has been proposed as a means of providing sufficient energy to facilitate nitrogen retention without compromising organ function or outcome.

Nitrogen retention increases with higher energy intakes but the effect is blunted as energy delivery increases above 60% of actual requirements. It has therefore been argued that providing energy intakes greater than 60% does not improve the efficacy of nutritional support.[8] Hypocaloric regimens aim to provide 50% to 60% of target energy intakes but 100% of protein requirements. The theory is that in overweight or obese patients the energy deficit caused by restricting energy intake will be compensated for by the mobilization of endogenous fat.

Hypocaloric regimens in obese ICU patients, providing 50% of measured energy expenditure, have been associated with reduced ICU length of stay, decreased duration of antibiotic therapy and a trend towards a decrease in the number of days of mechanical ventilation.[9] In the absence of indirect calorimetry, it has been suggested that the ideal body weight or an adjusted body weight be used in predictive equations to avoid over-feeding. There is concern that using the ideal body weight of morbidly obese patients in equations will result in significant under-feeding (<50% of energy requirements) and therefore an adjusted body weight may be more appropriate.

To date, no reports in the literature have found any adverse effects with hypocaloric feeding, although some have failed to show benefit. It appears safe in overweight and obese patients but would be contra-indicated in malnourished patients with little or no body fat reserve.

Protein requirements

The primary goal of nutritional support in critical illness is to preserve lean body mass and function. However, seemingly adequate nutritional support, in the presence of a severe illness or injury, only attenuates the breakdown of lean tissue.[10]

Total body protein losses of 12.5% (1.5 kg) have been reported in severely septic patients during the first 10 days of the illness.[11] Approximately 70% of protein losses came from muscle, which has serious implications for patient recovery and rehabilitation. A retrospective study comparing different protein intakes in ICU patients demonstrated that lean tissue losses were minimized with a protein intake of 1.2 $g.kg^{-1}$ pre-morbid body weight.[10] Protein intakes of 1.2 $g.kg^{-1}.d^{-1}$ should be the aim in the general ICU population, but intakes >1.5 $g.kg^{-1}.d^{-1}$ may be needed in patients in negative energy balance or those with pre-existing malnutrition. In patients requiring continuous renal replacement therapy, higher protein intakes are needed to compensate for nitrogen losses via the filtering process.[12] Intakes up to 2.5 $g.kg^{-1}.d^{-1}$ have been suggested.[13]

Practical aspects of feeding critically ill, mechanically ventilated patients

Once a patient's nutritional requirements have been established, regardless of whether they were measured or estimated, consideration must be given to the timing, delivery route and type of feed that best meets the patient's needs. Nutritional support is not without adverse effects and risk, particularly in vulnerable critically ill patients. Enteral nutrition is associated with a significantly higher incidence of under-feeding, gastrointestinal intolerance and an increased risk of aspiration pneumonia. Parenteral nutrition has been associated with over-feeding, hyperglycaemia and an increased risk of infectious complications. Various factors influence the choice of enteral or parenteral nutrition, one of which must be the estimate of treatment benefit and risk of harm.

Timing

The optimal timing of nutritional support is unclear. There is increasing evidence that early feeding (<48 hours after ICU admission) may be beneficial,

		Delay
	Early	(within 7–10
Risk Factors	(within 72 hours)	days)
Age	Children	Adult
	Elderly	
Diagnosis	Chronic	Acute
Severity of	High	Low
illness		
Nutritional	Malnourished	Adequate
status	Obese	
Weight loss	Acute (Unintentional)	Slow
Previous	< 50% of normal	50%–75% of
nutritional		normal
intake		

Table 9.1 Patients who may benefit from early nutritional support

Adapted from Planas and Camilo[42]

although it is generally accepted that feeding should be deferred until patients are adequately resuscitated and haemodynamically stable (Table 9.1).

Early enteral nutrition during ICU admission (within 48 hours) has been associated with reduced hospital length of stay and a reduction in hospital mortality.[14] In addition, nutritional end-points are significantly improved when feeding is commenced early. Energy and protein intakes, percentage goal achieved and nitrogen balance are better if feeding is commenced at an early stage.

Feeding route

Enteral nutrition is the 'preferred' route for nutritional support in patients with a functioning gastrointestinal tract in the ICU. It is cheaper and more physiological but, more importantly, the presence of enteral nutrition within the gut may help preserve its immunological health and integrity.

Parenteral nutrition is the accepted standard of care for patients with a non-functioning gastrointestinal tract or severe ileus. Although the indication for parenteral nutrition appears to be clearly defined, in the intensive care setting it is often difficult to establish whether the gut is functioning adequately. The frequency of gastrointestinal dysfunction is variable but it is consistently associated with a reduction in the delivery of enteral nutrition and can lead to significant under-feeding.[15]

Enteral versus parenteral route

Woodcock et al.[16] compared enteral and parenteral nutrition in an acute hospital population, 60% of whom were in the ICU. To avoid the inappropriate use of parenteral nutrition in patients with a functioning gastrointestinal tract, only those in whom intestinal function was in doubt were randomized. Over-feeding was avoided and enteral nutrition and parenteral nutrition feeding regimens were isonitrogenous and isocaloric. No statistically significant difference in the incidence of septic complications between those given parenteral nutrition or enteral nutrition was found.[16]

Non-septic complications occurred more frequently in patients receiving enteral nutrition. These included complications related to the delivery system, of which displacement of the feeding tube was most common, and feed-related complications, such as diarrhoea and large nasogastric aspirates. It was therefore concluded that there was no evidence to confirm an advantage of enteral nutrition over parenteral nutrition in terms of septic morbidity.[16]

Evidence-based guidelines for nutritional support in mechanically ventilated critically ill adults[17] recommend that in patients with an intact gastrointestinal tract, enteral nutrition should be used in preference to parenteral nutrition. This is based on the fact that, when compared with parenteral nutrition, enteral nutrition was associated with a reduction in infectious complications, although the literature showed no difference in mortality between critically ill patients fed either enterally or parenterally.

Enteral nutrition plus parenteral nutrition

The reduction in infectious complications associated with enteral nutrition lead many ICUs to completely avoid the use of parenteral nutrition.

In short-stay, adequately nourished ICU patients, this change in practice was probably of little consequence. However, in critically ill patients fed exclusively via the enteral route, under-feeding is common, and in patients who remain on the ICU for prolonged periods or have poor nutritional status, under-feeding will undoubtedly impact their nutritional status and outcome. It has been suggested that the administration of small volumes of enteral nutrition supplemented by parenteral nutrition, may enable the protein and energy requirements of critically ill patients to be better met.[16] A study using a combination of enteral nutrition and parenteral nutrition to meet patients' nutritional requirements showed that nutritional markers (pre-albumin and retinol binding protein) corrected more rapidly, but that short-term clinical outcomes (ICU morbidity or length of stay) did not improve.[18] In contrast, Heyland et al.[19] reported a significant increase in mortality rate in patients receiving a combination of enteral nutrition and parenteral nutrition. This difference in mortality remained even when data of patients who had been over-fed – which is one possible explanation for the difference – were excluded. They recommended that parenteral nutrition not be started in critically ill patients until all strategies to maximize enteral nutrition delivery have been attempted.[17]

Pre- versus post-pyloric enteral nutrition

Intragastric feeding is the principle route of feeding in most ICUs. It is considered the simplest, least invasive and least expensive way to initiate early enteral nutrition. Despite gastrointestinal dysfunction contributing to under-feeding in patients receiving enteral nutrition, Heyland et al.[20] reported that 67% of mechanically ventilated patients were able to tolerate early intragastric feeding. However, there is some evidence of an association between the site of enteral feeding and nosocomial pneumonia,[21] though a causal relationship remains unproven.

Post-pyloric enteral feeding is often considered an effective way of reducing regurgitation and aspiration and therefore the risk of pneumonia. However, studies to support this assumption are limited. A meta-analysis, aggregating the data from seven randomized controlled trials, failed to demonstrate any significant clinical benefits with early post-pyloric feeding.[22] There was no difference in mortality, the proportion of patients with aspiration or pneumonia, the length of stay in ICU, the amount of nutrition delivered or the time to achieve feeding targets.[22] It has been recommended that in units where obtaining small bowel access is feasible, small bowel feeding should be used routinely.[17] However, the most recent meta-analysis suggests that there is no advantage to small bowel feeding as primary prophylaxis against nosocomial pneumonia, especially in patients with no evidence of impaired gastric emptying.[22]

Feeding protocols

Many ICUs use a feeding protocol to promote early and safe enteral feeding. Heyland et al.[23] confirmed the benefit of enteral feeding protocols when they reviewed the adequacy of nutritional support provision following the introduction of evidence-based feeding guidelines. ICUs that used such a feeding protocol had a higher adequacy of enteral nutrition than ICUs that did not. Their use has been shown to increase the number of patients receiving enteral nutrition and reduce the number receiving parenteral nutrition or not being fed at all. In a multi-centre study, their use was associated with a reduction in hospital stay and decrease in hospital mortality rate.[14]

Gastric residual volumes

The majority of enteral feeding protocols rely on frequent checking of gastric residual volumes, which act as a marker of tolerance to feed. Elevated gastric residual volumes are assumed to reflect intolerance and have been associated with an increased risk of pulmonary aspiration and the development of pneumonia.[21] However, it has recently been suggested that gastric residual volumes may have very little clinical meaning.[24] Determination of the true risk of aspiration of enteral feed is difficult. Although some degree of aspiration undoubtedly occurs with enteral nutrition in critically ill patients, aspiration of oropharyngeal secretions occurs at least as often if not more frequently than that of gastric contents.

There has been much debate over the level of aspirate that should be used to determine tolerance and many protocols use 150 to 250 mL as an arbitrarily designated cut-off value. However, cut-off values of this magnitude are well within the range of what would be expected for normal physiology[25] and undoubtedly lead to inappropriate cessation of enteral feeding. McClave *et al.*[24] compared the success of enteral feeding and the risk of aspiration and regurgitation in ICU patients using either a 200- or 400-mL aspirate cut-off in their feeding protocol. The incidence of aspiration and regurgitation was similar between the groups. Recommendations were that feeds should not be stopped for gastric residual volumes below 400 to 500 mL in the absence of other signs of intolerance and that clinicians should be encouraged to look for a trend of gradually increasing gastric residual volumes, with abrupt cessation of feeds being reserved for those patients with overt regurgitation and aspiration.[24]

Delayed gastric emptying

Gastric stasis may be overcome by the regular administration of prokinetic agents. Metaclopramide and erythromycin are the most frequently used prokinetic drugs. Only one randomized trial of motility agents has evaluated their effect on clinically important end-points (pneumonia, length of stay and duration of mechanical ventilation), but it failed to demonstrate any significant treatment effect.[26] General recommendations are that meta-

Table 9.2 Most-frequently reported reasons for cessation of enteral feeding
GI intolerance (e.g. high GRVs and vomiting)
Airway management (e.g. tracheostomy)
Procedures (investigations and surgical intervention)
Problems with enteral access (e.g. tube blockage or removal)
GRV: gastric residual volume

clopramide should be used as a first line therapy because there are concerns that the routine use of erythromycin may result in antibiotic resistance.

Interruptions to feed

Unintentional under-feeding is common in the ICU. The unpredictable nature of critical illness and the medical management of these patients frequently lead to disruption in the delivery of nutritional support, especially enteral nutrition (Table 9.2).

As a result of these frequent interruptions, patients may receive as little as 40% of their prescribed feed.[19] The negative energy balances that accumulate during these interruptions in feeding have been associated with increased rates of infectious complications, although a recent study failed to demonstrate any significant impact on clinical outcome (i.e. length of stay and mortality).[27] Two-thirds of feed cessations have been attributed to avoidable causes.

Immunonutrition

The optimum energy and protein intakes of critically ill patients are unclear, so attention has focused on the quality of nutrients provided rather than the overall quantity. Several nutrients (e.g. glutamine, arginine and omega (n)-3 fatty acids) have been shown to influence immunologic and inflammatory responses in humans. The inclusion of these nutrients, singly or in combination, in nutritional support regimens is referred to as 'immunonutrition'.

Glutamine

Glutamine is a conditionally essential amino acid during periods of stress and is essential for maintaining intestinal function, immune response and amino acid homeostasis. It is also an important metabolic fuel for intestinal enterocytes, lymphocytes and macrophages and for metabolic precursors such as purines and pyrimidines. Glutamine is normally abundant in plasma, but during critical illness demand exceeds supply and plasma and tissue levels are readily depleted. A low plasma glutamine concentration on admission to the ICU is an independent risk factor for mortality.[28] Recent mechanistic research reveals that glutamine serves as a vital signalling molecule in critical illness, regulating the expression of many genes related to metabolism, signal transduction, cell defence and repair and to activate intracellular signalling pathways. In a comprehensive meta-analysis, glutamine supplementation in surgical patients was associated with a significant reduction in infectious complications and shorter hospital stay.[29] In critically ill patients, glutamine supplementation was associated with a statistically significant reduction in mortality in critical illness.[30] These data show that the greatest benefits are seen in patients receiving higher dose glutamine ($>0.3\,\mathrm{g.kg^{-1}.d^{-1}}$) administered via the parenteral route.[29,30] Glutamine given via the enteral route appears to have only modest treatment effects[17] and then only in specific patient groups. On this basis, North American guidelines[17] recommend that enteral glutamine should only be considered in trauma and burn patients, and that there is insufficient evidence to support routine glutamine supplementation in other critically ill patients. Intravenous glutamine is recommended for patients requiring parenteral nutrition support.[17]

Arginine

Arginine, like glutamine, is a conditionally essential amino acid. Arginine supplementation has been shown to accelerate wound healing and improve nitrogen balance, up-regulate immune function and modulate vascular flow.[31] It promotes the proliferation of fibroblasts and collagen synthesis and is important in maintaining the high-energy phosphate requirements for ATP synthesis.[31] It is also an important component of the urea cycle. The exact mechanisms are not known, but it promotes the secretion of anabolic hormones such as insulin and growth hormone and is the substrate for nitric oxide synthesis.

Omega-3 fatty acids

The type and amount of dietary lipid has been shown to modify the immune response during critical illness.[32] The lipid component of commercially available enteral and parenteral feeding formulas has traditionally been based on soybean oil, which is rich in the n-6 fatty acid called *linoleic acid*. Linoleic acid is the precursor of arachidonic acid which, in cell membrane phospholipids, is the substrate for the synthesis of biologically active compounds (eicosanoids) including prostaglandins, thromboxanes, and leukotrienes. These compounds can act as mediators in their own right, but they also act as regulators of processes such as platelet aggregation, inflammatory cytokine production and immune function. In contrast, fish oils containing long chain n-3 fatty acids, such as eicosapentaenoic acid and docosahexaenoic acid, have been shown to have anti-inflammatory effects.[32] When fish oil is provided, n-3 fatty acids are incorporated into cell membrane phospholipids, partly at the expense of arachidonic acid. Fish oil decreases production of pro-inflammatory prostaglandins such as PGE_2 and of leukotrienes such as LTB_4. In so doing, n-3 fatty acids can potentially reduce platelet aggregation and can modulate inflammatory cytokine production and immune function.[32]

A large number of studies incorporating fish oil into enteral formulae have been conducted in intensive care and surgical patients. In a randomized controlled multicentre trial, patients with adult respiratory distress syndrome (ARDS), who received an enteral formula supplemented with n-3 fatty acids and high levels of anti-oxidants (Oxepa; Abbott Laboratories, Illinois, USA), demonstrated a reduction in the numbers of leukocytes and neutrophils in the alveolar fluid and improvements in arterial oxygenation and gas exchange. Consequently, the duration of mechanical ventilation and ICU length of stay were both reduced.[33] In addition, fewer patients in the intervention group developed new organ failures although there was no difference in overall mortality.[33]

The benefit of intravenous fish oil supplementation in a mixed ICU population has also recently been reported.[34] This was an open-label multi-centre trial in which patients received parenteral supplementation with a 10% fish oil emulsion (Omegaven; Fresenius-Kabi AG, Homberg, Germany). Dose-dependent effects on survival, length of ICU and hospital stay, and antibiotic usage were evaluated. Benefits were both dose- and primary diagnosis-dependent. Mortality was reduced in patients with abdominal sepsis, multiple trauma and head injury at fish oil doses between 0.1 and $0.2\,g.kg^{-1}.d^{-1}$. There was an inverse relationship between fish oil dose and length of stay. In patients with abdominal sepsis or peritonitis, 0.23 g fish oil.$kg^{-1}.d^{-1}$ was associated with the shortest length of stay. Antibiotic usage was reduced[34] with fish oil supplementation between 0.15 and $0.2\,g.kg^{-1}.d^{-1}$.

Immune modulating mixes (IMM)

Several immune modulating mixes (IMM), which contain a combination of n-3 fatty acids, arginine, glutamine, anti-oxidants and nucleotides, are currently commercially available. Unfortunately, before the development of these formulas, extensive pre-clinical and clinical trials of each nutrient as a single dietary supplement were never performed. In addition, studies to examine the possible interactions between these nutrients, which were once

combined in IMM, are lacking. Despite the absence of this seemingly essential information, various IMMs were developed and have been used in clinical trials in critically ill patients. One consistent finding of these studies is that IMM do not appear to benefit all patient groups.

This may be explained by the heterogeneity in the immune response mounted by critically ill patients. The response to severe illness or injury typically features both pro-inflammatory and anti-inflammatory components, and the predominance of one of these components over the other may be associated with adverse outcomes. Thus, in a heterogeneous critically ill population, n-3 fatty acids may be beneficial in those with excessive pro-inflammatory responses, whereas arginine alone might even be harmful.[35] In patients with immune dysfunction, an immunostimulant like arginine might be beneficial. In patients with a balance of pro-inflammatory and anti-inflammatory immune responses, a combination of immunonutrients may be most appropriate.

When a meta-analysis of studies using IMM in critically ill patients was performed, the overall treatment effect was consistent with no effect on mortality, infectious complications or length of stay.[36]

Based on the available evidence, clinical practice guidelines recommend that diets supplemented with arginine and other immunonutrients not be used in critically ill patients.[17] At present, research is insufficient to make absolute recommendations regarding the amount and use of specific micro-nutrients and macro-nutrients in critically ill patients. This suggests that the way forward is to test single nutrients in large-scale, well-designed, randomized trials of homogenous patient populations. Prior to doing so, we first need to understand the optimal dose of such nutrients in different disease states.

Intensive insulin therapy

An acute state of insulin resistance characteristically accompanies the metabolic derangements associated with sepsis and injury, although the exact mechanisms precipitating this response remain unclear. Insulin resistance and hyperglycaemia often occur secondary to raised endogenous production or exogenous provision of insulin antagonists (e.g. noradrenaline, adrenaline, cortisol and glucagon). Pro-inflammatory cytokines are also thought to play a key role in the development of insulin resistance. Insulin resistance can be correlated directly with the severity of illness and determines the speed of recovery.

Van den Berghe et al.[37] produced a significant reduction in ICU morbidity and mortality by the aggressive use of insulin to maintain normoglycaemia. Favourable outcomes were attributed to the tight control of blood glucose levels between 4.4 and 6.1 mmol.L^{-1} compared with a control group where the target blood glucose was 10.0 to 11.1 mmol.L^{-1}. Benefits were greatest in patients who remained on the ICU for more than five days. Van den Berghe et al.[38] reviewed their data and concluded that the favourable effects of good blood glucose control on outcome were related to the glucose control itself and not to the effects of insulin.

On the basis of this study, it has been recommended that glycaemic control with intensive insulin therapy become the standard of care for the critically ill. However, the study has several limitations, not least that patients were recruited from only a single centre and there was a predominance of cardiac surgery patients in the study population. More recently a similar study was reported in medical ICU patients.[39] Compared with conventional insulin therapy, intensive insulin therapy was associated with improvements in renal function, duration of mechanical ventilation and discharge from ICU and from the hospital.[39] Again, benefits were greatest in those remaining on the ICU for more than five days. In contrast to the findings in surgical ICU patients, intensive insulin therapy did not decrease bacteraemia or reduce mortality in the medical population.[39] It is not entirely clear

why insulin therapy was less beneficial in medical patients. Compared with the surgical cohort, the medical patients were sicker, and since both studies show that the benefits of intensive insulin therapy accumulate over time, higher early mortality might be expected to dilute any potential mortality benefit. In addition, sepsis is a frequent cause of admission to a medical ICU and may explain why intensive insulin therapy was unable to reduce the incidence of bacteraemia in the medical patients studied.

Despite the many benefits associated with intensive insulin therapy, some authors argue that there is insufficient evidence to make a grade A recommendation for its routine application in ICU patients and that the results of ongoing, larger, multi-centre studies should be awaited.[40] In the clinical setting, the increased incidence of hypoglycaemia associated with intensive insulin therapy is of great concern and undoubtedly hinders the widespread acceptance of intensive insulin therapy protocols. Indeed, in their medical cohort, Van den Berghe et al.[39] found the incidence of hypoglycaemic morbidity (mean blood glucose concentration of 1.8 mmol.L^{-1}), was increased during intensive insulin therapy. Using logistic regression analysis, hypoglycaemia was identified as an independent risk factor for death.[39] In a recent editorial, Cryer[41] concluded that until a favourable benefit-to-risk relationship is established in rigorous clinical trials, euglycaemia is not an appropriate goal during critical illness.

Conclusion

Critically ill, mechanically ventilated patients are difficult to feed, not least because their optimum macronutrient and micronutrient requirements have yet to be determined. Despite the lack of definitive trials demonstrating clinically meaningful benefit from nutritional support, there is strong evidence that malnutrition is associated with a worse outcome. In addition, under-feeding and over-feeding have had undesirable consequences.

The use of various 'immune enhancing nutrients', particularly glutamine and the tight control of blood glucose using insulin, may represent novel therapies to improve the nutritional support and outcome of our sickest patients.

FURTHER READING

* Shikora SA, Matindale RG, Schwaitzberg SD (Eds). *Nutritional considerations in the Intensive Care Unit. Science, rationale and practice.* Iowa: Kendall/Hunt Publishing Company, 2002.

WWW RESOURCE

www.criticalcarenutrition.com

REFERENCES

1. Barr J, Hecht M, Flavin KE *et al*. Outcomes in critically ill patients before and after the implementation of an evidence-based nutritional management protocol. *Chest.* 2004;125(4):1446–57.

2. Cerra FB, Benitez MR, Blackburn GL *et al*. Applied nutrition in ICU patients. A consensus statement of the American College of Chest Physicians. *Chest.* 1997;111(3): 769–78.

3. Flancbaum L, Choban PS, Sambucco S *et al*. Comparison of indirect calorimetry, the Fick method, and prediction equations in estimating the energy requirements of critically ill patients. *Am J Clin Nutr.* 1999; 69(3):461–6.

4. Barak N, Wall-Alonso E, Sitrin MD. Evaluation of stress factors and body weight adjustments currently used to estimate energy expenditure in hospitalized patients. *J Parenter Enteral Nutr.* 2002;26(4):231–8.

5. Ireton-Jones C, Jones JD. Improved equations for predicting energy expenditure in patients: the Ireton-Jones Equations. *Nutr Clin Pract.* 2002;17(1):29–31.

6. Frankenfield D, Smith JS, Cooney RN. Validation of two approaches to predicting resting metabolic rate in critically ill patients. *J Parenter Enteral Nutr.* 2004;28(4): 259–64.

7. Klein CJ, Stanek GS, Wiles CE, III. Overfeeding macronutrients to critically ill adults: metabolic complications. *J Am Diet Assoc.* 1998;98(7):795–806.

8. Elwyn DH, Askanazi J, Kinney JM *et al*. Kinetics of energy substrates. *Acta Chir Scand Suppl.* 1981;507:209–19.

9. Dickerson RN, Boschert KJ, Kudsk KA *et al*. Hypocaloric enteral tube feeding in critically ill obese patients. *Nutrition.* 2002;18(3): 241–6.

10. Ishibashi N, Plank LD, Sando K *et al*. Optimal protein requirements during the first 2 weeks after the onset of critical illness. *Crit Care Med.* 1998;26(9):1529–35.

11. Streat SJ, Beddoe AH, Hill GL. Aggressive nutritional support does not prevent protein loss despite fat gain in septic intensive care patients. *J Trauma.* 1987; 27(3):262–6.

12. Frankenfield DC, Reynolds HN. Nutritional effect of continuous hemodiafiltration. *Nutrition.* 1995;11(4):388–93.

13. Scheinkestel CD, Kar L, Marshall K *et al*. Prospective randomized trial to assess caloric and protein needs of critically ill, anuric, ventilated patients requiring continuous renal replacement therapy. *Nutrition.* 2003; 19(11–12):909–16.

14. Martin CM, Doig GS, Heyland DK *et al*. Multicentre, cluster-randomized clinical trial of algorithms for critical-care enteral and parenteral therapy (ACCEPT). *CMAJ.* 2004; 170(2):197–204.

15. Engel JM, Muhling J, Junger A *et al*. Enteral nutrition practice in a surgical intensive care unit: what proportion of energy expenditure

is delivered enterally? *Clin Nutr*. 2003;22(2): 187–92.

16. Woodcock NP, Zeigler D, Palmer MD *et al.* Enteral versus parenteral nutrition: a pragmatic study. *Nutrition*. 2001;17(1):1–12.

17. Heyland DK, Dhaliwal R, Drover JW *et al.* Canadian clinical practice guidelines for nutrition support in mechanically ventilated, critically ill adult patients. *J Parenter Enteral Nutr*. 2003;27(5):355–73.

18. Bauer P, Charpentier C, Bouchet C *et al.* Parenteral with enteral nutrition in the critically ill. *Intensive Care Med*. 2000; 26(7):893–900.

19. Heyland DK, Schroter-Noppe D, Drover JW *et al.* Nutrition support in the critical care setting: current practice in Canadian ICUs – opportunities for improvement? *J Parenter Enteral Nutr*. 2003;27(1):74–83.

20. Heyland D, Cook D, Winder B *et al.* Do critically ill patients tolerate early intragastric enteral nutrition? *Clinical Intensive Care*. 1996;7(2):68–73.

21. Mentec H, Dupont H, Bocchetti M *et al.* Upper digestive intolerance during enteral nutrition in critically ill patients: frequency, risk factors, and complications. *Crit Care Med*. 2001;29(10):1955–61.

22. Ho KM, Dobb GJ, Webb SA. A comparison of early gastric and post-pyloric feeding in critically ill patients: a meta-analysis. *Intensive Care Med*. 2006;32(5):639–49.

23. Heyland DK, Dhaliwal R, Day A *et al.* Validation of the Canadian clinical practice guidelines for nutrition support in mechanically ventilated, critically ill adult patients: results of a prospective observational study. *Crit Care Med*. 2004;32(11):2260–6.

24. McClave SA, Lukan JK, Stefater JA *et al.* Poor validity of residual volumes as a marker for risk of aspiration in critically ill patients. *Crit Care Med*. 2005;33(2):324–30.

25. Lin HC, Van Citters GW. Stopping enteral feeding for arbitrary gastric residual volume may not be physiologically sound: results of a computer simulation model. *J Parenter Enteral Nutr*. 1997;21(5):286–9.

26. Yavagal DR, Karnad DR, Oak JL. Metoclopramide for preventing pneumonia in critically ill patients receiving enteral tube feeding: a randomized controlled trial. *Crit Care Med*. 2000;28(5):1408–11.

27. Dvir D, Cohen J, Singer P. Computerized energy balance and complications in critically ill patients: an observational study. *Clin Nutr*. 2006;25(1):37–44.

28. Oudemans-van Straaten HM, Bosman RJ, Treskes M *et al.* Plasma glutamine depletion and patient outcome in acute ICU admissions. *Intensive Care Med*. 2001;27(1): 84–90.

29. Novak F, Heyland DK, Avenell A *et al.* Glutamine supplementation in serious illness: a systematic review of the evidence. *Crit Care Med*. 2002;30(9): 2022–9.

30. Wischmeyer PE. The glutamine story: where are we now? *Curr Opin Crit Care*. 2006;12(2): 142–8.

31. Suchner U, Heyland DK, Peter K. Immune-modulatory actions of arginine in the critically ill. *Br J Nutr*. 2002;87 Suppl 1:S121–32.

32. Calder PC. n-3 fatty acids, inflammation, and immunity – relevance to postsurgical and critically ill patients. *Lipids*. 2004;39(12): 1147–61.

33. Gadek JE, DeMichele SJ, Karlstad MD *et al.* Effect of enteral feeding with eicosapentaenoic acid, gamma-linolenic acid, and antioxidants in patients with acute respiratory distress syndrome. Enteral Nutrition in ARDS Study Group. *Crit Care Med*. 1999;27(8):1409–20.

34. Heller AR, Rossler S, Litz RJ *et al*. Omega-3 fatty acids improve the diagnosis-related clinical outcome. *Crit Care Med*. 2006;34(4): 972–9.

35. Ochoa JB, Makarenkova V, Bansal V. A rational use of immune enhancing diets: when should we use dietary arginine supplementation? *Nutr Clin Pract*. 2004;19(3):216–25.

36. Heyland D, Dhaliwal R. Immunonutrition in the critically ill: from old approaches to new paradigms. *Intensive Care Med*. 2005;31(4): 501–3.

37. Van den Berghe G, Wouters P, Weekers F *et al*. Intensive insulin therapy in critically ill patients. *N Engl J Med*. 2001;345(19): 1359–67.

38. Van den Berghe G, Wouters PJ, Bouillon R *et al*. Outcome benefit of intensive insulin therapy in the critically ill: Insulin dose versus glycemic control. *Crit Care Med*. 2003;31(2):359–66.

39. Van den Berghe G, Wilmer A, Hermans G *et al*. Intensive insulin therapy in the medical ICU. *N Engl J Med*. 2006;354(5):449–61.

40. Angus DC, Abraham E. Intensive insulin therapy in critical illness. *Am J Respir Crit Care Med*. 2005;172(11):1358–9.

41. Cryer PE. Hypoglycaemia: the limiting factor in the glycaemic management of the critically ill? *Diabetologia*. 2006;49(8):1722–5.

42. Planas M, Camilo ME. Artificial nutrition: dilemmas in decision-making. *Clin Nutr*. 2002;21(4):355–61.

Chapter 10

Mechanical ventilation in asthma and chronic obstructive pulmonary disease

DAVID TUXEN AND MATTHEW T. NAUGHTON

Introduction

Mechanical ventilation of the patient with severe asthma or chronic obstructive pulmonary disease (COPD) has unique problems not routinely encountered in the more common critically ill patient without significant airflow obstruction (Table 10.1). These problems can lead to ventilator-induced morbidity and mortality if not recognized or managed appropriately. Improved out-patient management of both asthma and COPD and more widespread use of non-invasive ventilation (NIV) have resulted in a decreased requirement for invasive mechanical ventilation for both asthma and COPD.[1] This has resulted in both the selection of more difficult patients who require mechanical ventilation and a decreased familiarity with the problems associated with ventilation of patients with severe airflow obstruction.

Safe patient management requires understanding of the mechanism of these problems and strategies to avoid and manage them.

Pathophysiology of airflow obstruction during mechanical ventilation

The majority of critically ill patients do not have significant asthma- or COPD-related airflow obstruction and therefore have complete exhalation of their inspired tidal volume during the expiratory time

Table 10.1 Problems associated with significant airflow obstruction
• Static and dynamic hyperinflation due to gas trapping
• Hypotension and, less commonly, circulatory collapse with electro-mechanical dissociation
• Ventilation-induced tension pneumothoraces
• The need for specific strategies to reduce work of breathing
• Lactic acidosis and acute necrotizing myopathy

available, usually two to four seconds. As a result, at the end of expiration, the lungs return to their passive relaxation volume referred to as the functional residual capacity (FRC). In such patients, the FRC is at or below the normal volume because varying degrees of lung collapse are usually present (Figure 10.1). An expiratory reserve capacity is present by actively continuing expiration after passive exhalation is complete. The minimum achievable lung volume is determined by chest wall mechanics, with all ventilated lung units still communicating with the central airways.

This is not true in patients with airflow obstruction where the lungs are subject to both static and dynamic hyperinflation. In both asthma and COPD, airway narrowing predominates in the intra-pulmonary airways where the airway calibre is proportional to the lung volume. Because of this, airway diameter is increased at high lung

Core Topics in Mechanical Ventilation, ed. Iain Mackenzie. Published by Cambridge University Press.
© Cambridge University Press 2008.

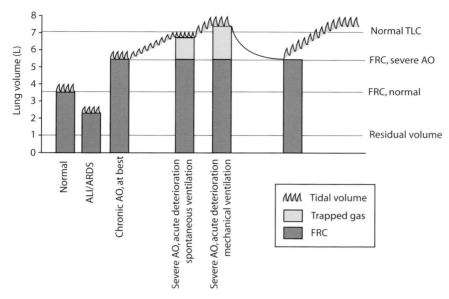

Figure 10.1 Comparison of lung volumes in patients with normal lungs, acute lung injury, and severe airflow obstruction both spontaneously ventilating and during mechanical ventilation.

In normal lungs, normal FRC is reached at the end of tidal ventilation (Vt), no further lung volume reduction occurs with prolonging expiratory time and a significant expiratory reserve capacity (ER Cap) remains available for expiratory effort to reach the minimum achievable lung volume (Min Vol). In acute lung injury (ALI), all these volumes are present but reduced. In severe airflow obstruction (Severe AO), end-tidal lung volume is elevated above FRC by trapped gas (Vtrap) that could be exhaled if a longer expiratory time (1–2 minutes) could occur to reach the Min Vol. This Min Vol (the FRC in severe AO) is also significantly elevated by airway closure. During spontaneous ventilation (spont vent) in severe AO, tidal ventilation cannot exceed the normal total lung capacity (TLC) but during mechanical ventilation, increased minute ventilation and ventilatory pattern can easily elevate end-inspiratory lung volume well above TLC.

volumes but diminishes progressively as lung volume decreases until the airways eventually close. Two consequences follow from this.

First, gas remains trapped in the lung by this airway closure at the end of prolonged expiration (up to two minutes) when all expiratory airflow has ceased, causing an increase in FRC that is referred to as *static hyperinflation*. In practice, such prolonged expiration can only be achieved with a period of apnoea during mechanical ventilation with the patient paralyzed.[2,3] In severe airflow obstruction, this elevation of static FRC may be up to 50% above normal (Figure 10.1). The degree of static hyperinflation depends primarily on the severity of airflow obstruction.

Second, slow expiratory airflow results in an inability to complete exhalation of the inspired

tidal volume during the expiratory time available (Figure 10.1), resulting in a progressive increase in the volume of gas trapped in the lungs by the onset of each successive breath,[2,3] a phenomenon referred to as *dynamic hyperinflation*. This causes a progressive increase in lung volume until an equilibrium point is reached where all the inspired tidal volume can be expired in the expiratory time available. This equilibrium point occurs because, as lung volume increases, so too does elastic recoil pressure and small airway calibre, both of which increase expiratory airflow. During spontaneous breathing, this equilibrium point cannot exceed total lung capacity because the patient is incapable of inspiring above this volume (Figure 10.1). However, during mechanical ventilation total lung capacity can easily be exceeded, with a significant risk of hypotension[1] and pneumothorax. Dynamic hyper-inflation depends primarily on three factors: the severity of airway obstruction, the inspiratory tidal volume and the time allowed for expiration.[4] Expiratory time obviously depends both on respiratory rate and I:E ratio.

Both static and dynamic hyperinflation will occur in proportion to the severity of airflow obstruction, and both will decrease as airflow obstruction improves. In addition, dynamic hyperinflation is dependent on the ventilatory pattern, so the ventilator settings can directly influence the risk of dynamic hyperinflation arising.

Clinical presentations

Asthma. Precipitators of an exacerbation of asthma leading to mechanical ventilation include allergen exposure, anxiety, and viral or bacterial lower respiratory tract infection. Up to 40% of exacerbations have no clear precipitant. Bacterial lower-respiratory tract infection is an uncommon precipitant of acute severe asthma and antibiotics are usually not required.[5]

Two clinical patterns of presentation have been recognized: acute severe asthma and hyperacute asthma. Patients presenting with acute severe asthma are presenting as an acute deterioration on a background of poorly controlled asthma. It is not uncommon for the deterioration to have occurred over a number of days, or longer, and the patients may have had prior medical presentations during that period.[6,7] They usually have significant airflow obstruction when stable and are therefore deteriorating from a poor baseline. Because of the significant component of chronic disease, these patients

commonly respond slowly to bronchodilators and steroids and require mechanical ventilation when they become exhausted.

Hyperacute asthma is a less common presentation that is seen predominately in males who have relatively normal baseline respiratory function with minimal airflow obstruction but marked bronchial hyperreactivity.[8] These patients may have a striking allergy history (e.g. nuts, seafood, food colourings or medications) that they may have unknowingly consumed to precipitate their bronchospasm. They may progress from baseline to fulminant asthma requiring ventilatory support over hours and sometimes minutes. Left untreated, these patients are at risk of a cardiorespiratory arrest but may also respond rapidly over hours to bronchodilator therapy.

Acute asthma can also be usefully classified on the basis of the degree of airflow obstruction into mild, moderate and severe categories[9] (Table 10.2).

COPD. Patients with COPD who require ventilatory support usually have significantly compromised lung function (e.g. $FEV_1 < 50\%$ of predicted) that is longstanding with a worsening of airflow obstruction or lung function precipitated by a lower respiratory tract infection, pneumonia, heart failure, a pulmonary embolus, surgery or a chest or abdominal injury that interferes with sputum clearance. These patients present with increasing dyspnoea and wheeze, with or without fever, and increased sputum production. On examination, the clinical signs include accessory muscle use, pursed lipped breathing, tachypnoea, and respiratory distress. Hypercapnia may be present.

Smoking is the most common risk factor for COPD as well as being a potent risk factor for atherosclerosis and, consequently, stroke and ischaemic heart disease. Patients with COPD who have ischaemic heart disease commonly have systolic heart failure,[10] while those without ischaemic heart disease commonly have diastolic dysfunction, secondary to hypoxic and tachycardia-induced

---

[1] During positive pressure mechanical ventilation, the lowest intrathoracic pressure occurs at the end of expiration, and in the absence of either static or dynamic hyperinflation this pressure is normally zero. However, with airflow obstruction, the end-expiratory pressure rises in proportion to the end-expiratory volume. Some of this pressure is transmitted to the heart and great vessels, and if significantly elevated, can reduce venous return, cardiac output and blood pressure. This effect is referred to as 'respiratory tamponade'.

Table 10.2 Classification of asthma on clinical criteria. Pulsus paradoxus when present indicates severe asthma but is an unreliable clinical sign

	Mild	Moderate	Severe
Conscious state	Alert and relaxed	Anxious	Difficulty sleeping, agitated, delirious
Speech	Sentences	Phrases	Words
Accessory muscles	Nil	Mild	Significant sitting upright
Wheeze	Moderate	Loud	Loud or silent
Pulse rate (beats.min^{-1})	<100	100 to 120	>120
Peak expiratory flow[a]	>80%	60 to 80%	<60%
PaCO$_2$ (kPa)	<6	<6	>6

a: Percent predicted for height and age.

ventricular stiffness, as well as respiratory 'tamponade',[11] Patients with COPD are also prone to life-threatening tachyarrhythmias.[12]

Medical management

In both asthma and COPD, full active management with bronchodilators and adjunctive therapies should be undertaken to avoid or minimize the need for ventilatory assistance.

Standard therapy

Oxygen delivered by face mask to achieve arterial haemoglobin saturations of 94% to 96% is appropriate in patients without evidence of chronic hypercapnia, which would include most patients with asthma and some with COPD. In patients with chronic hypercapnia or where oxygen-induced hypercapnia is known or suspected (usually those with severe chronic COPD), arterial haemoglobin saturations of 88% to 94% are safer. Oxygen may induce hypercapnia in a number of ways,[13] including (1) loss of hypoxic respiratory drive, (2) increased dead space,[2] (3) anxiolysis and promotion of sleep with a resultant reduction in

minute ventilation, and (4) the Haldane[3] effect. Furthermore, if oxygen is delivered to the patient using a variable performance mask or nasal cannulae, the reduction in peak inspiratory flow that accompanies a reduction in respiratory drive results in an increase in the fractional inspired oxygen concentration, creating a positive feedback loop for the suppression of respiratory drive by the mechanisms previously mentioned.

Inhaled salbutamol and other short-acting beta-2 adrenergic agonists are routinely used to alleviate bronchoconstriction. They are more effective in asthma than COPD. Inhaled salbutamol can be delivered by metered-dose inhaler via a 'spacer' device if the asthma severity is mild to moderate or,

[2] Blood flow to poorly ventilated lung units is normally minimized by hypoxic vasoconstriction. Supplemental oxygen increases the alveolar oxygen tension in these poorly ventilated lung units, reversing the hypoxic vasoconstriction and thus allowing a larger proportion of the pulmonary blood flow to pass through these poorly ventilated lung units.

[3] Although only 7% to 8% of the carbon dioxide in mixed venous blood is transported in chemical combination with haemoglobin (see Chapter 7), this fraction delivers just over 30% of the carbon dioxide released into alveolar gas. The reason for this is that oxyhaemoglobin is less able to buffer hydrogen ion than deoxyhaemoglobin, and therefore as the haemoglobin becomes oxygenated in its passage past the alveolus, hydrogen ions are released by the haemoglobin. These hydrogen ions then react with the chemically combined carbon dioxide (held as carbamate) to release carbon dioxide. The reverse of this process, the conversion of oxy-haemoglobin to deoxy-haemoglobin in the tissue capillaries, allows the deoxy-haemoglobin to 'pick up' comparatively large quantities of carbon dioxide. However, if less haemoglobin becomes deoxygenated in its passage through the tissues because the patient is receiving supplemental oxygen, less carbon dioxide will be transported away from the tissues, causing the partial pressure of carbon dioxide in the tissues to rise.

if severe, can be delivered as a nebulized aerosol.[4] In patients with severe airflow obstruction, salbutamol is commonly given hourly or even continuously in very severe cases, reducing to four-hourly as the clinical state improves or in clinically mild cases. In asthma, high-flow oxygen can be used, but in COPD, high-flow air is usually required to avoid oxygen-induced hypercapnia. Because narrowing of the small airways is due to the triad of smooth muscle contraction, mucosal oedema and mucus plugging, salbutamol can only reverse one factor. This explains the 'ceiling effect' to the salbutamol dose-response, where an increase in dose fails to yield further bronchodilatation but increases the risk of adverse effects such as lactic acidosis.

Inhaled anti-cholinergic drugs such as ipratropium bromide cause bronchodilatation by reducing vagal tone on the airways and by reducing mucus production. They are more effective in COPD than asthma but are routinely used in both conditions in severe cases. As with salbutamol, anti-cholinergic drugs can be delivered by metered-dose inhaler and spacer device or nebulizer, can be combined with salbutamol, and delivered using high-flow oxygen or air.

Intravenous steroids are used routinely in both disorders to reduce inflammation, and associated mucosal oedema. Although intravenous steroids are commonly used early in both conditions, there is little evidence that they are more effective given intravenously than orally; however, their onset of action may be more prompt when commenced intravenously. In asthma, they should be continued until the patient's wheeze has largely abated and their lung function, as reflected in measurement of peak flow, has returned to normal. In COPD steroids should be continued for 3 to 10 days. There appears to be no benefit of continuing steroids for longer than 10 days in patients with COPD, at which point the risk of their adverse effects, such as

insulin resistance, myopathy and peptic ulcer disease, outweigh their benefit. Inhaled steroids have been shown to be effective in long-term management of both asthma and COPD and are commonly used after an acute exacerbation. Their role in acute exacerbations is less clear, although it is likely that they may facilitate dose reduction of parenteral steroids and thereby reduce side effects. Budesonide 1 mg nebulized 12-hourly can be commenced in the first 24 hours in ventilated patients.

Lactic acidosis

Lactic acidosis is a recognized complication of moderate to high dose intravenous beta-2 adrenergic agonist therapy, although it may very occasionally be seen with inhaled therapy as well. Lactic acidosis commonly arises during the first 4 to 24 hours of salbutamol infusion, with plasma concentrations of lactate reaching 10 to 12 $mmol.L^{-1}$ when high dose infusions (>10 $\mu g.min^{-1}$) are used. The appearance of a low or decreasing blood bicarbonate concentration is suggestive of lactic acidosis, which should be confirmed by the measurement of blood lactate concentrations. Lactic acidosis can compound a respiratory acidosis or worsen acidosis when $PaCO_2$ values are improving. Lactate levels usually fall rapidly when the infusion rate is reduced or ceased. Also, high lactate levels will usually resolve during the second 24 hours of continued infusions. Lactic acidosis does not usually occur with intermittent nebulized salbutamol but can occur with continuous nebulized salbutamol over several hours.

Lactic acidosis does not appear to be harmful in its own right, but it can compound respiratory acidosis, increase dyspnoea, respiratory distress and fatigue and has been reported to precipitate respiratory failure.[14] In patients with cerebral oedema from ischaemic brain injury as a result of respiratory arrest, it can increase intracranial pressure.

The mechanism by which these drugs cause an increase in the blood concentration of lactic acid is

---

[4] Usually 2.5 or 5 mg.

not clear, but it is not thought to be the result of tissue hypoxia. Fortunately, the development of lactic acidosis does not have prognostic implications in asthma.

Optional therapies

The rationale for adding intravenous salbutamol infusion to continuous or frequently inhaled salbutamol is based upon the premise that some lung units may be so bronchoconstricted that inhaled salbutamol cannot reach them. In practice, and based upon clinical trials, the addition of intravenous salbutamol, or adrenaline, is rarely additive.

The theoretical advantages of aminophylline in COPD or asthma are an augmentation of cardiac and respiratory muscle strength and diuresis. However, because it is a relatively weak bronchodilator with significant side effects such as nausea, tachyarrhythmias and insomnia, and a narrow therapeutic window, its use is frequently limited and there is little advantage to be had.

In patients with unresponsive airflow obstruction due to asthma, 1.2 to 2.0 g of magnesium sulphate infused over 20 minutes is worth considering. Correction of any additional electrolyte disturbance is also important.

The oral cysteinyl leukotriene modifiers zafirlukast, montelukast and pranlukast block the breakdown of arachidonic acid and prevent the formation of bronchoconstrictors leukotriene C_4, D_4 and E_4 in mast cells and eosinophils. They are particularly helpful in patients with aspirin-induced asthma, and as protection from exercise-induced asthma and asthma related to eosinophilic inflammation. Their role in acute life-threatening asthma is not known.

Sodium cromoglycate and nedocromil sodium are inhaled preparations which appear to block IgE-mediated mediator release. Their effect in severe life-threatening asthma is minimal. They are usually used as a steroid-sparing agent in children.

Table 10.3 Contra-indications to non-invasive ventilation

- Inadequate airway protection (decreased level of consciousness or unconscious)
- Vomiting
- Sputum retention and inadequate cough
- Hypoxia not responding to CPAP and high-flow O_2

Non-invasive ventilation (NIV)

In acute exacerbations of COPD, non-invasive ventilation (NIV) has been shown to reduce the requirement for mechanical ventilation, decrease hospital stay and reduce mortality (see Chapter 3).

NIV has a well-established role in COPD and is now used more frequently than invasive mechanical ventilation.[15] NIV is also very effective in acute cardiogenic pulmonary oedema[16] which may co-exist with COPD (which will be discussed later).

Although there is good observational evidence for the use of NIV in acute severe asthma[17] and a brief randomized trial in acute mild to moderate asthma,[18] its role in acute severe asthma has never been established in randomized trials. With improvements in the community management of asthma, which has resulted in a sharp decline in the need for ventilatory assistance, it is unlikely that the role of NIV in asthma will ever be established in randomized trials. Despite this, its use in severe asthma is widely accepted.

The indications for the use of non-invasive ventilation in the two conditions are similar, namely (1) acute hypercapnia, (2) respiratory distress due to airflow obstruction or (3) hypoxia refractory to mask oxygen. Contra-indications to NIV are presented in Table 10.3.

NIV may be delivered by nasal mask, face mask, circumferential face mask or by a ventilation hood. In acute exacerbations, face or circumferential masks are usually preferred rather than nasal masks because higher pressures can be used. Importantly, it should be appreciated that circuits for NIV have

Table 10.4 Usual setting for non-invasive ventilation

	Minimum	Maximum
IPAP (cm H$_2$O)	10	20
EPAP (cm H$_2$O)	5	12.5

IPAP: inspiratory positive airway pressure.
EPAP: expiratory positive airway pressure. Referred to as positive end-expiratory pressure (PEEP) during conventional mechanical ventilation or continuous positive airway pressure (CPAP) if there is no inspiratory assistance.

a single limb, with expired gases being vented from a small orifice at the patient end of the circuit (see Chapter 3).

The choice and fit of interface are important factors in determining how well NIV is tolerated because these factors contribute directly to comfort, the risk of skin injury, the extent of air leak and the generation of claustrophobia. Masks that allow supplemental oxygen, nebulizer administration and concurrent nasogastric feeding are preferable.

Although continuous positive airway pressure (CPAP) alone reduces the work of breathing in airflow obstruction, additional inspiratory pressure support is commonly used. In practice, the maximum inspiratory pressure that can be consistently achieved is rarely much more than 20 cm H$_2$O with 5 cm H$_2$O expiratory positive airway pressure (EPAP) (see Table 10.4).

Although NIV could theoretically increase lung volumes to unsafe levels, in practice hypotension and pneumothorax are very uncommon. This is probably because significant negative intrathoracic pressures are still generated during inspiration, offsetting any reduction in venous return, and maximum airway pressures remain below a safe limit (25 cm H$_2$O). Mask leak usually occurs with pressures above 25 cm H$_2$O.

EPAP and inspiratory positive airway pressure (IPAP) should be titrated to maximize patient comfort and reduce work of breathing. Oxygen should be titrated to a peripheral haemoglobin oxygen saturation (SpO$_2$) target of 94% to 96% or 88% to 94% when chronic hypercapnia is present. The probability of chronic hypercapnia is increased in the presence of moderate to severe obesity, *cor pulmonale*, previous hypercapnia or elevated blood concentrations of bicarbonate on presentation in the absence of diuretic use.

NIV is usually used for short-term ventilatory support (2 to 48 hours) to allow time for bronchodilators and other therapies to improve lung function and reduce the work of breathing. Invasive mechanical ventilation should be considered in patients who fail to show signs of improvement after 24 to 48 hours.

Mechanical ventilation

Mechanical ventilation is not usually instituted until aggressive medical therapy and NIV have failed, or in patients for whom NIV is contra-indicated. In both asthma and COPD, invasive mechanical ventilation is also indicated where there is an inability to adequately clear lower respiratory secretions with or without NIV, usually in patients with COPD.

Asthma. An experienced clinician should, if possible, undertake intubation in patients with severe asthma as the risks of an adverse outcome are increased in anxious and inexperienced hands. Intravenous access, if not already established, is required to administer hypnotics and muscle relaxants but is also essential for the volume resuscitation that is almost invariably required. Induction of anaesthesia should be achieved using judicious doses of drugs, with consideration given to the use of ketamine in preference to propofol because ketamine causes less hypotension and has the added advantage of causing bronchodilatation. It shouldn't be forgotten that prolonged or aggressive administration of beta-2 adrenergic agonists can cause significant hypokalaemia, which if circumstances allow should be corrected before endotracheal intubation. In patients with severe asthma,

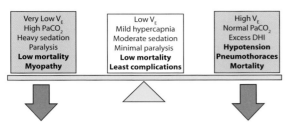

Very Low V_E	Low V_E	High V_E
High $PaCO_2$	Mild hypercapnia	Normal $PaCO_2$
Heavy sedation	Moderate sedation	Excess DHI
Paralysis	Minimal paralysis	**Hypotension**
Low mortality	**Low mortality**	**Pneumothoraces**
Myopathy	**Least complications**	**Mortality**

Figure 10.2 Comparison of the ill effects of excessive ventilation and excessive hypoventilation in mechanically ventilated patients with severe airflow obstruction and the need to achieve a balance between these levels of ventilation. DHI: dynamic hyperinflation.

severe hypercapnia as well as high levels of respiratory distress and respiratory drive are usually present both before and after intubation. Because of airflow obstruction, high peak airway pressures are commonly also present after intubation. For these reasons, a high minute ventilation to reduce hypercapnia and satisfy the patient's respiratory drive, and long inspiratory times to reduce inspiratory flow rates and reduce airway pressures seem logical. However, these ventilatory settings can cause major adverse effects in the patient with severe asthma. Both high minute ventilation and short expiratory times contribute to dynamic hyperinflation with the risk of hypotension and pneumothoraces and has been shown in case series to be associated with a higher mortality.[19] However, although a very low minute ventilation, to minimize dynamic hyperinflation, will eliminate these problems this is usually at the expense of heavy sedation and paralysis, with a high risk of severe prolonged myopathy.[4] Thus a balance between these two approaches should be attempted (Figure 10.2).

At the commencement of ventilation high levels of sedation are often required with or without 1 or 2 bolus doses of a neuromuscular blocking agent (NMBA) to safely establish mechanical ventilation.[4] Ventilation should be initiated with a low tidal volume (≤ 8 mL.kg^{-1}) and a low respiratory rate (8 to 10 breaths.min^{-1}) to ensure that minute ventilation remains ≤ 115[2,3,4] mL.kg^{-1}.min^{-1}

(≤ 8 L.min^{-1} for a 70-kg adult). The inspiratory flow rate should be ≥ 80 L.min^{-1} with an inspiratory time no greater than one second to allow at least four seconds for expiration. The plateau pressure should be measured during a 0.4-second pause following a single breath only. If the blood pressure is low or the central venous pressure high, the effect of disconnection from the ventilator for one minute or two minutes ventilation with a marked rate reduction should be observed. If the plateau pressure is greater than 25 cm H_2O or there is a significant haemodynamic improvement with the manoeuvres described, then the baseline ventilation rate should be decreased. If the plateau pressure is low and blood pressure is satisfactory, then ventilatory support can be increased by either a modest increase in the tidal volume or a modest reduction in the expiratory time, or both.

High peak airway pressures are a consequence of airflow obstruction and high inspiratory flow rate and do not reflect alveolar pressures. Decreasing the inspiratory flow rate with a constant tidal volume and ventilatory rate will decrease peak airway pressure, but the associated reduction in expiratory time will promote dynamic hyperinflation and cause an increase in alveolar pressures that may be unsafe.[2]

Arterial blood gas analysis should be performed regularly. The ventilator rate or tidal volume should not be increased in response to hypercapnia because this also can lead to dynamic hyperinflation. Creatine kinase levels should be measured daily to alert to possible muscle injury (discussed later).

Either volume- or pressure-controlled ventilation may be used as long as the above criteria are met, although in our practice volume-controlled ventilation is preferred.

During volume-controlled ventilation with a short inspiratory time, high peak inspiratory pressures are generated by the high inspiratory flow rates. This is of no concern providing the plateau pressure remains below 25 cm H_2O[3,20] to minimize dynamic hyperinflation. A plateau pressure above 25 cm H$_2$O should prompt a reduction in either tidal volume or ventilator rate, or both, to reduce minute ventilation and dynamic hyperinflation. High peak inspiratory pressures should not be treated by reducing inspiratory flow rate as this will exacerbate dynamic hyperinflation and may cause a dangerous rise in plateau pressure.[2]

In the presence of severe airflow obstruction and a short inspiratory time, pressure-controlled ventilation set to a conventionally 'safe' airway pressure limit of 25 to 30 cm H$_2$O will deliver unnecessarily small tidal volumes. If the pressure limit is set above this to ensure the delivery of more reasonable tidal volumes, then as the airflow obstruction improves this will result in the delivery of excessively large tidal volumes and dangerously high alveolar pressures.

Positive end-expiratory pressure (PEEP) should not be used during controlled ventilation as high levels of intrinsic PEEP will be present and extrinsic PEEP will further increase lung volume.[21]

When airflow obstruction improves, dynamic hyperinflation and plateau pressure will decrease and the ventilatory rate can be increased safely to reduce hypercapnia. At this stage, sedation can be reduced and spontaneous ventilation with low-level pressure support ($\leq$15 cm H$_2$O) can be commenced.

COPD. Patients with severe COPD can have all the complications of dynamic hyperinflation and myopathy; however, unlike patients with severe asthma, patients with an exacerbation of COPD usually only require a moderate amount of ventilatory support. Most can be commenced in volume- or pressure-controlled synchronized intermittent mandatory ventilation (SIMV) mode at a ventilator rate of 6 to 12 breaths.min^{-1} with minimal sedation and no paralysis to allow spontaneous ventilation (Table 10.5). Spontaneous breathing can usually be commenced soon after intubation and should be encouraged by reducing the ventilator rate, adding pressure support of 8 to 16 cm H$_2$O

Table 10.5 Suggested initial mechanical ventilator settings for patients with asthma and chronic obstructive pulmonary disease (COPD)

	Asthma	COPD
Mode	VCV	SIMV[a]
Rate (breaths.min^{-1})	8 to 10	10 to 12
V$_T$ (L.kg^{-1})	$\leq$8	$\leq$8
$\dot{V}_E$ (L.min^{-1}.kg^{-1})	$\leq$115	$\leq$115
$\dot{V}_I$ (L.min^{-1})	70 to 85	70 to 85
I:E	>1:3	>1:3
T$_E$ (s)	$\geq$4	$\geq$4
P$_{plat}$ (cm H$_2$O)	<25	<25
PEEP[b] (cm H$_2$O)	0	5 to 8
Sedation	Usually heavy	Usually mild
NMBA[c]	Minimize*	Rarely required
Spontaneous ventilation	Discourage	Encourage
Course	Await improvement	CPAP[d] ASAP

a: Synchronized intermittent mandatory ventilation.
b: Positive end-expiratory pressure.
c: Neuromuscular blocking agents.
d: Continuous positive airway pressure.

and PEEP of 5 to 8 cm H$_2$O to reduce the work of breathing.

Work of breathing is high for many reasons in airflow obstruction. One reason is that sufficient inspiratory effort must be made to negate the positive alveolar pressure present at the end of expiration (intrinsic PEEP) before inspiratory flow can commence. CPAP is used to reduce that effort by providing a positive airway pressure approximately equivalent to the intrinsic PEEP so that inspiratory flow will commence earlier and with less effort. For this reason, it may be valuable to measure intrinsic PEEP (the airway pressure during transient end-expiratory airway occlusion) and setting the extrinsic PEEP to a similar level. Some patients with severe airflow obstruction have a rapid inspiratory flow requirement that may exceed the ventilator's delivery during pressure support on standard settings. Such patients may benefit from an increased rise time.

Acute necrotizing myopathy

Acute necrotizing myopathy is now a well-recognized complication of patients requiring mechanical ventilation for acute severe asthma,[22,23] and is occasionally seen in patients with COPD. It is believed to be due to the combination of neuromuscular blocking agents and parenteral steroids. While neuromuscular blocking agents are believed to be primarily responsible, it has also been reported in patients with severe asthma receiving steroids and very deep sedation.[24] Acute necrotizing myopathy presents as weakness that usually becomes apparent when neuromuscular blockade is discontinued and sedation weaned. Weakness is both proximal and distal, with reduced or absent reflexes and intact sensation. Weakness can involve both facial and respiratory muscles. The consequences can range from mild weakness to functional quadraparesis. Acute necrotizing myopathy can commence in the first 24 hours, delay weaning from mechanical ventilation, prolong ICU and hospital stay and require rehabilitation. Although weakness will eventually resolve in most patients, patients with very severe myopathy can remain significantly disabled at 12 months.

Acute necrotizing myopathy can be recognized early by rising creatine kinase levels which may range from normal to 10 000 U.L^{-1}. Electromyography is always abnormal. It shows a myopathic pattern, but experience is required for its interpretation because some features can suggest neuropathy. Muscle biopsy is usually not required but if performed will show a characteristic pattern of severe non-uniform myonecrosis with vacuolation and a striking absence of inflammatory infiltrate that is commonly seen in other types of myositis.

There is no specific treatment, and avoidance is the best approach. Neuromuscular blocking agents should be avoided or confined to one or two bolus

---

Table 10.6 Assessment of muscular function

- Peripheral muscle strength parallels the respiratory muscle strength. Observing a patient's capacity to move limbs against gravity is a useful bedside test.
- Assessing the duration of time a patient is capable of maintaining independent ventilation is helpful.
- Assessing a patient's capacity to cough independently is useful (even with tracheostomy).
- Most patients suitable for weaning can raise their limbs against gravity, maintain ventilation independently for >30 minutes and can cough effectively.

---

doses. Infusions should only be used in exceptional circumstances. Steroids should be used in conservative doses, commencing with hydrocortisone 200 mg every 6 hours for a 70-kg adult, with dose reductions commencing after 24 to 48 hours. Inhaled steroids should commence during the first 24 hours to aid reduction of the parenteral steroid requirement. Nutrition and active mobilization should commence as soon as possible.

Clinical assessment of patients with post-ventilation myopathy can be difficult, because many are bed-bound with tracheostomies following a prolonged period of ventilatory support, muscle disuse, high-dose steroids, muscle relaxants, co-existent medical illness and infection or inflammation. Weaning from ventilatory support via a tracheostomy may be dependent upon muscle strength (Table 10.6).

Circulatory collapse

When dynamic hyperinflation is excessive, resulting in end-inspiratory lung volumes near or above total lung capacity, mild hypotension is common. Because lung volumes are large in asthma, unlike acute lung injury, alveolar pressures as low as 25 cm H_2O can significantly elevate mediastinal pressures and cause mild cardiac tamponade, especially if mild hypovolaemia is present.[20] Hypotension is associated with elevated oesophageal and central venous pressure.[2,20] Elevated pulmonary

Table 10.7 Management of haemodynamic instability in patients with severe airway obstruction who require mechanical ventilation

	Mild hypotension	Severe hypotension or EMD arrest
Tidal volume	Low	Low
Inspiratory time	Short	Short
Expiratory time	Long	Very long (2 to 6 breaths.min^{-1} with a PaCO$_2$ >13 kPa[26,27,28,29,30,31])
Fluid loading	Moderate	Marked
Inotropic support	Not required	Yes
ICP	Not required	May be appropriate if patient has suffered a cardiorespiratory arrest prior to mechanical ventilation

Notes

Persistent hypotension or high ICP as a result of hypercapnia consider helium/oxygen mixture[32] or extra-corporeal membrane oxygenation[33] (ECMO).

EMD: electro-mechanical dissociation

vascular resistance due to increased alveolar pressure may also be contributory. In a smaller number of patients severe hypotension, or circulatory collapse with apparent electromechanical dissociation, may occur. This may be due to (1) excessive minute ventilation,[25] (2) unusually severe airflow obstruction so that even 'safe' ventilation causes excessive dynamic hyperinflation,[26] or (3) pneumothorax either as a primary cause of hypotension or as a consequence of 1 or 2 above.

The most common cause of hypotension in a patient with airflow obstruction is dynamic hyperinflation, especially shortly after commencing or changing mechanical ventilation. Whether mild or severe hypotension is present, dynamic hyperinflation can be diagnosed or excluded as a cause by the 'apnoea test', which involves disconnection from the ventilator for at least one minute, followed by resumption of ventilation at a much lower rate[26] (Table 10.7).

Pneumothorax

In patients with severe airflow obstruction, pneumothoraces can arise as a result of (1) excessive dynamic hyperinflation, (2) insertion of central venous access, especially subclavian, or (3) needle thoracostomy for suspected pneumothorax. During mechanical ventilation, such pneumothoraces are always under tension in severe asthma and usually under tension in COPD. This is because the lung does not collapse and the airflow obstruction itself acts as a one-way valve. Small airways expand during inspiration allowing continued air leak and collapse during expiration. This often results in considerable tension with hypotension despite only small or moderate lung collapse on chest radiograph. On occasion, large cysts or bullae are evident on plain chest radiograph and their differentiation from a pneumothorax may be difficult. Concave attachment of the pleura to the chest wall and a similar appearance before and after mechanical ventilation suggest a bulla rather than a pneumothorax, but this may require confirmation with high resolution computerized tomography.

During volume-controlled ventilation, a tension pneumothorax on one side will redistribute ventilation to the contra-lateral lung, thereby worsening its dynamic hyperinflation and risking bilateral tension pneumothoraces with potentially fatal consequences. Clinical diagnosis is often difficult because a tension pneumothorax can be hard to distinguish from excessive dynamic hyperinflation. Both result in hyperinflated, hyper-resonant, lungs with poor air entry. Tracheal shift and asymmetry of breath sounds may also be difficult to diagnose with confidence.

With mild to moderate hypotension, the best course of action is to reduce the ventilatory rate to reduce dynamic hyperinflation and protect the contralateral lung, initiate modest fluid loading and request an urgent chest radiograph. If the radiograph confirms a pneumothorax, a small intercostal catheter should be inserted using blunt dissection only.

A similar course of action is appropriate with severe hypotension, although the intercostal catheter should be placed on the side of the suspected pneumothorax without waiting for radiographic confirmation. Insertion of an intravenous cannula through the chest wall to relieve a suspected tension pneumothorax is hazardous. If a tension pneumothorax is not present, the needle will penetrate the hyperinflated lung and will cause a tension pneumothorax.

If a patient in extremis requires or has had intravenous cannulae inserted through the chest wall, then intercostal catheters should be inserted as soon as possible because pneumothoraces will be present.

Subclavian central venous catheters should be avoided in patients with severe airflow obstruction.

Follow-up

Mechanical ventilation for asthma or an exacerbation of COPD is a life-threatening event and identifies the patient with a high risk of a future deterioration that could result in a repeated episode of mechanical ventilation or death.[27,28] For this reason, patients with either asthma or COPD should receive maximal medical therapy[29] and pulmonary rehabilitation[30] following an episode of mechanical ventilation. Regular follow-up should include regular spirometry, a plan for the management of deterioration and the institution of prevention strategies.

Conclusion

Prevention, early active medical therapy and NIV remain the best ways to manage severe airflow obstruction. Mechanical ventilation should be avoided unless it is unsafe not to do so. If mechanical ventilation is required, care should be taken to assess and minimize excessive dynamic hyperinflation, its complications, myopathy and lactic acidosis.

REFERENCES

1. Crummy F, Naughton M. Non-invasive positive airway pressure ventilation for acute respiratory failure: justified or just hot air? *Int Med J*. 2007;37:112–18.
2. Tuxen D, Lane S. The effects of ventilatory pattern on hyperinflation, airway pressures, and circulation in mechanical ventilation of patients with severe airflow obstruction. *Am Rev Respir Dis*. 1987;136:872–9.
3. Tuxen D, Williams T, Scheinkestel C *et al*. Use of a measurement of pulmonary hyperinflation to control the level of mechanical ventilation in patients with severe asthma. *Am Rev Respir Dis*. 1992;146(5): 1136–42.
4. Douglass J, Tuxen D, Horne M *et al*. Myopathy in severe asthma. *Am Rev Respir Dis*. 1992;146(2):517–19.
5. Little F. Treating acute asthma with antibiotics – not quite yet. *N Engl J Med*. 2006; 354:1632–4.
6. Jalaludin B, Smith M, Chey T *et al*. Risk factors for asthma deaths: a population-based, case-control study. *Aust NZ J Public Health*. 1999;23:595–600.
7. Sturdy P, Butland B, Anderson H *et al*. Deaths certified as asthma and use of medical services: a national case-control study. *Thorax*. 2005;60:909–15.
8. Wasserfallen J, Schaller M, Feihl F *et al*. Sudden asphyxic asthma: a distinct entity?

Am Rev Respir Dis. 1990;142:108–11.

9. Guidelines for preventing health-care-associated pneumonia, 2003 recommendations of the CDC and the Healthcare Infection Control Practices Advisory Committee. *Respir Care*. 2004; 49(8):926–39.

10. Baum G, Schwartz A, Llamas R *et al*. Left ventricular function in chronic obstructive lung disease. *New Eng J Med*. 1971;285:361–5.

11. Serizawa T, Vogel M, Apstein C *et al*. Comparison of acute alterations in left ventricular relaxation and diastolic stiffness induced by hypoxia and ischemia. *J Clin Investig*. 1981;68:91–102.

12. McNicholas W, Fitzgerald M. Nocturnal deaths among patients with chronic bronchitis and emphysema. *BMJ*. 1984; 289:878.

13. Malhotra A, White D. Treatment of oxygen induced hypercapnia (letter). *Lancet*. 2001; 357:884.

14. Tobin A, Santamaria J. Respiratory failure precipitated by salbutamol. *Intern Med J*. 2005;35(3):199–200.

15. Mehta, Hillsurname, S. Noninvasive ventilation. *Am J Respir Crit Care Med*. 2001; 163:540–77.

16. Hill K, Jenkins SC, Philippe DL *et al*. High-intensity inspiratory muscle training in COPD. *European Respiratory Journal*. 2006; 27(6):1119–28.

17. Meduri G, Abou-Shala N, Fox R. Noninvasive face mask mechanical ventilation in patients with acute hypercapnic respiratory failure. *Chest*. 1991;100:445–54.

18. Soroksky A, Stav D, Shpirer I. A pilot prospective, randomized placebo-controlled trial of bilevel positive airway pressure in acute asthmatic attack. *Chest*. 2003;123: 1018–25.

19. Tuxen D. Mechanical ventilation in asthma. In: Evans T, Hinds C, eds. *Recent Advances in Critical Care Medicine Number 4*. London, Churchill Livingstone. 1996:165–89.

20. Williams T, Tuxen D, Scheinkestel C *et al*. Risk factors for morbidity in mechanically ventilated patients with acute severe asthma. *Am Rev Respir Dis*. 1992;146(3): 607–15.

21. Tuxen D. Detrimental effects of positive end-expiratory pressure during controlled mechanical ventilation of patients with severe airflow obstruction. *Am Rev Respir Dis*. 1989; 140:5–9.

22. Douglass J, Tuxen D, Horne M *et al*. Acute myopathy following treatment of severe life threatening asthma (SLTA). *Am Rev Respir Dis*. 1990;141:A397.

23. Griffin D, Fairman N, Coursin D *et al*. Acute myopathy during treatment of status asthmaticus with corticosteroids and steroidal muscle relaxants. *Chest*. 1992; 102:510–14.

24. Leatherman J, Fluegel W, David W *et al*. Muscle weakness in mechanically ventilated patients with severe asthma. *Am J Respir Crit Care Med*. 1996;153:1686–90.

25. Kollef M. Lung hyperinflation caused by inappropriate ventilation resulting in electromechanical dissociation: a case report. *Heart Lung*. 1992;21:74–7.

26. Rosengarten P, Tuxen D, Dziukas L *et al*. Circulatory arrest induced by intermittent positive pressure ventilation in a patient with severe asthma. *Anaes Int Care*. 1990;19: 118–21.

27. Chu C, Chan V, Lin A *et al*. Readmission rates and life threatening events in COPD survivors treated with non-invasive ventilation for acute hypercapnic respiratory failure. *Thorax*. 2004;59:1020–5.

28. Marquette C, Saulnier F, Leroy O *et al.*
     Long-term prognosis of near-fatal asthma.
     Am Rev Respir Dis. 1992;146:76–
     81.

29. Pauwels R, Buist AS, Calverley P *et al.* Global
     strategy for the diagnosis, management and
     prevention of chronic obstructive pulmonary
     disease. NHLBI/WHO Global Initiative for
     Chronic Obstructive Lung Disease (GOLD)
     Workshop Summary. *Am J Respir Crit Care
     Med.* 2001;163:1256–76.

30. Goldstein R, Gort E, Stubbing D *et al.*
     Randomized controlled trial of respiratory
     rehabilitation. *Lancet.* 1994;344:
     362–8.

31. Corbridge T, Hall J. The assessment and
     management of adults with status
     asthmaticus. *Respir Crit Care Med.* 1995;
     151(2):1296–1316.

32. Gluck E, Onorato D, Castriotta R.
     Helium-oxygen mixtures in intubated
     patients with status asthmaticus and
     respiratory acidosis. *Chest.* 1990;98:693–8.

33. Shapiro M, Kleaveland A, Bartlett R.
     Extracorporeal life support for status
     asthmaticus. *Chest.* 1993;103:1651–4.

Chapter **11**

Mechanical ventilation in patients with blast, burn and chest trauma injuries

WILLIAM T. McBRIDE AND BARRY McGRATTAN

Blast injuries

The recent increase in terrorist bomb attacks on urban civilian targets in Europe and the USA has emphasized the need for all relevant health provision team members to become familiar with the pathophysiology and treatment of the resulting injuries. Despite this, many surgeons and intensivists have little direct experience treating blast lung injuries.[1]

The physics of explosions

Explosive devices instantaneously transform the explosive material into a highly pressurized gas, releasing energy at supersonic speeds (high order explosives) or subsonic speeds (low order explosives). High order explosives include Semtex, trinitrotoluene (TNT) and dynamite. Low order explosives include pipe bombs, petrol bombs or blasts caused by aircraft or motor vehicles used as missiles. The net result of any explosion, however, is the blast wave that travels out from the epicentre of the blast.[2]

The blast wave rapidly reaches a peak (3 to 5 atmospheres) and then slowly (2 to 3 minutes) declines to sub-atmospheric pressure. The physical characteristics of the blast wave may be described in terms of velocity, wavelength and amplitude. It is the amplitude of the blast wave that principally deter-

mines the severity of the resulting lung injury. When compared with an explosion in an open space, an explosion within a confined space, such as inside a bus or a train, will have a blast wave that is amplified and more prolonged, resulting in injuries of greater severity and mortality.

The blast wind should be distinguished from the blast wave. The former is the flow of superheated air from the explosion site and can cause superficial burns and internal scalds to the upper airways.

Moving outward from the radius of the explosive, three areas of diminishing primary blast injury have been described (Figure 11.1). The area nearest to the explosion where all victims are instantly killed is called 'the lethal zone'. Beyond this is the 'L-50' limit where 50% of victims will be instantly killed and beyond this is the injury zone in which death does not occur as a result of the primary blast wave, although victims may still sustain significant injury. It is the victims of the L-50 and injury zones who are likely to suffer from blast lung injury[3] (Figure 11.2).

Primary, secondary, tertiary and quaternary injuries

PRIMARY INJURY

As the high-pressure blast wave expands outward at the speed of sound, it interacts with the body, particularly air-containing pockets causing rapid

Core Topics in Mechanical Ventilation, ed. Iain Mackenzie. Published by Cambridge University Press.
© Cambridge University Press 2008.

210

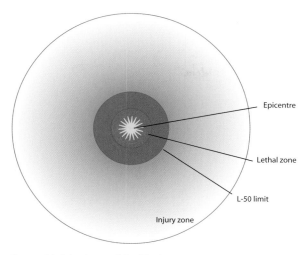

Epicentre

Lethal zone

L-50 limit

Injury zone

Figure 11.1 Anatomy of the blast zone.

compression. As the blast wave passes, there is rapid expansion of these compressed gas pockets causing secondary 'explosions' within gas-containing organs such as the lung, ear and bowel.[2]

As far back as the eighteenth century, respiratory problems were noted among sailors in the British navy who were thought to have been standing too close to a firing canon. The condition was attributed to an adverse effect arising from 'the wind of the shot'. Following World War I, 'air concussion' was described as a specific condition affecting blast victims, although its pathophysiology was not understood.

If the pressure wave hits fluid-containing tissue such as alveolar capillaries, which are relatively non-compressible compared with the relatively compressible gas-filled alveoli, this leads to a pressure differential between the alveolar capillaries and the alveolar spaces and causes fluid to move from the high pressure within the capillaries to the lower pressure within the alveoli. Fluid and blood accumulate within the alveolar spaces, a process which is further enhanced by breaches in alveolar capillary integrity caused by the blast wave itself. Massive rupture of capillaries and extravasation of red cells leads to release of haemoglobin

that is subsequently oxidized to methaemoglobin. This interacts with lipid hydroperoxides to produce ferryl-haemoglobin. This potent oxidant induces tissue damage directly by peroxidation reactions and indirectly by depleting intra-pulmonary anti-oxidant reserves (ascorbate, vitamin E, glutathione). By these and other mechanisms, the clinical picture of worsening respiratory distress rapidly develops.

Tears in small airways under immense pressure may lead to a unique form of air embolism due to alveolar pulmonary venous fistulae through which air passes directly to the pulmonary veins and rapidly to the systemic circulation. Air emboli in the coronary circulation can cause ischaemic changes on the ECG, arrhythmias and sudden death. Indeed, victims who die close to the scene of an explosion may have minimal outward injury but may have succumbed to a coronary artery air embolism. Air embolism of the cerebral vessels may contribute to transient neurological deficit and initial confusion in blast victims.[2]

SECONDARY INJURY

This refers to injuries sustained by the blast wind propelling solid matter into the patient. For example, dust and falling masonry may be blown into the patient's airways causing initial life-threatening obstruction.

TERTIARY INJURY

If the patient is caught in the blast wave and blown into solid matter, tertiary injury may ensue.

QUATERNARY INJURY

This refers to scalds caused by flames, heat or hot gases. This includes external burns or internal burns to upper airway caused by the blast wind.[4] This chapter focuses on blast injuries.

Diagnosis of blast injuries

Blast injury is a clinical diagnosis based on the presence of respiratory difficulty and hypoxia

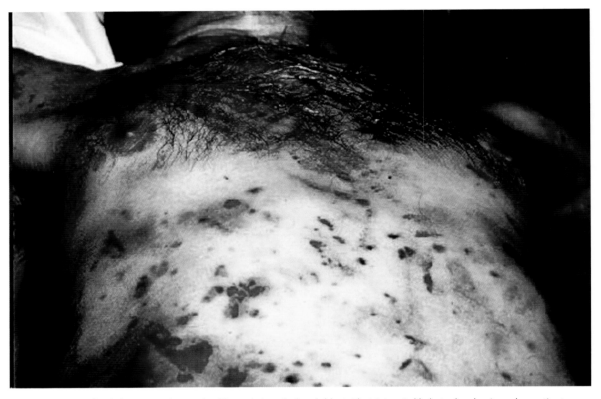

Figure 11.2 Superficial chest wounds sustained by a victim of a bomb blast. Blast injury is likely to develop in such a patient.

with or without obvious external injury to the chest.

The incidence of blast injuries

The wide range in reported incidence of blast injuries among survivors of bombings (see later discussion) reflects the effects of the environment in which the blast took place and the characteristics of the blast wave. In a review of the published literature addressing 220 bombing incidents world wide between 1969 and 1983, there were 3357 casualties and 2934 immediate survivors (87%), of whom 881 (30%) required hospitalization. Of the immediate survivors, 18 (0.6%) had blast lung and 40 (1.4%) ultimately died. Among those who survived the initial blast but then died in hospital, only 3.7% had blast lung, with 52% of these deaths being mainly attributed to head injury.[5] In

contrast to this all-inclusive survey of explosions, bomb blasts in an enclosed space generate a higher amplitude of blast wave and result in a higher incidence of blast injuries. Thus a bus explosion had an incidence of acute respiratory distress syndrome (ARDS) of 33% in immediate survivors,[6] and in a series of bombings in Israel (one in a shopping centre and two in buses) 5.6% of victims presented with blast injuries.[7] Similarly, following a terrorist bomb attack in a packed waiting room of a train station in Bologna, Italy, 9 of 107 bomb victims (8.4%) sustained blast injuries.[8] It should be remembered that variation in the reported incidence of blast injuries may be reflected in the definition of *victim*. For example, in an analysis of 1532 victims of terrorist bombings, only two primary blast lung injury cases were found,[9] but many of these 'victims' suffered emotional trauma only, with the result that the proportion of patients with blast injuries seemed small. Nevertheless, the increasing trend in recent years for bombs being detonated within an enclosed space highlights the importance of early diagnosis and treatment of blast injuries in survivors.

Blast injuries may present as acute hypoxia on admission or may develop over 12 to 24 hours following injury.

Primary blast injuries may cause injuries requiring urgent intervention in the emergency room. Unilateral or bilateral pneumothoraces should be suspected and treated. These arise from disruption of the alveolar integrity by the blast wave.[2] For example, of 15 patients who survived explosions in 2 buses in 1986, 7 presented with bilateral pneumothoraces and 2 with unilateral pneumothorax.[6] A clinically detectable pneumothorax with severe dyspnoea or signs of tension pneumothorax should not await chest radiography before chest drain insertion.

A sucking chest wound also requires immediate care. Disruption of the chest wall leads to an immediate pneumothorax. A conscious patient may discover that breathing is easier if he or she holds her arm over the defect. Emergency treatment involves a square dressing placed over the defect taped down on three edges to allow egress of air but not ingress of air during inspiration, thus allowing negative intra-pleural pressure during inspiration and lung expansion of the affected side. Definitive treatment requires emergency surgical repair of the chest wall.

A bronchopleural fistula may become apparent in the emergency room if a chest drain continues to bubble with expiration in the spontaneously breathing patient. In these patients a bronchopleural fistula is often self-limiting, but it may be persistent in those requiring mechanical ventilation. In one series, a clinically significant bronchopleural fistula occurred in 33% of patients with blast injuries.[6]

Table 11.1 Classification of blast lung injuries			
	Mild	Moderate	Severe
PaO$_2$:FiO$_2$ ratio (kPa)	>27	8 to 27	<8
Lung infiltrates	Localized	Diffuse (unilateral or bilateral)	Bilateral
Pneumothorax	No[5]	Yes/No	Yes

All victims of blast injury should have a chest radiograph. However, in a mass casualty situation clinical findings may have to guide treatment if the hospital radiography resources are overwhelmed. When a chest radiograph is available, bilateral lung opacities are common and have been reported in up to 80% of patients.[6] This may frequently have a 'butterfly' pattern that can arise from direct pulmonary parenchymal injury caused by the blast wave.[1]

The severity of the blast injuries on presentation to the emergency room has been graded into mild, moderate and severe injury based on an initial evaluation of alveolar arterial oxygen gradient, presence of chest radiograph infiltrates and evidence of barotrauma (Table 11.1).

Presenting signs of blast injuries

As with all trauma situations, the basic principles of immediate resuscitation apply.[1] However, in addition, the admitting physician should be aware of transient myocardial ischaemic changes and neurological deficits with confusion linked to air embolism. Common respiratory symptoms may include shortness of breath, chest pain (anginal or pleuritic), cough (secondary to inhaled dust and debris) or haemoptysis reflecting lung parenchymal or tracheo bronchial injury.[2]

---

[1] Well described in the American Trauma and Life Support (ATLS) courses.

Table 11.2 Key elements in the immediate management of blast lung injury

- High-flow oxygen
- Airway management
- Tube thoracostomy
- Mechanical ventilation

Table 11.3 Some causes of the acute respiratory distress syndrome (ARDS)

Direct lung injury	Indirect lung injury
Pneumonia	Sepsis/SIRS
Aspiration	Pancreatitis
Near-drowning	Transfusion-related
Inhalation of smoke/chemicals	Severe burns or trauma
Blast injury	

Immediate examination should be made for signs of cyanosis, breach of chest wall integrity, asymmetrical breathing pattern or loss of breath sounds.

Tube thoracostomy for relief of tension pneumothorax or dyspnoea due to bilateral pneumothorax should not await a chest radiograph. Nevertheless, at an opportune time a chest radiograph will help grade the severity of the blast lung injury.[2]

Treatment

There are four key elements to the immediate management of blast lung injury (Table 11.2). All patients with actual or suspected blast injuries should have supplemental oxygen provided as soon as practicable. Airway problems arise frequently in the emergency room, such as from loss of consciousness secondary to injury or air embolism, from airway oedema secondary to internal burns or scalds, or from haemoptysis.

Insertion of a chest drain – that is, tube thoracostomy – is mandatory in the setting of pneumothoraces. It is recommended prior to general anaesthesia or air transport to avoid tension pneumothorax in an environment where such a complication may be difficult to treat.

Mechanical ventilation may be required if ventilatory failure is imminent but may be unavoidable in patients who require general anaesthesia for treatment of other bomb-related injuries such as limb surgery. The decision to ventilate the patient should be weighed against the immediate risk of alveolar rupture and air embolism. Accordingly, if intubation and mechanical ventilation is required, it is important to avoid excessive airway pressures.

Long-term ventilatory strategy

The emergency conditions attending a response to a bomb blast injury, as well as the stresses on the team caring for multiple victims, make highly impractical the possibility of carrying out randomized controlled trials to assess optimal ventilatory strategy in such emergency situations. Information on optimal ventilatory modes in such patients relies on reports from centres that have cared for such patients. Nevertheless, advances in recent years in optimizing ventilatory modes of patients with acute lung injury (ALI) and ARDS has guided ventilation management in blast injuries patients.

We will therefore consider recent advances in ventilation strategies for ALI/ARDS and describe how this has been applied in the treatment of the severe blast injuries patient.

Ventilation in ARDS

The acute respiratory distress syndrome is a severe form of acute lung injury in which there are diffuse, bilateral pulmonary infiltrates on chest radiography and the $PaO_2:FiO_2$ (PF) ratio is less than 26.7 kPa. The chest radiograph appearance can be identical to that of cardiogenic interstitial pulmonary oedema, so the clinician must be confident that he is not dealing with left ventricular failure. ARDS may result from direct or indirect lung injury (Table 11.3).

Principles of ventilation in ARDS

Although chest radiographs in ARDS patients tend to show widespread lung disease, high-resolution

CT scanning has demonstrated areas of normal, consolidated and over-distended areas of lung. The consolidated areas do not participate in gas exchange and are mostly situated in the dependent areas of the lung. It has been demonstrated that some of these consolidated areas can be recruited using positive pressures with a resulting improvement in gas exchange. This can be maintained with the use of an adequate positive end-expiratory pressure (PEEP).

The ARDS lung typically has a markedly reduced compliance, such that the patient must work hard to breathe spontaneously and the clinician must ventilate at higher pressures to maintain normal gas exchange. Ventilation at higher pressures will unfortunately cause damage to the normal or over-distended areas of lung. These areas will then become abnormal, overall gas exchange will be worsened and lung compliance reduced even further.

The physician's difficulty in the management of the ARDS patient is to balance protection of the normal or over-distended lung with recruitment of the collapsed and consolidated areas. Another problem is that the high concentrations of oxygen required for these patients may be damaging to the ARDS lung. Studies have been carried out looking at protective modes of ventilation in ARDS.

Modes of ventilation in ARDS

Studies of ARDS patients undergoing mechanical ventilation have looked at various combinations of low-volume ventilation with normal or elevated PEEP. The importance of lung recruitment was shown by Amato et al. in 1998.[10]

The ARDSNet trial[11] looked at two groups of patients with ARDS. The first group was ventilated with tidal volumes of 12 mL.kg^{-1} predicted body weight with plateau airway pressures under 50 cm H_2O. The second group was ventilated at tidal volumes of 6 mL.kg^{-1} predicted body weight with plateau pressures under 30 cm H_2O. Survival was significantly greater in the second group, and the

trial was stopped early. This study changed the practice of physicians around the world, but its findings have been challenged as the control group patients were not ventilated according to widespread practice at the time. However, other studies failed to show benefit with low-volume, low-pressure ventilation in ALI/ARDS.[12, 13, 14] These seemingly contradictory findings were the subject of a meta-analysis by Eichacker et al. in 2002.[15] These authors looked at five studies where ALI/ARDS patients were randomized to either a low-pressure, low-tidal volume group or a higher-pressure, higher-tidal volume control group and compared the results. Two studies, referred to as the beneficial studies,[10, 11] showed benefit with the lower tidal volume, lower pressure treatments as compared with the controls. In contrast, three of the studies, referred to as the non-beneficial studies, found no benefit with the lower-pressure, lower-tidal volume treatments, with an insignificant decrease in survival odds ratio in the lower-tidal volume groups.[12, 13, 14] Eichacker showed that the apparent disparity in outcomes could be attributed to the widely differing levels of tidal volume and airway pressures in the so-called 'higher-pressure, higher-tidal volume, control group' used in the five studies. In particular, in the two studies claiming benefit for low-volume, low-tidal volume treatments, the control groups were subjected to a tidal volume of 10 to 12 mL.kg^{-1}, which is higher than most centres would now routinely use. This prompted the suggestion that the survival benefit observed with the lower tidal volumes (5 to 7 mL.kg^{-1}) merely reflected an increased mortality in the control group rather than an improvement with the lower-tidal volume group. By contrast, in the three 'non-beneficial' groups, the control patients were subjected to what are the routinely used tidal volume levels in ALI/ARDS patients (8 to 9 mL.kg^{-1}), while the treatment group was subjected to very low tidal volumes of 5 to 7 mL.kg^{-1}. Failure of benefit in the very low-tidal volume group compared with 7 to

9 mL.kg^{-1}, they argued, may show that lowering tidal volumes to less than 7 mL.kg^{-1} requires further evidence before widespread application because the increased arterial partial pressure of carbon dioxide (PaCO$_2$) and decreased pH may lead to haemodynamic disturbances and a need for muscle relaxation and sedation to ensure patient comfort, interventions that could be unhelpful in long-term care.

These observations led Eichacker to advance the hypothesis that plateau pressures between 28 and 32 cm H$_2$O are optimal for ALI/ARDS patients, with mortality increasing in patients ventilated below or above these ventilatory parameters. However, mortality seems to increase more markedly with pressures over 32 cm H$_2$O than under 28 cm H$_2$O.

More recently, Hager and Krishnan found that inspiratory plateau pressures of 30 to 35 cm H$_2$O are not safe, although they could not identify a safe upper limit for plateau pressures in patients with ALI/ARDS.[16]

With regard to the use of PEEP, physicians have been worried that the adverse cardiovascular effects of increased PEEP outweigh the benefits. The ARD-SNet group studied the effects of low versus high PEEP and found no difference in outcomes between the two groups.[17] However, Amato *et al.*[10] and Villar *et al.*[18] found significant improvement in mortality by using low-tidal volume ventilation with PEEP set 2 cm H$_2$O above the lower inflection point of the patient's compliance curve (plotted using a super-syringe or by serial ventilator measurement at different tidal volumes). It should be noted that the study by Villar *et al.* had a sicker cohort of ARDS patients. A summary of the steps to be taken in setting a ventilator for a patient with ARDS is set out in Table 11.4.

How these methods have been used successfully in blast injuries patients

Many patients with blast injuries go on to develop ARDS. In the Pizov series, 33% of patients developed ARDS.[2, 6] It is reasonable therefore to treat all

Table 11.4 A summary of steps to be taken in setting a ventilator for the patient with the acute respiratory distress syndrome (ARDS)

- Recruit the lung to open collapsed or consolidated areas.[19]
- Set PEEP at an appropriate level for that particular patient's lung as determined by compliance curve assessment (see earlier). This will usually be between 10 and 18 cm H$_2$O.
- Set the FiO$_2$ to the minimum required to produce a PaO$_2$ above 8.5 kPa or SaO$_2$ above 90%.
- Set the ventilator so that the tidal volume or inspiratory pressure are such that plateau pressures do not exceed 32 cm H$_2$0.

patients with moderate to severe initial blast injuries as at high risk of ARDS and use lung protective ventilation methods, as described above, by reducing lung pressures and tolerating a degree of hypercapnia. Several reports highlight the usefulness of this.[1, 7]

As far back as 1998, Sorkine *et al.* highlighted the importance of avoiding high peak inspiratory pressures (PIP), allowing permissive hypercapnia in severe blast injuries. They managed a series of 17 severe blast injuries patients (10 enclosed space and 7 open space explosions), using volume-controlled, synchronized intermittent mandatory ventilation such that

- If PIP exceeded 40 cm H$_2$O, the tidal volume was decreased to maintain PIP under 40 cm H$_2$O.
- Once arterial pH fell below 7.2, the respiratory rate was increased in increments of 2 breaths.min^{-1} until the arterial pH exceeded 7.25. At pH greater than 7.2, no attempt was made to control PaCO$_2$.

Four patients required increased ventilator rate because of pH less than 7.2. They had PaCO$_2$ tensions of 12.4 $\pm$ 1.6 kPa. There was no evidence that the respiratory acidosis arising from such permissive hypercapnia had contributed to renal, hepatic or haematological abnormalities.

Overall, this therapy was effective. Although all patients had low PF ratios as well as pulmonary compliance on admission to the ICU, the PF ratio as well as pulmonary compliance increased gradually up to day six.

Although the authors reported some evidence of ventilator-induced pulmonary barotrauma, the overall survival rate of 88% (15/17) suggested that limiting PIP in a volume-controlled mode is beneficial in blast injuries.[7]

Other methods employed in severe blast injuries include high-frequency jet ventilation, independent lung ventilation, nitric oxide and extracorporeal membrane oxygenation (ECMO). In the ECMO patients, mortality is high.[6]

Judicious fluid administration is an essential component in the management of blast lung injury.[2, 6] In particular, alveolar membranes damaged by the blast wave have increased capillary permeability with the result that over-zealously administered fluid will readily accumulate in the alveolar spaces, further compromising lung function. This is a particular hazard in patients requiring fluid resuscitation for other injuries such as severe limb trauma. In such patients, the initial butterfly pattern of the chest radiograph seen on presentation may over several hours become more pronounced.[1]

Systemic effects of blast injuries

An overall inflammatory response may ensue with electrolyte and coagulation disturbances. In five patients with severe blast injuries in a bus explosion, three out of five developed disseminated intravascular coagulation and four out of five developed significant hypokalaemia (2.2 to 2.9 mmol.L^{-1}) that was responsive to emergency replacement therapy.[20]

Outcomes from blast injuries

Most patients survive mild and moderate blast injuries with severe blast injuries carrying a high mortality.[6] Timely diagnosis and correct treatment result in excellent outcome, at least in the mild

to moderate severity group.[1] It is quite remarkable that for those who survive long term, sequelae are rare, with one 12-month post-injury survey of 11 blast injury survivors showing no pulmonary abnormality.[21] The patients were aged 28 $\pm$ 9.8 years and sustained multiple injuries in addition to the lung injury for which 10 required mechanical ventilation and 6 required chest drainage with ICU admissions lasting 11.8 $\pm$ 9 days and overall hospital stay of 32.4 $\pm$ 27.3 days. One year later, physical examinations, lung function tests and progressive cardiopulmonary exercise examinations showed that none had any pulmonary-related disability.[21]

Burns

Smoke, hot gas, or chemical inhalation injury are the most common cause of acute deterioration in lung function in burn injury patients and should always be suspected. Usually, such injuries are of chemical origin, and if these patients are compared with burn injury patients who did not sustain smoke inhalation injury, a 20% to 70% increased mortality in the smoke inhalation patient is observed.[22]

Incidence and pulmonary complications

A review of clinical and radiological findings in 64 smoke inhalation victims without cutaneous burns indicated that initial *clinical* signs help predict severity of injury and ICU course.

For example, if at initial presentation to the emergency room there were soot deposits in the oropharynx, or the presence of dysphonia or rhonchi, then there was a significant prolongation of ICU stay.

Moreover, dysphonia and rhonchi correlated with positive bacteriological sputum sampling in the first 24 hours, which in turn correlated with prolonged mechanical ventilation. Interestingly, initial chest radiograph signs did not correlate with severity of the clinical course.

Of the 64 patients, 35 required mechanical ventilation (mean 101 hours; range 8 to 648 hours) with 3.1% eventually dying from progressive respiratory failure.[23]

As with internal burns incurred in the blast wind as discussed earlier,[4] upper airway obstruction may rapidly evolve requiring acute intervention to secure the airway. This should be particularly suspected if burn marks are seen in the internal mucous membrane of the mouth and nose. If a blast injury is not involved, then concerns of air embolism attending immediate intubation and ventilation of the blast-injured patient are less pronounced.

If the burn involves the chest wall, care should be taken not to compromise chest wall compliance due to overly tight bandaging of the area. Later, as chest burn healing commences, scar tissue with contraction of body surface tissues can reduce lung expansion with risks of secretion retention and chest infection.

Patients with large burns sustain a massive inflammatory response that can be associated with systemic capillary leakage involving alveolar membrane leakiness. This, in combination with hypoalbuminaemia, can be associated with a rapidly evolving acute lung injury superimposed on any direct injury caused by smoke or chemical inhalation.[22]

Treatment

The principle of ventilatory management of the burn injury patient involves providing oxygen therapy for all burn patients and observing for the occurrence of upper airway obstruction. Should there develop acute upper airway obstruction or deterioration in oxygenation then intubation and ventilation are required. Adequate fluid resuscitation and prevention and treatment of infection are indirect measures that preserve pulmonary function.

Outcomes are improved with rapid resuscitative treatments. This should begin in the pre-hospital environment on arrival at the scene of the emergency crew. Gueugniaud described a care pathway

---

Table 11.5 Care pathway for burn patients (after Gueugniaud 1997)

- Pre-hospital care includes
  - Fluid loading with 2 mL.kg^{-1} for each % surface area burned over the first six hours
  - Sedation and analgesia
  - Prevention of hypothermia
  - Ventilatory support for acute airway obstruction or respiratory distress, extensive burn over 60% of total body surface area, carbon monoxide intoxication, tracheobronchial thermal injury and blast injury
- Care in a general hospital before transfer to a burn centre includes
  - Evaluation of burn and associated injuries
  - Ongoing fluid resuscitation
  - Perform initial emergency local treatment with sterile coverage or vaseline gauze
  - Possible escharotomies
  - Emergency treatment of other injuries
- Care in the burn centre includes
  - Ongoing hypovolaemia management with treatment of later hyperdynamic circulation
  - Definitive care of burned areas: escharatomies, skin grafts, skin substitution therapies
  - Optimizing tissue perfusion and oxygen delivery to burned tissues, as well as to healthy organs. This will involve attention to blood loss as escharotomies are often associated with rapid and large volume blood loss, which is particularly significant in children
  - Maintenance of sedation and analgesia (ICU manipulations may be very painful)
  - Prevention and treatment of infection
  - Maintenance of nutrition

---

for such patients beginning at the pre-hospital environment (Table 11.5): on arrival in the local hospital the patient should be stabilized, followed by transfer to the specialist burns unit where definitive treatment is carried out.[24] If burns patients develop ALI/ARDS, the ventilatory strategies discussed earlier apply.

Chest trauma

Pathogenesis

Pulmonary contusion is a common lesion occurring in patients sustaining severe blunt chest trauma.

Alveolar haemorrhage and parenchymal destruction are maximal during the first 24 hours after injury and then usually resolve within 7 days.

Diagnosis

The diagnosis of traumatic lung injury is usually made clinically with confirmation by chest radiography. The chest computed tomography scan is highly sensitive in identifying pulmonary contusion and may help predict the need for mechanical ventilation. Respiratory distress is common after lung trauma, with hypoxaemia and hypercapnia greatest at about 72 hours. Although management of patients with pulmonary contusion is supportive, pneumonia and adult respiratory distress syndrome with long-term disability occur frequently.[25]

Ventilation in blunt thoracic trauma

Blunt thoracic trauma can result in significant morbidity in injured patients. Both chest wall and the intrathoracic visceral injuries can lead to life-threatening complications if not anticipated and treated. Blunt thoracic trauma is also a marker for associated injuries, including severe head and abdominal injuries.[26]

LUNG CONTUSIONS

The passage of a shock wave through the pulmonary tissue leads to microscopic disruption at the alveolar–air interface. Alveolar haemorrhage and pulmonary parenchymal damage ensues, becoming maximal at 24 hours and usually resolving over the following week. Severe pulmonary contusion may rapidly lead to respiratory dysfunction due to ventilation perfusion mismatch in the injured area

of lung. Complications include pneumonia, ARDS and empyema.

A ventilatory strategy aimed at reducing risk of ARDS in these patents is important and applies as described earlier for blast and burn injuries. However, in 2002 the addition of lung recruitment manoeuvres (open lung concept) was suggested as being helpful.[27] Later, Schreiter applied in chest trauma patients low tidal volumes (≤ 6 mL.kg^{-1}) and positive end-expiratory pressure (PEEP, 5 to 17 cm H_2O) together with briefly applied high inspiratory pressures (mean 65, range 50 to 80 cm H_2O) for opening up collapsed alveoli. Then, external and internal PEEP was used to keep open the recruited lung units. Intrinsic PEEP was maintained by pressure-cycled high-frequency inverse-ratio ventilation^2 and maintained for 24 hours. At that time, the authors assessed the suitability of commencing ventilatory weaning by temporarily reducing respiratory rate to allow a fall in total PEEP. If, following this intervention, the PF ratio was less than 40 kPa, weaning was deferred, but if the ratio was greater than 40 kPa, weaning commenced. The authors described how lung recruitment significantly increased PF ratios as well as decreased atelectasis.[28]

Some centres use bronchoscopically guided bronchoalveolar lavage as a routine treatment in patients with severe traumatic lung contusions. The rationale is that this clears blood clots and secretions reducing infective and inflammatory related secondary lung injury.

REFERENCES

1. Avidan V, Hersch M, Armon Y *et al*. Blast lung injury: clinical manifestations, treatment, and outcome. *Am J Surg*. 2005;190(6):927–31.
2. Sasser SM, Sattin RW, Hunt RC *et al*. Blast lung injury. *Prehosp Emerg Care*. 2006;10(2): 165–72.

---

^{2} 80 breaths.min^{-1} inspiratory:expiratory ratio 2:1.

3. McBride WT. Chest trauma. In: Gosh S, Latimer RD, eds. *Thoracic Anaesthesia: Principles and Practice*. Oxford, Butterworth-Heinemann. 1999:174–88.

4. Ryan J, Montgomery H. The London attacks – preparedness: Terrorism and the medical response. *N Engl J Med*. 2005;353(6):543–5.

5. Frykberg ER, Tepas JJ, 3rd edn. Terrorist bombings. Lessons learned from Belfast to Beirut. *Ann Surg*. 1988;208(5):569–76.

6. Pizov R, Oppenheim-Eden A, Matot I *et al*. Blast lung injury from an explosion on a civilian bus. *Chest*. 1999;115(1):165–72.

7. Sorkine P, Szold O, Kluger Y *et al*. Permissive hypercapnia ventilation in patients with severe pulmonary blast injury. *J Trauma*. 1998;45(1):35–8.

8. Brismar B, Bergenwald L. The terrorist bomb explosion in Bologna, Italy, 1980: an analysis of the effects and injuries sustained. *J Trauma*. 1982;22(3):216–20.

9. Hadden WA, Rutherford WH, Merrett JD. The injuries of terrorist bombing: a study of 1532 consecutive patients. *Br J Surg*. 1978;65(8): 525–31.

10. Amato MB, Barbas CS, Medeiros DM *et al*. Effect of a protective-ventilation strategy on mortality in the acute respiratory distress syndrome. *N Engl J Med*. 1998;338(6): 347–54.

11. The Acute Respiratory Distress Syndrome Network. Ventilation with lower tidal volumes as compared with traditional tidal volumes for acute lung injury and the acute respiratory distress syndrome. *N Engl J Med*. 2000;342(18):1301–8.

12. Stewart TE, Meade MO, Cook DJ *et al*. Evaluation of a ventilation strategy to prevent barotrauma in patients at high risk for acute respiratory distress syndrome. Pressure- and Volume-Limited Ventilation Strategy Group. *N Engl J Med*. 1998;338(6):355–61.

13. Brochard L, Roudot-Thoraval F, Roupie E *et al*. Tidal volume reduction for prevention of ventilator-induced lung injury in acute respiratory distress syndrome. The multicenter trail group on tidal volume reduction in ARDS. *Am J Respir Crit Care Med*. 1998;158(6):1831–8.

14. Brower RG, Shanholtz CB, Fessler HE *et al*. Prospective, randomized, controlled clinical trial comparing traditional versus reduced tidal volume ventilation in acute respiratory distress syndrome patients. *Crit Care Med*. 1999;27(8):1492–8.

15. Eichacker PQ, Gerstenberger EP, Banks SM *et al*. Meta-analysis of acute lung injury and acute respiratory distress syndrome trials testing low tidal volumes. *Am J Respir Crit Care Med*. 2002;166(11):1510–14.

16. Hager DN, Krishnan JA, Hayden DL *et al*. Tidal volume reduction in patients with acute lung injury when plateau pressures are not high. *Am J Respir Crit Care Med*. 2005;172 (10):1241–5.

17. Brower RG, Lanken PN, MacIntyre N *et al*. Higher versus lower positive end-expiratory pressures in patients with the acute respiratory distress syndrome. *N Engl J Med*. 2004;351(4):327–36.

18. Villar J, Kacmarek RM, Perez-Mendez L *et al*. A high positive end-expiratory pressure, low tidal volume ventilatory strategy improves outcome in persistent acute respiratory distress syndrome: a randomized, controlled trial. *Crit Care Med*. 2006;34(5):1311–18.

19. Gattinoni L, Caironi P, Cressoni M *et al*. Lung recruitment in patients with the acute respiratory distress syndrome. *N Engl J Med*. 2006;354(17):1775–86.

20. Melzer E, Hersch M, Fischer D *et al*. Disseminated intravascular coagulation and hypopotassemia associated with blast lung injury. *Chest*. 1986;89(5):690–3.

21. Hirshberg B, Oppenheim-Eden A, Pizov R *et al*. Recovery from blast lung injury: one-year follow-up. *Chest*. 1999;116(6): 1683–8.

22. Gartner R, Griffe O, Captier G *et al*. [Acute respiratory insufficiency in burn patients from smoke inhalation]. *Pathol Biol (Paris)*. 2002;50(2):118–26.

23. Hantson P, Butera R, Clemessy JL *et al*. Early complications and value of initial clinical and paraclinical observations in victims of smoke inhalation without burns. *Chest*. 1997;111 (3):671–5.

24. Gueugniaud PY. Management of severe burns during the 1st 72 hours. *Ann Fr Anesth Reanim*. 1997;16(4):354–69.

25. Cohn SM. Pulmonary contusion: review of the clinical entity. *J Trauma*. 1997;42(5): 973–9.

26. Wanek S, Mayberry JC. Blunt thoracic trauma: flail chest, pulmonary contusion, and blast injury. *Crit Care Clin*. 2004;20(1):71–81.

27. Schreiter D, Reske A, Scheibner L *et al*. [The open lung concept. Clinical application in severe thoracic trauma]. *Chirurg*. 2002;73(4): 353–9.

28. Schreiter D, Reske A, Stichert B *et al*. Alveolar recruitment in combination with sufficient positive end-expiratory pressure increases oxygenation and lung aeration in patients with severe chest trauma. *Crit Care Med*. 2004;32(4):968–75.

Chapter 12

Ventilatory support: extreme solutions

ALAIN VUYLSTEKE

Introduction

One of the extreme solutions for the management of ventilatory failure is to replace the lungs altogether, either by transplantation or by the use of machines. Once the transplant has been completed, the means used to support the new lungs are little different from those used for any other patient. This statement will be a surprise to some because the transplanted lung has necessarily suffered many injuries during transplantation: in practical terms, the question of how best to ventilate a sick lung encompasses the field of lung transplantation. However, transplantation can only be offered to a few patients with the highest chance of survival in order to avoid the waste of precious resources. In the context of severe respiratory failure, other solutions are therefore necessary to provide ventilatory support, either as a bridge to recovery or transplantation, or as long-term support in an increasingly elderly Western population. These solutions are based on various mechanical means that take over some of the lung functions. Despite great advances in technology, these new methods are at present only temporary, intensive and laborious in their implementation and are usually accompanied by a high morbidity and mortality.

This chapter will review some of the key clinical questions concerning the ventilation of the lung transplant recipient and mechanical support of the failing lung.

Lung transplantation

Lung transplantation involves removing one or two lungs from the thoracic cavity and replacing them with similar-sized lungs obtained either from a deceased person or sometimes, in the case of a living donor, only one lung or even part of one. It can be done at the same time as a heart transplant or even as part of a multiple solid organ (lung, heart, liver, kidney, gut) transplant.

As long as the heart is left in place, such operations can be performed without extracorporeal circulation. In this case, the anaesthetist has the problem of conducting single-lung anaesthesia in which the remaining lung is, by definition, poorly functioning and which during part of the operation will be the only means by which to effect gas exchange. The perioperative technique is very similar to that used for pneumonectomy but with a number of important exceptions. First, it may not actually be possible to maintain gas exchange using the remaining sick lung. Second, mechanical ventilation of the diseased lung(s) can cause major haemodynamic instability, most commonly by air being trapped in emphysematous lungs, leading to a decrease in the venous return and loss of cardiac output.

Core Topics in Mechanical Ventilation, ed. Iain Mackenzie. Published by Cambridge University Press.
© Cambridge University Press 2008.

In the immediate post-transplant period, concern is often focused on right ventricular function because of the potential for a significantly increased pulmonary vascular resistance from peri-transplant lung trauma and consequent right ventricular failure. In addition, an inflammatory response to transplantation can lead to the development of all grades of acute lung injury that may affect postoperative recovery. Finally, starting at the time of transplantation, pharmacological immunosuppression has to be continuously adjusted to balance the risks of infection or rejection.

Spontaneous breathing after lung transplant

In the post-transplant period, mechanical ventilation is not usually a problem, providing the large airway anastomoses remain intact and blood is not permitted to accumulate in the pleural cavity. Spontaneous ventilation, however, can be challenged by pain, sedation, diaphragmatic paralysis,[1] or the presence of either a haemo- or pneumothorax. Both continuous positive airway pressure (CPAP) and non-invasive ventilation (NIV) are commonly used in the early stages of recovery. The work of breathing is reduced by keeping the alveoli open, which is helpful if poor organ protection during transfer leads to impaired surfactant production or during episodes of rejection or infection.

Denervation of the lung affects some classical reflexes of interest to the physiologist[2, 3, 4] but has little, if any, impact on clinical management.

Challenges of transplantation

Lung transplantation is a challenging process for both clinician and patient alike. The clinician is challenged by pathophysiological derangements to the graft and the management of immunosuppression, which remains more art than science. The patient, on the other hand, is challenged not only physiologically by a major surgical procedure, but

also by psychological aspects of transplantation peculiar to the lung.[1] Strong social support is an important contributor to a successful outcome.

Despite careful selection and the utmost care, an acute lung injury type response is not uncommon and may arise in a number of ways, including poor mechanical ventilation of the donor, surgical injury during harvesting, poor organ perfusion or protection during transport, or surgical injury during implantation. One of the principle sources of parenchymal damage to the graft arises from acute lung injury arising from the process of lung retrieval. In this respect, new techniques are continuously being evaluated to reduce graft ischaemia between harvest and implantation, which include transportation of the lung on a rig which provides continuous ventilation and perfusion.[5]

Suture lines in the main airway

The large airway anastamoses – inter-bronchial in the case of a single lung transplant and inter-tracheal in the case of double lung transplantation – are at significant risk of ischaemia because the surgeon has to peel away the surrounding vessels in order to place the stitches. Positive pressure ventilation is therefore not usually to blame for *causing* an airway anastomosis leak in the first place but undoubtedly contributes to making a leak larger. If the patient is well enough to breathe spontaneously, mechanical support should be discontinued as soon as possible, but this might be impossible to achieve. Spontaneous closure of an anastomotic leak is unlikely to occur in the presence of positive airway pressure, whatever mode of ventilation is used. Under these circumstances, surgical repair is required, which includes wrapping the defect with a vascularized flap of muscle.

A more common response to perioperative injury than anastomotic break-down or dehiscence is

---

[1] For example, some patients may find it quite difficult to cope with the thought that they might be producing 'someone else's' phlegm.

anastomotic stenosis. This usually occurs several weeks after transplantation and requires treatment with dilation or stenting. While asymptomatic in some, in others this presents as respiratory distress as well as increasing the risk of distal infection.

Pleurodesis

When the donor lungs are well size-matched to the recipient's thoracic cavity, the lungs eventually adhere to the recipient's thoracic cavity. Nevertheless, it is not uncommon for the donor lungs to be oversized, and a lung reduction (i.e. lobectomy) can be performed without affecting the outcome. The main issue in a size mismatch between donor and recipient is the relative diameters of the airways that need to be anastomosed because this renders the operation even more challenging. If the lungs are too small, an increase in pulmonary resistance is likely to occur and the right ventricle may ultimately suffer. The visceral pleura also commonly weep, either as a result of surgical trauma, an inflammatory response, or left ventricular failure; and pleural effusions are not uncommon.

Immunosuppression

Because the entire cardiac output passes through the pulmonary microcirculation, the recipient of a lung transplant is more exposed to foreign antigens borne on the graft than in any other form of solid organ transplant. To avoid developing an immune response to these foreign antigens and rejecting the transplant, the recipient must be given a potent cocktail of immunosuppressant drugs (Table 12.1). Unfortunately the suppression of the immune system is not specific to graft antigens, rendering the recipient uniquely vulnerable to a wide range of pathogenic viruses, bacteria, fungi and protozoa. The management of the patient's immunosuppression is therefore a fine and continuous balance between too little, risking rejection, and too much, risking infection. To further complicate the issue, the clinical and laboratory features of infection and

Table 12.1 Some of the immunosuppressant drugs used to prevent rejection in lung transplantation

Drug	Effect
Methylprednisolone	Inhibits T-cell proliferation by rendering T_H cells unresponsive to interleukin-1 and therefore unable to produce the T-cell growth factor interleukin-2
Rabbit-derived anti-thymocyte globulin (R-ATG)	Antibodies directed against human T cells
Cyclosporine or tacrolimus	Calcineurin inhibitors that interfere with both T-lymphocyte signal transduction and interleukin-2 transcription
Mycophenolate mofetil	Inhibits inosine monophosphate dehydrogenase, the enzyme that controls the rate of synthesis of guanine monophosphate in the *de novo* pathway of purine synthesis used in the proliferation of B and T lymphocytes
Basiliximab or daclizumab	Monoclonal antibodies directed at the interleukin-2 receptors on T cells, which then prevent T-cell activation

rejection overlap to a significant degree, making it very difficult to distinguish between the two with confidence.

Aspiration

A striking finding in patients dying after a prolonged stay in critical care following lung transplantation is the high incidence of gastric content aspiration, often characterized as 'chronic'. This is readily distinguished from fatal large-volume aspiration on the basis of post-mortem histology. Short of feeding all these patients through a jejunostomy or equivalent, the only effective measure likely to decrease the incidence of this problem is to nurse the patient in as upright a position as possible at all times.

Double or single

Mechanical ventilation following single lung transplantation can be tricky because the native and transplanted lungs are likely to have a very different compliance and pulmonary vascular resistance. The simplest solution is to allow the patient to breathe spontaneously as soon as possible and then extubate them. If the patient cannot be allowed to breathe spontaneously – for example, because of surgical bleeding or poor pain control – then special techniques can be used. However, the need to resort to these techniques is strongly associated with a poor outcome.

Independent lung ventilation

By using a double-lumen endotracheal tube with the bronchial extension usually introduced in the native lung to avoid pressure on the fragile anastomosis, one can use two ventilators to ventilate each lung separately. Some ventilators afford this function as part of their complex software, in which case the two ventilators are connected to each other by a special communication cable with one ventilator designated as the 'master', to control and synchronize breath onset and termination, and the second designated as the 'slave'. Each ventilator can then be independently programmed to deliver different oxygen concentrations and different tidal volumes and can have different end-expiratory pressures. The rates will usually be similar or coupled, and this is termed *synchronous* independent lung ventilation. When the respiratory rate, tidal volume, inspiratory flow, positive end-expiratory pressure (PEEP), FiO_2 or ventilatory mode is different between the two lungs, the term *asynchronous* independent lung ventilation is applied. Asynchronous independent lung ventilation does not require specialized software packages and is considered to be less complicated than synchronous independent lung ventila-

tion. Outcome and safety are similar between the two techniques and, in practical terms, independent lung ventilation can be performed with any two machines[2] as long as the pressure can be regulated.

Right ventricular failure

While the lungs are at high risk of failure for multiple reasons, the astute clinician knows that the right ventricle (RV) is particularly at risk. A failing RV will be reflected in a decrease in cardiac output and increase in venous pressure, leading to multiorgan impairment. There is little evidence that any one particular technique of mechanical ventilation can alter the strain on the RV. Conversely, injurious ventilation can both precipitate and exacerbate RV failure.

Treating RV failure usually requires the use of a vasodilator to decrease both RV pre-load and after-load. The effect of positive pressure ventilation or PEEP on RV after-load, expressed as pulmonary vascular resistance, is unpredictable because of the complex interaction between alveolar pressure, hypoxic pulmonary vasoconstriction and oxygenation. Increased airway and alveolar pressures can lead to thinning and compression of pulmonary capillaries resulting in distension of the lung, decreased perfusion and increased pulmonary vascular resistance, ultimately impairing RV function. PEEP may also increase pulmonary vascular resistance. However, if expiration is prolonged, the decreased pulmonary perfusion may be offset by normal thoracic venous return during expiration with no effect on pulmonary vascular resistance. In the presence of lung injury and hypoxia, pulmonary vascular resistance will increase because of pulmonary hypoxic vasoconstriction. Mechanical ventilation may open up vasoconstricted capillary beds by improving oxygenation and therefore

---

[2] Including high-frequency oscillatory ventilation or high-frequency jet ventilation on one side.

improving pulmonary perfusion and pulmonary vascular resistance. When functional residual capacity is decreased at low lung volume, applying PEEP can potentially open up collapsed alveoli, recruiting intra-parenchymal vessels and in turn improving $\dot{V}/\dot{Q}$ matching. Therefore, in some patients positive pressure increases pulmonary vascular resistance, whereas in others its causes pulmonary vascular resistance to fall.

Intravenous vasodilators, such as glyceryl trinitrate or sodium nitroprusside, can worsen the situation by obtunding the hypoxic vasoconstrictive response and worsening hypoxia, leading to poorer RV function due to the resulting ischaemia. The ensuing vasodilatation can also decrease systemic blood pressure and coronary perfusion, leading to further RV ischaemia, despite a decrease in RV strain by a decrease in pulmonary vascular resistance. Inhaled vasodilators, however, reduce RV after-load without causing a deterioration in $\dot{V}/\dot{Q}$ matching because they are, by definition, only delivered to alveoli that are ventilated. Inhaled vasodilators often lead to a transitory improvement in $\dot{V}/\dot{Q}$ matching as observed by improved gas exchange. While nitric oxide was the 'gold standard', it appears that it might do more harm than good, and other agents such as nebulized iloprost[3] are now preferred. It is important to realize that initiating inhaled nitric oxide usually means prolonging ventilation times because it takes time to wean the nitric oxide off, and it can't be given effectively in an extubated patient.

Attention to detail is paramount in these situations, and there is no definite recipe for success. Understanding the mechanism in a specific patient is greatly facilitated by the use of both a pulmonary artery catheter, allowing measurement of pulmonary vascular resistance, and echocardiography, allowing evaluation of ventricular contractility

and ventricular filling. Further adjustments include monitoring and evaluating the need to maintain the acid-base equilibrium within physiological limits. Acidosis will impair cardiac function and decrease the effectiveness of inotropic support. Respiratory acidosis might have to be accepted as part of the ventilatory strategy or as an inevitable result of the underlying disease impairing carbon dioxide removal. Metabolic acidosis can be a result of low perfusion or oxygenation. Correction with bicarbonate can be beneficial in some situations, but if ventilation is impaired, the additional bicarbonate will combine with plasma hydrogen ions and increase carbon dioxide production. If the carbon dioxide is retained, the acidosis will only get worse.

Other methods of lung support

Extracorporeal membrane oxygenation (ECMO)

When the lungs have failed, and new ones are not immediately available, or a transplant is not suitable, it is possible to use extracorporeal membrane oxygenation (ECMO).[6] By diverting the blood outside the body and passing it through a device that allows gas exchange, gas exchange can be controlled relatively precisely. In the past, oxygen was simply bubbled through the blood. This was shown to be unsatisfactory because of problems including protein denaturation, blood trauma, coagulation defects and microembolization. Nowadays, gas exchange is affected across gas-permeable membranes with a surface area of 0.5 to 3 m^2. While the large surface area permits efficient gas exchange, it also provides a large surface for activating both inflammatory and haemostatic responses. Modern membranes have been designed to minimize these problems. Nevertheless, despite these technological advances, systemic anticoagulation is still required. Although these modern membranes are much more efficient than they were even 10 years ago, they still require very large blood flows to

---

[3] A synthetic analogue of prostaglandin PGI_2, more commonly referred to as *prostacyclin*, prepared as a solution for inhalation.

provide the necessary gas exchange, especially when the patient's metabolic demands have been increased by stress and sepsis. These large blood flows require very large efferent[4] and afferent[5] cannulae, with an inherent risk of bleeding at the insertion site and vessel wall damage.

The risks linked to the insertion of the cannulae, which in most cases can be inserted percutaneously, and the fact that these techniques work best in 'expert' hands, usually limits their availability to centres versed in cardiopulmonary bypass for surgical purposes. To date, these are usually only used as rescue therapies, and it is still unknown if ECMO is indicated in the treatment of adult patients. Major trials are under way to assess the efficacy of ECMO in adult patients. The answers may be as complex as the questions, and several trials will probably be required to ascertain if ECMO should or should not be offered and to define whether it should be introduced early or late in new therapeutic algorithms.

Interventional lung assist

Conventional ECMO uses pumps to draw blood from a large central vein, push it through the membrane oxygenator and return it under pressure to the patient's arterial circulation. A much simpler form of ECMO uses the patient's own blood pressure to provide the driving force, drawing blood from the patient's arterial system and returning it to their venous system. This has been made possible by advances in material engineering resulting in highly efficient membranes with very low resistance to blood flow,[7] such as the Novalung®.

These systems are easier to use than the classical ECMO circuit, but have a number of significant drawbacks. First, they offer only partial exposure of the blood to the gas flow and, although equipped with highly efficient membranes, can only be used to remove carbon dioxide, rather than oxygenate.

Second, because the device acts as a massive arterio-venous shunt it makes significant demands on the patient's cardiac reserve. This makes it unsuitable for patients with haemodynamic instability or those whose cardiac reserve is limited by poor left ventricular function or valve problems. Finally, the need for large-bore cannulae in the femoral artery and vein carries the risk of venous thrombosis and leg ischaemia. Anticoagulation or platelet inhibition is advisable in using these devices, and the manufacturer's recommendations should be adhered to. There have been reports of patients surviving with these devices in cases where anticoagulation was contra-indicated.

These systems can be used as a short-term measure in specific cases and initial results are encouraging, mainly when patients need to be transported. They have been used successfully to transport military casualties. Studies are however needed to confirm their benefit[8] because controversy regarding their true efficiency is emerging.[9]

What to do with ventilation of the lungs during extracorporeal support

The best form of mechanical ventilation when using extracorporeal circulation has not yet been identified. Ideally the lung should be rested,[10] but how to achieve this efficiently has not been established. In partial support, the lung still needs to participate in gas exchange. Great care must be taken in not further injuring lungs which are already very sick, but the means to achieve this are still controversial. Using low-pressure, low-tidal volumes and maintaining (some) alveoli open is a valuable objective.[11]

Artificial lungs

The quest for an artificial lung is ongoing. So far, various attempts have resulted in the development of devices, either intravascular or para-corporeal, that are efficient at removing carbon dioxide but very poor at oxygenation. These devices may be important for the growing number of older people

---

[4] Inserted into large central veins, such as the inferior vena cava.
[5] Inserted into the aorta or both femoral arteries.

presenting with chronic lung conditions, but their use is limited for patients with acute lung disease.

Technology is however catching up, and the first devices capable of both carbon dioxide removal *and* oxygenation have now been designed.[12] However, challenges remain and are mainly related to the anatomical constraints of placement in the body or in major blood vessels.

Partial liquid ventilation

A fascinating, if unconventional, mode of ventilation is liquid ventilation. Partial liquid ventilation, on which much of the existing research has concentrated, requires a partial filling of the lungs with perfluorocarbons (PFCs) and ventilation with conventional mechanical ventilators. PFCs are compounds derived from hydrocarbons by replacement of hydrogen atoms with fluorine. Short chain PFCs are gases, but longer chain PFCs are volatile liquids that are denser than water. PFCs are not absorbed from the lung but remain in the alveoli, splinting them open. Their high solubility for oxygen and carbon dioxide allows gas exchange to occur at the air–liquid interface as well as the alveolo-capillary membrane. Total liquid ventilation is equivalent to immersion in the PFC and has been demonstrated to be viable in animals. It is not as practical in humans because it requires a liquid-filled tube system that contains pumps, heater and membrane oxygenator to deliver and remove tidal volume aliquots of conditioned perfluorocarbons. The lungs are usually filled with a volume equivalent to functional residual capacity and ventilated with standard equipment.

The physico-chemical properties of PFCs, such as stability, biological inertness, low diffusion rate and high gas solubility make them ideal agents. However, there may be an issue of environmental contamination because PFCs are exhaled unchanged and remain inert for a very long time. In babies, some studies have shown that partial liquid ventilation can result in a dramatic improvement in lung compliance and oxygenation with a reduction in mean airway pressure and oxygen requirements. It has shown promise for lung lavage procedures, pulmonary image enhancement and pulmonary administration of drugs. There are no long-term side effects reported in the baby.[13]

There is no evidence from randomized controlled trials to support or refute the use of partial liquid ventilation in adults or children with ALI or ARDS,[14, 15] and adequately powered, high quality randomized controlled trials are still needed. Clinically relevant outcome measures should be assessed, especially duration of respiratory support, length of hospital stay and hospital survival, as well as long-term cognitive function, quality of life and survival.[14] It is intriguing that these studies have not yet been done because PFCs have been around for many years.

SUMMARY

Extreme solutions to ventilation support include lung transplantation and the use of mechanical devices. Sadly, none of these are providing a good solution as (1) transplantation is only available to a few, and (2) mechanical support is still facing many technological and physiological challenges.

Standard manoeuvres to support the failing lungs are required in supporting those patients, and there is to date no 'magic recipe' to save them all.

REFERENCES

1. Ferdinande P, Bruyninckx F, Van Raemdonck D *et al*. Phrenic nerve dysfunction after heart-lung and lung transplantation. *J Heart Lung Transplant*. 2004;23(1):105–9.

2. Mitrouska I, Bshouty Z, Younes M *et al*. Effects of pulmonary and intercostal denervation on the response of breathing frequency to varying inspiratory flow. *Eur Respir J*. 1998;11(4):895–900.

3. Iber C, Simon P, Skatrud JB, Mahowald MW *et al*. The Breuer-Hering reflex in humans. Effects of pulmonary denervation and hypocapnia. *Am J Respir Crit Care Med*. 1995;152(1):217–24.

4. Lofaso F, Simonneau G, Ladurie FL *et al*. Frequency of mechanical ventilation and respiratory activity after double lung transplantation. *Respir Physiol*. 1993;92(3): 319–27.

5. Steen S, Ingemansson R, Eriksson L *et al*. First human transplantation of a non-acceptable donor lung after reconditioning ex vivo. *Ann Thorac Surg*. 2007;83(6): 2191–4.

6. Lim MW. The history of extracorporeal oxygenators. *Anaesthesia*. 2006;61(10): 984–95.

7. Bein T, Weber F, Philipp A *et al*. A new pumpless extracorporeal interventional lung assist in critical hypoxemia/hypercapnia. *Crit Care Med*. 2006;34(5):1372–7.

8. Walles T. Clinical experience with the iLA Membrane Ventilator pumpless extracorporeal lung-assist device. *Expert Rev Med Devices*. 2007;4(3):297–305.

9. Zick G, Frerichs I, Schadler D *et al*. Oxygenation effect of interventional lung assist in a lavage model of acute lung injury: a prospective experimental study. *Crit Care*. 2006;10(2):R56.

10. Deslauriers J, Awad JA. Is extracorporeal CO_2 removal an option in the treatment of adult respiratory distress syndrome? *Ann Thorac Surg*. 1997;64(6):1581–2.

11. Ventilation with lower tidal volumes as compared with traditional tidal volumes for acute lung injury and the acute respiratory distress syndrome. The Acute Respiratory Distress Syndrome Network. *N Engl J Med*. 2000;342(18):1301–8.

12. Zwischenberger BA, Clemson LA, Zwischenberger JB. Artificial lung: progress and prototypes. *Expert Rev Med Devices*. 2006;3(4):485–97.

13. Sehgal A, Guaran R. Liquid ventilation. *Indian J Chest Dis Allied Sci*. 2005;47(3):187–92.

14. Davies MW, Fraser JF. Partial liquid ventilation for preventing death and morbidity in adults with acute lung injury and acute respiratory distress syndrome. *Cochrane Database Syst Rev*. 2004(4): CD003707.

15. Davies MW, Fraser JF. Partial liquid ventilation for preventing death and morbidity in paediatric acute lung injury and acute respiratory distress syndrome. *Cochrane Database Syst Rev*. 2004(4):CD003845.

Chapter 13

Heliox in airway obstruction and mechanical ventilation

HUBERT TRÜBEL

Heliox, a mixture of helium and oxygen, was used by Barach in New York for the first time in the treatment of asthma and upper airway obstruction[1] after its introduction to deep sea diving. Since then it has been used not only as a rescue medication in emergency situations for spontaneously breathing patients with airway obstruction but also as the driving gas for mechanical ventilators. The increasing interest in heliox is indicated by the rising number of publications in recent years (Figure 13.1). In this chapter, theoretical considerations, the application of heliox in non-intubated (e.g. with upper and lower airway obstruction) as well as in ventilated patients will be outlined, followed by a brief overview of potential risks, costs and future applications.

Theoretical considerations

In a medical setting, the inhaled gas mixture usually consists of air with a variable oxygen content up to a fractional inspired oxygen concentration (FIO_2) of 1.0 and in some cases with the addition of nitric oxide (NO) or other medications in small amounts. Heliox is a commercially prepared mixture of helium and oxygen.[1] Helium is a non-toxic, tasteless and odourless gas with a low solubility in

fatty tissue. It can be used up to a fractional inspired helium concentration (FIHe) of 0.79 with an FIO_2 of 0.21. Helium was first discovered in 1868 by the French astronomer Janssen and later that year identified by the Englishman Lockyer in the spectrum of the sunlight before its identification as an element in natural gas in 1895 by the British chemist Ramsay. Natural gas still remains the only source of today's helium supply. Its separation from other components of natural gas and its purification for use in patient care makes it expensive when compared with oxygen. Helium possesses physical properties that make it specifically suitable for an application in certain medical conditions like airway obstruction.

The flow pattern of a gas is dependent on the Reynolds number (RN):

$$\text{Reynolds number} = \frac{4}{\pi \cdot D} \times \frac{\rho \cdot \dot{V}}{\mu}. \quad (13.1)$$

Where ρ is the density of the inspired gas, $\dot{V}$ is gas flow, μ is gas viscosity, and D is the airway diameter. Under conditions in which the RN is below 2000, gas flow will most likely be laminar; with an RN between 2000 and 4000, the gas flow will have turbulent components (transitional gas flow); and with an RN above 4000, turbulent gas flow will prevail. With gas flow in a tube of a specific diameter, Equation 13.1 tells us that the RN, and therefore the chance of turbulent flow, is proportional to the

Core Topics in Mechanical Ventilation, ed. Iain Mackenzie. Published by Cambridge University Press.
© Cambridge University Press 2008.

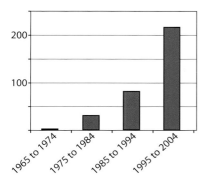

Table 13.1 Density and viscosity of different medical gases[4]

Gas	Density, ρ (kg.m^{-3})	Viscosity, μ (N.s.m^{-2})
Oxygen	1.33	20.1×10^{-6}
Nitrogen	1.17	17.9×10^{-6}
Helium	0.17	19.4×10^{-6}
20% oxygen, 80% nitrogen	1.20	18.3×10^{-6}
40% oxygen, 60% nitrogen	1.23	18.8×10^{-6}
20% oxygen, 80% helium	0.40	19.5×10^{-6}
40% oxygen, 60% helium	0.63	19.7×10^{-6}

density and flow of the gas but inversely proportional to the viscosity. In comparison to nitrogen, helium is seven times less dense (Table 13.1); this lower density reduces the chance of turbulent gas flow when heliox is used instead of air. Using special techniques, the profile of a turbulent gas flow can be visualized. This shows areas where flow is directed perpendicular or even at 180° to the principle axis of gas flow, thereby causing friction and hindering flow. Because a turbulent gas flow needs a higher driving pressure than a laminar one, the use of heliox will reduce the work of breathing in both ventilated and spontaneously breathing subjects alike and is therefore potentially rewarding. This concept only holds true when a turbulent gas flow can be changed to a transitional or even laminar flow by reducing its RN. The large airways down to the 5th or 6th generation are the most likely points where a turbulent gas flow is prevalent at all times. Currently, it is not known if the transition from turbulent to laminar flow occurs at this point or if it only occurs after the inspired gas has entered the bronchioles (after the 11th airway generation). If the latter is the case, the application of heliox in small airway disease, such as asthma or chronic obstructive lung disease (COPD), would be without benefit, which has been found by some[2] but not others,[3] possibly for different reasons. The branching pattern of the airways, the influence of age-dependent

factors on airway diameter and respiratory rate, and an incomplete understanding of the fluid dynamics make it difficult to predict the dominant gas flow pattern in an individual patient. Therefore, benefit from the use of heliox is also difficult to predict. Taking only the reduction in RN into account, conditions resulting in upper airway obstruction such as post-extubation laryngeal swelling, croup, or epiglottitis appear to benefit most from the application of heliox.

Besides its influence on RN, the density ρ of a gas also affects the driving pressure for a given gas flow under turbulent conditions[4, 5]:

$$\Delta P = C_t \cdot \rho \cdot \dot{V}^2, \qquad (13.2)$$

where ΔP is the pressure gradient driving gas flow, C_t is a constant, ρ is the density of the inspired gas, and $\dot{V}$ is the gas flow. This means that even with an entirely turbulent gas flow, a reduction in the density of the inspired gas mixture requires a smaller driving pressure to achieve the same inspiratory gas flow.[4]

Heliox also provides other benefits. For example, heliox-driven nebulizer treatment has been shown to improve the delivery of inhaled medications into small airways[6] due to optimal aerosol particle formation and deposition. Heliox has also been shown to enhance the elimination of carbon dioxide.[7] These additional factors may contribute to the effectiveness of heliox in patients with small airway disease. In summary, heliox can reduce the driving pressure needed to move a gas flow across the airways due to its low density. Further factors might also play a role in its effectiveness in small airway disease.

Application in non-intubated patients

Until recently, heliox was mainly viewed as a rescue medication in certain conditions affecting the upper and lower airway in which the gas could be delivered via face mask or nasal cannulae from a gas tank at the bedside in order to avoid mechanical ventilation. In general, disease originating from the calibre of the airways seems to be more amenable for the application of heliox than conditions that affect the pulmonary parenchyma. Because heliox is supplied in fixed proportions, the addition of oxygen for patients with increased oxygen requirements has usually required the modification of available gas blenders. Recently, commercially available blender devices have made it possible to add oxygen to achieve a controlled and accurate concentration of oxygen in heliox ranging from 21% to 99%. Physicians now have the option to titrate F_IHe to the need of the patient or to obtain maximum effect with minimal usage of gas.

As described earlier, heliox use in non-intubated patients seems to be of particular benefit in conditions affecting the larger airways. A large body of literature can be found with respect to the use of heliox in patients with upper airway obstruction, e.g. post-extubation stridor or viral croup.[8]

For lower airway obstruction, the literature is divided, with some authors finding evidence of benefit[6, 7, 9–11] and others not.[3, 12, 13] Since the effects of heliox are short-lived, some authors feel that a 'trial and error' approach is warranted, especially when performed in an intensive care setting where the adequate monitoring of vital signs is readily available.[14]

When using heliox in respiratory disorders, it is important to bear in mind the potential end-point.

For example, if a condition is likely to respond rapidly to therapeutic manoeuvres such as corticosteroids or irradiation for an anterior mediastinal lymphoma or an airway stent in a patient with a bronchial tumour, a clear indication for a trial of heliox can be seen. However, if intubation and mechanical ventilation seem unavoidable – for example, in a patient with respiratory failure because of a severe pulmonary infection or because of a defective respiratory drive – the use of heliox is unlikely to avoid the need for intubation and mechanical ventilation if those are the intended end-points of its use.

Besides the location of the airway obstruction, another crucial consideration is the mode of delivery to non-intubated patients. Since entrainment of room air will dilute the effective component, a tight-fitting non-rebreathing face mask[15] or even a face mask in combination with non-invasive ventilation system seems desirable. In certain circumstances, such as with non-co-operative patients or small children, this approach is not feasible and therefore heliox must be delivered by nasal cannula or head hood. According to some authors, an increased oxygen requirement ($F_IO_2 > 0.4$) is considered a contra-indication for the use of heliox even though prospective studies addressing this issue are lacking.[5] However, this may not be the case because heliox has been shown in a number of reports to reduce the F_IO_2 required to maintain high pulse-oximetry saturations.[16]

Application in ventilated patients

Since the care of ventilated patients necessitates the use of a ventilator, certain issues involved in the use of heliox as a component of the inhaled gas mixture have to be taken into account. First, since patients with oxygenation problems might need a higher F_IO2 than provided by heliox, the addition of supplemental oxygen will be needed at times. This gas mixture is analogous to the blending of oxygen in air during regular mechanical ventilation,

Table 13.2 The effect of heliox as the driving gas in different ventilators on displayed FIO_2 and V_T

Ventilator	Company	FIO_2 delivered/ FIO_2 set	V_T delivered/ V_T set
Servo 900C[19–22]	Maquet	1	>1
Servo 300[19,20,22]	Maquet	1	~1
Servo-i[23]	Maquet	1	<1
Veolar FT[20]	Hamilton	1	>1
Galileo[20]	Hamilton	1	>1
Evita 2[20]	Draeger	<1	>1
Evita 4[20,21]	Draeger	<1	≫1
Puritan-Bennett 7200[21]	Nellcor/Tyco	≫1	≪1
Inspiration[23]	eVent Medical	1	>1
Bird VIP[22]	Bird/Viasys	1	≫1
Bird VIP Gold[22]	Bird/Viasys	1	≫1
Bear 1000[21]	Bear Medical/ Viasys	≫1	≫1
Avea[a]	Viasys	1	1

[a] Information provided by Viasys Healthcare.

and indeed heliox is often delivered to the ventilator through the air inlet. The FiHe can vary between the maximum of 0.79 down to 0 in a patient with a large oxygen requirement. It is important to realize that the density of the resulting gas mixture will vary depending on the exact proportion of helium and oxygen.

Second, it should be remembered that because of the effect of helium in reducing the density of the inhaled gas mixture, the driving pressure required to deliver a given tidal volume will be less than when using oxygen in air (see Equation 13.2). Consequently, in a pressure-controlled mode of ventilation the delivered tidal volume will increase when switching from an air/O_2 mixture to a heliox/O_2 mixture, with the increase being proportional to the FiHe.

Third, ventilators using either a Fleisch-type pneumotachograph or a hot wire anemometer to measure gas flow and delivered tidal volume[2] will either under- or over-estimate both flow and volume[3]

when using a heliox/O_2 mixture (Table 13.2). When the fraction of helium (FiHe) and oxygen (FiO$_2$) are known, and therefore the density of the gas mixture is known, the correct tidal volume can be calculated. Some ventilators with a pneumotachograph have such an algorithm incorporated into their software. Most ventilators, however, do not have such an automated algorithm and the use of heliox with these machines puts the patient at risk of receiving higher tidal volumes than intended, possibly leading to volutrauma.

Finally, in most ventilators the delivered FIO_2 is calculated from the relative flows of the gases in

---

[2] By real-time calculation of the area under the flow/time profile.

[3] The Fleisch pneumotachograph estimates gas flow by measuring the pressure difference on either side of a fine

mesh. The pressure drop, however, is also dependent on the density of the gas mixture. With a heliox/O_2 mixture, the pressure drop across the mesh is much less than it would be for an air/O_2 gas mix at the same flow rate because of the much lower density of the heliox/O_2 mixture, causing the pneumotachograph to *under-estimate* the gas flow. A hot wire anemometer estimates gas flow by measuring the electrical resistance of heated wire. Because resistance is proportional to temperature and the temperature of the wire is inversely proportional to the gas flow (which cools it), gas flow can be estimated by changes in the electrical resistance of the wire. However, helium's thermal conductivity is six times higher than that of either oxygen or nitrogen and therefore a mixture containing helium will cool the wire much more effectively at any given flow, causing the hot wire anemometer to *over-estimate* the gas flow.

Table 13.3 Clinical trials of heliox in ventilated patients with chronic obstructive pulmonary disease (COPD) and asthma

First author	Year	n	Ventilator	Study duration	Outcome
				COPD	
Jolliet[24]	1999	19	Veolar	<1 hr	RR↓, V_T↑, $PaCO_2$?
Jaber[25]	2000	10	Horus	<1 hr	WOB↓, pH↑, $PaCO_2$↓
Tassaux[10]	2000	23	Servo 300, Veolar	2 hrs	iPEEP↓, trapped gas↓, P_{peak}↓, CO↔
Jolliet[26]	2003	10	Servo 300	2 hrs	iPEEP↓, P_{peak}↓, $\dot{V}/\dot{Q}$↔
Diehl[27]	2003	13	?	2 hrs	iPEEP↓, P_{peak}↓, WOB↓
Jolliet[18]	2003	123	Servo 300, Veolar		ICU and hospital LOS↓, fewer intubations
Lee[28]	2005	25	Servo 300	2 hrs	iPEEP↓, trapped gas↓, PP↓, CO↑
				Status asthmaticus	
Schaeffer[9]	1999	11	Servo 900c	1.5 hr	Aa-gradient↓
Abd-Allah[29]	2003	28	Servo 900c	71 hr	P_{peak}↓, pH↑, $PaCO_2$↓
Watremez[30]	2003	9	Servo 900c	<1 hr	WOB↓, P_{peak}↓, $\dot{V}/\dot{Q}$↔, pH↓, $PaCO_2$↑

Aa-gradient: alveolar–arterial partial pressure of oxygen gradient; CO: cardiac output; LOS: length of stay; $PaCO_2$: arterial partial pressure of carbon dioxide; P_{peak}: peak inspiratory pressure; PP: pulsus paradoxus, $\dot{V}/\dot{Q}$: pulmonary ventilation and perfusion; V_T: tidal volume; WOB: work of breathing.

the inspired gas mixture, rather than measured with a Clark type polarographic electrode. When heliox is used instead of air, the flow of heliox contributing to the gas mixture cannot be measured correctly (for the reasons mentioned earlier), leading to the calculated FIO_2 being either too high or too low. Table 13.2 summarizes bench studies of the ventilators that can deliver heliox and shows that most display incorrect values for V_T and FIO_2. Currently, only a few delivery systems are equipped with software that automatically corrects for the errors mentioned earlier, some of them being equipped for the ventilation of intubated patients (Avea® by Viasys, Inspiration® by eVent Medical) and two for non-invasive ventilation (Aptaér®-Heliox by GE Healthcare, Helontix® by Linde Gas Therapeutics). Other companies (Hamilton, Maquet, etc.) will enter the market with ventilators equipped to use heliox in 2008.

With the problems mentioned earlier and the hazards in mind, it is surprising that several authors using heliox with different ventilators could show positive short-term effects on different pulmonary and haemodynamic variables. A number of studies are summarized in Table 13.3. The focus in these studies was patients with lower respiratory disease with different degrees of bronchial obstruction. Among these studies is also one publication that could demonstrate the cost-effectiveness of heliox. Taken together, the studies that used heliox in ventilated subjects uniformly show positive effects on physiological parameters as well as clinical outcome, in contrast to the studies in non-intubated patients. This view is further supported by an animal study of acute lung injury that demonstrated a reduction in the inflammatory response using heliox compared with a nitrogen/O_2 mixture.[16] This study suggests that further work is required on the use of heliox, not only in diseases with airway obstruction but also in conditions with primarily injured lung tissue.

Potential risks and side effects

A major hazard associated with heliox is its use in the 'wrong' patient, either because of an inappropriate end-point (see earlier) or in a disease process in which airway obstruction is not the main problem, such as in a patient with a depressed respiratory drive. Especially in the latter case, both time and money can be wasted by not pursuing the correct therapeutic strategy.

Another risk that can be associated with the use of heliox is hypoxia. Therefore, when heliox is used it is mandatory to be able to deliver an accurately blended heliox/O_2 mixture and to monitor the patient for adequate oxygenation in an intensive care environment.[17] Separation of helium and oxygen in a heliox cylinder has been reported as a potential hazard,[17] but we could not find any evidence of separation when measuring the oxygen content of heliox cylinders over several months (unpublished data). Nevertheless, it seems only reasonable to measure F_IO_2, for example with an in-line polarographic electrode between the delivery system and the patient.

The thermal conductivity of heliox is much higher than any other medical gas.[4] Therefore, both the cooling of non-intubated patients or the overheating of intubated patients supplied with heated gas humidification should be considered as potential hazards. These problems have already been reported in deep sea divers[5] but have yet to be reported in the medical literature.

Another theoretical risk that has yet to be published is the delivery of too much bronchodilator when heliox is used as the driving gas for aerosol nebulization.

Taken together, the potential hazards of heliox appear to be rather small if certain precautions are taken, such as admission in an intensive care environment, and if careful monitoring is provided.

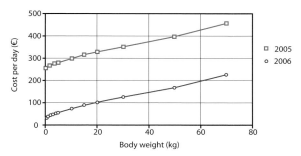

Figure 13.2 Daily cost of mechanical ventilation using heliox. Diagram showing additional cost when heliox is used as the ventilator's gas instead of room air with added oxygen during mechanical ventilation in patients of different sizes (Avea® by Viasys Health Care). Several factors, such as background flow, minute ventilation or leak, contribute to costs related to heliox. The lower line depicts the costs with a lower background flow implemented after 2006.

Cost considerations

Most Western countries face the problem of rising healthcare expenditure, and therefore a review on the use of an alternative treatment option such as heliox should also address considerations of cost. The price for a 50-L cylinder of compressed heliox at 200 atm (= 10 000 L) is given by Jolliet[18] as £137.[6] Heliox usage varies depending on a number of technical considerations such as ventilator function and bias flow as well as patient size (minute ventilation) and F_IHe. In Figure 13.2, the daily costs based on the reference by Jolliet[18] are calculated for different patients (from pre-term to adulthood using Avea® by Viasys Health Care). It can be seen that the costs are related to ventilator bias flow, as well as minute ventilation by the patient. With the development of new software that reduces the mandatory bias flow, a cost reduction occurs, but mechanical ventilation with heliox would still add about £99 in a 70-kg patient. If 10 L.min^{-1} heliox is provided by a non-rebreather face mask, the gas usage per day is around 14 400 L, which would add about £199 extra to the costs of the patient's care.

---

4 The thermal conductivity, κ, of air, nitrogen and oxygen is around 25 mW.m^{-1}.K^{-1}, whereas κ for heliox is just over six times higher at 153 mW.m^{-1}.K^{-1}.

5 Commercial divers who dive at great depths breathe a mixture of helium and oxygen in order to de-nitrogenate their bodies and avoid the risks of nitrogen narcosis.

6 Converted from the original figure of $275.

However, Jolliet et al.[18] demonstrated in their randomized controlled trial in adult patients with an acute exacerbation of COPD that heliox can actually help to save money if days on mechanical ventilation, re-intubation rate and length of stay are reduced. In their study, the savings amounted to £1 663 per patient,[7] with expenditure being lower in the heliox arm of the study.

Future prospects

Currently, the use of heliox in patients with respiratory problems has not been widely adopted despite a number of recent publications that show benefit in patients with upper and lower airway disease. Heliox inhalation in non-intubated patients is relatively simple but its use in ventilated patients is hampered by the lack of ventilators that can deliver heliox safely. Future developments should focus on ways to routinely apply heliox during mechanical ventilation, for example, as a commercially available add-on feature to conventional ventilators. Since its use can add significantly to healthcare costs, guidelines which give recommendations on the indications and use of helium-oxygen mixtures should be developed and rigorously evaluated. Hopefully, results such as those of Nawab et al.[16] could then be translated into benefits for patients. Moreover, in order to contain ICU costs, a heliox recycling system similar to the ventilatory circuits used during anaesthesia would be desirable. Currently, several companies are moving into the market. This might accelerate both technical and guideline development and could potentially reduce helium prices in the near future.

REFERENCES

1. Barach AL. Use of helium as a new therapeutic gas. *Proceedings of the Society for Experimental Biology and Medicine*. 1934;32: 662–4.

2. Hess DR. Heliox and noninvasive positive-pressure ventilation: a role for heliox in exacerbations of chronic obstructive pulmonary disease? *Respir Care*. 2006;51(6): 640–50.

3. Rodrigo GJ, Rodrigo C, Pollack CV et al. Use of helium-oxygen mixtures in the treatment of acute asthma: a systematic review. *Chest*. 2003;123(3):891–6.

4. Papamoschou D. Theoretical validation of the respiratory benefits of helium-oxygen mixtures. *Respir Physiol*. 1995;99(1):183–90.

5. Ho AM, Dion PW, Karmakar MK et al. Use of heliox in critical upper airway obstruction. Physical and physiologic considerations in choosing the optimal helium:oxygen mix. *Resuscitation*. 2002;52(3):297–300.

6. Kim IK, Phrampus E, Venkataraman S et al. Helium/oxygen-driven albuterol nebulization in the treatment of children with moderate to severe asthma exacerbations: a randomized, controlled trial. *Pediatrics*. 2005;116(5): 1127–33.

7. Martinon-Torres F, Rodriguez-Nunez A, Martinon-Sanchez JM. Nasal continuous positive airway pressure with heliox in infants with acute bronchiolitis. *Respir Med*. 2006;100(8):1458–62.

8. Duncan PG. Efficacy of helium-oxygen mixtures in the management of severe viral and post-intubation croup. *Can Anaesth Soc J*. 1979;26(3):206–12.

9. Schaeffer EM, Pohlman A, Morgan S et al. Oxygenation in status asthmaticus improves during ventilation with helium-oxygen. *Crit Care Med*. 1999;27(12):2666–70.

10. Tassaux D, Jolliet P, Roeseler J et al. Effects of helium-oxygen on intrinsic positive end-expiratory pressure in intubated and mechanically ventilated patients with severe chronic obstructive pulmonary disease. *Crit Care Med*. 2000;28(8):2721–8.

---

[7] Converted from the original figure of $3348.

11. Ho AM, Lee A, Karmakar MK *et al*. Heliox vs air–oxygen mixtures for the treatment of patients with acute asthma: a systematic overview. *Chest*. 2003;123(3):882–90.

12. Verbeek PR, Chopra A. Heliox does not improve FEV$_1$ in acute asthma patients. *J Emerg Med*. 1998;16(4):545–8.

13. Dorfman TA, Shipley ER, Burton JH *et al*. Inhaled heliox does not benefit ED patients with moderate to severe asthma. *Am J Emerg Med*. 2000;18(4):495–7.

14. Calzia E, Radermacher P. Helium in the treatment of respiratory failure: why not a standard? *Intensive Care Med*. Sep 2003;29(9): 1406–8.

15. Stillwell PC, Quick JD, Munro PR *et al*. Effectiveness of open-circuit and oxyhood delivery of helium-oxygen. *Chest*. 1989;95(6): 1222–4.

16. Nawab US, Touch SM, Irwin-Sherman T *et al*. Heliox attenuates lung inflammation and structural alterations in acute lung injury. *Pediatr Pulmonol*. 2005;40(6):524–32.

17. Fink JB. Opportunities and risks of using heliox in your clinical practice. *Respir Care*. 2006;51(6):651–60.

18. Jolliet P, Tassaux D, Roeseler J *et al*. Helium-oxygen versus air-oxygen noninvasive pressure support in decompensated chronic obstructive disease: A prospective, multicenter study. *Crit Care Med*. 2003;31(3):878–84.

19. Devabhaktuni VG, Torres A, Jr., Wilson S *et al*. Effect of nitric oxide, perfluorocarbon, and heliox on minute volume measurement and ventilator volumes delivered. *Crit Care Med*. 1999;27(8):1603–7.

20. Tassaux D, Jolliet P, Thouret JM *et al*. Calibration of seven ICU ventilators for mechanical ventilation with helium-oxygen mixtures. *Am J Respir Crit Care Med*. 1999;160(1):22–32.

21. Oppenheim-Eden A, Cohen Y, Weissman C *et al*. The effect of helium on ventilator performance: study of five ventilators and a bedside Pilot tube spirometer. *Chest*. 2001; 120(2):582–8.

22. Berkenbosch JW, Grueber RE, Dabbagh O *et al*. Effect of helium-oxygen (heliox) gas mixtures on the function of four pediatric ventilators. *Crit Care Med*. 2003;31(7): 2052–8.

23. Brown MK, Willms DC. A laboratory evaluation of 2 mechanical ventilators in the presence of helium-oxygen mixtures. *Respir Care*. 2005;50(3):354–60.

24. Jolliet P, Tassaux D, Thouret JM *et al*. Beneficial effects of helium:oxygen versus air:oxygen noninvasive pressure support in patients with decompensated chronic obstructive pulmonary disease. *Crit Care Med*. 1999;27(11):2422–9.

25. Jaber S, Fodil R, Carlucci A, *et al*. Noninvasive ventilation with helium-oxygen in acute exacerbations of chronic obstructive pulmonary disease. *Am J Respir Crit Care Med*. 2000;161(4 Pt 1):1191–200.

26. Jolliet P, Watremez C, Roeseler J, *et al*. Comparative effects of helium-oxygen and external positive end-expiratory pressure on respiratory mechanics, gas exchange, and ventilation-perfusion relationships in mechanically ventilated patients with chronic obstructive pulmonary disease. *Intensive Care Med*. 2003;29(9):1442–50.

27. Diehl JL, Mercat A, Guerot E, *et al*. Helium/oxygen mixture reduces the work of breathing at the end of the weaning process in patients with severe chronic obstructive pulmonary disease. *Crit Care Med*. 2003; 31(5):1415–20.

28. Lee DL, Lee H, Chang HW *et al*. Heliox improves hemodynamics in mechanically ventilated patients with chronic obstructive

pulmonary disease with systolic pressure variations. *Crit Care Med.* 2005;33(5):968–73.

29. Abd-Allah SA, Rogers MS, Terry M, Gross M *et al.* Helium-oxygen therapy for pediatric acute severe asthma requiring mechanical ventilation. *Pediatr Crit Care Med.* 2003;4(3): 353–7.

30. Watremez C, Liistro G, deKock M *et al.* Effects of helium-oxygen on respiratory mechanics, gas exchange, and ventilation-perfusion relationships in a porcine model of stable methacholine-induced bronchospasm. *Intensive Care Med.* 2003;29(9): 1560–6.

Chapter 14

Adverse effects and complications of mechanical ventilation

IAIN MACKENZIE AND PETER YOUNG

The adverse effects and complications of mechanical ventilation may arise from the artificial airway or from positive pressure ventilation and the drugs required to facilitate this. The occurrence of complications cannot be completely eliminated, but an appropriately managed intensive care unit will monitor the occurrence of complications and use this information to look for trends, to learn from the lessons that each complication can teach and as a quality assessment and quality assurance tool.

Intubation and the artificial airway

Immediate complications

Airway management and intubation in the operating department are performed under ideal circumstances with anaesthetists working in familiar, well-equipped surroundings supported by competent assistants on patients who, in the vast majority of cases, have been assessed and prepared for the procedure. Consequently, the complication rate is very low (Table 14.1). In contrast, airway management away from the operating department is often performed by non-anaesthetists, in more challenging locations, with little or no help, and on patients who, for the large part, need urgent airway management because of their poor or deteriorating condition. Not surprisingly, the complication rate in these patients is considerably higher (Table 14.1).

A significant contributory factor to the increased incidence of complications is the frequency of difficult intubation reported in these patients (Table 14.2), which is caused by the interaction between inexperienced operators and difficult circumstances (Figure 14.1).

Hypotension, hypoxia, cardiac arrest and death

The commonest reported immediate complications of intubation away from the operating department are severe hypotension and severe hypoxia, which occur in up to one in four patients. Hypovolaemia may be masked in patients with significant adrenergic drive arising from pain or fear. In these patients, the combination of a vasodilating hypnotic agent such as thiopentone, together with the loss of sympathetic tone brought about by unconsciousness, rapidly lead to profound hypotension.[1] In the elderly, who may have a slow circulation, inexperienced operators may be tempted into giving repeated doses of hypnotic in the mistaken belief that the initial dose has failed to have an effect, resulting in severe drug-related hypotension. In this regard etomidate is a reasonable choice even though it reduces adrenocortical steroid production for up

---

[1] It is said that on December 7, 1941 at Pearl Harbor more men lost their lives to thiopentone than were killed by the Japanese.

Core Topics in Mechanical Ventilation, ed. Iain Mackenzie. Published by Cambridge University Press.
© Cambridge University Press 2008.

Table 14.1 Incidence (%) of immediate complications of endotracheal intubation performed inside or outside the operating department

	Intubation in operating department	Intubation outside operating department
Severe hypotension	0.03[47]	26[48]
Severe hypoxia	NR	4.5[49], 26[48]
Oesophageal intubation	0.3[50], 0.5[51]	1[52], 4.6[48], 8[53], 9[54], 10[49]
Intubation of RMB	NR	4[53], 9[52]
Dental injury	0.03[55], 0.06[51]	2[52], 2.5[48, 54]
Aspiration	0.03[56], 0.05[57]	1.7[49], 2[58], 2.5[48], 4[53], 8[52]
Pneumothorax	Case reports only	1[52, 53]
Cardiac arrest	0.03[1]	1.6[48], 2[49]
Death	None[47], [50], [51]	0.13[49], 0.4[48], 3[53]b
Cases	1005[50], 17903[51]a, 40423[47], 53718[1], 185385[57], 215488[56]	150[54], 226[52], 253[48], 297[53], 3035[49]

a: No data on 302 laryngoscopies.
b: In 270 patients with a recordable blood pressure at the time of intubation.
RMB: right main bronchus.

Table 14.2 Incidence (%) of difficult endotracheal intubation depending on whether this was performed inside or outside the operating department

	Intubation in operating department	Intubation outside operating department
Serious difficulty	0.2[47], 0.8[50], 1.8[51]	8[53], 9[54], 12[48], 28[49]
Failure to intubate	None[50], 0.06[47], 0.3[51]	None[48, 53, 54], 0.4[49]
Abandoned	None[50], 0.16[51]	None[48, 53, 54]
Cases	1005[50], 17903[51] (b), 40423[47]	150[54], 253[48], 297[53], 3035[49]

to 48 hours. Ketamine, which is as cardiovascularly forgiving as etomidate without the effect on steroidogenesis, is under-used in this setting. This may be because the onset of unconsciousness is not as clear cut as with more commonly used hypnotics. The use of a muscle relaxant is desirable because it improves the conditions for intubation and abolishes the risk of coughing, straining or bucking, which can result in regurgitation as well as causing intracranial and intra-ocular pressures to increase. Suxamethonium is considered the drug of choice because of its rapid onset and short duration of action,[2] but has complications of its own. Muscle fasciculation causes elevation of intra-ocular and intra-abdominal pressure. The former can result in the extrusion of ocular content in patients with a penetrating eye injury; the latter can result in regurgitation of gastric content. Suxamethonium should be avoided in patients with a penetrating eye injury. Muscle depolarization is normally associated with a rise in plasma potassium concentration of less

[2] An 'intubating' dose of 1 mg.kg^{-1} causes muscle depolarization and relaxation in less than 60 seconds (depending on the speed of the circulation) and lasts no longer than 5 minutes.

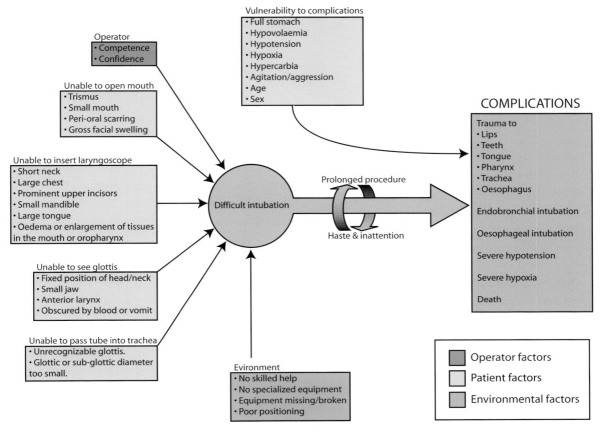

Figure 14.1 Interaction of factors linking difficult intubation to complications.

than 0.5 mmol.L^{-1}, but this effect may be significantly exaggerated in patients with either over-expression, or extra-junctional expression, of skeletal muscle acetylcholine receptors.[3] Rarely, muscle fasciculation can be followed by a failure of skeletal muscle relaxation, particularly in patients with myotonic dystrophy, which can make it impossible to open the patient's mouth. Following successful intubation, hypotension may then be aggravated by the reduction in venous return caused by positive pressure ventilation. Intubation-related hypotension can largely be prevented by ensuring that large-bore venous access has been secured

beforehand, that fluid resuscitation is in progress before the administration of any hypnotic and by using the appropriate drugs in measured doses.

While hypoxia may be the clinical problem that has precipitated the need for intubation, severe hypoxia *at the time of intubation* is almost invariably the consequence of poor manual ventilation with bag-valve-mask or prolonged attempts at intubation. Providing the risk of aspiration can be controlled with cricoid pressure and ventilation can be achieved non-invasively, the vast majority of patients can be supported until intubation has been successfully achieved or until help arrives. Failing to maintain adequate oxygenation *during* intubation also deprives the intubating clinician of noticing hypoxia that develops *after* intubation as a result

---

[3] Upper and lower motor nerve lesions, cerebral palsy, muscular dystrophy, tetanus, and three weeks to three months after severe burns.

Table 14.3 Signs to confirm correct placement of the endotracheal tube

- Low resistance to inflation
- Normal end-tidal carbon dioxide trace
- Normal and symmetrical movement of the chest wall
- Bilateral breath sounds on auscultation

Table 14.4 Risk factors for pulmonary aspiration

- Reduced level of consciousness from any cause
- Acute abdominal pathology
- Obesity
- Pregnancy

of inadvertent oesophageal or endobronchial intubation, or less commonly from a pneumothorax. Correct placement of the tube in the trachea is best achieved by noting its passage through the glottic opening. However, this is not always possible, so it is mandatory to confirm intratracheal placement by other means (Table 14.3).

Oesophageal intubation can occasionally be mimicked in patients with severe bronchospasm, following intubation of the right main bronchus, or with unilateral pulmonary pathology, but all of these should produce a normal end-tidal carbon dioxide trace. Following emergency intubation, particularly when an uncut endotracheal tube has been placed, the tip of the endotracheal tube may enter the right main bronchus in up to 10% of cases.[4] This causes an acute intra-pulmonary shunt with resultant hypoxaemia. If not rapidly recognized, this leads to left-sided lung collapse and right-sided hyperinflation with the risk of pneumothorax. The cuff portion of the tube should be passed only 3 to 5 cm beyond the cords. The tip of the tube should be at least 3 cm above the carina to prevent carinal stimulation or intermittent endobronchial intubation with ventilation. If there is any doubt as to the location of the tube, it should be removed and the patient re-intubated. The final confirmation of correct tube positioning is by inspection of a plain chest radiograph to ensure that the tip of the tracheal tube is midway between the carina and the larynx.

---

[4] This is more likely to occur in women, perhaps because of a shorter tracheal length.

The combination of hypoxia and hypotension, particularly the former,[1] contribute significantly to the 100-fold increased incidence of cardiac arrest, from which the outcome is often poor. The mortality associated with intubation outside the operating department is between 0.1% and 3%.

Regurgitation and aspiration

In general, aspiration of regurgitated gastric material is about 100-fold more common in patients who are intubated outside the operating department and occurs in 2% to 4% of cases, although there are specific patient groups who are particularly at risk (Table 14.4). This increased incidence is partly attributable to the patients, who by definition will be much more likely to have material in their stomachs. However, gastric insufflation by over-enthusiastic bag-valve-mask ventilation, together with poorly applied cricoid pressure, also make a substantial contribution. Correctly applied, cricoid pressure also serves to prevent the regurgitation of stomach content into the oropharynx.

The consequences of aspiration depend on the quantity and quality of the material aspirated.[2] Patients who are elderly, debilitated, or have been unwell for more than a couple of days are much more likely to have an altered oropharyngeal and stomach flora, which will then include respiratory tract pathogens such as *Staphylococcus aureus*, *Pseudomonas aeruginosa* and other Gram-negative enteric organisms. These patients are more likely to develop an aspiration pneumonia, and immediate therapy with empirical broad-spectrum antibiotics is appropriate. Younger, fitter patients whose illness is of sudden onset, such as with a drug overdose, are likely to have sterile gastric content. The injury in these patients arises from the acidity of the gastric content that causes a chemical burn of the tracheo-bronchial tree, an aspiration pneumonitis.[5] Only about 50 mL need be aspirated to cause significant injury, provided the material is sufficiently acid. In these patients, pulmonary function can deteriorate in a matter of minutes with pulmonary oedema and severe hypoxaemia (Figure 14.2). Initially, antibiotic therapy is not indicated in aspiration pneumonitis, although this should be considered in patients whose condition does not start to improve within 48 to 72 hours. Corticosteroids are of no benefit in either aspiration pneumonitis or aspiration pneumonia.

Other complications

There is no information on the incidence of direct patient injuries arising from intubation outside the operating department other than for dental damage that is reported to be between 50 and 80 times more common (Table 14.1). It is likely that the same applies to the incidence of other soft tissue injuries that are known to occur during intubation, such as injuries to the lips, tongue, fauces and pharynx. Although uncomfortable, these injuries are relatively minor, have no long-term sequelae and rarely lead to patient complaint. Damage to the larynx is the commonest site of injury during intubation that leads to litigation.

Oesophageal and tracheal perforations are fortunately rare and usually associated with difficult intubation or the use of rigid endotracheal tubes. This type of injury commonly presents with cervical surgical emphysema, but may progress to infection of the peri-tracheal fascia and mediastinitis. Tracheal perforations or tears that are less than 3 cm in length, situated in the upper half of the trachea, partial thickness, and not associated with evidence of mediastinitis can be managed conservatively by

placing the cuff of the endotracheal tube distal to the injury, minimizing airway pressures and empirical antibiotic therapy. Early surgical repair is indicated in all other cases. Oesophageal tears may initially be overlooked if mask ventilation applied after the injury is low-pressure and only produces small volumes of surgical emphysema. As with tracheal injuries, oesophageal tears can be managed conservatively or surgically, although the best approach remains controversial.

Damage to the cervical spine may occur during intubation in the operating department in non-trauma patients who have atlanto-axial instability, most notably patients with rheumatoid arthritis or Down's syndrome. The potential to cause cervical spinal cord damage during intubation is more keenly appreciated in trauma patients in whom the risk of causing serious injury is not merely theoretical.[3] Three steps are required to avoid causing serious spinal cord injury during tracheal intubation. First, the *potential* for instability of the cervical spine must be recognized. In the vast majority of cases, the history of trauma is evident and will often be advertised by the fact that the patient is wearing some form of cervical collar. The dangerous cases, however, are those where the trauma is not appreciated (Box 14.1). Second, proper preparation for tracheal intubation must be made, which includes assembling the right people and the right equipment. Third, the correct technique must be used, which consists of a rapid-sequence induction with cricoid pressure, removal or opening of the collar once the patient is immobilized and careful intubation using manual in-line stabilization without flexion or extension of either the head or neck. This is a challenging procedure and, where possible, should be performed by a senior anaesthetist with a particular interest in this type of problem.

The nasal route has largely fallen out of favour in the UK except for short-term use in very specific circumstances. Nasal intubation not

---

[5] Also referred to as *Mendelson's syndrome*.

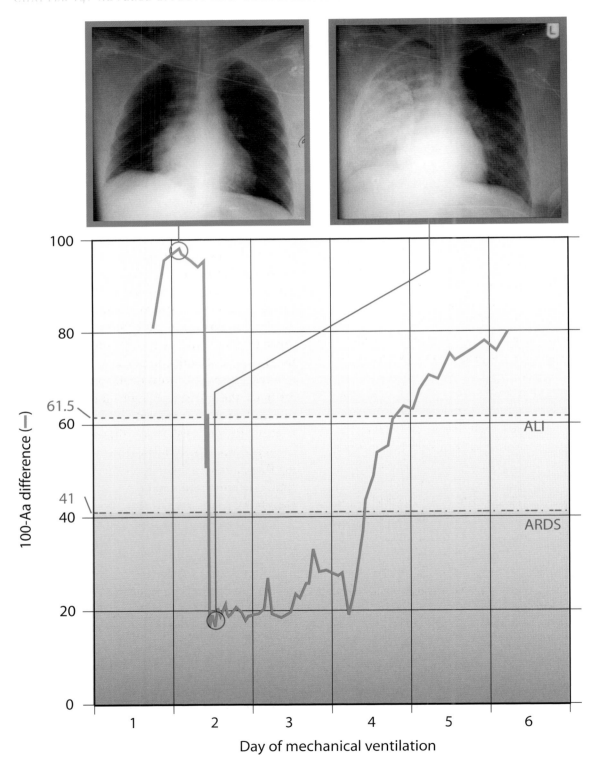

Figure 14.2 – Aspiration pneumonitis.

A young woman was admitted with a significant overdose of a tricyclic antidepressant and was therefore intubated and ventilated overnight. The following morning the sedatives were discontinued and she was extubated. However, instead of her level of consciousness gradually increasing, it gradually fell, and within an hour of extubation she had a generalized seizure, vomited and then had a cardiorespiratory arrest. She was immediately re-intubated, and although there was almost no residual material in her tracheobronchial tree, her pulmonary condition rapidly deteriorated. The figure shows the changes in her alveolar–arterial oxygen tension difference (subtracted from 100, see Chapter 6) over the six days she spent on intensive care together with a chest radiograph taken immediately prior to extubation (left) and a second radiograph taken within an hour of her aspiration (right).

Box 14.1

A 67-year-old man was admitted following a cardiac arrest at home that had complicated an acute myocardial infarction. He was intubated at the scene during the course of a relatively brief and successful resuscitation, and was admitted to intensive care for further management. After 48 hours of elective ventilation, the sedation was discontinued and although the patient was able to self-ventilate in a triggered mode of ventilation, he remained very poorly responsive, which was assumed to be the result of a severe hypoxic brain injury. Five days into his admission, one of the residents noticed that the patient was able to follow movements around the foot of the patient's bed with his eyes. A neurological examination confirmed intact cranial nerve function but complete absence of motor or sensory response in the limbs. A plain radiograph of the patient's neck showed a fracture dislocation of C2 on C3. On further enquiry, it emerged that the patient was found lying on the floor at the foot of a flight of stairs, which he had been descending when he had collapsed.

uncommonly provokes bleeding from trauma to the inferior turbinates, as well as causing abrasions to the posterior nasopharynx. In patients with basal skull fractures, nasal intubation can penetrate the skull base and enter the brain.

Reduction of immediate complications

Restricting acute airway management to staff who have the appropriate training, skill and experience reduces the risks of acute airway management problems. Acute airway management in critically ill patients should never be used as a training opportunity for staff who do not already possess this skill in straightforward cases, under optimal conditions. Apart from the operator, complications are also minimized by appropriate preparation in terms of both equipment and staff. Intensive care nurses only occasionally prepare for, and assist in, the process of intubation because the majority of patients admitted to intensive care have already been intubated. Familiarity with the process, drugs and equipment can be maintained by ensuring that all intensive care unit (ICU) staff receive regular refresher training in the operating theatre (Box 14.2).

Complications arising in the medium and long term

Injuries to the face, lips and oropharynx

In the absence of due care, prolonged intubation results in trauma to the lips or cheeks from the tube tie (Figure 14.3) and can provoke peri-oral herpes. Injuries to the tongue occasionally occur, particularly if the tongue becomes trapped between the endotracheal tube and the lower teeth. Pressure injuries to the palate and oropharynx are very uncommon.

Box 14.2 Scheme for minimizing complications during intubation outside the operating department

- Take your own equipment and drugs to the patient, including equipment to manage the difficult airway.
- If possible, take experienced help with you.
- If the patient has stridor, immediately call for senior anaesthetic help, and DO NOT ATTEMPT TO INTUBATE THE PATIENT YOURSELF unless the patient has stopped breathing.
- Establish large-bore venous access and initiate volume resuscitation unless there is unambiguous evidence of fluid overload (e.g. pulmonary oedema)
- Pre-oxygenate the patient.
- Establish appropriate monitoring.
- Call for help sooner rather than later if the patient looks like they may be difficult to intubate.
- In patients with hypotension consider giving 3 to 6 mg of ephedrine or 1 mg of metaraminol before administering the hypnotic.
- Always assume the patient has a full stomach. Use a rapid-sequence technique with the application of cricoid pressure.
- Use measured doses of hypnotic agents that have little or no hypotensive effect, such as midazolam, etomidate or ketamine.
- Use suxamethonium except in patients who might have hyperkalaemia, or within 1 and 6 weeks of severe burns or a neurological insult resulting in motor weakness.

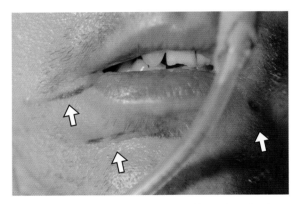

Figure 14.3 Abrasions to the face caused by endotracheal tube ties.

The arrows indicate abrasions caused by the tube ties.

Maxillary sinusitis and middle ear effusions

Maxillary effusions have been shown to develop in just over 20% of patients during 7 days of mechanical ventilation, even when both the endotracheal and gastric tubes are placed orally,[4] with the incidence increasing to 47% when the gastric tube is placed nasally,[5] and up to 95%[4] when both tubes are placed nasally. The positive association between effusion and a trans-nasal tube suggests that the former is related to the latter, although direct physical obstruction of maxillary sinus drainage is unlikely as the maxillary ostium lies in the hiatus semilunaris under the middle concha. Between 45%[4] and 71%[6] of these effusions become secondarily infected, most commonly with Gram-negative enteric organisms, and may contribute to the development of ventilator-associated pneumonia (see later discussion).

Middle ear effusions have been noted in up to 29%[7] and, as with sinus effusions, a proportion of these (22%) are infected. If these studies reflect the true incidence of middle ear effusion, which are likely to produce some degree of hearing impairment, this might contribute to the generation of fear, confusion and delirium in elderly intubated patients.

Pharyngo-laryngeal dysfunction

Post-extubation throat discomfort occurs in about 40% of patients and is similar regardless of the duration of intubation. Hoarseness, however, is reported in 52% of patients following short-term intubation but is reported in 70% of patients following prolonged intubation, an effect that is presumably related to the incidence of glottic oedema. These symptoms usually resolve within 24 to 48 hours. More prolonged symptoms would warrant direct inspection of the larynx. Injuries to the recurrent laryngeal nerve have been reported, but are extremely rare.

Swallowing is a complex reflex that depends on intact oral and pharyngeal sensation as well as motor control of the muscles of the pharynx, larynx and upper oesophagus. Even relatively short periods of orotracheal intubation result in significant slowing of the reflex mechanism (Figure 14.4) that remains abnormal for over 7 days. In one study, 13 of 82 (15.8%) patients who had been intubated for at least 4 days did not have a gag reflex on the day of extubation.[8] An abnormal swallowing reflex puts the patient at risk of aspiration. This was seen to occur at post-extubation FEES[6] examination in 36% of younger patients[9] (mean age 50 years) and 52% of elderly patients (mean age 75 years) intubated for at least 48 hours. Moreover, the incidence of *silent* aspiration was 20% in the younger patients and 36% in the older ones.[9] Repeated examinations showed that these abnormalities improved more rapidly in the younger patients. The optimum diagnostic strategy for detecting these swallowing disorders remains unclear because the sensitivity of FEES appears to be operator dependent, but is a more practical investigation than a videofluoroscopic contrast swallow, which is the 'gold

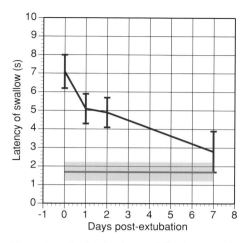

Figure 14.4 Swallowing latency following more than 24 hours of orotracheal intubation.

The latency is the time delay between providing a stimulus to swallow, which in this case was the instillation of 0.25 mL of 0.9% saline into the nasopharynx, and the detection of electromyographic activity in the sub-mental region. The value for non-intubated patients with a nasogastric tube was 1.7 ± 0.5 seconds and is represented by the dark green line and pale green error zone. The values for the 34 patients were measured on the day of extubation, and then on days 1, 2 and 7. They are plotted here as the mean with the error bars representing the standard error of the mean. From data presented in de Larminat V *et al. Crit Care Med.* 1995;23(3):486–90.

standard'. However, for a proportion of patients, there is little doubt that the early detection of post-extubation aspiration followed by appropriate dietary modifications or 'nil by mouth' would be life-saving.

Swallowing problems in patients with tracheostomy are discussed in Chapter 17.

Laryngeal injuries

Despite the fact that the most common types of endotracheal tube are made from thermolabile polyvinyl chloride (PVC) and soften at body temperature, the posterior margin of the glottis remains at risk for developing ulcers. Studies in dogs suggest that the risk of glottic injury increases during the first seven days of intubation, but then loses any particular relation with time. Simply on the basis

6 FEES, fibreoptic endoscopic evaluation of swallow.

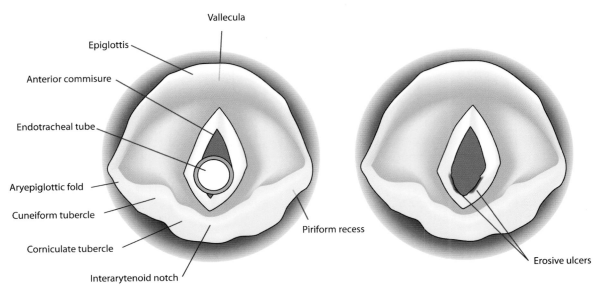

Figure 14.5 Laryngeal damage.

Laryngeal inlet showing position of tracheal tube (left), and the resulting position of erosive ulcers on the cartilaginous part of the true vocal folds.

of anatomy, it is unclear whether a canine model can adequately reproduce the situation in man, and in patients there are additional factors that may contribute to the risk of injury, such as co-existent shock, sepsis, or hypoxia. Prospective evaluation in 82 patients intubated for at least 4 days has shown that the vast majority of patients (94%) acquire some degree of glottic injury by the time they are extubated or receive a tracheostomy.[8] In 93% of cases, ulcers were present on either side of the posterior commisure where the endotracheal tube exerts pressure against the cartilaginous part of the true vocal folds (Figure 14.5), and in 51% of cases, this was accompanied by moderate or severe swelling of adjacent structures. Of those with laryngeal damage, 63% were healed by 4 weeks, and 82% by 8 weeks, but up to 6% of these lesions may result in stenosis of the posterior commisure.[10] Quite distinct from either healing or scarring, these ulcers can also give rise to granulation tissue. Granulomas have been reported to occur in 7% of patients intubated for four or more days,[8] although the inci-

dence may be higher in patients who have failed attempts at extubation.

Tracheal injuries

Tracheal damage from prolonged cuff over-inflation is believed to be much less of a problem with the introduction of high-volume, low-pressure cuffs in the late 1960s, although analysis of the cumulative caseload at a single academic cardiothoracic centre in the US would seem to belie this contention (Figure 14.6). Certainly severe tracheal damage continues to be reported, but in the absence of thorough, systematic, prospective studies, the true incidence of mild and moderate tracheal injuries remains speculative. There is little question that *concerns* about tracheal injury have largely subsided, and despite the clear evidence implicating cuff pressure in the aetiology of tracheal injuries, the routine measurement of cuff pressure in UK intensive care practice is still not universal. Mild injuries such as tracheal ulcerations, oedema and sub-mucosal haemorrhages are likely to be quite common but

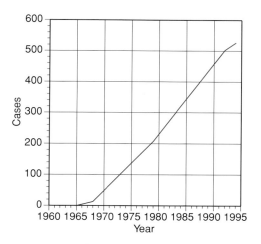

Figure 14.6 Incidence of tracheal stenosis.

Cumulative number of patients treated for tracheal stenosis at the Department of Thoracic Surgery of the Massachusetts General Hospital, Boston, USA, between 1965 and 1994.

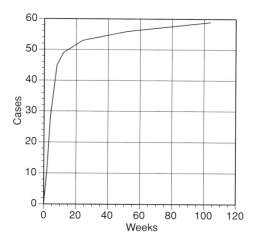

Figure 14.7 Plot showing the cumulative number of patients diagnosed with tracheal stenosis with the passage of time following extubation.

In a series of 59 patients diagnosed with post-tracheostomy tracheal stenosis, 50% of the cases were diagnosed within 1 month of de-cannulation and 90% of the cases were diagnosed within 6 months. Some cases, however, remained un-detected for 2 years. From Andrews MJ and Pearson FG. *Br J Surg.* 1973;60(3):208–12.

usually resolve without complications. The incidence of tracheal dilatation is unknown but appears to be both relatively uncommon and associated with prolonged intubation. Tracheal stenosis is potentially the most severe complication although this depends on whether the stenosis is clinically apparent or not. Very rarely an early stenosis may be the cause for persistent extubation failure, but these lesions usually become apparent some time after extubation as the patient's clinical condition improves. The stenosis may arise at the site of the cuff (50%) or at the site of the tracheostomy (35%), but in the remaining 15%, the cause of the stenosis is unclear. When the stenosis is less than 5 mm in diameter, patients present with stridor at rest, but those with less severe lesions only develop stridor or dyspnoea on exertion. As a significant proportion of the patients who develop this problem will have pre-existing cardiorespiratory disease, these symptoms may be ascribed to the latter, causing a substantial delay in the diagnosis (Figure 14.7). The diagnosis may be confirmed by computed tomography, but bronchoscopy is always needed to confirm the nature and extent of the lesion and to plan the optimum management strategy. While many patients require tracheal reconstruction, with a 2.4% mortality in one very large series,[11] this is not an option in those that remain ventilator-dependent or who have severe intercurrent disease. In these patients, conservative management with repeated broncho-scopic dilatation, laser treatment, cryotherapy or placement of a self-expanding metallic stent may be an option.

Unplanned extubation

Unplanned extubation describes any episode in which the tracheal tube is unintentionally withdrawn from the trachea and includes both *self-extubation*, where the tracheal tube is dislodged or removed by the patient, and *accidental extubation*, where the tracheal tube is dislodged by members of staff. The incidence of self-extubation is about 8%, while that of accidental extubation is just over 1% of all ventilation episodes. These events are quite distinct because they occur for different reasons in different types of patients and therefore have quite different consequences. Self-extubation is associated with both agitation and physical restraint and is more likely to occur in patients whose sedation is being reduced as part of a weaning strategy. As a consequence, these patients are much less likely to require re-intubation. However, accidental extubation is an event that occurs during patient care or transfer, without any association with weaning. As a consequence, these patients are much more likely to be deeply sedated or even paralysed, and are much more likely to require immediate re-intubation. Overall, patients who have an unplanned extubation spend longer in both the ICU and the hospital, but a recent case-controlled study has shown that those who require re-intubation have a significantly increased ICU and hospital mortality.[12]

It is not at all evident that self-extubation is a negative event, as it often appears to be a mechanism by which a patient who is ready for extubation can bring this fact to the attention of the staff. This suggests that clinical judgement is poor at predicting a patient's readiness for extubation, and even objective predictors of successful extubation have been shown to have poor sensitivity and a high false-negative rate.

The consequences of accidental extubation, although less common, are much more serious and much more likely to result in cardiac dysrhythmias, pulmonary aspiration, severe hypoxia, cardiac arrest and death. In patients with tracheostomy tubes, accidental de-cannulation is particularly serious as the problem may not be immediately apparent to the staff (see Box 17.1). Covert extubation can also occur in patients with an endotracheal tube, but the consequences of delayed detection are much less severe because the dislodged tube can still ventilate the patient, albeit with a significant leak. There is no data on the risk factors specifically associated with accidental extubation, but given the negative patient outcome, further study in this area is clearly desirable.

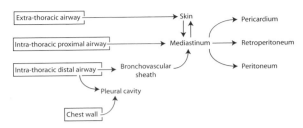

Figure 14.8 Movement of gas arising from the airway or chest wall along tissue planes to cause the manifestations of barotrauma.

Pulmonary complications of mechanical ventilation

Barotrauma

Rupture of the respiratory epithelium during positive pressure ventilation allows gas to escape into the lung parenchyma or pleural space. Gas entering the lung parenchyma tracks centrally along the bronchovascular sheath (pulmonary interstitial emphysema) to accumulate in the mediastinum (pneumomediastinum) from where the gas may enter the pericardium (pneumopericardium), the retroperitoneal space (pneumoretroperitoneum) or the peritoneal space (pneumoperitoneum; see Figures 14.8 and 14.9). If gas escapes from the distal airway and enters the pleural space, this results in a pneumothorax (Figure 14.10). Collectively these manifestations of escaped airway gas are referred to as *barotrauma*, a term which implies that excess airway pressure is fundamental to the mechanism, which is not always the case. Breach of the respiratory epithelium resulting in any of the manifestations of barotrauma can arise from trauma, iatrogenic or otherwise, and can also arise spontaneously in susceptible individuals (Table 14.5). It should not be forgotten that pneumomediastinum could also arise from damage to the oesophagus.

In the absence of extrinsic trauma or intrinsic failure of the lung tissue, ventilator-associated barotrauma is usually the result of the alveolar epithelium being over-stretched, which cannot occur in the absence of high airway pressures. However, high

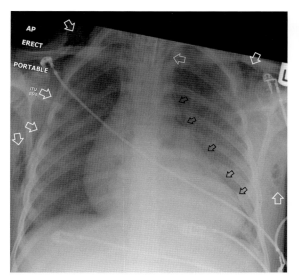 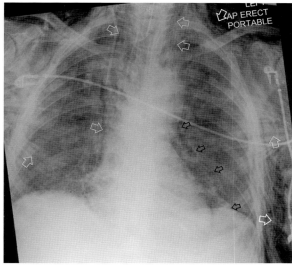

Figure 14.9 Radiographic appearance of barotrauma.

White arrows indicate subcutaneous gas, which is apparent clinically as 'surgical emphysema'. Pink arrows show mediastinal structures that have been delineated by the presence of gas, indicating pneumomediastinum. Black arrows delineate the pericardium, which normally cannot be distinguished from the cardiac silhouette, indicating the presence of gas within the pericardial cavity (pneumopericardium). On the left, this is quite subtle, and therefore easily missed. On the right, this is so gross that it too might easily be missed. Blue arrows, only present on the radiograph on the right, show gas delineating the fibres of pectoralis major muscle.

airway pressures do not necessarily result in over-stretching. Neither high pressures nor alveolar over-distension are required when the alveolar epithelium disintegrates as part of a pathological process, for example with necrotizing pneumonia or pulmonary vasculitis.

With the exception of pneumothorax, which is discussed later, none of the other manifestations of barotrauma are of particular clinical significance, although very occasionally surgical emphysema can threaten an unprotected airway and pneumomediastinum or pneumopericardium can lead to haemodynamic compromise. Active management is not necessary in the majority of cases, which resolve spontaneously. Where active decompression is thought to be indicated, there are reports that this can be achieved by the subcutaneous placement of either conventional chest tubes or, more elegantly, using large-bore intravenous cannulae with spirally placed side-holes.

The incidence of pneumothorax in patients receiving mechanical ventilation is now (2006) about 3% having been 14% in 1992, with just under half (44%) from mechanical ventilation alone. In many cases, pneumothorax is detected by routine radiology in high-risk patients, such as those with trauma or following central venous cannulation. However, small, stable and clinically silent pneumothoraces run the risk of being over-looked because of the subtlety of the radiographic appearances. This is particularly true of anterior pneumothoraces in the supine or semi-recumbent patient that are only visible as a reduction in the radiographic density in the affected hemi-thorax. Alternatively, a pneumothorax may be detected in the course of investigating a deterioration in respiratory function. About 30% of pneumothoraces continue to accumulate gas and develop sufficient pressure to cause significant cardiorespiratory compromise or collapse (Table 14.6), a 'tension'

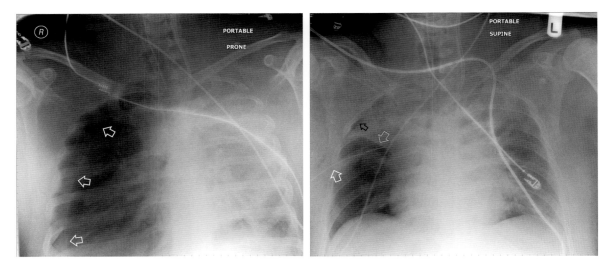

Figure 14.10 Pneumothorax before (left) and after (right) insertion of chest drain.

On the left, the presence of a right-sided pneumothorax is indicated by the visible lung edge (white arrows) lateral to which there are no lung markings. Although the right hemi-thorax is clearly less dense (darker) than the left, the lucency of the lung-free margin is less than normal because (1) the radiograph was taken in the prone position and (2) there was a considerable amount of fluid in the right hemi-thorax. Note the very horizontal position of the ribs, especially of the right hemi-thorax, indicating the presence of significant tension. This patient was in peri-arrest.

After needle decompression of the tension pneumothorax, a large-bore right-sided chest drain was inserted (white arrow) which drained 500 mL of serous fluid. The right lung has not quite fully expanded (black arrow), and from the angulation of the horizontal fissure (pink arrow) it is now evident that the right upper lobe is partially collapsed. The left hemi-thorax remains uniformly denser (whiter) than the right, suggesting the presence of a significant pleural effusion, as there was on the right.

pneumothorax. Under these circumstances, needle decompression should not be postponed for radiological confirmation (Box 14.3), and this should then be followed by insertion of a chest drain (Box 14.4). It is currently recommended that in patients receiving positive pressure ventilation, all radiologically confirmed pneumothoraces should be drained to avoid the risk of tension pneumothorax, although there is no data on the risk of this happening with small pneumothoraces detected as an incidental finding on routine radiology. Small-bore wire-guided catheter drainage is likely to be adequate for a simple pneumothorax, with the drain angled to run posteriorly into the apex of the pleural cavity. In patients who also need blood or fluid drained from the pleural cavity or who may have a substantial air leak a large-bore drain is preferable, and in this case, the drain should be angled

basally. Correct intra-pleural placement is suggested by bubbling in the underwater seal system and respiratory swings of the water level within the drain tip but should be confirmed by radiography. In most cases, lung expansion is completed within 48 hours of insertion, and provided that there is no air leak, the drain will stop bubbling but continue to swing. After a further 24 hours, the drain can be removed without clamping.

If 48 hours after chest drain insertion the lung has not fully re-expanded or the drain continues to bubble, the patient is considered to have a bronchopleural fistula. In this situation, a narrow-bore catheter should be replaced by a larger drain, and the drainage system connected to low-pressure (<20 cm H_2O) high-volume suction. At the same time, the ventilation strategy should be altered to minimize the pressure gradient across the leak

Table 14.5 Causes of barotrauma

- Thoracic trauma
  - Penetrating thoracic injuries (knife, bullet, shrapnel, glass, etc.)
  - Deceleration injuries → tracheal or bronchial transection
  - Blunt thoracic trauma → rib fractures → penetration of lung
  - Blast injuries
- Iatrogenic thoracic or airway trauma
  - Central venous access insertion
  - Chest drain insertion
  - Surgery to the lung or major airways
  - Intubation
  - Trans-bronchial biopsy
  - Surgery to the mouth (dental extractions), throat (tonsillectomy) or nose (sinus surgery)
  - Brachial plexus nerve block
- Excess airway pressure
- Failure of lung parenchyma
  - Bullous emphysema
  - Necrotizing pneumonia
  - Pulmonary vasculitis
  - *Pneumocystis jirovecii* pneumonia
  - Spontaneous pneumothorax
- Oesophageal damage
  - Spontaneous rupture (Booerhave's syndrome)
  - Iatrogenic perforation
  - Foreign body
  - Ulcer or chemical burns

Table 14.6 Clinical features of tension pneumothorax

- Hypoxaemia
- Increased airway pressure in volume-targeted ventilation or decreased tidal volume in pressure-targeted ventilation
- Decreased air entry into affected side associated with hyper-resonance on percussion
- Tracheal deviation away from the affected side
- Hypotension, tachycardia, raised central venous pressure and decreased cardiac output

Box 14.3 Emergency needle decompression of a suspected tension pneumothorax

In the mid-clavicular line of the affected side, palpate two rib spaces below the clavicle. Keeping your finger in the intercostal space in the mid-clavicular line, insert a large intravenous cannula perpendicularly to the skin immediately below your finger until it reaches the anterior surface of the third rib. With a syringe on the end of the cannula, advance the cannula over the top of the rib while aspirating, and continue advancing until the syringe suddenly aspirates air as it enters the pleural space. Holding the needle and syringe in place, advance the cannula fully and then remove the needle and syringe. If the patient has a tension pneumothorax, you should then hear gas escaping through the cannula. Proceed immediately to insert a chest drain on this side.

consideration should be given to more specific techniques for reducing the leak, such as independent lung ventilation (see Chapter 12), targeted bronchial obstruction, or high frequency oscillation (see Chapter 6). Tissue repair is maximized by ensuring optimum nutrition and the aggressive treatment of pulmonary and pleural sepsis. In some patients, surgical closure may be an option and these very difficult cases are best managed in collaboration with respiratory physicians and thoracic surgeons.

Ventilator-associated pneumonia (VAP)

Contrary to what might be expected from a device that provides an 'air-tight' seal, the cuff of a high-volume, low-pressure, tracheal tube does not provide a water-tight seal (see Figure 4.13) and allows repeated micro-aspiration of material that accumulates above the cuff in the subglottic space (see Figure 4.19). Initially, this material will contain typical upper respiratory tract flora, but within

(Table 14.7). In leaks that show no sign of abating after a further 48 to 72 hours, particularly in patients with inflammation or necrosis at the leak,

Box 14.4 Insertion of a chest drain (adapted from the BTS guidelines)

Preparation: Consider the sedation and analgesic requirements and correct coagulopathy or platelet defects. Consider antibiotic prophylaxis in trauma. Review the chest radiograph or CT scan (except in the case of tension pneumothorax) and consider the differential diagnosis (1) between a pneumothorax and bullous disease and (2) between collapse or consolidation and a pleural effusion.

Drain size: Many clinicians now use small catheters (10 to 14 F) because these are often as effective as larger bore tubes and are better tolerated by the patient. If the air leak exceeds the capacity of the catheter then a larger bore tube should be inserted. Large bore tubes (28 to 30 F minimum) are required for an acute haemothorax to assist in the assessment of continuing blood loss.

Positioning: Position supine and slightly rotated, with the ipsilateral arm behind the patient's head to expose the 'safe triangle' in the axilla bordered by the anterior border of the latissimus dorsi, the lateral border of the pectoralis major muscle, a line superior to the horizontal level of the nipple and an apex below the axilla. The most common site for chest tube insertion is in the mid-axillary line through the 'safe triangle' to avoid the internal mammary artery. For apical pneumothoraces, the second intercostal space in the mid clavicular line may be chosen. If a loculated pleural collection requires drainage, the position of insertion will be dictated by the site of the locule as determined by imaging and the procedure should be performed by an experienced operator, for example, a thoracic surgeon.

Insertion: Use aseptic technique. Air or fluid should be needle aspirated and if none is forthcoming then further imaging is required (such as bedside ultrasonography). The incision should be made just above and parallel to a rib and should be slightly bigger than the tube.

(1) Blunt dissection (large-bore drains): A Spencer-Wells clamp is used to dissect a path through the chest wall by opening the clamp, thereby separating the muscle fibres. This track should be explored with a finger into the thoracic cavity to ensure there are no underlying organs that might be damaged at tube insertion.

(2) Seldinger technique (small-bore drains): A needle and syringe are used to identify air or pleural fluid. A guidewire is then passed and the tract enlarged using dilators. A small-bore tube is then passed into the thoracic cavity along the wire.

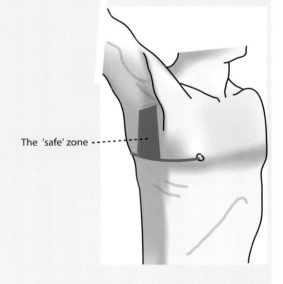

The 'safe' zone - - - - - - - - -

Briefly disconnect from the ventilator prior to insertion to avoid lung injury.

Insertion of a chest tube should never be performed with substantial force since this risks sudden chest penetration and damage to intrathoracic structures.

Tip Position: This should be aimed apically for a pneumothorax or basally for fluid; however, an effectively functioning drain should not be repositioned because of its radiographic position.

Secure drain: Connect to drainage system. Use '1' silk and avoid purse string sutures. Support the tube to prevent kinking. Perform a chest radiograph.

Table 14.7 Manoeuvres to reduce air leak across a bronchopleural fistula

- Minimize minute ventilation (decrease tidal volume and respiratory rate)
- Minimize inspiratory time (increase inspiratory flow rate, increase I:E ratio)
- Encourage spontaneous ventilatory effort
- Minimize positive end-expiratory pressure (PEEP)
- Exploit positional reductions in leak
- Minimize resistance to expiratory gas flow (bronchoconstriction, bronchial mucosal oedema)

Table 14.8 Clinical criteria for the diagnosis of ventilator-associated pneumonia

- New or progressive radiological infiltrate and
- Two of the following:
  - Fever over 38 °C
  - White cell count < 4 or >11 $\times$ 10^9 cells.mm^{-3}
  - Purulent tracheal secretions

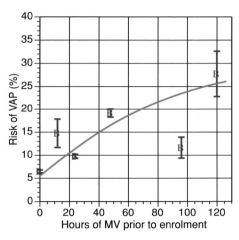

Figure 14.11 Risk of developing ventilator-associated pneumonia (VAP).

Risk of developing VAP reported in prospective cohort and non-randomized studies in patients mechanically ventilated (MV) for a minimum number of hours prior to enrolment, shown with 95% confidence intervals for the proportions calculated. Data from Safdar N *et al. Crit Care Med.* Oct 2005;33(10):2184–93. From left to right, 15 studies (24 628 patients) contributed to the point at 0 hours, 1 study (521 patients) to the point at 12 hours, 7 studies (14 194 patients) to the point at 24 hours, 13 studies (7548 patients) to the point at 48 hours, and 1 study each at 96 hours (764 patients) and 120 hours (314 patients).

micro-aspiration can lead to ventilator-associated pneumonia.

Data from 38 prospective cohort and non-randomized studies collated by Safdar and colleagues (Figure 14.11) suggests that the risk of developing VAP increases with time, being around 6% at the onset of mechanical ventilation and increasing to 20% in those ventilated for 72 hours or more. Pooled data[13] from case-controlled studies suggests that each episode of VAP lengthens the duration of intensive care by 6.1 days at an estimated additional cost of £4 996[7] per case. The effect on outcome is less evident, although it is likely that VAP doubles the risk of death in the intensive care unit but not thereafter.[13]

Diagnosis

The diagnosis of VAP is usually considered when there are signs of systemic sepsis, such as fever and raised inflammatory markers, together with evidence implicating the lungs, such as an abnormal chest radiograph, purulent tracheal aspirates and an elevated alveolar–arterial oxygen difference (Table 14.8). Unfortunately, this combination of features is not uncommon in mechanically ventilated patients and can arise from a wide range of clinical conditions other than VAP. Using stricter clinical criteria risks missing the diagnosis in some patients, while using more relaxed criteria will inevitably result in the inappropriate administration of antibiotics with the risk of generating antibiotic resistance. Examination and culture of lower

5 days of hospitalization the oropharynx becomes colonized by atypical bacteria, including antibiotic resistant strains of *Staphylococcus aureus, Pseudomonas aeruginosa*, Acinetobacter or Enterobacter species. In the context of a patient who is immunocompromised by severe intercurrent illness and who cannot cough effectively to clear secretions, this

---

[7] Calculated from the original figure of $10 019.00 US, equivalent to 7 378.85 Euros.

Table 14.9 Quantitative criteria for the diagnosis of ventilator-associated pneumonia from respiratory tract samples

	New antibiotics in previous 72 hours?	
	No	Yes
Endotracheal aspirate	$\geq 10^6$ cfu.mL^{-1}	$\geq 10^4$ cfu.mL^{-1}
Bronchoalveolar lavage	$\geq 10^4$ or 10^5 cfu.mL^{-1}	$\geq 10^3$ cfu.mL^{-1}
Protected brush sample	$\geq 10^3$ cfu.mL^{-1}	$\geq 10^2$ cfu.mL^{-1}

cfu: colony-forming unit.

respiratory tract samples not only confirms the diagnosis, but also allows therapy to be appropriately focused. These samples can be obtained either by endotracheal aspiration, bronchoalveolar lavage or protected brush sampling, and these should be accompanied by the culture of blood in all patients and pleural fluid in those with an effusion. Where possible, these investigations should precede empirical antibiotic therapy. Microbiological analyses of the respiratory tract samples are reported either semi-quantitatively or quantitatively,[8] depending on the resources and enthusiasm of the local microbiology department (Table 14.9). However, semi-quantitative reports differentiate poorly between colonization and infection,[9] resulting in the overuse of antibiotics. To some extent, this can be redeemed if the antibiotic therapy is reviewed in the light of the patient's response following 72 hours of treatment (Figure 14.12). Careful post-mortem examination

[8] A semi-quantitative report would describe the organisms isolated and describe whether their growth was light (+), moderate (++) or heavy (+++), while a quantitative report would give the number of each organism, referred to as a *colony-forming unit*, per mL of the original specimen, expressed to the nearest factor of 10, e.g >10^4 cfu.mL^{-1}.

[9] In contrast to blood or cerebrospinal fluid, the isolation of bacteria from the respiratory tract of a patient who is unwell does not *necessarily* mean that the organism is causing an infection even though this organism would not normally be found in the respiratory tract in health. This is because during severe illness the mouth, pharynx and upper respiratory tract rapidly become colonized with Staphylococci and Gram-negative enteric bacteria.

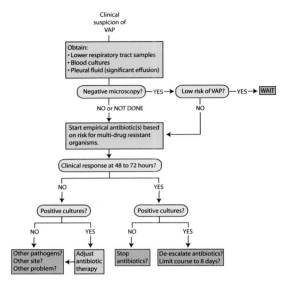

Figure 14.12 Management strategy for suspected cases of ventilator-associated pneumonia (VAP).

Based on the joint guidelines of the American Thoracic Association and Infectious Diseases Society of America. *Am J Respir Crit Care Med.* Feb 15 2005;171(4):388–416.

of the lungs of patients with VAP show that foci of infection are frequently multiple and heterogeneous in both physical location and 'maturity', with a predilection for dependent lung zones. This explains the lower sensitivity of protected brush sampling, which can only draw material from a single sub-segmental bronchus. In contrast, bronchoalveolar lavage allows material to be sampled from a much larger volume of lung. Where the skills necessary to perform bronchoscopic sampling are not available, both bronchoalveolar lavage and protected brush sampling can both be performed 'blindly' but at the expense of a reduction in sensitivity. Invasive approaches, blind or otherwise, are associated with temporary deteriorations in gas exchange but with few other complications of note.

Treatment

In the absence of risk factors for infection caused by an antibiotic-resistant pathogen (Table 14.10), initial treatment with a single agent active against

Table 14.10 Risk factors for antibiotic-resistant infection

- Residential care
- Antibiotic therapy in preceding 90 days
- Home wound care
- Family member with antibiotic-resistant organism
- Chronic dialysis
- High local prevalence of resistant organisms
- Two or more days as an in-patient in previous 90 days
- Five or more days in hospital this admission
- Immunosuppressed

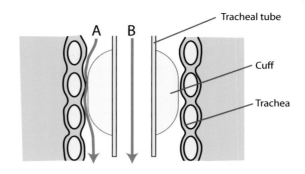

Figure 14.13 Contamination routes for the lower respiratory tract in the acquisition of ventilator-associated pneumonia.

A: The para-cuff route, with endogenous contaminants pooling in the secretions above the cuff in the sub-glottic space arising from the oropharynx, stomach, nose and sinuses.

B: The trans-luminal route, with exogenous contaminants coming from the surfaces of the endotracheal tube, catheter mount, suction equipment, nebulizer equipment, and ventilator circuit.

the most likely organisms such as *Streptococcus pneumoniae*, *Haemophilus influenzae*, *Staphylococcus aureus* and antibiotic-sensitive Gram-negative enteric bacilli is indicated. Suitable agents might include a third-generation cephalosporin or a quinolone. Where there is a chance that the infection might be due to a resistant organism such as metnicillin-resistant *Staphylococcus aureus* (MRSA), *Pseudomonas aeruginosa*, *Klebsiella pneumoniae* or species of Acinetobacter, triple therapy with an agent active against MRSA, such as vancomycin,[10] and two broad-spectrum agents such as an anti-pseudomonal carbapenem[11] or beta-lactam[12] together with either an aminoglycoside[13] or an anti-pseudomonal fluoroquinolone[14] should be considered. The specific choice of agent will depend on the local sensitivity patterns, and if these are not known by the prescriber, then a discussion with the local microbiologists is likely to be helpful. After 48 or 72 hours of treatment, the management strategy should then be reviewed in light of the patient's response, and the specific antibiotic sensitivities of the organisms isolated (Figure 14.12).

Prevention

The presence of a cuffed tracheal tube has the dual effect of allowing pathogens originating from either the patient's oropharynx (endogenous) or the internal surfaces of the endotracheal tube and ventilator circuit (exogenous, Figure 14.13) increased entry to, as well as decreased clearance from, the lower respiratory tract. Both routes have been shown amenable to strategies aimed at reducing the risk of VAP, and these are discussed later (Table 14.11). Of course, one of the most obvious ways of reducing the risk of VAP is to avoid tracheal intubation in the first place, and indeed in selected patients non-invasive ventilation is an option that should be exploited. For the majority, intubation is unavoidable. As discussed previously, intubation away from the operating department environment is associated with a significant risk of aspiration, and indeed it has been suggested that prophylactic antibiotics should be prescribed after these intubations. Rather than treating possible aspiration with antibiotics, which is not endorsed by either the American[14] or European[15] guidelines, it is preferable to reduce the chances of

---

[10] 15 mg.kg^{-1} every 12 hours, trough levels 15 to 20 µg.mL^{-1} .
[11] Imipenem (1 g every 8 hours) or meropenem (1 g every 8 hours).
[12] Piperacillin/tazobactam (4.5 g every 6 hours).
[13] Amikacin (20 mg.kg^{-1} daily, trough level <4 to 5 µg.mL^{-1}), gentamicin (7 mg.kg^{-1} daily, trough level <1 µg.mL) or tobramycin (7 mg.kg^{-1} daily, trough level <1 µg.mL^{-1}).
[14] Ciprofloxacin (400 mg every 8 hours) or levofloxacin (750 mg daily).

Table 14.11 Measures for preventing ventilator-associated pneumonia

Measure	ATS/IDSA[14] (2005)	Canadian[20] (2004)	ESICM[15] (2001)
Avoidance of intubation or re-intubation	Yes	–	Yes
Post-intubation antibiotics	No	–	No
Regular cuff pressure measurement	Yes	–	Yes
New cuff design	–	–	–
Sub-glottic suction	Yes	Yes	No
Avoidance of supine position	Yes	Yes	Yes
Avoiding transfers	–	–	–
Kinetic beds	–	Yes	–
Sucralfate for stress ulcer prophylaxis		No	NR
Selective decontamination of the digestive tract	No	NR	Yes
Avoidance of gastric distension	–	–	–
Oral decontamination	No	–	–
Oral intubation	Yes	Yes	Yes
Orogastric tubes	Yes	–	–
Hand hygiene and infection control	Yes	–	Yes
Cohorting of staff	–	–	–
Isolation of patients with multi-drug-resistant pathogens	Yes	–	–
Avoid understaffing	Yes	–	–
Avoid overcrowding	–	–	–
Breathing circuit changes weekly or less	–	Yes[15]	Yes
Closed suction systems	–	Yes[16]	No
Avoidance of hot water humidification systems	No	Yes	No
Prevention of circuit condensate entering airway	Yes	–	–
Reducing the duration of mechanical ventilation	Yes	–	–
Early tracheostomy	–	NR	–
Avoidance of neuromuscular blocking agents	Yes	–	Yes
Microbiological surveillance	Yes	–	–

–: not discussed.
NR: no recommendation possible on the available evidence.
ATS: American Thoracic Society.
IDSA: Infectious Disease Society of America.
ESICM: European Society of Intensive Care Medicine.

aspiration, and other intubation-related complications, by having this procedure performed under optimum conditions as discussed above. Within the intensive care unit itself, two of the most common reasons for urgent tracheal intubation are following accidental or failed extubation. Because both of

these are the consequence of staff actions and can be reduced by the implementation of appropriate practices and procedures, their incidence should be routinely monitored as a measure of quality assurance.

Endogenous route

The current design of high-volume, low-pressure tracheal tube cuffs develop folds when inflated within the tracheal lumen that allow liquid

---

[15] In fact, the Canadian guidelines recommend a circuit change if it becomes visibly soiled.
[16] On the basis of cost.

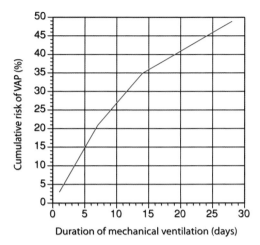

Figure 14.14 Cumulative risk of developing ventilator-associated pneumonia (VAP) with the duration of mechanical ventilation.

The cumulative risk suggests that all patients mechanically ventilated for 79 days will develop VAP.

material to seep through into the lower airway[16] (see Figure 4.13). The aspirated material may arise from a number of sources, including the oropharynx, stomach, mouth, nose and sinuses, and accumulates above the cuff in the sub-glottic space (see Figure 4.19). In a multivariate analysis of large case series, the failure to maintain cuff pressure above 20 cm H_2O was independently associated with an increased risk of VAP[17] (relative risk 4.23, 95% confidence interval 1.12 to 15.92), and regular measurement of cuff pressure has been recommended by a number of organizations.[17] Despite this, and the simplicity of the intervention, routine measurement of cuff pressures is still not performed in some

intensive care units in the UK. Continuous automated cuff pressure controllers are available and in a recent study reduced clinical VAP from 29% to 22%, although this did not reach statistical significance. Two new designs of cuff have recently been introduced aimed at eliminating cuff folds. The Microcuff™ endotracheal tube[18] has a very thin polyurethane high-volume cuff which is cylindrical in shape and in a laboratory evaluation effectively eliminated leakage past the cuff.[18] The LoTrach™ tube[19], in contrast, has a low-volume low-pressure silicone cuff that has been calibrated to deliver a tracheal wall pressure of 25 to 30 cm H_2O when the internal cuff pressure is maintained at 74 to 79 cm H_2O using a constant-pressure inflation device. The LoTrach tube has been shown to significantly reduce leakage past the cuff in both laboratory and clinical evaluations. The impact of either of these new cuff designs on the incidence of VAP has yet to be evaluated.

Some models of endotracheal and tracheostomy tube[20] allow material collected above the cuff to be aspirated through additional suction channels. A recent meta-analysis of 5 randomized studies showed that sub-glottic suction reduced the incidence of VAP by almost 50%, although the effect was most evident for pneumonia occurring within the first week of intubation.[19] Excluding one study, in which the mean duration of mechanical ventilation was less than 48 hours, sub-glottic suction also resulted in a reduction in the duration of both mechanical ventilation and length of stay in the intensive care unit.

Because aspiration of gastric content is believed to be a contributory mechanism to the development of VAP, a number of interventions have been aimed at reducing both the risk of regurgitation as well as the bacterial load in the regurgitated material. Nursing

[17] The joint guidelines of the American Thoracic Society and the Infectious Diseases Society of America. From Guidelines for the management of adults with hospital-acquired, ventilator-associated, and healthcare-associated pneumonia. *Am J Respir Crit Care Med.* 2005;171(4):388–416 and guidelines written by the European Task Force on Ventilator-Associated Pneumonia on behalf of the European Society of Intensive Care Medicine. From Torres A, Carlet J. Ventilator-associated pneumonia. European Task Force on ventilator-associated pneumonia. *Eur Respir J.* 2001;17(5): 1034–45.

[18] Kimberley-Clark Health Care, Roswell, Georgia, USA. See www.kchealthcare.com/microcuff/.
[19] LMA International SA, Henley, UK.
[20] Hi-Lo™ Evac (Mallinckrodt), LoTrach (LMA International)

the patient with the torso at 45° to the horizontal has been shown to reduce the incidence of VAP, but achieving this accurately and persistently in clinical practice is almost impossible for a number of reasons. First, it appears not to be widely appreciated that the angulation that matters is that between the patient's torso and the horizontal rather than that between the head of the bed and the horizontal. These are not equivalent. Second, clinical staff have been shown to significantly overestimate the angle achieved, and so tend to *aim* for a torso position that is 50% too supine. Third, maintaining a 45° angle is difficult, especially in a patient who is restless. Nevertheless the avoidance of a supine position is one of the few unanimous recommendations of the American,[14] Canadian[20] and European[15] guidelines.

There are occasions when it is necessary to lay the patient completely supine, such as for diagnostic or therapeutic imaging and surgical procedures. These are the situations most commonly associated with patient transfer, which has been shown in two studies to be independently associated with an increased risk for VAP. Whether this association is causal or not is unclear, but clearly unnecessary patient transfers should be avoided wherever possible.

A number of studies have looked at the effect of beds that provide continuous side-to-side tilt, also known as *kinetic therapy*. A recent meta-analysis has confirmed a significant effect of this on reducing the incidence of VAP[21] (odds ratio 0.38, 95% confidence interval 0.28 to 0.53). Kinetic therapy is suggested as a consideration in the Canadian guidelines. However, these beds are not suitable for some patients, not tolerated by others, and have significant cost implications.

Gastric content in health is normally maintained relatively sterile by the low gastric pH, but the stomach is rapidly colonized by Gram-negative enteric organisms following hospitalization, and all the more so if gastric pH is increased by histamine receptor antagonists or proton pump inhibitors admin-

istered as stress ulcer prophylaxis. In the case of stress ulcer prophylaxis, there is a choice between agents that increase gastric pH and therefore the risk of VAP, but which are more effective at reducing stress-related gastric haemorrhage, or sucralfate that is less effective at preventing bleeding but which increases the risk of VAP. Neither the European[15] nor the American[14] guidelines make a recommendation, although there is some evidence that the outcome from gastric haemorrhage is poorer than that from VAP, favouring agents that increase gastric pH.[22] An alternative approach is to administer powerful broad-spectrum but non-absorbable antibiotics into the gastrointestinal tract to eliminate the potentially pathogenic organisms, often referred to as *selective decontamination of the digestive tract* (SDD). Where the background incidence of multi-drug-resistant organisms is low, this approach has been very effective in reducing both the incidence and consequent mortality of VAP, and indeed is an approach endorsed by the European guidelines.[15] However, in many countries the background incidence of highly resistant organisms such as MRSA, vancomycin-resistant enterococci and certain strains of *Acinetobacter baumanii*, *Klebsiella pneumoniae* and *Pseudomonas aeruginosa* is high (such as the UK and the US). In this context, SDD rather than reducing VAP may encourage the emergence of these strains and should only be used in selected populations. As gastropharyngeal reflux is thought to be a contributing mechanism to the generation of VAP, it seems logical to minimize the chances of this happening, which might reasonably include measures to avoid large gastric volumes such as reducing the use of opiates and anticholinergic agents, use of prokinetic agents and post-pyloric feeding. However, none of these interventions has been evaluated for efficacy and they are not mentioned in any of the recent guidelines.

Besides the stomach, endogenous contamination of aspirated material can arise from organisms that colonize the mouth, nose and sinuses. Although dental plaque is estimated to harbour about 500 species of micro-organism at a density of 10^8 per mm^3, respiratory tract pathogens are rarely isolated from healthy adults. In contrast, about 60% of patients have respiratory pathogens in their dental plaque on the day of admission to intensive care. Under normal circumstances, both plaque load and the prevalence of respiratory pathogen colonization increase with the duration of mechanical ventilation. In up to 76% of cases of VAP, the pathogens identified in plaque are also cultured from the lung. There are three possible sources for these organisms. First, it is possible that respiratory pathogens are in fact normal members of plaque flora but suppressed to undetectable numbers by a number of mechanisms operating in good health, such as the secretion of saliva, which contains numerous antibacterial proteins[21] and maintains an elevated oral pH, normal processes of oral hygiene, and substrate competition by the normal non-pathogenic oral flora. Second, these pathogens may reach the mouth by sequential colonization from the lower gastrointestinal tract, eventually reaching the mouth in material regurgitated from the stomach. Third, they may enter the mouth from the hospital environment as contaminants on the surface of equipment or on the hands of caregivers. While not all cases of VAP are derived from the aspiration of pathogens from the mouth, oral disinfection with chlorhexidine has been shown to reduce the incidence of VAP (relative risk 0.56, 95% confidence interval 0.39 to 0.81) in a recent meta-analysis,[23] but the data on oral antibiotics remains inconclusive.

Infected nasal secretions are another source of pathogens that can reach the lower respiratory tract following micro-aspiration. The risk of developing radiological maxillary sinusitis (RMS) after 7 days of ventilation is *much* greater in patients with naso-tracheal intubation compared to orotracheal intubation[4] (odds ratio 73.5, confidence interval 7.42 to 728.2), a finding that also applies to feeding tubes. However, the relationship between radiological maxillary sinusitis and VAP is unproven because the only randomized controlled trial (RCT) to date failed to control for the presence of RMS at randomization, later shown to be present in 59% of patients on admission to ICU.[4] Although the incidence of VAP in patients randomized to nasotracheal intubation was greater, this did not reach statistical significance (odds ratio 2.03, 95% confidence interval 0.88 to 4.72).[24] Rouby and colleagues' finding of a significantly increased risk of VAP with *infectious* maxillary sinusitis (IMS) compared to *sterile* maxillary sinusitis (SMS) (odds ratio 2.7, 95% confidence interval 1.17 to 6.24)[4] is consistent with this as the risk of IMS presumably increases in proportion to the risk of RMS.

Exogenous route

Undoubtedly, horizontal transmission[22] is a significant source of VAP in mechanically ventilated patients with the introduction of pathogens either into the mouth or nose, or into the airway itself by contamination of the breathing circuit or other respiratory equipment. This route of transmission tends to become highlighted during outbreaks involving organisms with memorable names,[23] or memorable antibiograms,[24] but occurs constantly. Simple infection control measures, such as hand

---

[21] Such as lysozyme, lactoferrin, lactoperoxidase, immuno-globulins, proline-rich proteins, cystatins, histatins, Von Ebner gland proteins, secretory leukocyte proteinase inhibitor, fibronectin and chromogranin A.

[22] Patient-to-patient transmission of pathogens by caregivers.

[23] For example, *Burkholderia cepacia*.

[24] The antibiogram is the pattern of antibiotic sensitivity that is reported by the microbiology laboratory when a pathogen has been isolated. Fortunately, resistance to multiple antibiotics remains the exception rather than the rule, and certain species of bacteria are typically resistant to certain types of antibiotic only. A broad or unusual resistance pattern makes a particular strain of organism uniquely recognizable, briefly exposing the otherwise occult occurrence of horizontal transmission.

hygiene, are endorsed by the North American and European guidelines, but these documents largely overlook the important contribution that can be made by other measures, including the cohorting of staff, isolation of infected patients and the avoidance of both understaffing and overcrowding.

Opening of the breathing circuit contributes to the development of VAP in two ways. First, the loss of positive end-expiratory pressure significantly accelerates the leak of material past the cuff, increasing the risk of endogenous infection. Second, it allows the inner surfaces of the circuit and endotracheal tube to become contaminated, increasing the risk of exogenous infection. A number of interventions require that the breathing circuit be opened, including breathing circuit changes, and tracheobronchial suction using an open technique. The evidence from both prospective randomized trials and cohort studies suggests that reducing the frequency of breathing circuit changes certainly does not increase the risk of VAP and indeed may very well reduce it. Circuits should therefore only be changed when visibly soiled; if routine changes are felt necessary, these should be no more often than weekly, or even less often. In contrast, the type of suction system does not appear to have an impact on the incidence of VAP, although in patients who are dependent on positive end-expiratory pressure (PEEP), the closed system may be preferable.

The warming and humidification of inspired gases is important in preventing both heat loss and the inspissation of tracheobronchial secretions but there have been concerns that hot-water humidifiers might increase the risk of VAP compared to heat-and-moisture exchange filters. Ten randomized trials comparing the incidence of VAP between the two humidification techniques have been published since 1990, of which eight were available for the meta-analysis in 2005 which concluded that the risk was indeed lower for the heat-and-moisture exchange filters[25] (relative risk 0.69, 95% confidence interval 0.51 to 0.94), especially for patients

requiring 7 or more days of mechanical ventilation. However, in two subsequent studies that randomized 750 patients between them, the benefit in favour of heat-and-moisture exchange filters is not significant, and adding these data to the previous studies broadens the confidence interval to include 1 (relative risk 0.83, 95% confidence interval 0.67 to 1.03). Bearing in mind the large difference in cost between the two systems, it would seem prudent to reserve the use of hot-water humidifiers to situations where aggressive humidification is indicated.

Regardless of the type of humidification, the internal surface of the endotracheal tube rapidly becomes colonized with upper respiratory flora and coated with expectorated sputum. Both the sputum coating and a bacterially-derived biofilm, secreted under certain conditions, form a protective environment that can harbour large numbers of bacteria. These can then be transferred to the lower respiratory tract with each ventilator cycle or during suctioning. Physical removal of this biofilm has been achieved with an inflatable silicone rubber 'razor', and clinical evaluation is awaited. More conventionally, the efficacy of antibacterial coatings on the endotracheal tube surface, such as chlorhexidine or silver, are currently being evaluated in patients.

The risk of developing VAP is particularly high during the first week of ventilation when it increases by 3% per day, but then the risk only increases by 2% per day for the second week, and then 1% per day thereafter[26] (Figure 14.14). This would suggest that techniques designed to reduce the duration of mechanical ventilation might reduce the risk of developing VAP. This has been hard to prove because the studies evaluating techniques for reducing the duration of mechanical ventilation, such as protocols and sedation breaks, have not enrolled sufficient patients to detect the expected reduction in VAP rate. Nevertheless, minimizing the duration of mechanical ventilation is common sense, and is recommended in the North American

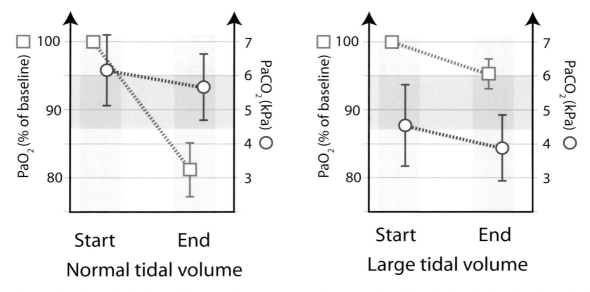

Figure 14.15 Change in arterial partial pressure of oxygen expressed as a percentage of baseline in patients undergoing surgical procedures under general anaesthesia with positive pressure ventilation.

The left panel is from nine patients ventilated with 'normal' tidal volumes, resulting in arterial partial pressures of carbon dioxide ($PaCO_2$) at the top end or just above the reference interval, shaded in green. The arterial partial pressure of oxygen (PaO_2) falls in these patients by a mean of 16.8% (SD 5.7%).

The right panel is from nine patients receiving supra-physiological tidal volumes, resulting in a $PaCO_2$ at the bottom end or just below the reference interval, shaded in green. The PaO_2 falls in these patients by a mean of 4.8% (SD 2.3%).

Both the initial and final $PaCO_2$ are significantly different between the groups (ANOVA, p = 0.005 and 0.0003 respectively), as is the PaO_2 drop (ANOVA, p <0.0001). Figure and statistics based on data presented in Bendixen HH, Hedley-White J, Laver MD. *N Engl J Med.* 1963;269:991–6.

guidelines.[14] Where prolonged tracheal intubation is required, a tracheostomy may reduce the risk of developing VAP, although the evidence on this is conflicting. A more definitive answer is likely to be provided by the UK TracMan study.

Ventilator-associated lung injury

Although the first commercially available, integrated, automated, blood gas analyser was not marketed until 1973,[25] the measurement of blood pH, and blood oxygen (PO_2) and carbon dioxide (PCO_2) tension at the bedside, rather than as a laboratory technique, became possible with the development of electrochemical methods of measurement at the end of the 1950s. Shortly afterward, in

1963, a group at the Massachusetts General Hospital in Boston measured arterial blood gases in patients undergoing surgical procedures under general anaesthesia with positive pressure ventilation, and found that patients that had been ventilated with supra-physiological tidal volumes maintained their oxygenation, while patients ventilated with 'normal' tidal volumes did not[27] (Figure 4.15). They concluded 'large tidal volumes, by providing continuous hyperinflation, protect against an increase in the variable shunt'. Aware of the dangers of hyperoxia (see later discussion) and uncertain of the role of PEEP, large tidal volumes became established as a method of maintaining oxygenation in patients receiving mechanical ventilation. Indeed, they became such an established method that during the mid to late 1960s, reports emerged of

[25] ABL1, Radiometer, Copenhagen.

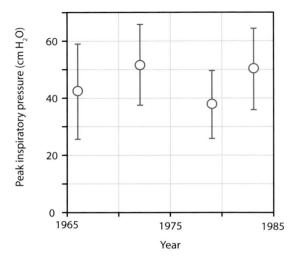

Figure 14.16 Peak inspiratory pressures in patients receiving mechanical ventilation reported in the literature between 1965 and 1985.

Calculated from data in *J Clin Invest*. 1966;45(10):1543–54; *Scand J Respir Dis*. 1972;53(3):149–60; *Anesthesiology*. 1979;50(3):185–90 and *Crit Care Med*. 1983;11(2):67–9.

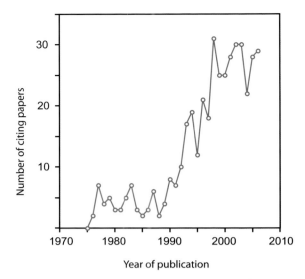

Figure 14.17 Number of papers citing Webb & Tierney (See Reference 29).

complications from hypocapnia and respiratory alkalosis including cardiac dysrhythmias, shock, seizures, and neurological disturbances. Rather than reduce tidal volumes, solutions proposed included the addition of 5% carbon dioxide to the inspiratory gas mixture, nomograms for the addition of equipment deadspace, and the invention of devices to provide variable deadspace. Concerned that these high inspiratory pressures might be damaging, Webb and Tierney published a paper in 1974 that examined the effect of peak inspiratory pressures of up to 45 cm H_2O on the lungs of normal rats.[28] Much to their surprise, they found that mechanical ventilation with these pressures, which were in common use in patients at the time (Figure 14.16), was in fact rapidly lethal in rats. Although their findings had a significant impact on their own clinical practice, it remained largely ignored by other clinicians but did provoke further work on the subject in animals. However, the accumulating animal data were sufficiently convincing to cause a group of clinicians in Christchurch, New Zealand, to adjust

their clinical practice in the latter part of 1980s. By 1990, they were able to show an unexpectedly low mortality in their patients ventilated with limited inspiratory pressures,[29] which seems to have sparked much more widespread interest in the issue (Figure 14.17). By the end of the decade, the effect of high inspiratory pressures had been examined in four prospective randomized controlled trials,[30,31,32,33] although without reaching a common conclusion. The issue was largely settled in 2000 with the publication of the ARDSnet[26] study, a collaborative study involving a consortium of 20 academic institutions in the United States.[34] In this study, patients with acute lung injury requiring mechanical ventilation were randomized to a 'traditional' tidal volume of 12 mL.kg^{-1} (n = 429)[27] with plateau pressures ≤50 cm H_2O or 'low' tidal volumes of 6 mL.kg^{-1} (n = 432) with a plateau pressure ≤30 cm H_2O. Recruitment was terminated early because of a significant difference

[26] Acute respiratory distress syndrome network (ARDSnet), a consortium of North American hospitals collaborating on clinical trials of ARDS therapies.

[27] Body weight predicted by sex and height.

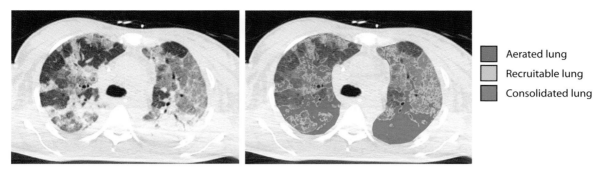

Aerated lung
Recruitable lung
Consolidated lung

Figure 14.18 Computerized tomography of a patient with acute respiratory distress syndrome (ARDS, left), which can be divided into three zones (right); normally aerated lung (green), recruitable lung (amber), and consolidated lung (red).
Computerized tomogram courtesy of Dr Simon Finney, Royal Brompton and Harefield NHS Trust.

in hospital mortality (31% versus 39.8%) in favour of the low-tidal volume group (p = 0.007). This study has established that mechanical ventilation has an impact on outcome; in this case, as a result of pulmonary damage from excess tidal volumes.

Volume or pressure?

Although the ARDSnet study was framed primarily in terms of a target inflation volume and it is now clear that the mechanism of damage is longitudinal stress on over-inflated pulmonary tissue, ventilation to a target *volume*, however small, does not guarantee that damage is not being done. This is because the lungs of patients with lung injury are not homogenous, but have areas of normal lung, areas of consolidation and areas of recruitable lung (Figure 14.18). This means that the volume of lung available for ventilation cannot be estimated on a mL.kg^{-1} basis or even by ensuring that the end-inspiratory lung volume is kept within normal limits; the prevention of over-distension can *only* be guaranteed by ensuring that inspiratory pressures are maintained at values that would not cause over-distension in lung tissue of normal compliance (Figure 14.19).

Pathophysiology

The pathophysiological details of ventilator-induced lung damage have largely been investigated in animal models, for obvious reasons. Two distinct

processes have been identified, which occur initially in sequence: an acute phase characterized by interstitial and pulmonary oedema and surfactant dysfunction, followed by a sub-acute phase characterized by inflammation.

Acute oedema occurs through the combined effects of increased filtration and increased permeability. The transcapillary hydrostatic pressure, which is the pressure responsible for driving fluid out of the extra-alveolar pulmonary vessels, is increased in two ways. First, it is increased by a drop in the interstitial pressure around the extra-alveolar vessels resulting from (1) increased surface tension secondary to surfactant dysfunction, and (2) stretching open of the interstitial space by the lung over-inflation (Figure 14.20). Second, it is increased by an increase in extra-alveolar hydrostatic pressure which occurs in response to the decreased calibre of intra-alveolar vessels caused by the raised alveolar pressure.

Surfactant dysfunction arises from a number of possible mechanisms. In the short term, surfactant release from type 2 alveolar cells is enhanced by high-volume ventilation, but the increased surface area changes of the alveoli increases the rate at which surfactant is 'milked' into the conducting airways and eventually exceeds the rate of production. In addition, high tidal volume ventilation increases the conversion of 'large aggregate' surfactant into

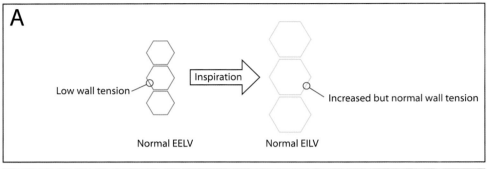

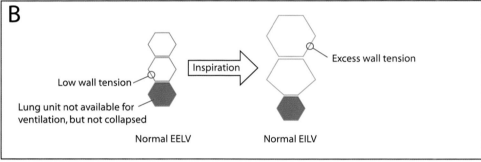

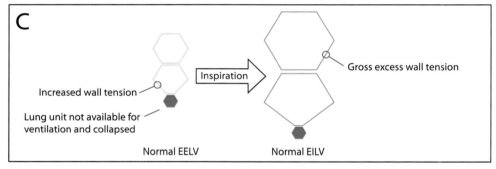

Figure 14.19 Effect of inspiration of a 'normal' tidal volume on alveolar wall stress.

Panel A depicts a lung with normal end-expiratory lung volume (EELV) and low alveolar wall tension into which is delivered a 'normal' volume breath, resulting in a 'normal' end-inspiratory lung volume (EILV) with modestly increased alveolar wall tension.

In panel B, a proportion of the lung units are not available for ventilation, but have not collapsed. This means that at the normal EELV the wall tension in the functional alveoli is not raised. However, in this situation a 'normal' tidal volume is now delivered into fewer alveoli. This means that although the EILV is still 'normal', the functioning alveoli are over-expanded and have excess wall tension.

In panel C, which represents the more usual situation, the non-functioning lung units have collapsed. In this situation if the EELV is to remain 'normal', the functional lung units have to be larger than usual, and even at end-expiration have increased wall tension. Now a normal tidal volume results in a gross increase in alveolar wall tension, even though the EILV is 'normal'.

the inactive 'small aggregate' form. Finally, residual surfactant is rapidly inactivated by plasma proteins that leak into the alveoli.

The permeability of both the capillary endothelium and the alveolar epithelium is increased by a number of mechanisms, ranging from the generation of both intracellular and intercellular gaps, which is separation of these cells from the underlying basement membrane, to complete loss of capillary endothelial cells and alveolar type 1

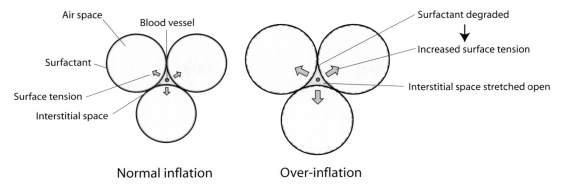

Figure 14.20 Effect of surfactant degradation and alveolar over-inflation on interstitial pressure.

The diagram on the left represents a pulmonary interstitial space with a central blood vessel surrounded on three sides by air spaces lined by surfactant. Under conditions of over-inflation (right) the interstitial pressure is reduced by being 'stretched' open by the adjacent air spaces, as well as a significant increase in the air space surface tension caused by surfactant degradation.

epithelial cells. Ultimately, the basement membrane itself may give way, leading to alveolar haemorrhage. Alveolar type 2 cells, which usually occupy the alveolar corners appear to be relatively spared in this process.

Increases in intracellular calcium concentration arising from breaches in the cell membrane provoke the mobilization, coalescence and exocytosis of intra-cytoplasmic 'patches' of lipid vesicles at the site of damage to the cell membrane. Cellular deformation is sensed by molecules that are positioned at the junction between the cell's cytoskeleton and the trans-membrane connectors to adjacent cells and tissues, and which trigger a number of other processes involved in cellular remodelling and repair. These include the activation of genes involved in paracrine signalling, resulting in the production of factors such as transforming growth factor (TGF-β1) and basic fibroblast growth factor, as well as genes involved in the synthesis of fibronectin, collagen and matrix metalloproteinases.

Whether the responses mentioned previously are also directly responsible for the activation of pro-inflammatory genes, or whether their activation arises secondary to cell necrosis and the exposure of basement membrane, or whether both mechanisms operate, remains to be elucidated. Regardless,

it is now clear that the sub-acute response to stretch injury is an inflammatory response that draws neutrophils to the lung parenchyma and macrophages to the alveolar air spaces, and that this process is exacerbated by hyperoxia. The inflammatory process produces cytokines that can be detected in lung lavage, which may then 'spill over' into the systemic circulation to cause organ damage at other sites. It has been suggested, but remains to be proved, that ventilation-induced pulmonary-derived inflammatory mediators might be responsible for the multiple organ failure seen in patients with severe lung injury.

The role of lung mechanics

Detection of the end-inspiratory lung pressure or volume at which over-distension is occurring would be useful, as it would allow clinicians to set the upper pressure or volume limits for non-injurious mechanical ventilation. Inspection of the static inflation pressure-volume curve from functional residual capacity to vital capacity, which can now be measured on some modern ventilators, often shows an upper inflection, which is said to mark the end of alveolar recruitment or the beginning of lung over-distension (Figure 14.21). However, the exact significance of the upper inflection point is not known, the pressure-volume curves are awkward and

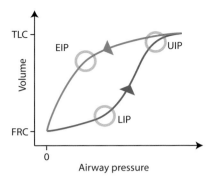

The blue line indicates paired measurements of inflating pressure plotted against lung volume from functional residual capacity (FRC) to total lung capacity (TLC). In order to avoid the effect of resistance to gas flow, the measurements should be made by the sequential introduction of a small, known, volume of gas (50 to 100 mL) followed by a brief pause to allow the airway pressure to settle to its true value. Mechanical ventilators actually measure the *quasi*-static inflation pressure/volume curve because they measure pressures during a constant low-flow insufflation and ignore the effect of resistance to gas flow. An 'ideal' inflation pressure-volume has a lower inflection point (LIP) and an upper inflection point (UIP), but in practice these points cannot always be identified. The physiological significance of the LIP and UIP remain disputed.

The deflation limb (green) of the pressure-volume traces a different contour, reflecting the fact that the lung has hysteresis. As with the inflation limb, an ideal deflation limb has an inflection which is known as the expiratory inflection point (EIP), and which is said to represent the onset of alveolar collapse.

time-consuming to measure, and there is no evidence that using the upper inflection point is any more effective than using the lowest possible inflating pressure. At the low-volume end of the static inflation pressure-volume curve is the lower inflection point[28] (LIP, Figure 14.21), which for a long time was thought to represent the end of alveolar recruitment. Besides the fact that there is now good evidence that alveolar recruitment occurs throughout the inflation phase, there remains consider-

[28] Sometimes referred to in the literature as 'P$_{flex}$'.

able uncertainty about the events at a cellular level which constitute 'alveolar recruitment' and that are responsible for the transition from a lower compliance to higher compliance state. The currently accepted view regards this to be due to the opening of alveoli, predominantly in the dependent parts of the lung, that have collapsed under the combined effects of the weight of overlying oedematous lung, and of surfactant degradation. However, this view has been challenged. Studies in animals suggest that ventilation in which the LIP is repeatedly crossed is injurious, and this damage can be avoided by setting PEEP above the LIP. In fact, evidence that this is the case in humans is lacking. Thus the ARDSnet comparison of high PEEP versus low PEEP, in which there was no outcome difference between the groups, did not select the high PEEP on the basis of the LIP,[35] and the two clinical studies that *have* selected high PEEP on the basis of the LIP[30,36] also used lower tidal volumes in the high PEEP group, making it impossible to isolate the effect of the higher PEEP from that due to the lower tidal volume. Besides the LIP, which is on the inspiratory limb of the pressure-volume curve, there is also an inflection on the deflation limb that is sometimes called the 'expiratory inflection point' or 'closing volume' that often occurs at a lower pressure than the LIP, but at a greater lung volume (Figure 14.21). On the basis that this inflection is caused by an increase in the rate of alveolar collapse, it is believed by some that PEEP should be set at or above the EIP following a recruitment manoeuvre, although to date the EIP has been substituted for optimal SpO$_2$ in clinical studies.

Although not formally recognized as such, recruitable lung is in fact present in two forms: a *tidally* recruited form and a *potentially* recruitable form. The potentially recruitable lung is that part of the lung which is not opened by the pressure excursions of normal ventilation but which can be opened by a high-pressure 'recruitment manoeuvre'. Many such manoeuvres have been

Table 14.12 Questions that remain to be answered about recruitment manoeuvres and positive end-expiratory pressure

Recruitment Manoeuvres	Positive end-expiratory pressure (PEEP)
Which recruitment manoeuvre is best, and does it depend on the lung pathology?	How should we set PEEP?
What proportion of patients are recruitable when they are first intubated?	
Does this depend on the lung pathology?	
Does a patient's 'recruitability' change with time? If this is so, does this also depend on the lung pathology?	
How often does a patient need to be recruited, and what does this depend on?	
Does maintaining a patient optimally recruited alter the course of their lung disease?	
Is lung recruitment harmful? Are there any patients who should not have their lungs recruited?	

described in the literature, and have been shown in both animals and man to improve lung mechanics and oxygenation. Furthermore, identifying the critical closing pressure on the deflation limb of the pressure-volume curve (Figure 14.21) allows PEEP to be set at a pressure that is often lower than the LIP. Because many questions remain to be answered about recruitment manoeuvres (Table 14.12,) they should be used selectively, but routine use cannot yet be endorsed.

Ventilator-induced diaphragmatic damage (VIDD)

Diaphragm inactivity caused by mechanical ventilation results in a significant reduction in diaphragmatic strength that arises independently of the effects of anaesthetic agents and neuromuscular blocking drugs, and worsens with the duration of mechanical ventilation. Atrophy, remodelling of fibres, structural injury and oxidative stress have all been implicated as potentially causative. Attenuation of VIDD has been achieved by anti-oxidant treatment, which reduces proteolysis, and by use of a triggered mode of ventilation rather than continuous mandatory ventilation in order to maintain muscle activity. VIDD may contribute to the many

factors causing failure to wean in patients undergoing mechanical ventilation.

Oxygen toxicity

The survival benefit of mechanical ventilation with lower tidal volumes demonstrated by the ARDSnet study[34] serves as a useful reminder that clinical interventions may be contributing to both morbidity and mortality. The potential for harm is formally acknowledged for drug therapy in the 'therapeutic ratio', which is the ratio between toxic and therapeutic concentrations. In this sense, oxygen is no different from any other drug.

Oxygen's toxicity to both plant and animal life was appreciated very shortly after its discovery in the 1770s but was not systematically investigated until Paul Bert's work in the 1870s and J. Lorrain Smith's work in the late 1890s. From animal studies, it is evident that oxygen's toxicity is a function of both the inhaled partial pressure and the duration of exposure. In a hyperbaric environment, pure oxygen causes seizures, but at atmospheric pressure it has effects on the lung and circulation. Normobaric hyperoxia has also been shown to suppress erythropoeisis and decrease systemic oxygen consumption. All of these effects can be reproduced in

Table 14.13 Markers of oxygen damage in patients with the acute respiratory distress syndrome (ARDS)

- Increased hydrogen peroxide in exhaled gas
- Increased lipid peroxidation products in exhaled gas
- Decreased plasma concentrations of thiol groups
- Increased carbonyl formation in plasma proteins
- Increased oxidized glutathione in lung lavage fluid
- Oxidatively modified α-1-proteinase inhibitor in lung lavage fluid

animals, and indeed the smaller (or younger) the animal, the more susceptible they are to oxygen toxicity. The prior presence of pulmonary inflammation renders the animal even more sensitive. Evidence supporting the hypothesis that oxygen's toxicity is mediated by the generation of free radicals comes from experiments in which the formation of free-radicals has been either enhanced or suppressed, with the effect of either accelerating or delaying, respectively, the animal's death.

There is little direct evidence of pulmonary oxygen toxicity in patients receiving high inspired oxygen concentrations because of respiratory failure. However, given the fact that toxicity has been demonstrated in normal animal and human lungs, and animal data has shown that pulmonary inflammation sensitizes the lung to oxygen's toxic effects, it is likely that a similar effect would be seen in humans. Indeed, there is plenty of indirect evidence of significant oxidant damage in patients with ARDS (Table 14.13). Hyperoxia increases the activity of nuclear factor κB (NF-κB), which, in turn, increases the expression of many key mediators of inflammation such as IL-1β, IL-6, IL-8 and TNFα. Conversely, the anti-oxidant N-acetyl-L-cysteine reduces the activation of NF-κB and the neutrophilic alveolitis in a lipopolysaccharide model of acute lung injury.

Unnecessary oxygen therapy has been shown to increase the mortality in patients following mild to moderate stroke[37] and in patients with myocardial infarction there was a tendency for both a higher mortality and more tachydysrhythmias.[38] In critically ill patients, a number of outcome prediction models such as APACHE II,[29] MPM[30] and SAPS II[31] have found that outcome is negatively correlated with the ratio of the arterial partial pressure of oxygen (PaO_2) to the fractional inspired oxygen concentration (FiO_2), the so-called P:F ratio. Similarly, analysis of the distribution of PaO_2 and FiO_2 in survivors and non-survivors of ICU admission from the British Intensive Care Society's APACHE II data base shows no significant difference between the two groups in terms of PaO_2 but a significantly higher FiO_2 in those who died[39] (Figure 14.22). Of course, proof of association is not proof of causation, and a reasonable explanation for these observations is that patients with more severe lung disease, who are therefore more likely to die, require a higher FiO_2 to achieve clinically acceptable oxygenation. However, interventions that have yielded significant improvements in oxygenation, such as inhaled nitric oxide, prone ventilation, or increased PEEP, have all failed to deliver a survival benefit, perhaps because of the negative effects of hyperoxia.

So what is safe?

Studies in *healthy* human subjects have failed to detect any harmful effects from the normobaric inhalation of 50% oxygen. However, there is no data on the 'safe' concentration of oxygen in patients with lung disease, and on the basis of the effect that pulmonary inflammation has on oxygen toxicity in animals (see earlier discussion), it would be reasonable to conclude that this would be less than 50%. In view of this, it is probably more useful to consider any oxygen concentration above 21% as potentially toxic in patients with lung inflammation in order

---

29 Acute Physiology and Chronic Health Evaluation II.
30 Mortality Prediction Model.
31 Simplified Acute Physiology Score II.

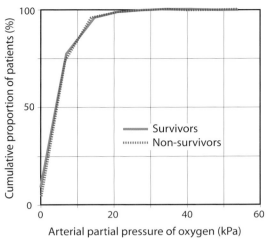 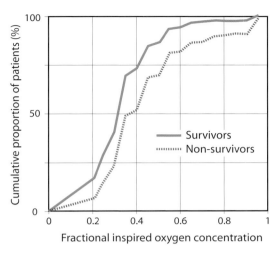

Figure 14.22 Distribution of the lowest arterial partial pressure of oxygen (left) and highest fractional inspired oxygen concentration (right) in the first 24 hours of intensive care between survivors and non-survivors to hospital discharge.

Data from the UK's APACHE II database. Figure adapted from Young JD. Hypoxemia and mortality in the ICU. In: Vincent J-L, ed. *Yearbook of Intensive Care and Emergency Medicine*. Berlin: Springer-Verlag; 2000:858.

to encourage the delivery of an FIO_2 that just meets clinically acceptable oxygenation targets.

Of course, in this context the next question is, 'What is the lowest acceptable arterial oxygen saturation or PaO_2?' Although there is no clear answer to this question, it is interesting to note that humans are able to live permanently at altitudes in the region of 5500 metres, where the arterial partial pressure of oxygen would be around 2.9 kPa. Although some of the effects of this low PaO_2 would be offset in the long term by physiological adaptations,[32] this nonetheless suggests that the traditional view that a PaO_2 under 8 kPa is unacceptable is probably not appropriate.[33] For each patient, the clinician will need to balance the harm of too little oxygen against the harm of too much, perhaps titrating the FIO_2 down until it is no more than 30% or there is functional evidence of hypoxia, such as confusion or a rising blood lactate concentration.

[32] Increased haematocrit, increased red cell concentrations of 2,3-diphosphoglycerate, increased respiratory rate, increased renal bicarbonate loss and increased organ capillary density.
[33] In neonatal practice it is not unusual to manage infants with saturations of around 60%.

Extra-pulmonary effects of mechanical ventilation

Cardiovascular system

During positive pressure ventilation, the pressure excursions within the airways, alveoli, lung parenchyma, pleural cavity and mediastinum are opposite to those that occur during normal breathing. As the heart lies within the mediastinum, the pressures within the cardiac chambers are influenced by fluctuations in airway pressure (although this is attenuated to varying degrees by the compliance of the intervening tissues of the lung parenchyma, mediastinal pleura, mediastinum and pericardium) and this has a detectable effect on cardiac performance.

Venous return

The flow of blood from the extrathoracic systemic veins to the right atrium is passive and depends on the steepness of the pressure gradient between the two. During both spontaneous ventilation and positive pressure ventilation, the increase in thoracic volume compresses the abdominal contents, causing intra-abdominal pressure to rise and with this, the pressure within the large intra-abdominal veins. Although this has no effect on the pressure within the extrathoracic veins above the diaphragm, the overall effect on the extrathoracic systemic veins is to cause a small increase in pressure during inspiration (Figure 14.23). However, intrathoracic pressure, and therefore right atrial pressure, falls during inspiration in spontaneous ventilation but rises during positive pressure ventilation.[34] The result is that inspiration increases venous return during spontaneous ventilation but decreases venous return during positive pressure ventilation.

Although mean right atrial pressure is increased during positive pressure ventilation, the pressure difference between the cavity of the right atrium and the tissue surrounding it, known as the *transmural pressure*, actually *falls*, because of the even greater increase in the pressure around the right atrium (Figure 14.24). Because atrial transmural pressure is one of the physiological mechanisms for estimating intravascular volume, the fall in atrial transmural pressure is interpreted as an abrupt loss of volume, activating compensatory mechanisms, which include a sharp reduction in the release of atrial natriuretic peptide, and increases in the circulating concentrations of vasopressin, renin, angiotensin and aldosterone. Together with the reduction in cardiac output that is also caused by positive pressure ventilation (see later discussion), these mechanisms combine to produce reductions in renal blood flow,

glomerular filtration rate and urine output, together with increases in the renal re-absorption of sodium and water.

Right ventricular performance

As a consequence of the reduction in venous return with positive pressure ventilation, right ventricular stroke volume also falls. Right ventricular performance is also dependent on the right ventricular after-load represented by the pulmonary vascular resistance, which is affected by lung volume.

Pulmonary vascular resistance

Lung volume has a strong influence on pulmonary vascular resistance through two independent mechanisms, one physical, the other physiological. On the physical side, the pulmonary vessels are thin-walled compared to systemic arteries, and their diameter depends on the pressure that surrounds them. Smaller pulmonary arterioles, capillaries and venules run within the alveolar septa and can effectively be considered as intra-alveolar vessels that are exposed to alveolar pressure. The remaining vasculature is effectively extra-alveolar and sits within the pulmonary parenchyma where it is subject to the distending tension normally present at normal lung volumes. At high lung volumes, the extra-alveolar vessels are held widely open by the increased stretching force within the pulmonary parenchyma, but the intra-alveolar vessels are compressed by the high alveolar pressures, resulting in an increase in pulmonary vascular resistance (Figure 14.25). At low lung volumes, the parenchymal stretch diminishes, allowing the extra-alveolar vessels to narrow and pulmonary vascular resistance to increase. In addition, at low lung volumes the physiological mechanism also becomes effective through alveolar closure and atelectasis. As the alveolar partial pressure of oxygen falls within the poorly ventilated lung units, which is in contrast to systemic arterioles under these conditions, pulmonary arterioles constrict as a means of optimizing ventilation and

---

[34] The rise in vascular pressures caused by positive airway pressure is proportional, but not identical, because of the dissipation of pressure between the two compartments caused by the compliance of intervening tissue. Even in patients with normal respiratory system compliance, only 20% to 25% of the airway pressure is transmitted to the vascular compartment. Thus the addition of 12 cm H_2O of PEEP, for example, would only be expected to cause a 3-cm H_2O water rise in central venous pressure, at most. In patients with poor respiratory system compliance, who might require high levels of PEEP, the proportional transmission of airway pressure to the vascular compartment will be much less and may be undetectable.

SPONTANEOUS VENTILATION

POSITIVE PRESSURE VENTILATION

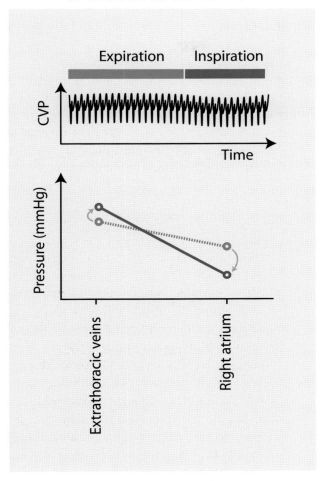

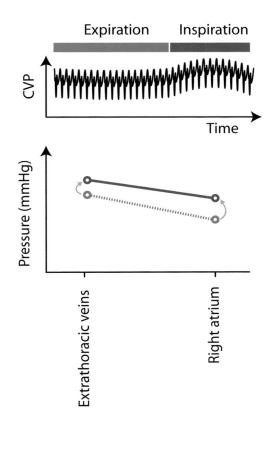

Figure 14.23 Effect of positive pressure ventilation on venous pressures.

perfusion. Thus at low lung volumes, extra-alveolar vessels narrowing is compounded by intra-alveolar vasoconstriction in response to local hypoxia, with both contributing to an increase in pulmonary vascular resistance (Figure 14.25).

Left ventricular performance

The reduction in right ventricular stroke volume that accompanies the institution of positive pressure ventilation inevitably results in a fall in left ventricular stroke volume and cardiac output. However, the increase in intrathoracic pressure trans-

mitted to the left ventricle results in an increase in the end-diastolic ventricular pressure. Therefore, the difference between the left ventricular end-systolic and end-diastolic pressures is reduced, and with it the work-load imposed on the left ventricle (Figure 14.26). In patients with normal cardiac function, the reduction in cardiac pre-load has a predominating effect, resulting in a marked fall in cardiac output (Figure 14.27). In patients with cardiac failure, however, the reduction in pre-load and after-load can result in significant improvements in cardiac function.

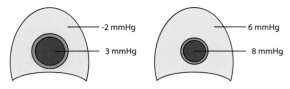

Figure 14.24 Effect of positive pressure ventilation on right atrial distension.

The atrial transmural pressure, which is the difference between the pressure in the right atrial cavity and the pressure of the tissue surrounding the right atrium (intrathoracic pressure), determines right atrial distension. During spontaneous ventilation, right atrial pressure is low, but the mean intrathoracic pressure around the right atrium is negative. In contrast, during positive pressure ventilation, the mean intrathoracic pressure rises considerably more than the right atrial pressure, which means that although the right atrial pressure *increases*, the atrial transmural pressure actually *decreases*, and the volume of the right atrium falls.

Gastrointestinal system

MOUTH, OESOPHAGUS, STOMACH AND SMALL INTESTINE

Physical damage to the mouth and oesophagus have been discussed earlier,[35] as have the changes to the oral flora.[36] Erosive oesophagitis has been found in 30% to 50% of patients ventilated for more than 48 hours, and together with duodenal ulceration is the most common cause for significant upper gastrointestinal haemorrhage. Although gastric tubes contribute to the damage, both by facilitating gastroesophageal reflux and causing mechanical irritation, gastroesophageal reflux occurs even in the absence of a gastric tube because of the high prevalence of very poor lower oesophageal sphincter tone.[40] Both opiates and adrenergic agonists undoubtedly contribute to this. While acid-suppression therapy may reduce oesophagitis caused by acid reflux, it will not prevent the oesophageal damage caused by duodenogastroesophageal reflux, which in one study was detected in

---

[35] See 'Other complications' under 'Intubation and the artificial airway' in this chapter.
[36] See 'Endogenous route' under 'Ventilator-associated pneumonia, Prevention' in this chapter.

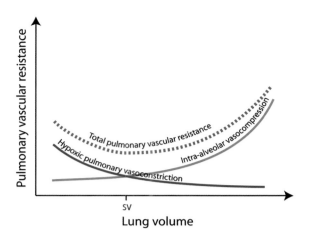

Figure 14.25 Effect of changes in lung volume on the contributory components to total pulmonary vascular resistance.

48% of the patients examined.[41] In the absence of gastric acid, reflux of duodenal content may cause oesophageal damage through the action of trypsin, which is normally inactivated by gastric acid or by unconjugated bile acids generated from their conjugated form by gastric bacterial overgrowth. It is perhaps not coincidental, therefore, that bacterial colonization of the stomach is more likely in patients with gastric stasis, and in this study the severity of oesophagitis was correlated with the gastric residual volume. The degree to which duodenogastric reflux or disturbances of gastric and bowel motility can be ascribed to mechanical ventilation or associated therapy as opposed to any of the myriad associated conditions requiring mechanical ventilation, remains to be clarified. However, opioids and adrenergic agonists are almost invariably prescribed in mechanically ventilated patients for patient comfort, sedation and bronchodilatation, and are known to interfere with gastrointestinal motility, as are oedema and electrolyte disorders which arise in response to signals generated by increased intrathoracic pressure. The strong independent association between positive pressure ventilation and upper gastrointestinal haemorrhage

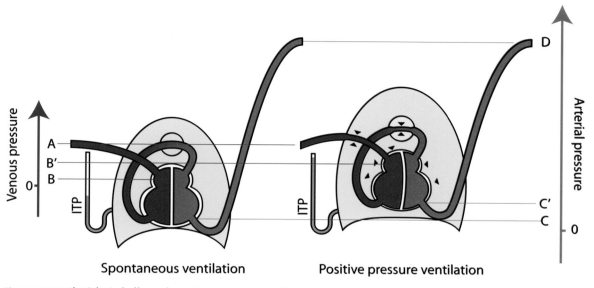

Figure 14.26 Physiological effects of positive pressure ventilation.

from gastric erosions or ulcers is likely to be due to a combination of factors, including stress, and decreased gastric mucosal protection secondary to a fall in splanchnic blood flow.

Large bowel

Constipation and abdominal distension are commonly associated with patients receiving positive pressure ventilation and are most likely to be caused by the same factors that cause motility problems in the small bowel.

Liver and gallbladder

The liver is unique in having a dual blood supply, with 50% to 55% of the oxygen supply coming from the portal venous blood and 45% to 50% coming from the hepatic artery. As discussed above, positive pressure ventilation causes a reduction in cardiac output that is further reduced by PEEP. While the cerebral and renal circulations are able to autoregulate, this is not so for the splanchnic circulation as a whole, and so reductions in cardiac output result in proportionally greater reductions in portal venous flow.[42] However, reductions in portal

flow are compensated by increases in hepatic arterial flow in a manner described as the 'hepatic arterial buffer response', which attempts to maintain total hepatic perfusion. In addition, the liver is sensitive to 'downstream' pressure changes in the right atrium and supra-hepatic inferior vena cava, and hepatic engorgement has been documented in animals following the institution of positive pressure ventilation with PEEP. Prolonged periods of positive pressure ventilation with high mean intrathoracic pressures have been associated with venous ischaemia, resulting in elevations in serum transaminases and hyperbilirubinaemia. This is unlikely to be seen where lung-protective ventilation strategies are used. Nevertheless, even with an intact hepatic arterial buffer response and reasonable tidal volumes, mechanical ventilation is able to reduce hepatic blood flow sufficiently to cause measurable reductions in drug clearance.

Renal function

In addition to a renal response to the reduction in cardiac output and mean arterial pressure described previously, the institution of mechanical ventilation is also immediately accompanied by a reduction in urine output as a result of the fall in the transmural pressure of the right atrium. This causes a reduction in the secretion of atrial natriuretic peptide and activation of both the renin-angiotensin-aldosterone system and pituitary vasopressin secretion.

Neurological function

Acute effects

The cerebral circulation is sensitive to the arterial partial pressure of carbon dioxide ($PaCO_2$), responding to hypocapnia by vasoconstriction and to hypercapnia by vasodilatation. Cerebral vasoconstriction reduces cerebral blood flow, and by reducing the intra-cerebral blood volume results in a fall in intra-cerebral pressure. In patients at risk of raised intra-cranial pressure, deliberate hyperventilation to achieve a $PaCO_2$ of around 4 kPa can therefore be used as an additional control measure. In these patients, inadvertent hypoventilation leading to intra-cranial hypertension may result in either a poorer neurological outcome, or in some cases might actually precipitate trans-tentorial herniation[37] and death. The benefits of hyperventilation on intra-cranial pressure must be balanced with the detrimental effects on blood flow of cerebral vasoconstriction with excessive $PaCO_2$ reduction.

Although PEEP is transmitted to the central venous pressure and therefore contributes to a reduction in cerebral perfusion pressure,[38] only a modest fraction of the applied PEEP is actually transmitted in patients with normal pulmonary compliance (20% to 25%), and even less in patients with poor pulmonary compliance. In truth, the impact that positive pressure ventilation and PEEP has on cerebral perfusion is mediated through the reduction in cardiac output rather than any increases to venous pressures and is readily cor-

rected by an increase in circulating volume or, where necessary, the use of vasopressors.

Sleep

Normal sleep involves two quite distinct brain states: light and deep non-rapid eye movement (NREM) sleep and rapid eye movement (REM) sleep. On average, an adult is asleep for about 8 hours during which the brain cycles between sleep states with periods of REM sleep occurring every 90 to 120 minutes. Overall, about 50% of the total sleep time (TST) is spent in stage 2 NREM, 25% in REM sleep and 10% to 15% in deep (stages 3 and 4) NREM, also called slow-wave sleep (Figure 14.28). Although the function of sleep is still unknown, both the quality and quantity of sleep are important. Sleep deprivation and sleep fragmentation in both animal and human studies cause a range of adverse effects including accelerated protein catabolism, defects in lymphocyte and neutrophil function, loss of the normal circadian rhythm of neurohypohyseal secretion, and carbohydrate intolerance, in addition to the neuropsychiatric side effects including daytime somnolence, poor mood and reduced motivation. Although total sleep time may not be universally decreased in mechanically ventilated patients, sleep architecture is grossly disturbed, with loss of the diurnal sleep/wake cycle and significant reductions in the duration of deep NREM and REM sleep with little or no sleep consolidation (Figure 14.29). While critical illness and the intensive care unit environment have to take some of the blame, there is little doubt that mechanical ventilation, per se, is also responsible (Table 14.14).

Psychological morbidity

The intrinsically unpleasant nature of tracheal intubation and positive pressure ventilation inevitably require the administration of sedatives or analgesics or both, and occasionally neuromuscular blocking agents. The neurological complications of these drugs, particularly when used by continuous

---

[37] Known colloquially as 'coning'.
[38] Cerebral perfusion pressure = *mean arterial pressure – central venous pressure*.

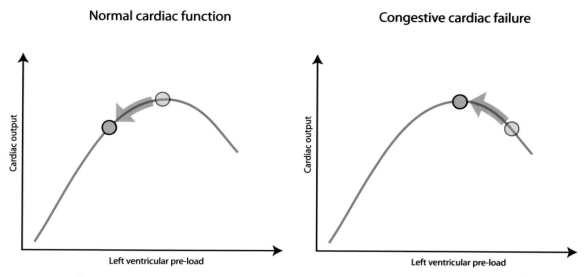

Normal cardiac function

Congestive cardiac failure

Figure 14.27 Effect of reduced pre-load on cardiac output.

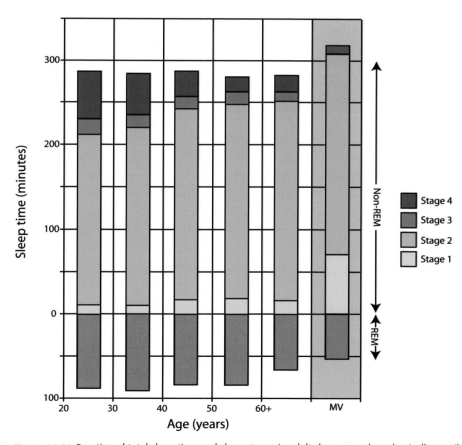

Figure 14.28 Duration of total sleep time and sleep stages in adults by age, and mechanically ventilated patients.

Table 14.14 Mechanisms by which mechanical ventilation disrupts sleep

- Noise disruption
  - Ventilator alarms (inappropriate thresholds, delayed alarm inactivation)
  - Humidifier alarms
- Disruption by nursing interventions
  - Airway suction
  - Nebulizer delivery
- Ventilation-related pharmacological disruption
  - Benzodiazepines (↓REM, ↓ deep NREM)
  - Opioids (↓REM, ↓ deep NREM)
  - Neuromuscular blocking drugs
- Ventilator mode
  - Pressure-support ventilation

Table 14.15 Objective indicators of withdrawal syndrome in patients receiving mechanical ventilation. The diagnosis of withdrawal can be made if two or more indicators are present in the context of reduction or discontinuation of an opioid or benzodiazepine

Opiates	Benzodiazepines
Tachycardia	Tremor
Hypertension	Nausea
Tachypnoea	Sweating
Sweating	Agitation
Agitation	Muscle aches or cramps
Diarrhoea	Seizure
Pupillary dilatation	
Lacrimation	
Rhinorrhoea	
Insomnia	
Nausea	
Fever	
Muscle aches or cramps	

infusion, include prolonged sedation, delirium, and neuromyopathy, which are discussed in Chapter 8, as well as withdrawal syndromes and an increased risk for long-term psychological disturbance, which are discussed later.

Repeated or continuous administration of some drugs can induce tolerance or dependence, or both. Tolerance to a drug is said to occur when progressively larger doses of the drug are required to achieve the same clinical end-point and may arise because of the induction of drug clearance mechanisms (pharmacokinetic tolerance), or because of decreasing effector-site activity because of receptor down-regulation, sub-cellular adaptation or induction of counter-regulatory mechanisms (pharmacodynamic tolerance). Dependence describes the triggering of a reproducible and characteristic constellation of effects (the withdrawal syndrome) following drug withdrawal or dose reduction that may be either psychological or physical. Benzodiazepines and opioids both induce tolerance and dependence, and prolonged use of either drug is associated with a characteristic withdrawal syndrome (Table 14.15). In one small study in adults, withdrawal syndrome occurred in 32% of the patients who spent more than seven days in intensive care. These

patients were younger, received mechanical ventilation for longer, had received higher mean doses of opioids and benzodiazepines and were more likely to have received propofol and neuromuscular blocking drugs.[43] Withdrawal syndromes are thought to be less likely with potent, short-acting opioids, but in fact have been reported for fentanyl, sufentanil and remifentanil. Indeed, in one hospital where remifentanil has largely replaced both propofol and morphine in order to provide 'analgesia-based' comfort, expenditure on clonidine to treat agitation has risen proportionally to the increased expenditure on remifentanil (Figure 14.30). There is very little information on the adverse consequences of the withdrawal syndrome in patients receiving mechanical ventilation, although it is likely that these might include re-introduction of the offending drug, leading to a prolongation of the need for ventilatory support, self-extubation, seizures (benzodiazepines) and cardiac consequences from the combination of tachycardia and hypertension in vulnerable patients. As the withdrawal syndrome

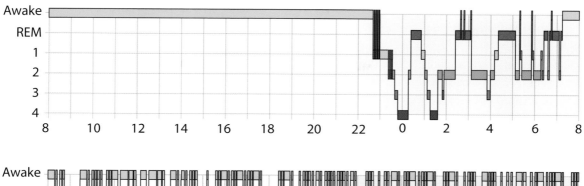

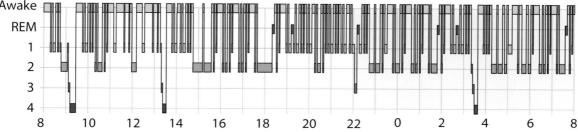

Figure 14.29 Twenty-four-hour hypnograms showing the typical duration and transition between sleep stages in a normal adult (above), and a patient receiving mechanical ventilation (bottom).

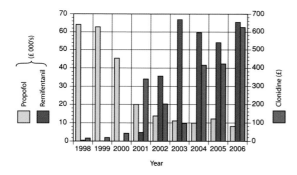

Figure 14.30 Annual expenditure on propofol, remifentanil and clonidine in one adult intensive care unit between 1998 and 2006.

to opioids is associated with rises in the plasma concentrations of β-endorphin, met-enkephalin, adrenocorticotrophin and cortisol, it is possible that changes in these hormones could be used to provide more information on the incidence and consequences of withdrawal.

The fact that mechanical ventilation, and in particular essential coincidental issues such as the tracheal tube, suctioning, communication prob-

lems and ventilator dependence, are believed to be unpleasant is based on an intuitive assessment corroborated by patients' reports. The traditional response has been to prevent patients from becoming aware of these events through the liberal use of sedatives, supplemented, where necessary, by analgesics. However, evidence is emerging that the incidence of unpleasant psychological sequelae of mechanical ventilation, such as anxiety, depression and the post-traumatic stress disorder, is actually *increased* in patients who have been prevented from laying down factual memories, even though the recollections are for unpleasant events.[44] One approach is to reduce 'sedative saturation' with daily sedation breaks, which has been shown not only to reduce the duration of mechanical ventilation,[45] but may also reduce the incidence of post-traumatic stress disorder.[46] An alternative approach is to switch the emphasis from sedation to analgesia, with the aim of increasing awareness and recollection, while minimizing or eliminating discomfort, so-called 'analgesia-based' sedation. Remifentanil, a potent and ultra-short acting 4-analidopiperidine[39] agonist at the μ-opioid receptor, is rapidly hydrolysed by plasma esterases to almost inactive metabolites. In combination with its potency, this theoretically gives the drug two important properties: organ-independent elimination and non-accumulation. This makes it the ideal opioid for providing analgesia-based sedation. However, specifically with respect to the psychological sequelae of mechanically ventilation, it is unlikely that an opioid-based regime will deliver the intended benefits because of the combined effects of dysphoria and the interference with the laying down of long-term memory caused by opioid-induced disruption of deep NREM and REM sleep.

REFERENCES

1. Braz LG, Modolo NS, do Nascimento P, Jr. *et al.* Perioperative cardiac arrest: a study of 53,718 anaesthetics over 9 yr from a Brazilian teaching hospital. *Br J Anaesth.* 2006; 96(5):569–75.

2. Marik PE. Aspiration pneumonitis and aspiration pneumonia. *N Engl J Med.* 2001; 344(9):665–71.

3. Muckart DJ, Bhagwanjee S, van der Merwe R. Spinal cord injury as a result of endotracheal intubation in patients with undiagnosed cervical spine fractures. *Anesthesiology.* 1997;87(2):418–20.

4. Rouby JJ, Laurent P, Gosnach M *et al.* Risk factors and clinical relevance of nosocomial maxillary sinusitis in the critically ill. *Am J Respir Crit Care Med.* 1994;150(3):776–83.

5. Bach A, Boehrer H, Schmidt H *et al.* Nosocomial sinusitis in ventilated patients. Nasotracheal versus orotracheal intubation. *Anaesthesia.* 1992;47(4):335–9.

6. Holzapfel L, Chastang C, Demingeon G *et al.* A randomized study assessing the systematic search for maxillary sinusitis in nasotracheally mechanically ventilated patients. Influence of nosocomial maxillary sinusitis on the occurrence of ventilator-associated pneumonia. *Am J Respir Crit Care Med.* 1999;159(3):695–701.

7. Lucks D, Consiglio A, Stankiewicz J *et al.* Incidence and microbiological etiology of middle ear effusion complicating endotracheal intubation and mechanical ventilation. *J Infect Dis.* 1988;157(2): 368–9.

8. Colice GL, Stukel TA, Dain B. Laryngeal complications of prolonged intubation. *Chest.* 1989;96(4):877–84.

9. El Solh A, Okada M, Bhat A *et al.* Swallowing disorders post orotracheal intubation in the elderly. *Intensive Care Med.* 2003;29(9): 1451–5.

10. Whited RE. Posterior commissure stenosis post long-term intubation. *Laryngoscope.* 1983;93(10):1314–18.

11. Grillo HC, Donahue DM, Mathisen DJ *et al.* Postintubation tracheal stenosis. Treatment and results. *J Thorac Cardiovasc Surg.* 1995;109(3):486–92; discussion 492–3.

12. Krinsley JS, Barone JE. The drive to survive: unplanned extubation in the ICU. *Chest.* 2005;128(2):560–6.

13. Safdar N, Dezfulian C, Collard HR *et al.* Clinical and economic consequences of ventilator-associated pneumonia: a systematic review. *Crit Care Med.* 2005; 33(10):2184–93.

14. Guidelines for the management of adults with hospital-acquired, ventilator-associated, and healthcare-associated pneumonia. *Am J Respir Crit Care Med.* 2005;171(4):388–416.

15. Torres A, Carlet J. Ventilator-associated pneumonia. European Task Force on ventilator-associated pneumonia. *Eur Respir J.* 2001;17(5):1034–45.

---

[39] Chemically related to fentanyl, alfentanil and sufentanil.

16. Seegobin RD, van Hasselt GL. Aspiration beyond endotracheal cuffs. *Can Anaesth Soc J.* 1986;33(3 Pt 1):273–9.

17. Rello J, Sonora R, Jubert P *et al.* Pneumonia in intubated patients: role of respiratory airway care. *Am J Respir Crit Care Med.* 1996;154(1):111–15.

18. Dullenkopf A, Gerber A, Weiss M. Fluid leakage past tracheal tube cuffs: evaluation of the new Microcuff endotracheal tube. *Intensive Care Med.* 2003;29(10):1849–53.

19. Dezfulian C, Shojania K, Collard HR *et al.* Subglottic secretion drainage for preventing ventilator-associated pneumonia: a meta-analysis. *Am J Med.* 2005;118(1): 11–18.

20. Dodek P, Keenan S, Cook D *et al.* Evidence-based clinical practice guideline for the prevention of ventilator-associated pneumonia. *Ann Intern Med.* 2004; 141(4):305–13.

21. Delaney A, Gray H, Laupland KB *et al.* Kinetic bed therapy to prevent nosocomial pneumonia in mechanically ventilated patients: a systematic review and meta-analysis. *Crit Care.* 2006;10(3): R70-R82.

22. Cook DJ, Reeve BK, Guyatt GH *et al.* Stress ulcer prophylaxis in critically ill patients. Resolving discordant meta-analyses. *JAMA.* 1996;275(4):308–14.

23. Chan EY, Ruest A, Meade MO *et al.* Oral decontamination for prevention of pneumonia in mechanically ventilated adults: systematic review and meta-analysis. *BMJ.* 2007;334(7599):889–900.

24. Holzapfel L, Chevret S, Madinier G *et al.* Influence of long-term oro- or nasotracheal intubation on nosocomial maxillary sinusitis and pneumonia: results of a prospective, randomized, clinical trial. *Crit Care Med.* 1993;21(8):1132–8.

25. Kola A, Eckmanns T, Gastmeier P. Efficacy of heat and moisture exchangers in preventing ventilator-associated pneumonia: meta-analysis of randomized controlled trials. *Intensive Care Med.* 2005;31(1): 5–11.

26. Cook DJ, Walter SD, Cook RJ *et al.* Incidence of and risk factors for ventilator-associated pneumonia in critically ill patients. *Ann Intern Med.* 1998;129(6):433–40.

27. Bendixen HH, Hedley-White J, Laver MD. Impaired oxygenation in surgical patients during general anaesthesia with controlled ventilation. *N Engl J Med.* 1963;269:991–6.

28. Webb HH, Tierney DF. Experimental pulmonary edema due to intermittent positive pressure ventilation with high inflation pressures. Protection by positive end-expiratory pressure. *Am Rev Respir Dis.* 1974;110(5):556–5.

29. Hickling KG, Henderson SJ, Jackson R. Low mortality associated with low volume pressure limited ventilation with permissive hypercapnia in severe adult respiratory distress syndrome. *Intensive Care Med.* 1990; 16(6):372–7.

30. Amato MB, Barbas CS, Medeiros DM *et al.* Effect of a protective-ventilation strategy on mortality in the acute respiratory distress syndrome. *N Engl J Med.* 1998; 338(6): 347–54.

31. Brochard L, Roudot-Thoraval F, Roupie E *et al.* Tidal volume reduction for prevention of ventilator-induced lung injury in acute respiratory distress syndrome. The Multicenter Trail Group on Tidal Volume reduction in ARDS. *Am J Respir Crit Care Med.* 1998;158(6):1831–8.

32. Brower RG, Shanholtz CB, Fessler HE *et al.* Prospective, randomized, controlled clinical trial comparing traditional versus reduced tidal volume ventilation in acute respiratory

distress syndrome patients. *Crit Care Med.* 1999;27(8):1492–8.

33. Stewart TE, Meade MO, Cook DJ *et al.* Evaluation of a ventilation strategy to prevent barotrauma in patients at high risk for acute respiratory distress syndrome. Pressure- and Volume-Limited Ventilation Strategy Group. *N Engl J Med.* 1998;338(6): 355–61.

34. Acute Respiratory Distress Syndrome Network. Ventilation with lower tidal volumes as compared with traditional tidal volumes for acute lung injury and the acute respiratory distress syndrome. The Acute Respiratory Distress Syndrome Network. *N Engl J Med.* 2000;342(18):1301–8.

35. Brower RG, Lanken PN, MacIntyre N *et al.* Higher versus lower positive end-expiratory pressures in patients with the acute respiratory distress syndrome. *N Engl J Med.* 2004;351(4):327–36.

36. Villar J, Kacmarek RM, Perez-Mendez L *et al.* A high positive end-expiratory pressure, low tidal volume ventilatory strategy improves outcome in persistent acute respiratory distress syndrome: a randomized, controlled trial. *Crit Care Med.* 2006;34(5):1311–18.

37. Rønning OM, Guldvog B. Should stroke victims routinely receive supplemental oxygen? A quasi-randomised controlled trial. *Stroke.* 1999;30:2033–7.

38. Rawles JM, Kenmure AC. Controlled trial of oxygen in uncomplicated myocardial infarction. *BMJ.* 1976;i:1121–3.

39. Young JD. Hypoxemia and mortality in the ICU. In: Vincent JL, ed. *Yearbook of Intensive Care and Emergency Medicine.* Berlin, Springer. 2000:239–46.

40. Nind G, Chen WH, Protheroe R *et al.* Mechanisms of gastroesophageal reflux in critically ill mechanically ventilated patients. *Gastroenterology.* 2005;128(3):600–6.

41. Wilmer A, Tack J, Frans E *et al.* Duodenogastroesophageal reflux and esophageal mucosal injury in mechanically ventilated patients. *Gastroenterology.* 1999;116(6):1293–9.

42. Winso O, Biber B, Gustavsson B *et al.* Portal blood flow in man during graded positive end-expiratory pressure ventilation. *Intensive Care Med.* 1986;12(2):80–5.

43. Cammarano WB, Pittet J-F, Weitz S *et al.* Acute withdrawal syndrome related to the administration of analgesia and sedative medications in adult intensive care unit patients. *Crit Care Mede.* 1998;26(4): 676–84.

44. Jones C, Griffiths RD, Humphris G *et al.* Memory, delusions, and the development of acute posttraumatic stress disorder-related symptoms after intensive care. *Crit Care Med.* 2001;29(3):573–80.

45. Kress JP, Pohlman AS, O'Connor MF *et al.* Daily interruption of sedative infusions in critically ill patients undergoing mechanical ventilation. *N Engl J Med.* 2000;342(20): 1471–7.

46. Kress JP, Gehlbach B, Lacy M *et al.* The long-term psychological effects of daily sedative interruption on critically ill patients. *Am J Respir Crit Care Med.* 2003;168(12): 1457–61.

47. Fasting S, Gisvold SE. Serious intraoperative problems – a five-year review of 83,844 anesthetics. *Can J Anaesth.* 2002;49(6):545–53.

48. Jaber S, Amraoui J, Lefrant JY *et al.* Clinical practice and risk factors for immediate complications of endotracheal intubation in the intensive care unit: a prospective, multiple-center study. *Crit Care Med.* 2006; 34(9):2355–61.

49. Mort TC. The incidence and risk factors for cardiac arrest during emergency tracheal

intubation: a justification for incorporating the ASA Guidelines in the remote location. *J Clin Anesth*. 2004;16(7):508–16.

50. Asai T, Koga K, Vaughan RS. Respiratory complications associated with tracheal intubation and extubation. *Br J Anaesth*. 1998;80(6):767–75.

51. Rose DK, Cohen MM. The airway: problems and predictions in 18,500 patients. *Can J Anaesth*. 1994;41(5 Pt 1):372–83.

52. Stauffer JL, Olson DE, Petty TL. Complications and consequences of endotracheal intubation and tracheotomy. A prospective study of 150 critically ill adult patients. *Am J Med*. 1981;70(1):65–76.

53. Schwartz DE, Matthay MA, Cohen NH. Death and other complications of emergency airway management in critically ill adults. A prospective investigation of 297 tracheal intubations. *Anesthesiology*. 1995;82(2): 367–76.

54. Benedetto WJ, Hess DR, Gettings E *et al*. Urgent tracheal intubation in general hospital units: an observational study. *J Clin Anesth*. 2007;19(1):20–24.

55. Fung BK, Chan MY. Incidence of oral tissue trauma after the administration of general anesthesia. *Acta Anaesthesiol Sin*. 2001;39(4): 163–7.

56. Warner MA, Warner ME, Weber JG. Clinical significance of pulmonary aspiration during the perioperative period. *Anesthesiology*. 1993;78(1):56–62.

57. Olsson GL, Hallen B, Hambraeus-Jonzon K. Aspiration during anaesthesia: a computer-aided study of 185,358 anaesthetics. *Acta Anaesthesiol Scand*. 1986;30(1): 84–92.

58. Mort TC. Emergency tracheal intubation: complications associated with repeated laryngoscopic attempts. *Anesth Analg*. 2004;99(2):607–13.

Chapter 15

Mechanical ventilation for transport

TERRY MARTIN

Introduction

The number of transfers of critically ill patients within and between hospitals has been continuously increasing throughout the entire evolution of intensive care medicine. This is mostly due to the development of highly technical and non-portable diagnostic devices, the escalating complexity of healthcare, the concentration of skills into specialized regional centres and, not uncommonly, a shortage of intensive care beds. The transfer or transport of critical care patients offer the most difficult challenges and require detailed planning, preparation, skill, knowledge and teamwork to achieve success. Even the transport of patients between two departments in one hospital can be hazardous. Arguably, the highest risk is that of ensuring a patent airway and adequate ventilation. This chapter discusses the process of transferring ventilated patients and examines portable ventilators in some detail.

Basic overview of ventilation for transfer or transport

Indications and contra-indications for transfer

Almost invariably, critical care patients are transferred or transported either to a higher level of clinical care or to a diagnostic procedure that will help direct future clinical management. The indica-

tions for transfer are therefore clinical and have the ultimate aim of delivering the patient to the most appropriate care or delivering the most appropriate care to the patient. On occasion, the number of patients requiring intensive care exceeds the number of beds available and a less critical patient may need to be transferred to create 'care space' for a new and unstable patient who is less fit for transport. Clearly, this transfer has no direct advantage for the patient, and under these circumstances the balance of risks and benefits is totally one sided. These 'non-clinical' transfers are often not easy to justify and present the most difficult ethical dilemmas. Contra-indications to transfer are presented in Table 15.1.

Risks and hazards of transportation

Critically ill patients have deranged physiology and require organ support and invasive monitoring. They tolerate poorly the effects of movement and vibration or changes in body temperature, and complications are not uncommon (Table 15.2). Audits suggest that 15% of patients arrive at the destination hospital with detrimental hypoxia or hypotension, and 10% have injuries or other problems not detected before transfer.

A study of 191 incident reports from intrahospital transfers in Australia[1] found that 39% of incidents identified problems with equipment and

Core Topics in Mechanical Ventilation, ed. Iain Mackenzie. Published by Cambridge University Press.
© Cambridge University Press 2008.

Table 15.1 Contra-indications to transfer

Inability to
- Maintain and protect a patient's airway during transport
- Provide adequate oxygenation or ventilation during transport using either manual (bag-valve) ventilation or the available portable ventilator
- Maintain acceptable haemodynamic performance during transport
- Adequately monitor patient cardiopulmonary status during transport

Table 15.2 Specific hazards and complications of transporting the mechanically ventilated patient

- Hyperventilation during manual ventilation may cause respiratory alkalosis, cardiac dysrhythmias and hypotension.
- Loss of PEEP or CPAP may result in hypoxaemia.
- Position changes may result in hypotension, hypercarbia or hypoxaemia.
- Tachycardia and other dysrhythmias have been associated with transport.
- Movement may cause disconnection from ventilatory support and respiratory compromise.
- Movement may result in accidental extubation.
- Movement may result in accidental removal of vascular access.
- Loss of oxygen supply may lead to hypoxaemia.
- Equipment failure can result in inaccurate data or loss of monitoring capabilities.
- Inadvertent disconnection of intravenous pharmacologic agents may result in haemodynamic instability.

61% identified patient management issues. Serious adverse outcomes occurred in 31% of these reports. These included major physiological derangement (15%), prolonged hospital stay (4%), physical or psychological injury (3%) and death (2%). Communication problems, inadequate protocols, inadequate servicing and poor training were prominent factors in equipment-related incidents. Errors of problem recognition and judgement, failure to follow protocols, inadequate patient preparation, haste and inattention were common management-related incidents. The authors conclude that intra-hospital transport poses an important risk to ICU patients and that it is reasonable to expect that inter-hospital transfers would offer even more opportunities for error and the sub-optimum performance of both equipment and staff.

Assessing the need for transfer

The need for the transfer should be assessed by the consultants in charge of the patient so that the risks of transport can be weighed against the potential benefits from the planned diagnostic or therapeutic procedure to be performed. In making the decision, the question arises: 'will information from this diagnostic procedure actually change the patient's management?' A number of authors[2, 3] have suggested that nearly two thirds of all transports for diagnostic studies fail to yield results that affect patient care, but these studies are now out of date and the current situation is unclear.

Equipment and procedures

The desirable characteristics of equipment for intra-hospital transfer are the same as those for inter-hospital transfers (Table 15.3).

The standard of patient monitoring during the transfer is essentially the same as that prior to transfer, although in some cases it may actually require increasing the monitoring. Modalities monitored depend on the condition of the patient and the likelihood of any deterioration. Minimum standard

Table 15.3 Criteria for transport equipment

- Robust
- Lightweight
- Portable
- Failsafe
- Battery powered with mains charging
- Fully compatible and modular
- Illuminated displays
- Visible and audible alarms
- User friendly

Table 15.4 Minimum standard monitoring modalities for a ventilated patient

- Pre-transfer blood gas analysis (long distance transports may require 'bedside' analysers)
- Pre-transfer NIBP 'cuff' pressure (to cross-check the invasive BP)
- Ventilator settings
  - Ventilation mode
  - Ventilation rate
  - Delivered tidal volume
  - Peak airway pressure
  - Peak end-expiratory pressure
- Oxygen saturation (pulse oximetry)
- End-tidal capnography
- Heart rate and electrocardiogram
- Blood pressure (preferably using arterial cannulation)

Table 15.5 Essential equipment

- Electrical charging units and leads
- Bag-valve mask device with oxygen reservoir
- Sufficient oxygen in lightweight cylinders
- Portable suction unit

monitoring modalities for a ventilated patient are presented in Table 15.4.

In addition to a compact multi-modality monitor, preferably with an integrated defibrillator, a number of other major items of equipment are also essential (Table 15.5). On long inter-hospital transfers, it is also advisable to carry spare ventilator tubing and appropriate hygroscopic condenser humidifiers as well as oxygen cylinder spare parts such as replacement regulators and Bodok seals. If the transfer is international, it is essential to carry oxygen piping to connect the ventilator to different types of wall terminal and cylinder outlets. Although terminal out-

lets have been standardized in the UK since 1978,[1] there is no worldwide standard and in some countries more than one type of outlet can be found. Multiple types of outlet can even sometimes be found in different departments of the same hospital. Small sections of oxygen pipe with different plug connections can be used to interconnect between ventilator and cylinder or wall-mounted outlets – for example, between self-closing Schraeder type outlets (such as BOC mark 1 or 2) to Ohmeda mark 4 or screw fittings.

Emergency airway management supplies should also be available. This includes anaesthetic drugs, stethoscope, laryngoscope, intravenous fluids, stylet, gum-elastic bougie, a selection of endotracheal tubes or tracheostomy accessories, if applicable, and a self-inflating bag and mask of appropriate size. These are best kept in a transport bag or located on the transfer trolley.

Depending on the destination of the transfer, the receiving facility may have monitoring equipment, a ventilator and gas supplies available. Provided these are frequently and regularly checked, a switchover after arrival is advisable to save on batteries and cylinder oxygen supply. Battery life on items not available at the destination can be prolonged if electric cables accompany the patient so equipment can be connected to the mains electricity supply for as long as possible.

Preparing the patient

From the perspective of ventilatory support, the simplest patients to prepare for transfer are those

---

[1] BS 5682, updated in 1984.

Box 15.1

Case 1

A 45-year-old mechanic was cutting open an empty fuel storage tank with an oxy-acetylene torch when residual vapour that was not known to be present ignited, causing a flash explosion. The mechanic, who was only wearing goggles and received serious burns to the head, face, upper chest and arms, was seen within 40 minutes of the incident in the emergency department of the local hospital. The patient was conscious and self-ventilating but in some pain. Intravenous access was secured with a central venous catheter in the femoral vein, and the patient then received intravenous opiate for his pain and was started on the Mount Vernon fluid resuscitation regime. Despite the presence of soot in the patient's nose, mouth and throat, his chest radiograph was normal and his arterial blood gases were entirely normal. Admission to the regional burns unit, which was two hours away by road, was agreed upon and in view of the severity of the patient's burns, he was transferred with one of the junior trainees from the emergency department. By the time the patient left the first hospital, the patient's face was beginning to swell, and after a further hour and a half on the road, the patient's upper airway was so compromised that the trainee decided to intubate the patient. The ambulance stopped in the side of the road where the trainee attempted to perform a rapid sequence intubation, which was unsuccessful.

Case 2

A 63-year-old alcoholic woman was admitted to a district general hospital with a history of haematemesis and melaena. Following appropriate volume resuscitation, endoscopy of the upper gastrointestinal tract was performed the day after admission, in which a number of oesophageal varices were banded. Views in the stomach were poor because of the large quantities of residual blood. Following discussion with the regional Hepatology Unit, it was decided to transfer the lady for further management. She had been haemodynamically stable for three days, but was now becoming rapidly more confused, agitated and both verbally and physically aggressive. To assist with the transfer, she was given a small dose of midazolam, which improved the situation dramatically. She was then transferred to the regional Hepatology Unit in the care of a paramedic crew. Because she was now sleeping, the ambulance crew travelled together at the front of the vehicle and were unable to intervene when the patient started to vomit. The patient aspirated large quantities of blood and died in the intensive care unit a week later.

that already have definitive airway management in place, either in the form of a trans-laryngeal tube or tracheostomy, and are receiving a mandatory mode of ventilation. Regrettably, these conditions are often lacking in one or other respect prior to many transfers, and therefore decisions need to be made about securing the airway or changing the mode of mechanical ventilation for the transfer.

Tracheal intubation is the safest and most effective technique for (1) providing respiratory support, (2) maintaining an open airway, (3) protecting the airway from aspiration, and (4) providing tracheo-

broncheal toileting. If there is *any* chance that the patient may need to have any of these benefits of tracheal intubation during the transfer, then it is essential that this is performed prior to transfer where the conditions are optimum and additional help is available (Box 15.1).

Infection control

Universal precautions should be rigorously observed[4] and all equipment should be disinfected between patients. Published recommendations (e.g. from the US Center for Disease Control and

Prevention) for control of exposure to tuberculosis and droplet nuclei should be implemented when a patient is known or suspected to be immunosuppressed, is known to have tuberculosis or has other risk factors for the disease.[5]

Intermediate information on transport ventilators

Oxygen supplies

The recent development of new lightweight portable oxygen cylinders made of carbon fibre[2] has been of great benefit to patient transportation. As well as being lighter than conventional metal cylinders, they are strong and resistant to corrosion. Cylinder technology is very important in long distance transfers, especially in aeromedical transportation. For instance, cylinders used in commercial aircraft must be approved and stored separately from the aircraft emergency oxygen supplies. It is vital to calculate the patient's oxygen requirements because, although taking too little can be a catastrophe, taking too much can be an expensive and greatly inconvenient error. Cylinder weight, even the new carbon fibre cylinders, and bulk are potential problems. It is therefore essential that all the cylinders carried are as near to full as possible at the start of the journey. Clearly, in aeromedical practice, cylinders need to be changed more frequently than in a hospital setting. In a hospital, it may be reasonable to allow a cylinder to get as low as to a quarter of its full contents before changing it, whereas in an aircraft the difficulty with cylinder changes in flight, as well as the bulk and weight issues, means that they are often changed on the ground if they are below three quarters full.

To address these issues, some air ambulance systems use oxygen concentrators or liquid oxygen containers when undertaking long distance transfers. The issues that apply to aircraft oxygen systems also apply to medical oxygen systems. Oxygen is classed by aviation authorities around the world as dangerous air cargo, and special arrangements must be made to carry or use it in flight.

With liquid oxygen (LOX) stores, it is now possible to provide flow rates sufficient enough to power ventilation equipment and suction devices without the need for heavy reducing valves and regulators. One litre of LOX stored at $-180\,^{\circ}$C will yield over 800 litres of gaseous oxygen. This expansion rate is almost seven times greater than can be achieved with pressurized gas in conventional cylinders at 1800 psi. LOX converters are lightweight insulated containers which may contain up to 25 litres of liquid. Insulation is never perfect and, as temperature rises, if oxygen is not being used, more gas is formed and pressure within the container increases. A relief valve will eventually vent this excess but, when calculating oxygen requirements, adjustments must be made to compensate for the fall in oxygen content which starts to occur about 10 hours after LOX cylinders are filled.

An alternative method of obtaining high concentrations of oxygen is to generate oxygen on board the aircraft. The best method involves the use of zeolite molecular sieve technology to adsorb nitrogen in compressed air. This effectively enriches the oxygen content as nitrogen is removed. Almost 100% inspired oxygen concentration can be achieved, but flow rates are not sufficient for gas-driven devices. The need for faster flow rates and the danger of compressor failure disrupting the major oxygen supply will always necessitate the carriage of supplemental oxygen cylinders or LOX stores.

Transport ventilators

The ideal transport ventilator should have the features listed in Table 15.6. Clearly, the best ventilator is the one that will reproduce the ventilatory needs of the individual patient in the intensive care unit. However, a compromise is almost always inevitable in the quest for portability, ruggedness, and power

---

[2] Sabre™ Full Wrap cylinders.

Table 15.6 Features of the ideal transport ventilator

- Compact, robust and lightweight
- Easy to understand with simple stepwise settings
- Clear display and settings with the display protected from damage
- Monitor airway pressure
- Disconnect alarm
- Clear illuminated visible and audible alarms
- Settings lockable or protected by a cover
- Powered by 12-volt DC and 110/240-volt AC supply with a long-lasting internal battery
- Mountings that can enable securing inside an ambulance or aircraft
- Approved for use at extreme temperature and altitudes, vibration and shock (drop tested)
- Provide internal PEEP from 0 to 20 cm H_2O
- Provide a FiO_2 from 0.21 to 1.0 if required
- Independent control of tidal volume and respiratory frequency
- Capability for continuous mechanical ventilation as in assist-control or intermittent mechanical ventilation
- Deliver a constant volume in the face of changing pulmonary impedance

or gas consumption. This 'quest for the best' has inevitably spawned a wide range of potential models as technology has progressed in recent years. In fact, the choice is so great now and the technical abilities and limitations of each so complex that the potential customer needs help in making a choice. These items are expensive and should last for several years, so it is important to make the right choice before making a purchase. Ventworld is a valuable resource with good data summaries of many of the modern ventilators.[3]

Simple mechanical ventilators, such as the original Dräger Oxylog and the Pneupac series (Ventipac, Parapac, etc.), require no electrical power supply because the motive force is supplied by pressure from the oxygen cylinder. This clearly has a great advantage in terms of negating the risk of electrical failure or battery exhaustion, but the disadvantages include inadequate alarms and the lack of more complex ventilatory modes, as well as greatly increased gas consumption. Primary missions, when patients are delivered from the site of injury or illness direct to hospital, do not require complex ventilatory modes. The same can be said

for the majority of intra- and inter-hospital transfers. In such cases, a patient requiring ventilation can be sedated (and preferably paralysed) and a mandatory mode, such as intermittent positive pressure ventilation (IPPV), can almost always be used. The main exception might be severe asthma where IPPV struggles to provide adequate inflation. Hand ventilation may then be the only suitable alternative en route.

In the tertiary transfer of a patient who may be partially weaned from a ventilator, it may be useful to have other ventilatory modes available. The commonest of these is continuous positive airway pressure (CPAP),[4] triggered modes such as pressure support (PS) or hybrid modes such as synchronized intermittent mandatory ventilation (SIMV). The other requisite feature is the ability to provide positive end-expiratory pressure (PEEP) with any mode. This can be done in some cases by use of extra circuit valves separate to the ventilator. It seems likely that the use of non-invasive ventilation, and in particular the use of mask CPAP, will become increasingly common modalities of support during transport. Mask CPAP can be particularly useful

---

[3] See http://www.ventworld.com.

[4] The only pure spontaneous mode. See Chapter 5.

for the cardiac pulmonary oedema patient and, of course, in paediatrics. At the time of this writing, there are several ventilators on the market which offer a good range of ventilatory modes, as well as durability, robustness and varying degrees of power economy and gas consumption.

In essence, transport ventilators can be divided into two basic groups. The first group is pneumatically driven ventilators that require high-pressure oxygen to drive the ventilator. No electrical power source is required. These ventilators tend to consume at least one litre of oxygen per minute to drive the ventilator. This one litre per minute of oxygen flow is lost for patient use and can add up to a substantial amount of oxygen during long distance transport.

The second group of ventilators generates tidal volume with electrically powered internal compressors. The benefit is that low-flow oxygen can be tapped into the ventilator inlet or directly into the patient circuit. These ventilators are the only ventilators that can be used on routine commercial airlines. It is important to know that most airlines will not allow these ventilators to be plugged into the aircraft electrical system. Sufficient source of external portable power is therefore essential during patient transport. Because of possible electromagnetic emissions generated by power-driven ventilators, operators of air ambulances and some aviation authorities will have an approved list of safe ventilators.

Examples of transport ventilators

The Breas PV403, Pulmonetic LTV1000, Newport HT50, Uni-Vent 754 and Puritan Bennett LP10 have been reviewed and compared in a recent study by an Australian aeromedical retrieval service.[6] Three of the most commonly used examples are compared here and in Table 15.7.

PULMONETIC LTV1000

The Pulmonetic LTV1000 is a popular modern electrically powered, computer-assisted transport and bedside ventilator. It is the size of a laptop computer and weighs only 5.7 kg. A useful interface makes the 'push-and-turn' operation of the LTV1000 easy to use and understand. Its sophisticated technology allows comprehensive management of ventilated breaths. The main cause of concern most often reported is the short battery life and the total and abrupt loss of ventilation and memory when power is lost.

DRÄGER OXYLOG 3000

The ubiquitous Dräger Oxylog 3000 is a user-friendly, portable, time-cycled, volume-constant, pressure-controlled ventilator that can provide a number of ventilation modes (Table 15.7). It also has the benefits of inspiratory hold, a gas consumption display, 100% oxygen breaths and a simple self-check system with easy on-screen instructions.

UNI-VENT EAGLE TM754

After a three-year study involving the transport of 125 ventilated patients by air ambulance with an average duration of transport of 10.6 hours, an unpublished report[5] confirms the Uni-Vent Eagle TM754 ventilator fulfills all the recommended criteria for a transport ventilator.

Manual Ventilation

Most anaesthetists who are given the option to ventilate manually would probably prefer to use a Waters bag (Mapleson C circuit) because of the 'feel' this allows the operator and the presence of a manually adjustable exhaust valve which can be used to add variable amounts of PEEP (Figure 15.1). However, the Waters system does not have a self-inflating bag and separate reservoir, hence its non-inflating bag also acts as a reservoir but empties quickly as it requires high oxygen flow to meet the needs of peak inspiration. In effect, the self-inflating bag-valve-mask or airway adjunct (e.g. the Ambu™

---

5 Van Reenan C, 2006. Unpublished correspondence.

Table 15.7 Comparison of three popular transport ventilators

	Pulmonetic LTV1000	Dräger Oxylog 3000	Uni-Vent Eagle TM754
Weight	6.1 kg	4.9 kg	5.8 kg
Dimensions	30 × 25 × 8 cm	28.5 x 18.4 × 17.5 cm	22 × 29 × 11.5 cm
AC supply	90 to 240 V ac	100 to 240 V ac	110 to 240 V ac
DC 12 volt compatible	11 to 15 V dc	10 to 32 V dc	Yes
Internal battery life	2 hours	4 hours	5 hours
Operating temp	+5 to +40 °C	−20 to +50 °C	−60 to +60 °C
Display	LED	Electro-luminescent	LCD
FIO_2 range	0.21 to 1.0	0.4 to 1.0	0.21 to 1.0
Tidal volume	50 to 2000 mL	50 to 2000 mL	Full range possible
Tidal volume stability at altitude	?	Up to 15 000 feet	Up to 25 000 feet
Respiratory rate settings	2 to 80	2 to 60	1 to 150
Peak inspiratory flow rate	$\leq$60 L.min^{-1}	$\leq$60 L.min^{-1}	$\leq$60 L.min^{-1}
PEEP	0 to 20 mbar	0 to 20 mbar	0 to 20 cm H_2O
Pressure support	0 to 60 mbar	0 to 35 mbar (relative to PEEP)	Yes
Spontaneous mode (CPAP)	0 to 20 mbar	Yes	Yes
Triggered mode	Yes, volume (ACV)	Yes, pressure	No
Hybrid mode(s)	SIMV	SIMV, BIPAP	SIMV, ACV
Mandatory mode(s)	IPPV	IPPV	No
Comprehensive alarm system	Yes	Yes	Yes

1mbar = 0.1 kPa = 1.0197 cm H_2O

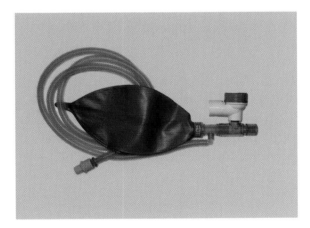

Figure 15.1 The Waters circuit.

resuscitators and their many 'me-too' copies) is the safest option because in the event of oxygen failure at least ventilation can continue using ambient air. This is not possible for the Waters system.

Advanced topics in difficult transfer and transport scenarios

As mentioned in the introduction to this chapter, inter-hospital transfers are becoming increasingly common, and outside of the hospital environment, there are few, if any, opportunities to make good any deficiencies that arise in transit. While a number of eventualities are unpredictable, running out of oxygen is not among them and can be avoided by some relatively straightforward calculations (Box 15.2).

Intra-hospital transfers to MRI scanners

Magnetic resonance imaging (MRI) is becoming commonplace in UK hospitals, and seriously ill and injured patients are often transferred from the emergency department or intensive care unit for urgent imaging. With the advent of magnets of increasing

Box 15.2 Calculating the amount of oxygen in litres required during transport

Flow rates depend on which ventilator is being used. For example, the original Dräger Oxylog 2000 uses a minimum of 1 L.min^{-1} plus 50% of the set minute volume in the 'air mix' mode (FiO$_2$ of 0.6) or 1 L.min^{-1} plus the set minute volume in the 'no air mix' mode (FiO$_2$ of 1.0).

Using the Uni-Vent 754 ventilator without use of a modified circle system, a flow rate of 2 L.min^{-1} can provide a FiO$_2$ of 0.38. A flow rate of 4 L.min^{-1} can provide a FiO$_2$ of 0.58. By using the modified circle system, a flow rate of 2 L.min^{-1} can provide a FiO$_2$ of at least 0.8.

To calculate the number of oxygen cylinders required, calculate the patient's minute volume ($\dot{V}$):

$$\dot{V} = V_T \times f, \tag{15.1}$$

where V_T is the tidal volume in litres and f is the respiratory rate in breaths.min^{-1}. Then do the following:

- add 1 L.min^{-1} for pneumatically driven ventilators,
- estimate the journey time (T_J) in minutes as accurately as possible and
- check the type of oxygen cylinders available for the journey and look up the volume of oxygen (litres) available in a full cylinder (see Figure 15.2 and Table 15.8).

Use the FiO$_2$ calculated or set on the ventilator.

Multiply the calculation by 1.5 to add a 50% reserve in case of unexpected delays or an increase in oxygen demand.

Round the answer up.

For pneumatically driven ventilators, use the following:

$$\text{Number of cylinders} = \frac{1.5 \times ((\dot{V} + 1) \times T_J \times F_{IO_2})}{\text{Cylinder volume}}.$$

For electrically driven ventilators, use the following:

$$\text{Number of cylinders} = \frac{1.5 \times (\dot{V} \times T_J \times F_{IO_2})}{\text{Cylinder volume}}.$$

Example. How many D-size oxygen cylinders (see Table 15.8) are required using the LTV 1000 (electrically driven) for a journey time of six hours in a patient with a tidal volume of 0.6 litres ventilated at 10 breaths per minute with an FiO$_2$ of 0.4?

$$\text{Number of cylinders} = \frac{1.5 \times (\dot{V} \times T_J \times F_{IO_2})}{\text{Cylinder volume}}$$

$$\text{Number of cylinders} = \frac{1.5 \times (0.6 \times 10 \times 360 \times 0.4)}{340} = 3.8.$$

Answer: It will take four full D-size cylinders.

strength, medical and other health workers have the potential for increased exposure to specific MRI hazards and concerns have also been expressed over patient safety, not least from equipment and items used or taken in to the scanner room.

There are three types of magnetic fields produced by MRI. Switched gradient fields and radiofrequency fields only exist within the confines of the magnet and present no real hazard. However, static fields extend beyond the confines of the magnet and

Table 15.8 Oxygen cylinders available in UK hospitals (See also Figure 15.2.)

	Weight (empty, kg)	Contents (litres)	Valve outlet pressure (bar)	Valve outlet connection
AZ	2.3	170	137	Pin-index
C	2.0	170	137	Pin-index
AD	3.7	400	4	6 mm firtree
CD	2.7	460	4	Schraeder/6 mm firtree
PD	4.8	300	137	Bullnose 5/8″ BSP
RD	4.1	460	4	Schraeder/6 mm firtree
D	3.4	340	137	Pin-index
E	5.4	680	137	Pin-index
F	14.5	1360	137	Bullnose 5/8″ BSP
HX	15.5	2300	4	Schraeder/6 mm firtree
ZX	10.0	3040	4	Schraeder/6 mm firtree
G	34.5	3400	137	Bullnose 5/8″ BSP
J	68.9	6800	137	Pin-index (side spindle)

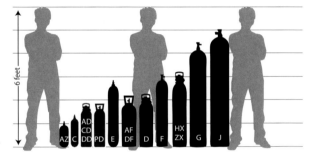

Figure 15.2 Comparative sizes and silhouettes of oxygen cylinders available in UK hospitals.

give a greater cause for concern. The field strength depends on the configuration and shielding of the magnet and decreases rapidly as the distance from the magnet increases.

The intense static magnetic field can be demonstrated by the attraction of ferromagnetic metals towards the bore of the scanner. Apart from the obvious dangers of being injured by unrestrained objects or by the movement (or malfunction) of any MRI incompatible implants within the body, short-term exposure represents no known health risk. There are, however, limitations on the types of equipment that can be used, including the ventilator. Therefore, the patient must be moved from the transfer ventilator to one which is free of ferromag-

netic components and hence is safe in the MRI environment. Penlon (Nuffield) manufacture an MRI compatible device. It is a time-cycled unit powered by medical air or oxygen at 340 to 410 kPa and has preset volume and flow rate for adult or paediatric patients.

Limitations on equipment that can be used safely in the scanner, and difficulty with monitoring consciousness level and the adequacy of airway patency when patients are in the bore of the scanner (especially from a remote location) all have major safety implications.

Aeromedical transportation

As discussed earlier, there are two major logistical issues that require important consideration when transporting ventilated patients over long distances. These are oxygen supply to the patient and power supply to the electrical equipment. When using a dedicated air ambulance, neither are real issues because most aircraft carry large stores of oxygen on board and have electrical systems that allow 110- to 240-volt power supply from the aircraft for the electrical equipment. However, the transport of ventilated patients on commercial airlines can offer considerable cost savings compared with transport on dedicated air ambulance aircraft, though oxygen supplies and power sources are limited. Most commercial airlines that do provide supplemental oxygen for patient transport can only supply continuous oxygen at fixed flow rates of 2 or 4 $L.min^{-1}$. Most airlines will limit the number of cylinders that they supply on any one flight due to availability of cylinders and limited storage space inside the cabin during a full flight. The total amount of oxygen provided and the maximum FiO_2 obtained at these limited low-flow rates may become limiting factors that prevent safe transport of stable ventilated patients on commercial airlines.

Practical solutions to the problem of reducing overall oxygen consumption and methods to increase the maximum FiO_2 delivered to the patient by using a modified version of the circle system[6] have been recently published.[6,7] The challenge when transporting ventilated cases over long distances is determining the amount of oxygen required to maintain adequate oxygenation for the whole duration of the journey. In order to do this, it is necessary to (1) know the predicted FiO_2 required at the cabin altitude to maintain a saturation above 90% and (2) have knowledge of the ventilator settings, breathing circuit setup and flow rates to deliver the required FiO_2. Finally, once the volume of oxygen required is known, it is important to check with the airline that this volume of oxygen can be supplied.

Calculating altitude-equivalent PaO_2 and FiO_2 requirements during transport

Helicopters and some smaller fixed-wing air ambulances are unpressurized, which means that the

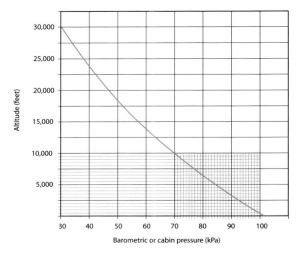

Figure 15.3 Barometric pressure at altitude.

To calculate the FiO_2 required to maintain haemoglobin saturation at a specific value. First, adjust the FiO_2 on the ground so that the patient's haemoglobin saturation is what you consider to be the minimum acceptable; this is the 'ground FiO_2'. Then using the graph, look up the in-flight cabin pressure from the in-flight cabin 'altitude'; this is the 'in-flight Pb'. Knowing the barometric pressure at ground level, 'ground Pb', which may not be sea level, the in-flight FiO_2 is calculated this way:

$$\text{in-flight } F_{IO_2} = \text{ground } F_{IO_2} \times \left(\frac{\text{ground } Pb - 6.3}{\text{in-flight } Pb - 6.3} \right).$$

For example, at sea level (ground $Pb = 101$ kPa), a patient requires an FiO_2 of 0.45 to maintain a haemoglobin saturation of 90%. From the graph it can seen that at a cabin 'altitude' of 6000 feet the cabin pressure will be 82.5 kPa. Therefore, to maintain the same haemoglobin saturation in flight the patient will require the following:

$$\text{in-flight } F_{IO_2} = 0.45 \times \left(\frac{101 - 6.3}{82.5 - 6.3} \right) = 0.45$$

$$\times \left(\frac{94.7}{76.2} \right) = 0.56.$$

The volume of oxygen required for the flight can then be calculated as in Box 15.2.

crew, passengers and patients on board are all subjected to the ambient pressure at the altitude the aircraft is flying. Commercial airliners and medium to large fixed-wing air ambulances are pressurized as they climb through the atmosphere. Pressurization systems are designed to offer a compromise between the physiological demands of the occupants and

---

[6] A circle system is a breathing circuit commonly employed during general anaesthesia in which the patient re-breathes their exhaled gas but with the carbon dioxide removed by passage through granules of soda lime. Because only a small proportion of the oxygen delivered in each breath is absorbed, a circle system only requires a very small oxygen supply to maintain a constant FiO_2. This makes a circle system very efficient.

the engineering demands of efficient and economic flight at higher altitudes. Modern pressurized aircraft therefore provide a 'normal' cabin pressure equivalent to an altitude of 6000 to 8000 feet above sea level. This is called the 'cabin altitude'. Healthy occupants of the aircraft will cope easily with a 'normal' cabin altitude, but oxygen dependant patients will require a higher FIO_2 to maintain an acceptable saturation. The more expensive option is to request that the cabin pressure is increased to a lower 'altitude-equivalent' pressure, but requesting a 'sea level' pressure has severe penalties on aircraft cruise altitude, speed, duration of flight and fuel consumption. Inevitably, an aircraft forced to fly at sea-level cabin altitude will take much longer to reach its destination and may even be delayed further by extra refuelling stops.

Due to increased altitude and subsequent decrease in ambient partial pressure, oxygen dependant patients will require a higher FIO_2 at normal pressurized cabin altitude to maintain an acceptable saturation. The minimal acceptable oxygen concentration might arguably be that which would give an alveolar PO_2 equivalent to that found at 8000 ft (2440 m), since normal individuals are unaware of any symptoms at that altitude. However, patients will generally have higher oxygen demands because of their pathology or treatment. The aim must therefore be to maintain alveolar PO_2 at their sea level equivalent, probably in the range 10.7 to 13.3 kPa (Figure 15.3).

FURTHER READING

- Martin TE. *Handbook of Patient Transportation*. 2001; Cambridge University Press.
- Martin T. *Aeromedical Transportation: A Clinical Guide*. 2006. Avebury.
- Branson RD, Campbell RS *et al.* AARC clinical practice guideline: transport of the mechanically ventilated patient. *Respiratory Care*. 1993;38:1169–72.

- DiLuigi, KJ. (2005). Transport ventilators: a guide for critical-care transportation, Aeromedical and prehospital operations. *Emergency Medical Services*. 34(1):67–70.

REFERENCES

1. Beckmann U, Gillies DM, Berenholtz SM *et al.* Incidents relating to the intra-hospital transfer of critically ill patients. An analysis of the reports submitted to the Australian Incident Monitoring Study in Intensive Care. *Intensive Care Med.* 2004;30(8):1579–85.
2. Indeck M, Peterson S, Smith J *et al.* Risk, cost, and benefit of transporting ICU patients for special studies. *J Trauma.* 1988;28(7): 1020–5.
3. Hurst JM, Davis K, Jr., Johnson DJ *et al.* Cost and complications during in-hospital transport of critically ill patients: a prospective cohort study. *J Trauma.* 1992;33(4):582–5.
4. Centers for Disease Control. (1988). Perspectives in disease prevention and health promotion update: universal precautions for prevention of transmission of human immunodeficiency virus, hepatitis B virus, and other bloodborne pathogens in health-care settings. *Morb Mortal Wkly Rep.* 1988;37(24): 377–88.
5. Dooley SW, Jr., Castro KG, Hutton MD *et al.* Guidelines for preventing the transmission of tuberculosis in health-care settings, with special focus on HIV-related issues. *MMWR Recomm Rep.* 1990;39(RR-17):1–29.
6. Lowes T, Sharley P. Oxygen conservation during long distance transport of ventilated patients. *Air Med J.* 2005;24(4):164–71.
7. Lowes T, Sharley P. Oxygen conservation during long-distance transport of ventilated patients: assessing the Modified Circle System. *Air Med J.* 2006;25(1):35–9.

Chapter 16

Special considerations in infants and children

ROB ROSS RUSSELL AND NATALIE YEANEY

Introduction

This book is intended for an audience whose main preoccupation is the care of adults, but it seems very appropriate to include a chapter on children. Until the early 1990s, it was not unusual for children in the United Kingdom to be managed on intensive care units for adults. With the development of neonatal intensive care units (NICUs), and more recently paediatric intensive care units (PICUs), this situation is now extremely rare. However, neither NICUs nor PICUs are available in every hospital, and children will continue to become ill, occasionally critically so, wherever they happen to be. Staff may therefore be called upon to manage infants or children with respiratory failure, often unexpectedly, at almost any time. In this chapter we will attempt to outline the major differences that need to be considered when faced with neonates and children who require mechanical ventilation. It is not a comprehensive text but more of a taster, looking at the anatomy, physiology and some particular examples of paediatric care.

Anatomy

Lung development occurs early in gestation, but maturation of the alveoli and surfactant production only commence in the third trimester, and this generally limits respiratory viability to infants of 23 weeks gestation or more. At this stage, the lungs are in the canalicular stage (17 to 27 weeks gestation), and the acinar gas exchange units are just beginning to form at the end of each terminal bronchiole. Production of surfactant only starts at 20 to 24 weeks gestation. Between 27 and 35 weeks gestation (saccular stage) alveolar development and septation occurs, increasing the pulmonary surface area considerably. However, compared to the adult lung, surface area remains greatly reduced. In the infant at term, surface area is about 3 m^2 compared to 70 m^2 in the adult, with only one tenth the number of small airways found in the adult.

When lungs in the early proliferating stages of development are forced prematurely into use, the incompletely formed thick-walled acinar units are much less compliant than the terminal airways, leading them to become over-distended. The junction between the terminal airway and alveolar duct is susceptible to shear stress and tearing, resulting in complications such as interstitial emphysema and pneumothoraces. In addition, the majority of babies that weigh less than 1500 grams develop a degree of respiratory distress syndrome, with surfactant deficiency leading to alveolar collapse and ventilation/perfusion mismatch. Both higher oxygen concentrations and higher alveolar opening pressures are needed to prevent hypoxia and metabolic acidosis in the baby. Over a few hours, cellular debris from injured lung epithelium and oedema

Core Topics in Mechanical Ventilation, ed. Iain Mackenzie. Published by Cambridge University Press.

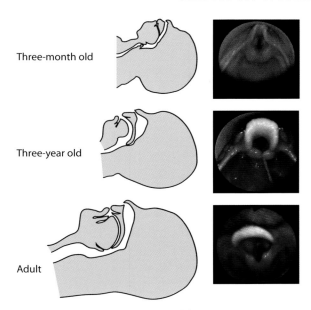

Three-month old

Three-year old

Adult

Figure 16.1 Comparative anatomy of the upper airway.

from capillary leak line the terminal bronchioles and alveolar ducts, further impeding alveolar oxygen uptake. The damage caused by oxygen toxicity and ventilation of immature lungs probably contributes to the altered lung structure seen in those that go on to develop chronic lung disease.

The upper airway

At birth, the shape and position of structures in the upper airway is quite different from that in adults. The head is proportionately much larger in the infant and child than in the adult and head control is, of course, poor in the infant. The tongue is relatively large and in a small mouth this can obstruct any view of the larynx. Once past the tongue, the epiglottis is also positioned differently. In the newborn, it lies at the level of the first cervical vertebra, higher and more anterior than in adults. It is also softer, 'U-shaped' and more prone to collapse from external pressure (Figure 16.1).

In practical terms this leads to a number of difficulties. Getting a good view of the larynx can be very difficult. In infants up to 12 months old, a laryngoscope with a straight blade and no side-flange is often preferred. It is advanced in the midline over the back of the tongue and over the anterior lip of the epiglottis. Pulling up then exposes the vocal cords by pulling the epiglottis forwards. In larger children and adults, the tip of the laryngoscope is placed in the vallecula in front of the epiglottis, which is pulled forwards. The soft larynx in the infant means that over-extension of the neck is likely to kink the airway and needs to be avoided; the head should be kept in the neutral position when examining the infant airway.

Moving down the airway, the shape of the larynx in the child below the age of about eight years is conical, with the narrowest part lying at the level of the cricoid cartilage. This is unlike the adult or older child where the shape is cylindrical, with the narrowest part therefore lying at the level of the vocal cords. As mentioned previously, it lies three to four cervical vertebrae higher than in the adult, giving a much more acute angle between the oropharynx and the glottis.

In older children and adults, foreign bodies passing beyond the vocal cords will pass down into the right or left main bronchus, allowing ventilation of the opposite lung. In small infants, however, objects can occlude the main airway at the cricoid cartilage and for this reason care must be taken not to push foreign bodies past the vocal cords. Finger sweeps of the mouth should not be undertaken in suspected foreign body aspiration (Figure 16.2). This is also one of the reasons that un-cuffed endotracheal (ET) tubes are used in small children, because the cuff would lie at the level of the cricoid, causing irritation and a risk of subsequent sub-glottic injury.

Chest wall

Chest wall mechanics comprise another important difference from adults. The newborn infant, especially if pre-term, has a much more compliant chest wall than an adult. This will tend to collapse inward during forced inspiration, reducing the effectiveness of the breath, and increasing the work of breathing.

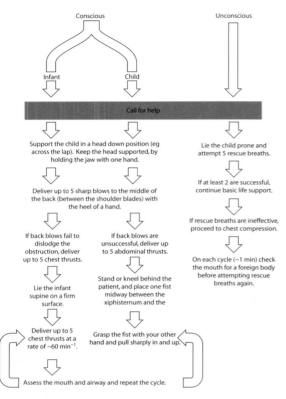

Figure 16.2 Algorithm for the management of upper airway obstruction in infants and children.

Infant diaphragms may be more resistant to muscle fatigue than adults, but significant chest wall deformity during breathing can add considerable work and can contribute to lung collapse during expiration, again increasing the work required to re-inflate them.

In children who have yet to learn to walk, the ribs are aligned horizontally relative to the spine and only develop a caudal slope once the child is walking. This means that the intercostal muscles cannot increase lung volume, and the infant's inspiratory effort is entirely dependent on its diaphragm.

The development of muscle fatigue is an important cause of respiratory failure in infants and children with significant pulmonary disease, such as severe bronchiolitis. Recognition of chest distortion, and thus the greater risk of fatigue, is important. Reduced energy stores (low glycogen and fat

stores) may cause infants to collapse rapidly as fatigue develops.

Cardiovascular system

There are also several important differences in the cardiovascular system. Before birth, oxygenation occurs in the placenta with only minimal blood flow through the lungs. At birth, the infant has a high pulmonary vascular resistance. As placental flow drops, systemic resistance rises. Increasing arterial partial pressure of oxygen causes a fall in pulmonary vascular resistance and closure of the ductus arteriosus that connects the pulmonary trunk to the descending aorta. These changes occur rapidly, probably over a period of hours in the normal infant. In some infants, particularly those that are pre-term, those with significant cardiac disease, or infants with a diaphragmatic hernia, these changes are interrupted. In these situations, pulmonary vascular resistance remains high, causing deoxygenated blood to cross the atrial septum from right to left. The ductus arteriosus may also stay open allowing for a significant shunt, usually from left to right. Significant cardiac disease will also alter blood flow.

In respiratory terms, the most significant problem seen here relates to persistent pulmonary hypertension of the newborn (PPHN). This is discussed later, but it can cause very substantial difficulties in ventilation and gas exchange. A number of congenital cardiac abnormalities may also present with pulmonary hypertension, and these infants will require specialist care from a cardiac centre.

Physiology

The most obvious physiological difference between adults and children is their size. This has implications for many aspects of respiratory support, but in practical terms it means that the child's size has to be incorporated into calculations of drug dosages, fluid volumes, tidal volumes, and endotracheal tube sizes, among others. There are several

Table 16.1 Some physiological comparisons between infants and children. Values given are approximate

	Neonate (term)	Infant (~1 year)	Child (~8 years)	Formula for calculation
Weight	3.5–4 kg	~10 kg	~25 kg	(Age + 4) × 2
ET tube size	3.0–3.5 mm	4.0–4.5 mm	6.0 mm	Age/4 + 4 (after 1 year)
Daily fluid requirement	Day 1: 60 mL.kg^{-1}	~1000 mL.d^{-1}	~1600 mL.d^{-1}	For first 10 kg: 100 mL.kg^{-1}
	Day 5: 120 mL.kg^{-1}	(40 mL.hr^{-1})	(64 mL.hr^{-1})	For second 10 kg: 50 mL.kg^{-1}
				For rest: 20 mL.kg^{-1}
Tidal volume (mL)	20–30	50	125	4–6 mL.kg^{-1}
Heart rate (beats.min^{-1})	110–150	100	70	
Respiratory rate (breaths.min^{-1})	40–60	30	20–25	
Systolic blood pressure (mm Hg)	>60	80–90	105	90 + (2 × age)

formulae and tables designed to help with these calculations (Table 16.1).

Size has important implications in the lungs as well. Airway resistance follows Poiseuille's law,

$$R = \frac{8 \cdot l \cdot \eta}{r^4} \qquad (16.1)$$

from which it follows that resistance (R) is inversely proportional to the fourth power of the radius (r) of the airway; halving the airway diameter will therefore increase resistance by 16-fold. It is important to recognize also that a 1-mm reduction in a 4-mm diameter airway (whether from oedema or the insertion of an endotracheal tube) will increase resistance three-fold, whereas in an adult a similar reduction in an 8-mm airway would only increase resistance by a factor of 1.7. This has significant implications in the small child who develops upper airway disease or requires intubation. For example, laryngotracheobronchitis (croup) causes swelling of the larynx and upper trachea, and in the older child this has little effect. In the infant it can give rise to a substantial increase in the work of breathing and may lead to fatigue and respiratory failure. Similarly, for the small infant who is intubated, the endotracheal tube can itself provide a noticeable increase in airway resistance, and therefore small infants (certainly those under one year of age) require

support, usually in the form of pressure support, when spontaneously breathing through an endotracheal tube.

Control of breathing

The infant's control of breathing is less developed than in the older child. The newborn is thought to be relatively insensitive to carbon dioxide,[1] particularly the pre-term infant, and this is important in the immediate post-natal period when respiration is primarily driven by hypoxia. However, this effect only lasts for about 15 minutes before the drive diminishes. The respiratory response to the arterial partial pressure of carbon dioxide is flatter in the newborn, and hypoxia shifts the curve to the right, as opposed to a left shift in adults.[2] This early hypoxic drive is importantly blunted by hypothermia, emphasizing the importance of warmth at this time. By three weeks of age, a pattern of sustained respiratory drive in response to hypoxia is seen. However, patterns of breathing remain more erratic. The pre-term infant will often display periodic breathing[1] with occasionally prolonged periods of apnoea that respond to treatment with

---

[1] Periodic breathing is a pattern of breathing where the depth of each breath will increase to a peak and then diminish. Each cycle of breaths (commonly about 10–15 breaths) will end in a brief pause of 2–10 seconds before the cycle repeats.

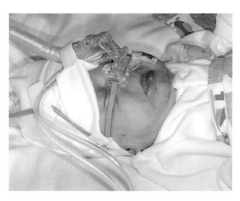

Figure 16.3 Infant receiving nasal continuous positive airway pressure (CPAP).

caffeine. Even the neonate at term may develop apnoea following anaesthesia. Infants less than 44 weeks corrected gestation[2] have an increased risk of post-operative apnoea of around 20% to 40% within the first 12 hours following anaesthesia. This risk is increased by anaemia and again, reduced by caffeine.[3] Apnoea is also seen in older infants with viral infections, particularly bronchiolitis and pertussis. There is some limited evidence that caffeine may help older infants with bronchiolitis.[4] In this condition, the apnoeas usually only occur during the first 48 hours and so ventilation may be avoidable if caffeine is administered.[4] Similarly, less invasive support, such as nasal continuous positive airway pressure (CPAP), may tide the child over until recovery begins (Figure 16.3).

Lung mechanics

The lung mechanics of children also differ from adults. Infants are unable to breathe through their mouths for the first weeks of life. Obstruction of the nose, whether through disease, such as choanal atresia, or obstruction from secretions or tubes placed through the nose, can cause significant difficulties for the self-ventilating infant.

Compared to adults, small children have a disproportionately small tidal volume of about 4 to 6 mL.kg^{-1} and together with a higher basal metabolic rate this gives them a significantly increased demand for alveolar minute volume (Table 16.1). This means that dead space ventilation is increased. Chest wall compliance is high in the newborn and gradually falls over the first two years of life to reach adult values.

Practical implications relate to the setting up of ventilation in children and the need for positive end-expiratory pressure (PEEP) in most clinical settings. A combination of the proportionately increased dead space ventilation, which makes the measured minute volume less closely related to the alveolar minute volume, and the increased metabolic demands per kilogram of weight of the child means that ventilation is usually set up by determining the tidal volume and adjusting the rate rather than setting a particular minute volume. A tidal volume of 5 to 8 mL.kg^{-1} is usually used, and the rate adjusted to control carbon dioxide elimination. The same concerns about volutrauma damage to the paediatric lung apply as they do in adults, and the tidal volume should be restricted wherever possible.

Because of their increased chest wall compliance, infants up to the age of about nine months maximize functional residual capacity (FRC) by shortening the expiratory time (TE) and 'braking' expiration, which may be heard as an expiratory grunt. Their faster respiratory rate also contributes to the maintenance of functional residual capacity. Mechanical ventilation abolishes these mechanisms, and maintenance of end-expiratory lung volume requires the use of PEEP.

One important difference is the relationship between FRC and closing volume, which is the lung volume at which airway collapse occurs. In children up to the age of about four years, closing volume is greater than FRC, which means that if a child makes a forced expiratory effort, as in screaming, part of

---

[2] In other words, 44 weeks from conception or 4 weeks after the expected delivery date.

the lung is able to collapse, creating a shunt and rapidly leading to cyanosis. This is the physiological basis of 'breath holding attacks', where small children can develop rapid cyanosis after minor injuries.

Ventilation and perfusion matching also varies between children and adults. Although the distribution of blood flow within the lung follows a similar pattern to adults, being primarily determined by gravity, ventilation patterns are different. As in the adult, ventilation is greater in the lower part of the lung, when upright, but in the supine or lateral position the non-dependent lung is better ventilated in children up to the age of about eight years.[5]

Consequently, manoeuvres to position a child 'good lung down' to improve ventilation/perfusion matching as would be reasonable in adults may worsen gas exchange in children. However, in children with acute lung injury there may still be benefits in prone positioning, as is seen in adult practice, in those that develop interstitial pulmonary oedema, although this was not supported by a recent randomized study.[6]

Specific situations

Neonatal

Neonatologists encounter a variety of pathological lung conditions including incompletely developed lungs, surfactant deficiency, pneumonia, meconium aspiration, congenital structural anomalies and bronchopulmonary dysplasia (chronic lung disease). Many of the current concepts in neonatal ventilation attempt to minimize damage to the delicate neonatal lung and can be applied to most babies with respiratory failure, regardless of their underlying lung disease.

General concepts

Several basic concepts can be applied to neonatal ventilation. First, the minimum support that results in adequate gas exchange is provided. Second, the

baby's work of breathing is minimized in order to optimize comfort and to free energy expenditure for growth and lung repair. Third, attention is focused on limiting sudden shifts and extremes of the arterial partial pressures of oxygen (PaO_2) and carbon dioxide ($PaCO_2$). Hypocapnia causes cerebral artery vasoconstriction and decreases oxygen delivery to the brain, while hypercapnia causes cerebral artery vasodilatation and increased cerebral blood flow that may contribute to intraventricular haemorrhage. While the above concepts are generally accepted to reduce lung and brain injury in the neonate, other approaches to ventilation such as the preferential use of continuous positive airway pressure in babies with the respiratory distress syndrome,[7] preferential use of high frequency oscillatory ventilation over conventional mechanical ventilation and use of the newer modalities of conventional ventilation remain controversial.

Permissive hypercapnia

Maintaining gas exchange with lower tidal volumes and higher ventilatory rates, while accepting $PaCO_2$ levels above the normal range of 4.5 to 5.8 kPa, should reduce the risk of ventilator-induced lung injury. It may also be of potential benefit in conditions like congenital diaphragmatic hernia in which there is lung hypoplasia. A Cochrane review[8] has compared a hypercapnic with a normocapnic strategy. Their data suggest that mild permissive hypercapnia, 6 to 8 kPa, was not associated with adverse outcome, but the benefits seen in clinical trials appear small, and a recent meta-analyis of neonatal ventilator strategies suggests the data remain ambivalent.[9]

Non-invasive ventilation and CPAP

By applying a constant distending pressure to the alveoli, CPAP recruits collapsed alveoli, increases lung volume, maintains FRC above the closing volume and results in a more regular pattern of breathing in the pre-term neonate.[10] CPAP is delivered through a device that maintains a positive pressure in a circuit that provides a continuous flow of humidified air at a flow of 5 to 10 $L.min^{-1}$. The patient interface consists of either nasal prongs, a mask fitted over the nose, or a nasopharyngeal tube (Figure 16.3). CPAP has the drawbacks of potentially causing nasal breakdown (at pressure points on the nose), abdominal distension from air forced into the gut or when high pressures are used, decreased venous return to the heart.

While it is known that CPAP can be used successfully following extubation and reduces the risk of reintubation,[7] the early use of CPAP as the sole respiratory support in premature babies with respiratory distress syndrome remains controversial. In one unit, the wide use of CPAP in neonates under 1500g, and the acceptance of a high $PaCO_2$, up to 8.5 kPa, has resulted in a reduction in chronic lung disease from 36% to 10%,[11] but a recent Cochrane review remained uncertain about the benefits,[12] and there has been some hesitancy in applying this approach widely because neurodevelopmental outcome data are limited.[13]

Conventional ventilation

Conventional ventilation in the neonate is usually administered in a pressure-controlled mode. The physiological problems of prematurity (as discussed earlier) give rise to poorly compliant lungs, and both high inflating pressures and high PEEP may be needed. Although some patients may be paralysed, there is good evidence that synchronizing the ventilator with the infant reduces morbidity associated with ventilation, in particular the risk of pneumothorax.

Recent advances in ventilators have now allowed the use of volume-controlled ventilation[3] but this is not yet common practice in view of the potential errors.

---

[3] Tidal volumes of only 3 to 4 mL may be needed for very small infants!

Pressure support is important in neonatal practice. Endotracheal tubes are very small, have a high resistance, and dead space is proportionately very high. Support pressures of 8 to 10 cm H_2O are often needed to overcome the added work of breathing. Respiratory rates are usually set at around 60 breaths a minute, with a short inspiratory time to prevent gas trapping and over-distension of the lungs.

Choanal atresia

This congenital condition may be caused by complete bony obstruction of the nasal choanae, or by membranous stenosis or obstruction. In severe cases, newborn infants (who are obligate nose breathers) develop respiratory distress shortly after birth. The diagnosis is often considered when attempts to pass a nasogastric tube are unsuccessful. It can be a medical emergency, and oral intubation followed by referral to a paediatric ear, nose and throat (ENT) surgeon is needed.

Congenital diaphragmatic hernia

In congenital diaphragmatic hernia, a developmental defect in the diaphragm allows displacement of the viscera into the chest. The severity of the lesion depends upon the extent of the muscular defect and the gestational timing of the intestinal herniation. Pulmonary hypertension is nearly always a feature of the disease process and the condition carries a high mortality rate.

Typically, only a rudimentary lung remains on the side of the defect and survival thus depends upon the degree of hypoplasia of the opposite lung. A mediastinal shift caused by the displaced intestine exacerbates the situation by compressing viable lung. Post-natal management of a baby with a known diaphragmatic hernia begins with placing an endotracheal tube as soon as possible after delivery to limit distension of the intestinal lumen by air. Ventilator management in the past focused on targeting alkalotic blood gas parameters in the range of pH 7.4 to 7.5, but the higher pressures required

Table 16.2 Treatment strategies for persistent pulmonary hypertension

Type	Proven therapies[a]	Potentially beneficial therapies	Unproven therapies
Pulmonary treatments	Oxygen surfactant for RDS, pneumonia, meconium aspiration syndrome	High frequency ventilation	Respiratory alkalosis
Pharmacologic treatments	Inhaled nitric oxide	–	Alkali infusion, tolazoline, other intravenous vasodilators
Cardiac support	Support of cardiac output with dopamine, fluid normalization of ionized calcium	–	–
Environmental strategies	–	Avoidance of noise, reduced light	Sedation
Rescue treatments	Inhaled nitric oxide, extracorporeal membrane oxygenation	–	–

[a]Efficacious in well-designed randomized trials
Table from Fanaroff and Martin,[27] with permission.

resulted in ventilator-induced lung injury. An approach to ventilation using lower tidal volumes and permissive hypercapnia has since been advocated by many referral centres. Routine administration of surfactant is not recommended in term newborns with congenital diaphragmatic hernia.[14] Surgery is usually delayed for a few days after birth until the pulmonary vascular bed is less reactive.

Persistent pulmonary hypertension

A rapid decrease in pulmonary vascular resistance mediated by lung expansion, oxygen, and endothelial factors, is central to the process of transition from fetal to extrauterine life. Failure of the pulmonary vasculature to dilate at birth is termed persistent pulmonary hypertension of the newborn (PPHN). PPHN can be a feature of a number of neonatal disorders, including lung hypoplasia, meconium aspiration syndrome, perinatal asphyxia, congenital diaphragmatic hernia (see earlier) and pneumonia. Even in the absence of these conditions, abnormalities in muscularization of the pulmonary arterioles or defects in endothe-

lial function can trigger PPHN. A constricted pulmonary vascular bed causes right ventricular cardiac pressures to remain high which in turn leads to the shunting of blood across the foramen ovale and ductus arteriosus. The resulting profound hypoxia can sometimes make it difficult to differentiate between PPHN and right-sided heart defects.

The treatment goals in PPHN are to manage any concurrent parenchymal lung disease and to selectively lower the pulmonary vascular resistance (Table 16.2). Therapies proven to improve the clinical course in PPHN include oxygen, fluid and inotropic support of cardiac output, normalization of ionized calcium, and inhaled nitric oxide. Because proteinaceous alveolar exudates may inactivate native surfactant in both pneumonia and meconium aspiration syndrome, treating this subset of newborns with surfactant is advisable. High frequency oscillatory ventilation may be of benefit to neonates with PPHN by optimizing lung volumes and thereby improving oxygenation.[15] Although alkolosis induces pulmonary vasodilatation, hyperventilation and continuous alkali infusions have not been proven to be of benefit in clinical trials. In practice, maintaining a pH between 7.4 and 7.45 for most newborns with PPHN seems reasonable. However, in conditions such as congenital diaphragmatic hernia in which there is significant lung hypoplasia, this practice may actually be detrimental. The use of intravenous vasodilatory drugs should be avoided since they cause systemic vasodilatation in addition to pulmonary vasodilatation, increasing the risk of compromised tissue perfusion.

The criterion for initiating inhaled nitric oxide is a failure to improve pulmonary vasodilatation despite ventilating with high concentrations of oxygen. A trial of inhaled nitric oxide is often considered when the oxygenation index[4] surpasses 20 or when the PaO_2 is less than 4 to 5.3 kPa on a fractional inspired oxygen concentration (FiO_2) of 1. In neonates, inhaled nitric oxide is usually started at a concentration of 20 parts per million (ppm). The potential toxic side effects of nitric oxide include increased blood concentrations of both methaemoglobin and nitrogen dioxide. Inhaled concentrations of nitric oxide of 80 ppm have been associated with oxidative injury to the pulmonary membranes. Neonates usually respond to nitric oxide within 30 to 60 minutes of commencing inhalation and the mean improvement in PaO_2 is 7 kPa. Unfortunately, around 40% of treated infants fail to respond to inhaled nitric oxide therapy.[16]

Conclusion

Unlike the use of surfactant, which has been proven to decrease neonatal mortality, many ventilatory approaches have not been conclusively shown to decrease either chronic lung disease or mortality. The overall incidence of chronic lung disease in the neonatal population has remained about the same,

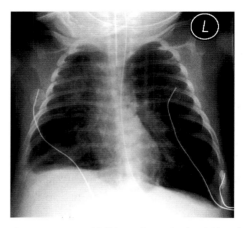

Figure 16.4 Bronchiolitis. Radiograph of a child with bronchiolitis showing areas of hyperinflation, especially the left lower lobe.

but it now occurs in smaller babies than previously survived.

The older child

Bronchiolitis

One of the commonest conditions that leads to a need for ventilation in small children is bronchiolitis, which can be caused by a number of viruses but is usually caused by respiratory syncitial virus (RSV). Every single infant within the first two years of life acquires an RSV infection and most develop mild symptoms of an upper respiratory infection. Approximately 0.5% require hospitalization and each winter around 2% to 5% of these will require admission to a PICU. As its name suggests, it is characterized by inflammation of the small airways, causing an obstructive problem and a wheezy child. Response to either salbutamol or ipratropium bromide may be limited, and respiratory support may be required for exhaustion or for apnoeas, which are not uncommon (Figure 16.4).

The first line treatment, especially for those infants with apnoea as the major feature, is often non-invasive nasal ventilation. This can be delivered

---

[4] Mean airway pressure (cm H_2O) $\times$ 100 $\times$ FiO_2/post-ductal PaO_2 (in mm Hg).

by specific devices (such as the Flow Driver), but effective nasal ventilation can also be delivered using a short endotracheal tube positioned in the back of the throat and above the cords through which gas is delivered using pressures of 5 to 10 cm H_2O (nasal CPAP). CPAP acts by holding the upper airways open, thereby reducing airway resistance and also stimulating respiratory effort. A Cochrane review of the technique in neonatal practice has demonstrated an advantage in the 'two prong' delivery systems.[7] In patients where non-invasive ventilation is inadequate, intubation may be needed. The ventilation strategy at this stage should be focused on adequate lung recruitment, limiting the inspired oxygen to below 60%, if possible. Despite the wheeze, infants usually respond better to moderate levels of PEEP (5 to 8 cm H_2O) because there is often associated atelectasis. There is some evidence that surfactant may be of benefit in severely ill children with bronchiolitis.[17] Paralysis may be needed, but many infants can be managed with sedation alone.

High frequency oscillatory ventilation

High frequency oscillatory ventilation (HFOV) is well established in neonatal practice having been in use for over two decades. In marked contrast to conventional ventilation, HFOV applies a high mean airway pressure (allowing lung recruitment), which is then oscillated at a rate between 3 and 15 Hz (180 to 900 breaths per minute). Pressure excursions at the tracheal tip (around 4.3 kPa or 44 cm H_2O) drop to around 0.5 kPa ($\sim$5 cm H_2O) in the trachea and proximal airway. Not surprisingly, the oscillation consequently only produces a tiny tidal volume. Gas exchange does not depend, therefore, on traditional tidal ventilation, but instead occurs between two streams of gas moving slowly in opposite directions: a peripheral stream, or sleeve, which is moving out of the lung, and a central stream, or core, which is moving into the lung. This form of

Table 16.3 Suggested starting frequencies for high frequency ventilation depending on patient weight

Weight	Initial frequency
<2 kg	15 Hz
2–12 kg	10 Hz
13–20 kg	8 Hz
21–30 kg	7 Hz
31–50 kg	6 Hz
>50 kg	5 Hz

gas exchange is known as 'augmented diffusion'.[18] The major advantage of HFOV probably lies in the ability to recruit non-compliant lung while minimizing volutrauma. HFOV is now well established in neonatal practice, especially in the management of infants with diaphragmatic hernia, and on PICU, and a number of adult studies are now appearing as HFOV is used in conditions such as acute respiratory distress syndrome (ARDS).[19]

Criteria for instituting HFOV are varied. For children or adults, a mean airway pressure > 18 to 20 cm H_2O, an FiO_2 >0.60 and a peak inspiratory pressure >35 cm H_2O should prompt consideration of the technique.[19, 20] Neonatal practice tends to have lower thresholds.[21] In brief, patients being transferred from conventional ventilation are generally started on HFOV using a mean airway pressure slightly higher than that being used on conventional ventilation at the time. The intention is to recruit atelectatic alveoli so that the lung moves on to the steep part of the compliance curve. The frequency used depends on patient size (Table 16.3) although considerable variation may be used. The size of the excursions of each breath (the 'power') is set as the ΔP,[5] and this is adjusted to ensure visible chest vibration, and then according to the $PaCO_2$. Mean airway pressure is generally increased until the FiO_2 required to achieve the target PaO_2 drops

---
[5] Pronounced 'delta' P.

below 0.60, indicating alveolar recruitment. A chest radiograph is often advisable after a few hours to ensure that the lungs are not over-distended. Once lung recruitment has been achieved, inspired oxygen requirements will often fall dramatically, but care must be taken not to reduce mean airway pressure too fast as de-recruitment can occur. Suction is usually managed using inline devices, and limited to avoid volume loss. Weaning may be managed on HFOV or by transferring back to conventional ventilation.

The results of high quality studies on the benefits of HFOV are contradictory. In situations where HFOV has been used as rescue therapy, there is limited evidence of clear benefit, although there is an increasing tendency to use HFOV electively and therefore earlier in certain cases.[21]

Ventilation for non-respiratory conditions

The critical upper airway

For many years the commonest cause of acute life-threatening airway obstruction in children was epiglottitis, but the development of a vaccine for *Haemophilus influenzae* type b has had dramatic effect on the incidence of this disease, which is now very rarely seen.[22] Although occasional cases of vaccine failure can occur, the commonest causes of acute airway obstruction now include severe laryngotracheobronchitis (croup) or trauma. Congenital causes, including laryngeal stenosis or web and tracheal stenosis, or acquired conditions (e.g. subglottic stenosis) are rare. In a patient with visible haemangiomata elsewhere, consideration of a laryngeal haemangioma is warranted.

In a critical situation, airway control is clearly the priority. The patient should be transferred (locally) to an environment suitable for intubation, preferably by an anaesthetist together with an ENT surgeon in case a tracheostomy is required. Induction of anaesthesia may be hazardous.

Where there is critical upper airway obstruction, the initial response should be to administer oxygen by face mask and keep the child calm and in a comfortable position. An experienced anaesthetist and ENT surgeon should be present, ideally in a theatre environment. Securing the airway is of paramount importance and should not be delayed while further procedures or investigations are performed. Direct examination of the epiglottis in the emergency department is not recommended because it may worsen airway obstruction in the case of epiglottitis. In addition, any painful procedure may distress the child and precipitate sudden loss of airway.

Once in theatre, the child is often most comfortable sitting on a parent's lap. The child is gently anaesthetized by administering slowly increasing concentrations of volatile anaesthetic agent in oxygen. Muscle relaxants are avoided to allow the child to continue breathing spontaneously and therefore to maintain his own airway. Once deeply anaesthetised, laryngoscopy can be performed and the trachea intubated. If it is not possible to intubate the trachea, the ENT surgeon should immediately perform a surgical airway.

Head injury

Following a head injury, children may require intubation or ventilation for several different reasons. Children with a reduced conscious level[6] may need a CT scan. Some children may have a depressed respiratory drive secondary to the head injury or to the administration of sedatives or analgesics. There may of course be associated lung injury, and for patients with raised intracranial pressure, control of $PaCO_2$ is an important part of maintaining adequate cerebral perfusion pressure, which should be kept in the low to normal range.[23] In the latter patient, PEEP is often not used in adult practice but is an important element of paediatric care.

---

[6] In our practice, a Glasgow Coma Score below 13.

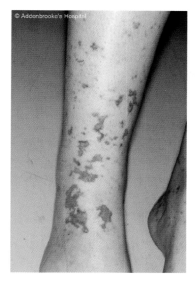

Figure 16.5 Meningococcal sepsis. Typical meningococcal rash, showing irregular, sharp-edged violaceous lesions.

Sepsis

In the severely ill child with sepsis, cardiovascular collapse is a major component of the presentation,[24] creating a high requirement for fluids (Figure 16.5). This, coupled with the capillary leak that these patients develop, means that they are at significant risk of developing pulmonary oedema. In this situation, patients will often become hypoxic and require ventilation. As with an adult in this condition, high PEEP may be needed to reverse the pulmonary oedema.

However, many guidelines on the management of severe sepsis in children now recommend elective intubation in any child who requires more than 40 mL.kg^{-1} resuscitation fluid. This will in part act as a precaution against the development of pulmonary oedema. It also helps off-load the heart, by allowing paralysis (and so reducing muscle metabolic demands) and sedation (similarly reducing cerebral demands).[7]

---

[7] See 'Early management of meningococcal disease in children' at www.meningitis.org.

Muscle weakness

There are a number of conditions in children that lead to muscle weakness, both in infants (e.g. spinal muscular atrophy) and older children (e.g. Duchenne muscular dystrophy). Children may therefore present with hypercapnia and require ventilation. Wherever possible, discussion with the child's paediatrician is important before instituting mechanical ventilation as in some cases this may be inappropriate. In many others, no such discussion is appropriate or possible. Non-invasive ventilation using a mask, or *cuirasse* ventilation, is often worth attempting because the chest is usually very compliant, and the technique can avoid intubation and a prolonged stay on PICU. Increasing numbers of these patients are receiving long-term non-invasive ventilation at home or in hospital.[25]

Mechanical and technical considerations

Humidification is the most important technical aspect of ventilation in children that may vary from adult practice. There is compelling evidence that a lack of humidification can increase the risk of tube obstruction and impair mucociliary clearance. Given the importance of maintaining maximal airway diameter and limiting any potential obstruction, humidification for all ventilated infants and children is essential.

Social aspects – families and consent

As with patients of all ages, a good understanding of consent issues is essential. In children this can be complicated in several ways. In the normal situation, consent will be given for 'minors' (children under the age of 16) by their parents. Increasingly, parents may be separated or divorced, and this needs to be considered when taking consent. Estranged fathers (and occasionally mothers) may or may not have legal rights to give consent for their children, and it is advisable to involve both parents wherever possible in the discussions. Children who are in care or who are fostered can give rise to particularly complex problems because the legal guardianship may lie with a variety of people, including Social Services, who are often not present when the child is brought in and may be difficult to contact.

Children who are 'Gillick competent' (and have a clear and mature understanding of the issues at stake and are able to make an informed choice) may also make decisions and give consent.[26] If this consent conflicts with that of their parents, then the child's opinion will often take precedence, and this can give rise to very complicated situations. Clearly, it is best if consensus can be achieved from all parties.

Staff involved in the ventilation of children also need to be aware of child protection issues. Recognition of features that may be seen in non-accidental injury such as a torn frenulum or other mouth trauma, and unusual bruises (e.g. external laryngeal bruising) should give rise to discussion about possible causes. Equally, any injuries caused during line insertion or intubation should be carefully documented so that an appropriate explanation is clearly stated.

SUMMARY

Although the majority of children who require mechanical ventilation are now seen in units that specialize in such care, many staff who may deal predominantly with adults may come across such children, especially in the acute situation. Understanding the physiological differences between adults and children, and knowing some of the common illnesses that precipitate such problems can help improve the care of these children. Children are not just small adults, but at the same time principles of care for the adult, put into practice with an understanding of the anatomical and physiological differences in the child, are usually appropriate and sensible. Good links with a supportive NICU or PICU

are also invaluable in establishing sensible and safe guidelines.

REFERENCES

1. Adamson SL. Regulation of breathing at birth. *J Dev Physiol.* 1991;15(1):45–52.
2. Rigatto H. Control of ventilation in the newborn. *Annu Rev Physiol.* 1984;46:661–74.
3. Liu LM, Cote CJ, Goudsouzian NG *et al.* Life-threatening apnea in infants recovering from anesthesia. *Anesthesiology.* 1983;59(6):506–10.
4. McNamara DG, Nixon GM, Anderson BJ. Methylxanthines for the treatment of apnea associated with bronchiolitis and anesthesia. *Paediatr Anaesth.* 2004;14(7):541–50.
5. Davies H, Helms P, Gordon I. Effect of posture on regional ventilation in children. *Pediatr Pulmonol.* 1992;12(4):227–32.
6. Curley MA, Hibberd PL, Fineman LD *et al.* Effect of prone positioning on clinical outcomes in children with acute lung injury: a randomized controlled trial. *JAMA.* 2005;294(2):229–37.
7. De Paoli AG, Davis PG, Faber B *et al.* Devices and pressure sources for administration of nasal continuous positive airway pressure (NCPAP) in preterm neonates. *Cochrane Database Syst Rev.* 2002(4):CD002977.
8. Woodgate PG, Davies MW. Permissive hypercapnia for the prevention of morbidity and mortality in mechanically ventilated newborn infants. *Cochrane Database Syst Rev.* 2001(2):CD002061.
9. van Kaam AH, Rimensberger PC. Lung-protective ventilation strategies in neonatology: what do we know–what do we need to know? *Crit Care Med.* 2007;35(3):925–31.
10. Saunders RA, Milner AD, Hopkin IE. The effects of continuous positive airway pressure on lung mechanics and lung volumes in the

neonate. *Biol Neonate*. 1976;29(3−4): 178−86.

11. Polin RA, Sahni R. Newer experience with CPAP. *Semin Neonatol*. 2002;7(5): 379−89.

12. Subramaniam P, Henderson-Smart DJ *et al*. Prophylactic nasal continuous positive airways pressure for preventing morbidity and mortality in very preterm infants. *Cochrane Database Syst Rev*. 2005(3): CD001243.

13. Wintermark P, Tolsa JF, Van Melle G *et al*. Long-term outcome of preterm infants treated with nasal continuous positive airway pressure. *Eur J Pediatr*. 2006.

14. Colby CE, Lally KP, Hintz SR *et al*. Surfactant replacement therapy on ECMO does not improve outcome in neonates with congenital diaphragmatic hernia. *J Pediatr Surg*. 2004;39(11):1632−7.

15. Kinsella JP, Truog WE, Walsh WF *et al*. Randomized, multicenter trial of inhaled nitric oxide and high-frequency oscillatory ventilation in severe, persistent pulmonary hypertension of the newborn. *J Pediatr*. 1997;131(1 Pt 1):55−62.

16. Finer NN, Barrington KJ. Nitric oxide for respiratory failure in infants born at or near term. *Cochrane Database Syst Rev*. 2006(4): CD000399.

17. Davison C, Ventre KM, Luchetti M *et al*. Efficacy of interventions for bronchiolitis in critically ill infants: a systematic review and meta-analysis. *Pediatr Crit Care Med*. 2004; 5(5):482−9.

18. Slutsky AS, Drazen JM. Ventilation with small tidal volumes. *N Engl J Med*. 2002;347(9): 630−1.

19. Derdak S. High-frequency oscillatory ventilation for acute respiratory distress syndrome in adult patients. *Crit Care Med*. 2003;31(4 Suppl):S317−23.

20. Gerstmann DR, Minton SD, Stoddard RA *et al*. The Provo multicenter early high-frequency oscillatory ventilation trial: improved pulmonary and clinical outcome in respiratory distress syndrome. *Pediatrics*. 1996;98(6 Pt 1):1044−57.

21. Courtney SE, Durand DJ, Asselin JM *et al*. High-frequency oscillatory ventilation versus conventional mechanical ventilation for very-low-birth-weight infants. *N Engl J Med*. 2002;347(9):643−52.

22. Slack MP, Azzopardi HJ, Hargreaves RM *et al*. Enhanced surveillance of invasive *Haemophilus influenzae* disease in England, 1990 to 1996: impact of conjugate vaccines. *Pediatr Infect Dis J*. 1998;17(9Suppl): S204−7.

23. Adelson PD, Bratton SL, Carney NA *et al*. Guidelines for the acute medical management of severe traumatic brain injury in infants, children, and adolescents. Chapter 12. Use of hyperventilation in the acute management of severe pediatric traumatic brain injury. *Pediatr Crit Care Med*. 2003;4(3Suppl): S45−8.

24. Welch SB, Nadel S. Treatment of meningococcal infection. *Arch Dis Child*. 2003;88(7):608−14.

25. Mellies U, Ragette R, Dohna Schwake C *et al*. Long-term noninvasive ventilation in children and adolescents with neuromuscular disorders. *Eur Respir J*. 2003;22(4):631−6.

26. Wheeler R. Gillick or Fraser? A plea for consistency over competence in children. *BMJ*. 2006;332(7545):807.

27. Fanaroff AA, Martin RJ. *Neonatal-Perinatal Medicine: Diseases of the Fetus and Infant*. 7th edn. London, Mosby, 2001.

Chapter 17

Tracheostomy

ABHIRAM MALLICK, ANDREW BODENHAM
AND IAIN MACKENZIE

Introduction

Although some authorities have suggested that Egyptian stone tablets from around 3600 BC depict tracheostomy, this remains speculative; however, indirect evidence of sporadic attempts at tracheostomy are suggested by Coelius Aurelianus's comment, writing in the fifth century AD, that it was a 'futile and irresponsible idea'. By the early seventeenth century, little had changed as Hieronymus Fabricius ab Aquapendente,[1] an anatomist and surgeon in Padua, called the operation a 'scandal'. Despite the use of tracheostomies by Marco Aurelio Severino[2] to save a number of lives during the 1610 diphtheria epidemic in Naples, there were only 28 successful procedures recorded between 1500 and 1833. Towards the end of this period, Pierre Bretonneau[3] published a description of diphtheria and reported the successful use of tracheostomy to relieve asphyxiation. By the 1850s, a survival rate of 27% was considered a success, and in Morrell Mackenzie's 1880 textbook on laryngology the issue of how a surgeon must determine 'whether the symptoms are sufficiently urgent to render the operation necessary' is addressed (Figure 17.1). Chevalier Jackson described the modern surgical tracheostomy in 1909, and until the introduction of positive pressure ventilation for respiratory failure as opposed to anaesthesia, tracheostomy remained a surgical procedure for bypassing glottic or supra-glottic airway obstruction, or was required as a consequence of laryngectomy.

This situation was transformed by the development of physician-led units specializing in the provision of respiratory support that arose from the polio epidemics of the late 1940s and early 1950s (see Chapter 20). For patients requiring respiratory support without general anaesthesia, trans-laryngeal intubation of the trachea was intolerable and the only intravenous sedative available in the early 1950s was thiopentone, which was awkward to administer by infusion.[4] For these patients, therefore, tracheostomy was a prerequisite for the provision of positive pressure ventilation.

Nowadays, most patients tolerate short-term trans-laryngeal tracheal intubation with few, if any, complications. For those who require more prolonged intubation, a tracheostomy may provide a number of advantages. This chapter outlines indications, timing, complications and techniques of tracheostomy.

---

[1] 1537–1619.
[2] 1580–1656.
[3] 1778–1862.

[4] Hydroxydione was introduced in 1955, propanidid in 1956 and methohexitone in 1957. The first benzodiazepine, chlordiazepoxide, was not introduced until 1961.

Core Topics in Mechanical Ventilation, ed. Iain Mackenzie. Published by Cambridge University Press.
© Cambridge University Press 2008.

Table 17.1 Indications for tracheostomy

- Primary
  - Trauma or surgery in the face/neck region
  - Severe glottic or supraglottic airway obstruction where trans-laryngeal intubation is considered too dangerous or too difficult (trauma, infection, malignancy), or where the airway obstruction is unlikely to resolve in a matter of days
- Secondary
  - Aid to weaning from assisted ventilation
  - Tracheal access to remove thick pulmonary secretions
  - Prevention of pulmonary aspiration (cerebrovascular accidents, Parkinson's disease, severe brain injury)
  - Long-term or life-long respiratory support (Guillain-Barré syndrome, tetanus, botulism, paralytic poliomyelitis, tick paralysis, cervical spinal cord injury, motor neurone disease, polymyositis, spinal muscular atrophy)
  - Long-term or life-long bypass of glottic or supraglottic airway obstruction (laryngeal or sub-glottic stenosis, bilateral recurrent laryngeal nerve palsy, severe sleep apnoea)

Table 17.2 Immediate management of life-threatening upper airway obstruction

1. Ensure that you, and those around you, remain calm. Patient distress can precipitate loss of the airway. Ensure that someone takes responsibility for summoning appropriate help and alerts the operating theatres.
2. If available, give the patient a helium/oxygen mixture to breathe.
3. Establish if the patient has any drug allergies.
4. Establish intravenous access as quickly and painlessly as possible. Do not give opiates or sedatives. If the airway obstruction might have an inflammatory component,[5] give corticosteroids (hydrocortisone 100 mg or dexamethasone 8 mg) and antihistamines (chlorphenamine 10 mg), and consider giving nebulized and intramuscular adrenaline.
5. Transfer to the operating theatre for further management.

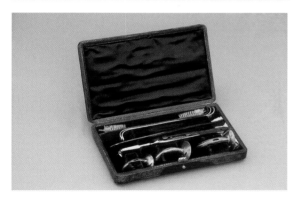

Figure 17.1 Percutaneous tracheostomy set from the last century.

Indications

A minority of patients are admitted to intensive care with a tracheostomy already in place, and in the majority of these cases the tracheostomy is sited in the operating theatre as a routine part of a surgical procedure involving the neck, oropharynx or face (Table 17.1). Much less commonly, patients present with life-threatening or rapidly worsening upper airway obstruction and require immediate management (Table 17.2). These cases are usually best managed in the operating theatre by an experienced anaesthetist who will decide whether trans-laryngeal intubation can be attempted (Figure 17.2).

More commonly, patients initially receive their ventilatory support via a trans-laryngeal tube and the decision to convert to a tracheostomy is based either on the obvious need for prolonged intubation, or when repeated attempts to wean from mechanical ventilation or multiple trials of extubation have been unsuccessful (Figure 17.3). Unfortunately, it is not always obvious in advance into which category a patient belongs (Table 17.3).

Risk:benefit ratio and timing

Trans-laryngeal and tracheostomy tubes provide exactly the same functions, namely (1) a tracheal seal for positive pressure ventilation, (2) a means of maintaining a patent airway, (3) a means of

---

[5] Anaphylaxis, infection, burns.

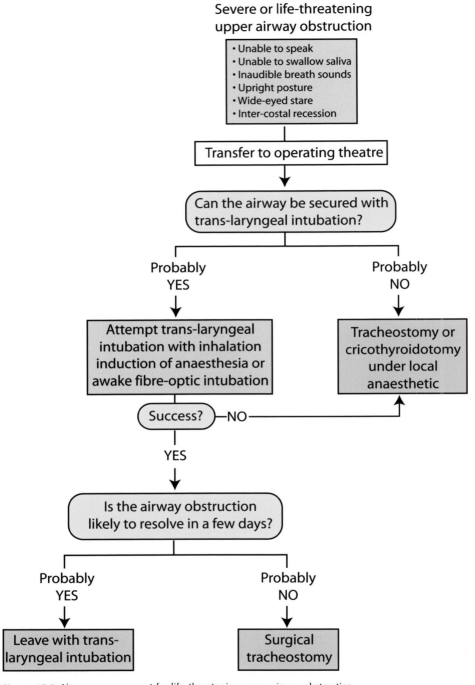

Figure 17.2 Airway management for life-threatening upper airway obstruction.

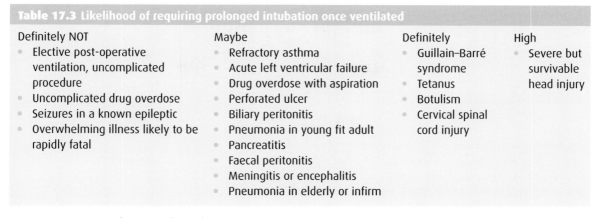

Table 17.3 Likelihood of requiring prolonged intubation once ventilated

Definitely NOT	Maybe	Definitely	High
• Elective post-operative ventilation, uncomplicated procedure • Uncomplicated drug overdose • Seizures in a known epileptic • Overwhelming illness likely to be rapidly fatal	• Refractory asthma • Acute left ventricular failure • Drug overdose with aspiration • Perforated ulcer • Biliary peritonitis • Pneumonia in young fit adult • Pancreatitis • Faecal peritonitis • Meningitis or encephalitis • Pneumonia in elderly or infirm	• Guillain–Barré syndrome • Tetanus • Botulism • Cervical spinal cord injury	• Severe but survivable head injury

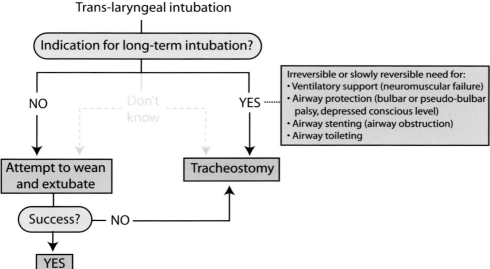

Figure 17.3 Decision tree for elective tracheostomy.

assisting with tracheobronchial toileting and (4) a moderately effective means of preventing pulmonary aspiration. Both have advantages and disadvantages (Table 17.4) that have evolved with the passage of time, influenced by developments in the materials used in the construction of the tubes, their design and the development of percutaneous techniques for performing tracheostomy at the bedside (Figure 17.4). Thus, in the 1950s, when the need for prolonged ventilatory support was first identified, trans-laryngeal intubation was used, if at all, simply as a short-term bridge prior to definitive

airway management in the form of a tracheostomy, as described in a 1957 *Lancet* editorial:[1]

In America a metal tracheotomy tube is used and the patient nursed in a tank respirator with a special device to hold the collar away from the tracheotomy tube. In Europe, however, most people favour a cuffed rubber tube, and convenient tubes have been designed for this purpose. Artificial respiration is then provided through it by intermittent positive pressure – the method introduced by Lassen.

Table 17.4 Pros and cons of tracheostomy compared to trans-laryngeal intubation

	Trans-laryngeal intubation	Tracheostomy
Insertion	Simple, very cheap, very low risk	Not simple, more expensive, low risk
Mouth care	More difficult	Easier
Access for tracheobronchial toilet	Reasonable	Excellent
Risk of secretion obstruction	Medium	Low
Risk of VAP	High	Lower
Comfort	Low	High
Requirement for sedation and analgesia	High	Low/none
Risk of damage to supraglottic structures	Yes	No
Risk of damage to larynx and vocal cords	Yes	No
Risk of damage to trachea	Yes	Yes
Frequency of accidental extubation	Low	Lower
Consequences of unplanned extubation	Low risk	Moderate risk
Patient communication	Poor	Easier
Phonation	Impossible	Possible
Work of breathing	Higher	Lower
Mobilization	Never	Sometimes
Co-operation with physiotherapy	Poor	Easier
Oral intake	Rare	Sometimes
Entry-site problems	Only for nasal route	Common
Neck scarring	Never	Uncommon
Can be managed in non-ICU setting	Rare	Frequently

VAP: ventilator-associated pneumonia

At this early time, prolonged trans-laryngeal intubation was not an option for two reasons. First, the cuffed endotracheal tubes that were available were made of red rubber, which provoked an inflammatory reaction in the airway when used for prolonged periods. Second, the technology and pharmacology for providing continuous intravenous sedation was not available.

In 1964, Portex introduced the first polyvinyl chloride (PVC) endotracheal tube with an integral cuff for anaesthesia, but the cuff was as thick as contemporary rubber cuffs, and even by 1966 one author tellingly commented: 'A word should also be added about special situations such as barbiturate poisoning where unconsciousness may last less than 48 hours. Here, *tracheostomy may be avoided* and respiration maintained through an orotracheal tube'.[2] However, the 1960s witnessed an inexorable increase in the number of patients requiring prolonged mechanical ventilation and with this came a mounting catalogue of tracheostomy-related complications. Kirby in 1970 commented: 'The use of tracheostomy and prolonged intermittent positive pressure ventilation (IPPV) in the care of patients with respiratory insufficiency has been accompanied by an increasing incidence of tracheal mucosal erosion, bleeding and tracheoesophageal fistula'.[3]

In the 1970s a range of strategies were evaluated in an effort to reduce these complications, including regular cuff pressure measurement, intermittent cuff deflation,[3] alternate inflation of double-cuffed tubes,[4] and the use of high-volume, low-pressure cuffs that had originally been

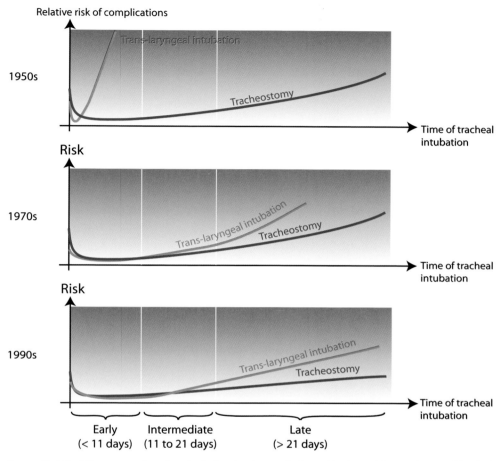

Relative risk of complications

1950s

Trans-laryngeal intubation

Tracheostomy

Time of tracheal intubation

Risk

1970s

Trans-laryngeal intubation

Tracheostomy

Time of tracheal intubation

Risk

1990s

Trans-laryngeal intubation

Tracheostomy

Time of tracheal intubation

Early (< 11 days) Intermediate (11 to 21 days) Late (> 21 days)

Figure 17.4 Evolution over various decades in the development of complications with trans-laryngeal intubation and tracheostomy.

described by Lomholt.[5] However, the pressure to proceed to tracheostomy was relieved to a significant extent by the availability of a number of intravenous sedatives and analgesics, including diazepam,[6] etomidate and althesin.[7] The addition of evidence that early tracheostomy increased airway colonization and the duration of intubation,[6] and reports of the safety of prolonged trans-laryngeal intubation,[7] meant that by the end of the decade the pendulum was swinging in favour of delayed tracheostomy. Indeed, by 1981 one group of authors concluded that 'the value of tracheotomy

when an artificial airway is required for periods as long as three weeks is not supported by data obtained in this study'.[8] As the tide was turning against tracheostomy, investigators began to explore the feasibility of prolonged nasotracheal intubation[9] as a way of making trans-laryngeal intubation more bearable, as was common in paediatric practice. Popularized in the early 1980s, it only took five years before reports started to emerge of serious problems associated with prolonged nasotracheal intubation in adults, most notably maxillary sinusitis.[10] This, combined with Ciaglia's description of a simple and elegant percutaneous technique,[11] a number of indisputable advantages to tracheostomy (Table 17.4) and a powerful

[6] First used in 1966.
[7] Both introduced into clinical practice in 1973.

financial incentive to perform tracheostomy in the United States[8] has meant that the last 15 years have been a period of uncertainty. A systematic review in 2005[13] could only identify five prospective clinical trials comparing early versus late tracheostomy, of which two were only quasi-randomized. Meta-analysis of the data from these studies was unable to confirm an effect of early tracheostomy in reducing the risk of either pneumonia or death, but did find a significant effect on the duration of mechanical ventilation and the length of stay in intensive care.[13] It is hoped that a prospective randomized trial being conducted in the UK (TracMan) between 2004 and 2009, which is aiming to recruit 1200 patients allocated to either early (days 1 to 4) or late (> day 10) tracheostomy will provide more definitive data on timing.

Complications

Complications of tracheostomy can be classified into perioperative, early and late (Table 17.5), with both the type and incidence of specific complications differing between surgical and percutaneous techniques.

Perioperative

As with any procedure the risks of intra-operative complications are as much a reflection on the training and supervision of the operator as they are of the procedure itself, and untangling these issues from the available literature is not straightforward. Furthermore, the risk of reported complications has to be applied to a specific clinical context where local expertise may be notable for its presence, or otherwise.

In many centres in the UK, surgical tracheostomy may only be performed in the operating theatre,[9] which inevitably requires that the patient be transferred there and back. Any intra-hospital transfer exposes the mechanically ventilated patient to additional risk. In the majority of patients, this additional risk is small, but becomes significant in the presence of complicating factors such as morbid obesity. With a surgical approach, intra-operative bleeding, either minor or major, is not usually a problem providing the surgeon is sufficiently experienced. In some centres, however, routine tracheostomy for ventilator-dependent patients is viewed as an ideal training opportunity, increasing both the duration of the procedure and the risk of surgical misadventure. Bleeding is generally less of a problem with percutaneous tracheostomy, although a number of fatal haemorrhages have been reported.

Cardio-respiratory arrest, prolonged or irretrievable loss of the airway, and death are all recognized complications of both surgical and percutaneous tracheostomy. Analysis of reports describing the surgical and percutaneous approaches suggests that these very serious perioperative events are very uncommon in patients undergoing percutaneous tracheostomy (<1%), *but ten times less common* in patients undergoing surgical tracheostomy.[15] While these data are indisputable, it is possible that these rates of serous adverse events have been influenced by early experience with the percutaneous technique, as suggested by Dulguerov *et al.*[14] A definitive answer to this question will require prospective long-term national audit.

Puncture of the endotracheal cuff can occur during either surgical or percutaneous tracheostomy

---

[8] In 1987 the Health Care Financing Administration of the United States, the body responsible for determining rates of reimbursement through the Prospective Payment System, added two new Diagnosis-Related Groups (DRGs) which applied to Major Disease Category 4: Respiratory System (MDC4). These DRGs applied to patients receiving mechanical support via a tracheostomy (474) or endotracheal tube (475), and added a reimbursement weighting of 11.9 and 3.2, respectively. Two years later the following comment was made: 'the weighting factor for DRG 474 was so high that there might be undue pressure placed on physicians to perform tracheostomies prematurely on these critically ill patients'.[12]

[9] In Dulguerov *et al.*'s 1999 review,[14] surgical tracheostomy was performed at the bed side in 66% of cases, while percutaneous tracheostomy was performed in the operating theatre in 16% of cases.

Table 17.5 Complications of tracheostomy performed for ventilatory support

	Surgical	Percutaneous
Perioperative (within 48 hours)		
Risks associated with move to OR	Yes	No
Minor bleeding	0.1%	0.1%
Major bleeding	Uncommon	Very rare
ET tube cuff puncture	Uncommon	More common
Needle damage to bronchoscope	–	Common
Ventilation problems	Uncommon	More common
Intracranial pressure	May rise	May rise
Tracheal damage	0.06%	0.5%
Oesophageal damage	Extremely rare	Rare
Creation of paratracheal passage	0.1%	1.6%
Pneumothorax/pneumomediastinum	0.8%	0.7%
Airway obstruction due to blood clot	Very uncommon	Rare
Convert to surgical	–	4.6%
Cardiorespiratory arrest	0.06%	0.3%
Death	0.03%	0.5%
Early postoperative (up to day 5)		
Surgical emphysema	0.2%	1%
Tension pneumothorax	Very uncommon	Rare
Persistent bleeding	Less common	Very uncommon
Dislodgement of tracheostomy tube	0.9%	0.5%
Late postoperative (day 6 onwards)		
Minor bleeding	2.5%	2%
Major bleeding	0.7%	0.4%
Stomal site infection	3%	1%
Difficulty swallowing (TT in place)	Common	Common
Difficulty swallowing (de-cannulated)	Common	Common
Subglottic/tracheal stenosis	0.3%	1%
Tracheo-oesophageal fistula	0.1%	0.2%
Tracheomalacia	?	?
Persistent tracheo-cutaneous fistula	?	?
Tethering of the trachea	–	Uncommon
Unsightly scar	1 to 5%	<1%

Data from Dulguerov et al.[14] and Durbin.[15]

Very common	common	less common	uncommon	very uncommon	rare	very rare	extremely rare
>25%	≥15%	≥5%	≥1%	≥0.1%	≥0.01	≥0.001	<0.001

and providing the operator has correctly identified the anatomical landmarks in the neck, responsibility lies with the person managing the airway. This problem can be averted by vigilance, timely retraction of the trans-laryngeal tube or, for patients undergoing percutaneous tracheostomy, by exchange of the trans-laryngeal tube for a laryngeal mask airway.[16] Endoscopic assistance during the procedure *may* reduce the incidence of posterior tracheal wall damage and tube misplacement and in many centres is regarded as mandatory, but there is insufficient published data to support this

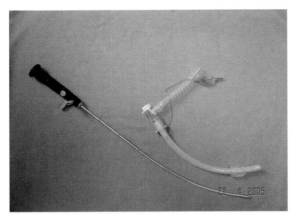

Figure 17.5 A modified curved Bonfils semi-rigid 5 mm fibrescope and tracheal tube with rubber cap to insert scope through.

assertion. Moreover, the presence of an endo-scope risks poorer ventilation, increasing the risk of hypoxia and hypercapnia, as well as needle dam-age to the instrument. While the latter is of no con-sequence to the patient, repairs are expensive. It should be appreciated that bleeding, distortion of structures and obstruction of the visual field with larger dilators may prevent visualization of dam-age until after it has occurred and the section of trachea adjacent to tracheostomy tube cannot be easily visualized after tube insertion. An alternative approach includes the use of a rigid metal cased, small-diameter scope, such as a Bonfils laryngo-scope[17] or an optical stylet (Figure 17.5).

Tracheal damage is more common with percuta-neous tracheostomy, including rupture or displace-ment of the tracheal rings, particularly in elderly patients with heavily calcified tracheal cartilage. Tear of the posterior tracheal wall is another seri-ous complication which may lead to the forma-tion of tracheo-oesophageal fistula or mediastini-tis. While reported as a complication of surgical tra-cheostomy this appears to be more common with certain types of percutaneous technique, such as the PercuTwist® and Ciaglia-pattern serial dilators. Experiments in cadavers suggest that a significant risk factor for this complication is retraction of the guidewire into the dilator, allowing the latter to dig into the posterior tracheal wall.[18] Both guidewire retraction and guidewire misplacement, which causes the creation of false passages, are effectively prevented by bronchoscopic visualization of the procedure.

Early and late

Pneumothorax and surgical emphysema usually become apparent within 24 to 48 hours of the procedure, are slightly more common in percuta-neous tracheostomies and do not usually cause a significant problem. Persistent bleeding, however, tends to be a feature associated with surgical tra-cheostomies, perhaps related to the fact that coag-ulopathy is a relative contra-indication for the per-cutaneous approach, and the stoma is bigger so no tamponade around the tube occurs.

A more common problem in the early post-tracheostomy phase is unplanned de-cannulation, especially if this is not immediately recognized (Box 17.1). With complete de-cannulation the air-way problem is obvious and should be managed by occluding the stoma and securing the airway using standard upper airway techniques, includ-ing bag-valve-mask ventilation or re-intubation of the trachea with an oral tube. Attempts to re-cannulate the tracheal stoma are almost certainly doomed to failure this soon after purcutaneous tra-cheostomy, because a definitive stoma tract will not have formed. Considerably more dangerous, particularly for the unwary, is unrecognized de-cannulation, which can occur when a patient with a large neck has a tracheostomy inserted that is too short. The combination of a significant increase in airway pressures, poor air entry and worsening surgical emphysema are pathognomonic for a dis-placed tracheostomy tube, which should be imme-diately removed. Removing the tracheostomy tube and reverting to standard airway management will inevitably solve the problem if the tracheostomy tube is displaced, may solve the problem if the

Box 17.1

A 63-year-old lady with a background history of non-insulin-dependent diabetes, obesity and smoking-related chronic pulmonary disease was admitted with a severe community-acquired pneumonia. After 12 days of mechanical ventilation, she underwent a surgical tracheostomy and was returned to the intensive care unit with size 8 Portex Blue-line tracheostomy tube, where ventilation was continued with synchronized intermittent mandatory ventilation (SIMV). In the early hours of the following morning, the nurse was alerted by the ventilator's alarm, which indicated high airway pressures and a low minute volume, and this was shortly followed by the monitor alarm, indicating low peripheral haemoglobin oxygen saturation. The nurse disconnected the patient from the ventilator and attempted to manually ventilate the patient with a self-inflating bag attached to the patient's tracheostomy, only to find that the tracheostomy appeared to be blocked. Help was summoned, and assuming that the tracheostomy tube had become blocked by blood from the recent tracheostomy, an attempt was made to remove the obstruction by suction. The suction catheter could only be passed with great difficulty, and did not aspirate blood or secretions or relieve the airway. An anaesthetic trainee arrived shortly after and was able to ventilate the patient with extreme difficulty, at which point it was noted that the patient was developing progressively worsening surgical emphysema. At this point, the consultant was called in from home. By the time the consultant arrived 15 minutes later, the surgical emphysema was so severe that the patient's mouth could not be opened to insert a laryngoscope, and the patient died. A post-mortem examination revealed that the tip of the tracheostomy tube, which was too short to lie in the correct position, was lying anterior to the tracheal lumen.

tracheostomy tube is blocked (the blockage may be below the tracheostomy) and reduces the differential if neither of these are the case.

Stomal infections are common following surgical tracheostomy and may produce significant quantities of purulent secretions that can cause maceration of adjacent skin. In patients with an adjacent surgical wound, such as a median sternotomy, the stomal infection can spread to involve the sternum or mediastinum, resulting in significant morbidity, mortality and a prolonged hospital stay. For this reason, many cardiothoracic surgeons prefer their patients to have a percutaneous tracheostomy.

Tracheo-innominate artery[10] fistula is an uncommon but life-threatening complication that is usually fatal unless treatment is instituted immediately. Many causes have been implicated including pressure necrosis from high cuff pressure, tra-

cheal wall trauma and perforation from a mal-positioned tube tip, low tracheal incision and prolonged tracheostomy. Any significant or repeated bleeding occurring from three days to six weeks after tracheostomy should be considered to be a tracheo-innominate artery fistula unless proven otherwise. Smaller herald bleeds may precede this complication and should prompt formal exploration in the operating theatre in case a major bleed is precipitated. Immediate control of the haemorrhage may be achieved by over-inflation of the tracheostomy cuff, or by compressing the artery between a gloved finger and the deep surface of the manubrium. Definitive treatment requires median sternotomy and bypass of the artery.

Damage to the posterior tracheal wall either during tracheostomy or as a consequence of cuff pressure can cause a tracheo-oesophageal fistula, and should be excluded in patients with

---

[10] Also called *the brachiocephalic artery*.

persistent bronchorrhoea, repeated aspiration pneumonia, persistent failure to pass a swallowing assessment or symptoms of aerophagia. The diagnosis can be made by careful bronchoscopic examination of the de-cannulated trachea together with oesophagoscopy. Surgical repair is required as without this the condition is invariably fatal.

While long-term complications appear to be uncommon, the incomplete follow-up and lack of consistent definitions of outcome measurements in the available randomized controlled trials make conclusions difficult to draw. However, uncontrolled studies have found that clinically relevant tracheal stenosis is uncommon in percutaneous tracheostomy when performed by experienced operators.[19,20] Tracheal stenosis can occur at, or either side of the stoma, at the level of cuff, and at the tip of the tube. The main reason for development of stenosis appears to be mucosal ischaemia. Most stenoses tend to be asymptomatic unless they reduce the tracheal lumen by more than 50%. Tracheal stenosis caused by percutaneous tracheostomy may be significantly closer to the vocal cords compared to surgical tracheostomy making tracheal resection and end-to-end anastomosis very difficult.[21] This provides a strong argument for ensuring appropriate levels of stoma formation using endoscopy during percutaneous tracheostomy. The introducer needle should be ideally passed between the second and third tracheal rings or one space lower. However, needle insertion below the fourth tracheal ring poses a risk of tube erosion into adjacent blood vessels.

The ability to swallow without aspirating depends on an intact swallowing mechanism that has both neural and muscular components. The swallowing reflex is initiated by the sensation of food or fluid against the oropharynx, which causes the reflex contraction of pharyngeal muscles which serve to close the nasopharynx, lift the trachea, close the glottis and drop the epiglottis over the laryngeal inlet. At the same time, the cricopharyngeal sphincter relaxes, allowing the passage of the bolus into the proximal oesophagus. Aspiration can result from disorders of sensory or motor nerves, central processing, neuromuscular transmission, muscle function or loss of movement of glottic structures. With a tracheostomy, tracheal elevation may be restricted, preventing the epiglottis from descending over the laryngeal inlet and allowing contamination of the pyriform recesses and laryngeal ventricles. Furthermore, while the cricopharyngeal sphincter may relax appropriately, the bolus may be prevented from dropping into the proximal oesophagus by the presence of the tracheostomy tube and its cuff. There is little data on the frequency of swallowing disorders in patients with a tracheostomy; the information available suggests a rate of 7% in the short term[22] (up to 10 days), and 50%[23] in the long term (over 1 month), but the frequency in the medium term (10 days to 1 month) is unknown. Clinical evidence of aspiration (coughing) is likely to be an insensitive indicator, and although risk factors for aspiration have been identified, there has been no attempt to formulate a predictive tool for identifying these patients. Currently, the 'gold-standard' evaluation is a videofluoroscopic swallow, but this can usually only be done in the radiology department. Bedside evaluation depends on clinical assessment by a speech and language therapist[11] supplemented, where available, by a fibreoptic endoscopic evaluation of swallow (FEES). Many centres attempt to evaluate swallowing with a variant of the 'Evans blue dye test', in which blue food dye is added to orally presented food or fluid. While the value of a positive test is clear, the value of a negative test is uncertain because there is evidence of a high false-negative rate. Patients who require positive airway pressure[12] have to be evaluated with an inflated tracheostomy

---

[11] A speech pathologist in the USA.
[12] Either in the form of continuous positive airway pressure (CPAP), or inspiratory support.

Table 17.6 Comparison between surgical and percutaneous tracheostomy		
	Surgical	Percutaneous
Administrative hindrance	Moderate to high	Low
Delay between decision and procedure	May be prolonged	None
Cost	High	Low
Skilled intensivists	Not required	Required
Absolute contra-indications	Haemodynamic instability	Haemodynamic instability
	Severe hypoxaemia	Severe hypoxaemia
	Severe coagulopathy	Severe coagulopathy
Relative contra-indications	Recent median sternotomy	Children under 12
		Difficult anatomy
		Previous neck surgery or radiotherapy
		Difficult intubation
		Cervical spine injury
		Raised intracranial pressure
		Infection or burn at the insertion site

tube cuff, whereas other patients should be evaluated with their cuff deflated.

Tracheostomy techniques

Since 1985, clinicians have been able to choose between surgical or percutaneous tracheostomy and these techniques are compared in Table 17.6. As experience with the percutaneous approach increases, the list of contra-indications is being constantly eroded, and there are now reports in the literature describing the successful use of this approach in patients with obesity, coagulopathy or even as an emergency procedure. Ultrasound imaging of the neck prior to tracheostomy (Figure 17.6) allows the anatomy of the anterior neck structures to be identified, particularly the location of blood vessels and the depth and angulation of the trachea.[24] This information may contribute to the risk to benefit analysis between surgical and percutaneous tracheostomy.

Surgical tracheostomy

Conventional surgical tracheostomy is usually performed by ear, nose and throat (ENT), or maxillofacial surgeons, although in some centres

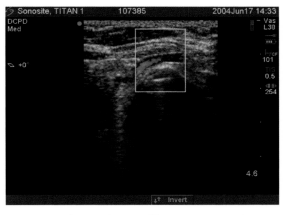

Figure 17.6 Ultrasound image of large ectatic carotid artery in front of the trachea.

cardiothoracic or neurological surgeons routinely perform the procedure. A transverse skin incision is made between the lower border of the cricoid cartilage and suprasternal notch. The strap muscles are retracted laterally to expose the underlying thyroid isthmus and the trachea (Figure 17.7). The thyroid isthmus is either retracted cephalad or divided exposing the tracheal rings. A window is made in the trachea that is most commonly centred on the third tracheal ring (Figure 17.8). An alternative is the so-called Björk flap. A flap incision hinged to

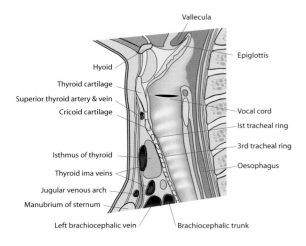

Figure 17.7 Sagittal section of the neck.

Note that the trachea does not lie parallel to the surface of the neck, but is angled posteriorly as it enters the thorax. Note also the close relationship of the brachiocephalic trunk (innominate artery) just above the manubrium.

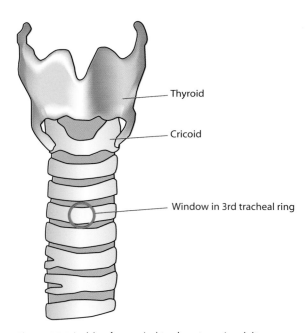

Figure 17.8 Incision for surgical tracheostomy in adults.

the fourth tracheal ring is created. The flap is then sutured to the skin, thereby creating a clear path from skin to the trachea. It is supposed to create a safe track if accidental de-cannulation occurs, but may cause problems if the suture pulls out or if the stoma is too deep for the flap to reach the skin. Flaps floating free will cause problems and if pushed into the trachea may heal as a stenosis and should therefore be removed or resutured. The tracheostomy tube is then placed under direct visualization. The open technique at the bedside performed in some institutions does not differ in any way to open technique in the operating theatre. This procedure done at the bedside is more difficult because lighting, operating on a wide bed and other facilities are suboptimal.

Percutaneous tracheostomy

Although originally described in 1955[25] percutaneous tracheostomy was never a serious alternative to the formal surgical technique until Pasquale Ciaglia described his dilatational technique in 1985,[11] since then a number of alternative techniques have been described (Table 17.7). All of the techniques use a guidewire to guide dilatation of the anterior tracheal wall either from outside in or from inside out (trans-laryngeal). A tracheostomy tube loaded over a loading dilator is then inserted through the stoma. Several clinical trials have compared these techniques without any method being shown to be conclusively superior.[26] Operator experience and patient selection are crucial determinants of complications.

PRACTICALITIES

Two operators are required, one to perform the tracheostomy and the other to provide general anaesthesia, manage the airway, and handle the endoscope. The procedure should ideally be performed during normal working hours to ensure the supervision and support from senior staff members and other specialists if required.

At least 30 minutes prior to the procedure, nasoenteric feed should be stopped, the stomach emptied by aspiration and the nasogastric tube left on

Table 17.7 Types of percutaneous tracheostomy

Year	Author	Sets	Seldinger	Dilator	Dilatation direction
1985	Ciaglia[11]	UltraPerc™ (Portex)	Yes	Serial dilatation using smooth plastic dilators	Outside-in
1990	Griggs[27]	Griggs Forceps Technique (Portex)	Yes	Forceps	Outside-in
1997	Fantoni[28]	Translaryngeal Tracheostomy (Tyco Healthcare)	Yes	Integral to tracheostomy tube	Inside-out
2000	Byhahn[29]	Ciaglia Blue Rhino™ (Cook Critical Care) UltraPerc™ (Portex), Experc™ (Tracoe)	Yes	Single dilator adaptation of the Ciaglia technique	Outside-in
2003	Westphal[30]	PercuTwist™ (Rüsch)	Yes	Single screw-threaded plastic dilator	Outside-in
2005	Zgoda[31]	Not available	Yes	Balloon	Neither

free drainage. Following the induction of general anaesthesia, the patient is given a single dose of muscle relaxant[13] and ventilated in a mandatory, volume controlled, mode with 100% oxygen. The patient is positioned supine so that the chin and sternal notch are in a straight line, with the head extended by removing the pillow and placing a soft roll under the patient's shoulders. The superior and inferior borders of the thyroid cartilage, cricoid cartilage and first three tracheal rings are identified by palpation and marked. The skin is prepared with antiseptic solution and the neck draped to maintain a sterile field. The area of incision is infiltrated with up to 20 mL of lidocaine 1% with adrenaline 1:200 000. The second operator then aspirates the trachea, mouth and oropharynx, and under direct laryngoscopy aspirates the laryngopharynx and glottic opening. An assistant deflates the cuff of the trans-laryngeal tube, which is then either withdrawn so that the cuff lies immediately subglottic and the cuff is re-inflated, or the tube is exchanged for a laryngeal mask airway. The patient is then reconnected to the ventilator. The second operator then visualizes the cricoid cartilage with the endoscope. At this point, it is sometimes instructive to dim the room lights and check that the light from

the endoscope can be seen trans-illuminating the patient's neck.

A small transverse incision[14] is made in the midline of the patient's neck over the space between the first and second or the second and third tracheal rings. The subcutaneous tissue is bluntly dissected using a pair of curved forceps. An introducer needle with cannula is inserted midline into the trachea, between the 2nd and 3rd tracheal rings, ideally under endoscopic guidance. Intratracheal needle position can also be confirmed by air aspiration or capnography when endoscopy is not available.

A 'J-tipped' guidewire is passed through the cannula after the introducer needle has been removed. A guide catheter is advanced over the guidewire, followed by dilatation of the stoma by a series of plastic dilators, a single dilator or forceps. Finally, the tracheostomy tube, pre-loaded onto a dilator of the appropriate size, is advanced over the guidewire and guide catheter into the tracheal lumen. The latter two are removed, leaving the tracheostomy tube in place. The distal airway is aspirated with a sterile suction catheter to remove any blood, then the cuff is inflated until no air leak is heard. The cuff pressure should not exceed 25 cm H_2O (18 mmHg).

[13] Commonly atracurium at 0.5 mg.kg^{-1}.

[14] Between 11 mm for a size 6 tube, and 17 mm for a size 10.

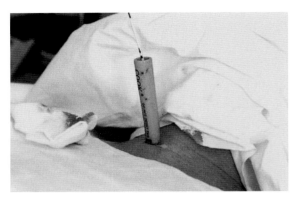

Figure 17.9 Stomal dilatation using Blue Rhino dilator (Cook) passed over a guidewire and plastic stiffner with the black mark at skin level.

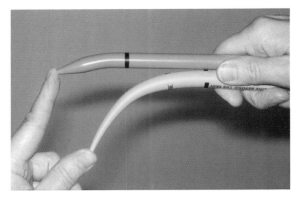

Figure 17.10 Comparison of the single step Blue Rhino dilator (lower) with the original serial dilator (lower) (36 Fr), both Cook products.

Note the different taper and softer more flexible material of the former.

It is important that this is checked regularly to prevent complications of tracheal mucosal damage, stenosis and tracheo-oesophageal fistula. The tube should be tied in securely.

SINGLE DILATOR TECHNIQUES

In an attempt to minimize the risk of tracheal damage, a number of manufacturers have introduced a single-step dilatation technique based on Ciaglia's orginal method. The single dilator (Figure 17.9) has a hydrophilic coating which, when wet, reduces friction and thus allows smooth, rapid, dilatation of the tracheal stoma. This minimizes the time during which dilators obstruct the airway, reducing the risk of hypercapnia and hypoxia. Moreover, the dilator tapers to a more flexible tip, which will bend at the required angle to follow the direction of the guidewire down the trachea (Figure 17.10). Use of this technique avoids the aerosolization of blood and secretions as dilators are changed, and the continuous tamponade effect reduces bleeding during the procedure.

Choice of tracheostomy tube

There is a wide range of tracheostomy tubes commercially available that vary with respect to material (polyvinyl chloride, polyurethane, silicone or metal), cuff (none, standard, low-profile or high-volume), length, inner cannula, fenestrations and other special features. The anatomy of a tracheostomy tube is shown in Figure 17.11.

MATERIAL

The commonest type of tracheostomy tube is made from polyvinyl chloride (PVC), which is cheap, inert, smooth and becomes malleable at body temperature (thermolabile). Polyurethane tubes are generally a little more expensive, but do not lose their rigidity at body temperature. With both PVC and polyurethane tubes, the lengths of the neck, bending section and stem are fixed, and with these tubes it is important to ensure that the patient is fitted with the right size of tube (Figure 17.12).

Silicone tubes are very flexible, invariably presented with a reinforcing metallic spiral embedded in the wall of the tube, and usually longer than standard tubes. Being flexible along their entire length, these tubes have no pre-defined bending section and therefore conform to any variation in tracheal depth or tracheal anatomy. In addition, the flanges on these tubes can usually be moved to any position along the neck of the tube. The silicone has a slightly 'sticky' surface and these tubes do not allow

SIDE VIEW   FRONT VIEW

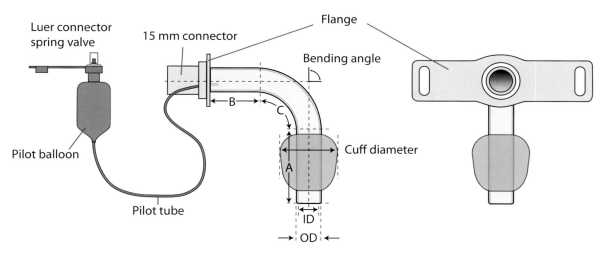

Figure 17.11 Anatomy of a tracheostomy tube.

A. The stem, also called the distal or vertical section.

B. The neck, also called the proximal or horizontal section.

C. The bending section.

The angle between the axis of the neck and stem is referred to as the bending angle, and in many designs of tube this is 90°. Because the axis of the trachea is not parallel to the skin surface of the neck (see Figure 17.12), a larger bending angle bending (100° to 110°) allows the axis of the stem to lie in the same axis as the trachea with the flange held flat against the skin of the patient's neck.

Fixed-length tracheostomy tubes are available in a range of sizes defined, for endotracheal tubes, by the internal diameter (ID). There is a variation in the length and curvature of a particular manufacturer's tubes as the ID changes. There is also considerable variation between manufacturers. Thus if difficulty is experienced with malposition of a tracheostomy tube, then there should be consideration of a change in size (ID) or tube type.

the easy passage of a bronchoscope. Unfortunately, adjustable flange tracheostomy tubes do not have the advantage of inner cannulae.

Silver tubes (e.g. silver Negus) are used by patients with long-term or permanent stomas and can be custom-made. These tubes do not have a cuff but may have a low-profile inner cannula with or without an integral flap that acts as a speaking valve. An inner cannula with a standard 15 mm catheter mount connector is available for patients who require intermittent (nocturnal) respiratory support. These tubes offer the airflow advantages of thin walls and theoretically the antibacterial effect of silver. With the general move to disposable equip-

ment and reports of tube fractures these are now less frequently used.

CUFF

Cuffed tubes provide a degree of airway protection and facilitate intermittent positive-pressure ventilation. Disadvantages are risk of excessive cuff pressure, difficulty in swallowing and inability to phonate. High-volume, low-pressure cuffs reduce the incidence of cuff-related mucosal damage by providing a wider surface area of the trachea for the pressure to be dissipated. The cuff pressure should not exceed 25 cm H_2O (18 mmHg) to reduce the risk of complications. Some long-stemmed

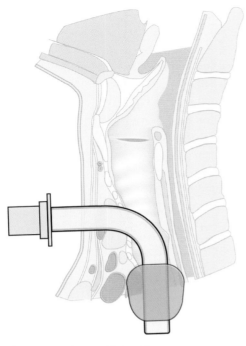 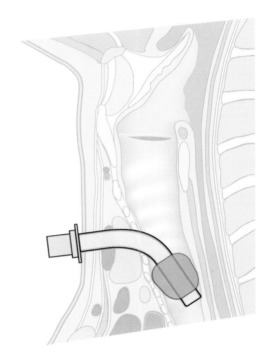

Figure 17.12 Incorrect tube sizing.

On the left, the neck length of the tracheostomy tube is too long for the tracheal depth, forcing the anterior rim of the tube tip against the anterior tracheal wall. Note the close approximation of the brachiocephalic trunk (innominate artery). This position may result in the tube eroding into the artery, with catastrophic consequences.

On the right, the neck length of the tracheostomy tube is too short for the depth of the stoma, forcing the posterior rim of the tube tip against the posterior tracheal wall. In this position the patient is at risk of developing a tracheo-oesophageal fistula.

tracheostomy tubes are fitted with two cuffs, which are meant to be inflated alternately. This is designed to reduce the incidence of cuff-related tracheal damage, but has yet to be validated. In contrast to endotracheal tubes,[15] *un-cuffed* tubes are commonly used in self-ventilating patients who need assistance with secretion clearance, and may be used in combination with a speaking valve to allow speech and improve the cough. Un-cuffed tubes may occasionally be used to provide some degree of respiratory support (even though they have a large leak) but do not protect the airway from aspiration.

LENGTH

Tubes with a pre-formed bending section can be lengthened at either the neck or stem sections

---

[15] In adults. Un-cuffed tubes are standard in paediatric practice.

(Figure 17.13), or may have a flange that can be positioned at any point along the tube for patients whose trachea is deeper than usual below the skin and soft tissues in the neck (e.g. obese patients). The depth of the stoma should be considered at the outset, during the insertion procedure and by visualizing the tube position within the trachea at endoscopy via the glottis and through the tube. It should be appreciated that standard tubes have a relatively short neck.

DOUBLE CANNULA

Many manufacturers now provide a replaceable inner cannula to enable regular cleaning of the lumen. This reduces the likelihood of blockage and reduces re-inoculation of this material into the tracheobronchial tree with inspiration and with the

LONG-NECKED TUBE

LONG-STEMMED TUBE

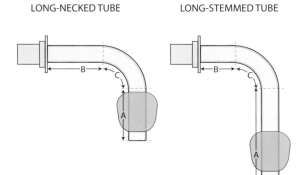

Figure 17.13 Variations in tracheostomy tube length.

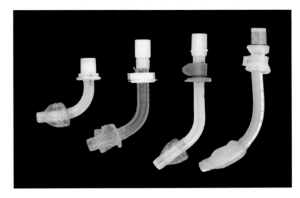

Figure 17.14 Different size 8 tracheostomy tubes with flange and pilot tubes removed for clarity.

passage of suction catheters. Tracheostomy tubes with an inner tube may remain in place up to 30 days or more.

FENESTRATIONS

A fenestration is a single large hole or series of smaller holes situated in the outer curve of the bending section of the tracheostomy tube that allows the free passage of gas between the laryngeal inlet above and the tracheobronchial tree below. The tracheostomy tube should be of the appropriate size for the patient so that the fenestration lies completely in the trachea. Incorrectly positioned fenestrations can cause subcutaneous emphysema. These tubes may be cuffed or un-cuffed. If the

tracheostomy tube has an inner cannula, there may be a choice (dependent on manufacturer) of having a fenestrated inner cannula or an un-fenestrated inner cannula. Thus a cuffed, fenestrated tracheostomy tube with a choice of fenestrated or non-fenestrated inner cannula can be used with the cuff inflated or deflated (effectively cuffless) and as a fenestrated or non-fenestrated tube.

SPEAKING VALVES AND CAPS

In the process of weaning from mechanical ventilation, it is desirable for patients to breathe across their larynx and pharynx. This may help to normalize mucosal sensation and may improve swallowing. By allowing apposition of the vocal cords, it also enables the patient to clear their own secretions by coughing. In patients with sufficient strength, coughing is a more effective mechanism to mobilize secretions from the chest than blind tracheal suctioning. Simply deflating the cuff (following the cuff deflation guidelines described earlier) and capping the tracheostomy tube permits ventilation around the tube, albeit at the expense of increased resistance to inspiration and expiration. A speaking valve is a simple light-weight, one-way valve that can be used instead of a cap. With the cuff deflated, the patient draws breath through the tracheostomy valve and then exhales around the deflated cuff and through the fenestrations, through her glottis and out through her mouth and nose in the normal way. Although the patient can cough and speak, the tracheostomy partially obstructs tracheal gas flow and adds to the work of breathing. Because the upper airway is bypassed on inspiration, patients should receive warmed, humidified gases via a tracheostomy mask when a speaking valve is used.

Role of cricothyroidotomy or mini-tracheostomy

A small diameter (4 mm ID), un-cuffed tube can be inserted percutaneously via the cricothyroid membrane following skin infiltration with local anaesthetic. This facilitates treatment of sputum retention by providing an access for regular suction of respiratory secretions. This technique has also been used in the emergency management of upper airway obstruction. Limitations of the mini-tracheostomy kit include small-bore suction, inability to provide CPAP and positive-pressure ventilation. There is no cuff to provide airway protection.

Aftercare

Meticulous skin care at the stoma site has been suggested to decrease bacterial contamination and the inflammatory response leading to granulation tissue. Adequate humidification, tracheal suctioning and physiotherapy are essential to avoid obstruction of tracheostomy tubes (see Chapter 4). The obstruction of tracheostomy tubes can be static because of thick tenacious secretion or dynamic because of partial obstruction by the membranous posterior wall encroaching on the tracheostomy tube lumen. The degree of dynamic obstruction appears to increase when the intrathoracic pressure increases. Dynamic obstruction can be prevented by a properly designed tube with optimum length and angle to ensure tracheostomy tube positioning within the trachea.

For tracheostomy tubes with inner cannulae, regular removal for cleaning is important to maintain tube patency. Tubes without inner cannulae should be exchanged every 7–14 days, or more frequently if secretions build up, to avoid the risk of progressive hypoxia and possibly cardio-respiratory arrest. Removal of the tracheostomy tube may be required if suctioning fails to clear the obstruction. In the short term, spontaneously breathing patients will usually manage to breathe through their own airway. If the tracheostomy is more than one week old, the stoma is generally well established to allow early tube replacement, if required.

For patients dependent on assisted ventilation, re-intubation by the oral route may be needed in

Table 17.8 Mandatory bedside equipment for patients with a tracheostomy

- Tracheostomy tubes (same size as *in situ* and one size smaller)
- Tracheal dilators
- Suction unit, catheters and gloves
- Self-inflating bag-valve-mask device and tubing
- 10-mL syringe for cuff inflation or deflation
- Standard intubation equipment
- An oxygen supply

the interim if difficulties occur in replacing the tracheostomy tube.

When caring for a tracheostomy patient, appropriate airway equipment should always remain with the patient (Table 17.8). De-cannulation is discussed in Chapter 18.

REFERENCES

1. Long-continued artificial respiration (editorial). *Lancet*. 1957;i:417.
2. Adler RH. The surgeon in a respiratory intensive care unit. *Dis Chest*. 1966;50(3): 248–53.
3. Kirby RR, Robison EJ, Schulz J. Intermittent cuff inflation during prolonged positive-pressure ventilation. *Anesthesiology*. 1970; 32(4):364–6.
4. Salpekar PD. Double-cuff endotracheal tube. *Br Med J*. 1971;3(5773):525.
5. Lomholt N. A new tracheostomy tube. I. Cuff with controlled pressure on the tracheal mucous membrane. *Acta Anaesthesiol Scand*. 1967;11(3):311–18.
6. El-Naggar M, Sadagopan S, Levine H *et al*. Factors influencing choice between tracheostomy and prolonged translaryngeal intubation in acute respiratory failure: a prospective study. *Anesth Analg*. 1976;55(2): 195–201.

7. Vogelhut MM, Downs JB. Prolonged endotracheal intubation. *Chest*. 1979;76(1):110–11.

8. Stauffer JL, Olson DE, Petty TL. Complications and consequences of endotracheal intubation and tracheotomy. A prospective study of 150 critically ill adult patients. *Am J Med*. 1981;70(1):65–76.

9. Via-Reque E, Rattenborg CC. Prolonged oro- or nasotracheal intubation. *Crit Care Med*. 1981;9(9):637–9.

10. Willatts SM, Cochrane DF. Paranasal sinusitis: a complication of nasotracheal intubation. Two case reports. *Br J Anaesth*. 1985;57(10):1026–8.

11. Ciaglia P, Firsching R, Syniec C. Elective percutaneous dilatational tracheostomy. A new simple bedside procedure; preliminary report. *Chest*. 1985;87(6):715–19.

12. Plummer AL, Gracey DR. Consensus conference on artificial airways in patients receiving mechanical ventilation. *Chest*. 1989;96(1):178–80.

13. Griffiths J, Barber VS, Morgan L *et al*. Systematic review and meta-analysis of studies of the timing of tracheostomy in adult patients undergoing artificial ventilation. *BMJ*. 2005;330(7502):1243–7.

14. Dulguerov P, Gysin C, Perneger TV *et al*. Percutaneous or surgical tracheostomy: a meta-analysis. *Crit Care Med*. 1999;27(8): 1617–25.

15. Durbin CG, Jr. Early complications of tracheostomy. *Respir Care*. 2005;50(4): 511–15.

16. Cattano D, Abramson S, Buzzigoli S *et al*. The use of the laryngeal mask airway during guidewire dilating forceps tracheostomy. *Anesth Analg*. 2006;103(2):453–57.

17. Buehner U, Oram J, Elliot S *et al*. Bonfils semirigid endoscope for guidance during

percutaneous tracheostomy. *Anaesthesia*. 2006;61(7):665–70.

18. Trottier SJ, Hazard PB, Sakabu SA *et al*. Posterior tracheal wall perforation during percutaneous dilational tracheostomy: an investigation into its mechanism and prevention. *Chest*. 1999;115(5):1383–9.

19. Sue RD, Susanto I. Long-term complications of artificial airways. *Clin Chest Med*. 2003;24(3):457–71.

20. Norwood S, Vallina VL, Short K *et al*. Incidence of tracheal stenosis and other late complications after percutaneous tracheostomy. *Ann Surg*. 2000;232(2): 233–41.

21. Raghuraman G, Rajan S, Marzouk JK *et al*. Is tracheal stenosis caused by percutaneous tracheostomy different from that by surgical tracheostomy? *Chest*. 2005;127(3):879–85.

22. Bonanno PC. Swallowing dysfunction after tracheostomy. *Ann Surg*. 1971;174(1): 29–33.

23. Elpern EH, Scott MG, Petro L *et al*. Pulmonary aspiration in mechanically ventilated patients with tracheostomies. *Chest*. 1994;105(2): 563–6.

24. Hatfield A, Bodenham A. Portable ultrasonic scanning of the anterior neck before percutaneous dilatational tracheostomy. *Anaesthesia*. 1999;54(7):660–3.

25. Shelden CH, Pudenz RH, Freshwater DB, *et al*. A new method for tracheotomy. *J Neurosurg*. 1955;12(4):428–31.

26. Bardell T, Drover JW. Recent developments in percutaneous tracheostomy: improving techniques and expanding roles. *Curr Opin Crit Care*. 2005;11(4):326–32.

27. Griggs WM, Worthley LI, Gilligan JE *et al*. A simple percutaneous tracheostomy technique. *Surg Gynecol Obstet*. 1990;170(6):543–5.

28. Fantoni A, Ripamonti D. A non-derivative, non-surgical tracheostomy: the translaryngeal method. *Intensive Care Med.* 1997;23(4):386–92.

29. Byhahn C, Lischke V, Halbig S *et al.* Ciaglia blue rhino: a modified technique for percutaneous dilatation tracheostomy. Technique and early clinical results. *Anaesthesist.* 2000;49(3):202–6.

30. Westphal K, Maeser D, Scheifler G *et al.* PercuTwist: a new single-dilator technique for percutaneous tracheostomy. *Anesth Analg.* 2003;96(1):229–32.

31. Zgoda MA, Berger R. Balloon-facilitated percutaneous dilational tracheostomy tube placement: preliminary report of a novel technique. *Chest.* 2005;128(5): 3688–90.

Chapter 18

Weaning, extubation and de-cannulation

IAIN MACKENZIE

Although mechanical ventilation is a life-saving intervention, it is associated with a number of complications and has its own mortality (see Chapter 14). Because the risk of complications increases with the duration of mechanical ventilation, it is important not to prolong the duration of mechanical ventilation unnecessarily. The process of withdrawing mechanical ventilation is commonly referred to as 'weaning', but in the literature the term has acquired two distinct meanings, having been described as either (1) the process of gradually decreasing ventilatory support to return the work of breathing back to the patient or (2) a means of determining when patients have the ability to be safely liberated from the ventilator. Much of the available literature on weaning in fact refers to the second definition; furthermore, much of this work is difficult to interpret because successful *extubation* has been used as the end-point to assess *ventilator independence*. These are not synonymous because it is possible for a patient to be capable of self-ventilation without being ready for extubation. In this chapter, therefore, the term 'weaning' refers only to the process of returning the work of breathing back to the patient. Determining readiness for extubation or de-cannulation is dealt with as a separate issue.

The majority of patients admitted to a general ICU do not stay very long and their stays account for only a small proportion of the bed-days (Figure 18.1).

Conversely, patients who require prolonged periods of mechanical ventilation may be in the minority, but they consume a large part of the unit's capacity. The proportion of this time that is spent weaning is often quoted as 40%,[1] but this figure is deceptive. For patients requiring short periods of mechanical ventilation, for example 24 or 48 hours, weaning and extubation can often be accomplished in less than an hour, which represents between 2% and 4% of the total duration of mechanical ventilation. Patients who require more than seven days of mechanical ventilation will often spend many days or even weeks in the process of weaning. For this small group of patients, weaning accounts for a much larger proportion of the total duration of mechanical ventilation, perhaps as much as 60% to 70%. For this reason, a small decrease in the duration of mechanical ventilation in these patients, resulting from more effective weaning, can generate significant and very worthwhile resource savings.

When should weaning be initiated?

For most patients, who require only short periods of mechanical ventilation, the time at which weaning is initiated has little or no impact on the duration of weaning. For the remainder, in whom prolonged support is anticipated because of the severity of their condition or the nature of their co-morbidities, weaning has traditionally been delayed until the

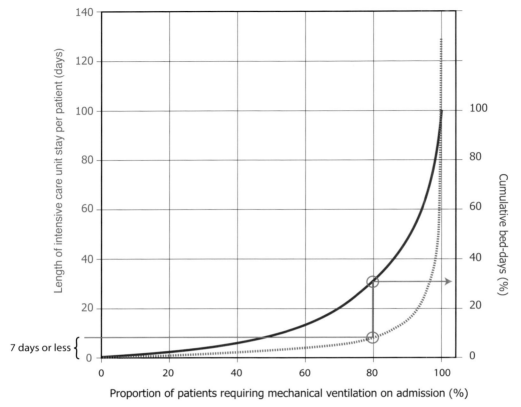

Figure 18.1 Length of stay per patient (green) and cumulative proportion of bed days (blue) for patients admitted to a mixed medical and surgical intensive care unit who required mechanical ventilation.

Of the 355 admissions that required mechanical ventilation, 79.3% stayed in the intensive care unit for 7 days or less but only accounted for 29.8% of the total bed-days. The remaining 20.7% of the admissions stayed in the ICU for between 8 and 129 days, but accounted for 70.2% of the bed-days.

Data from the John Farman Intensive Care Unit, Addenbrooke's Hospital, Cambridge, for the period 9 Jan 2005 to 31 Aug 2006.

patient's physiology has returned to normal. In a few of these patients, such as those with severe hypoxic respiratory failure, suppression of the patient's respiratory efforts with deep sedation or neuro-muscular blockade can sometimes be the only way to achieve acceptable oxygenation, particularly if high-frequency oscillation or prone ventilation are required. However, in the absence of such a clear indication (Table 18. 1) the wisdom of prolonged respiratory muscle 'rest' is now open to question. Diaphragm inactivity caused by mechanical venti-lation results in a significant reduction in diaphrag-matic strength that worsens with the duration of

mechanical ventilation and has been referred to as 'ventilator-induced diaphragmatic dysfunction' (VIDD; see also Chapter 14). VIDD is attenuated by the use of a triggered mode of ventilation rather than continuous mandatory ventilation. These data sug-gest that the return of spontaneous respiratory ac-tivity, using either a hybrid or triggered mode of ven-tilation, should be attempted as early as possible (Box 18.1).

What is the *first* stage of weaning?

Un-assisted spontaneous ventilation has two indis-pensable requisites: firstly, the ability to initiate

Table 18.1 Indications for suppressing respiratory activity with deep sedation, muscle relaxants or hyperventilation

	Deep sedation	Muscle relaxation	Hyperventilation
1. Severe hypoxic respiratory failure requiring			
a) High-frequency oscillation	✓	(✓)	✗
b) Prone ventilation	✓	(✓)	✗
c) Permissive hypercapnoea	✓	(✓)	✗
d) Inverse-ratio ventilation	✓	(✓)	✗
2. Severe bronchospasm requiring			
a) Long expiratory time	✓	(✓)	✗
b) Permissive hypercapnoea	✓	(✓)	✗
3. Raised intracranial pressure requiring			
a) Therapeutic hyperventilation	✓	✗	✓
b) Therapeutic hypothermia	✓	✓	✗
4. Therapeutic suppression of muscle contraction or movement because of			
a) Unstable spinal injury	✓	✓	✗
b) Reconstructive surgery that could be disrupted by movement	✓	✓	✗
c) Tetanus	✓	✓	✗
d) Rabies	✓	✓	✗
5. Unilateral lung pathology requiring independent lung ventilation	✓	(✓)	✗
6. Bronchopleural fistula requiring high frequency oscillation	✓	(✓)	✗

rhythmic inspiratory effort, and secondly the muscular strength and stamina to maintain tidal ventilation. Although *both* are required, spontaneous ventilation is impossible in the absence of a respiratory rhythm generated by the brain and an intact neural connection between the brain and the respiratory muscles (Figure 18.2). For weaning to start, therefore, every patient must *first* demonstrate the ability to generate rhythmic inspiratory effort. The establishment of a spontaneous

Box 18.1 What's wrong with suppressing respiratory effort?

Anyone who has had a leg immobilized for a couple of days will appreciate how quickly unused muscles weaken and atrophy. The same, it would appear, holds true for respiratory muscles. Although the currently available evidence is derived from animals (rats, rabbits, piglets, baboons), it is evident that mechanical ventilation results in both disuse atrophy, which causes a reduction in the cross-sectional area of the muscle fibre, as well as a reduction in intrinsic strength. These effects are synergistic and result in a significant reduction in the maximum force that the respiratory muscles can generate. This has an immediate impact on a patient's capacity to self-ventilate because susceptibility to fatigue is inversely related to maximum force.[7] The animal data suggest that the duration of ventilation required to elicit this effect depends on the animal species studied, being only one day in rabbits but three days in piglets.

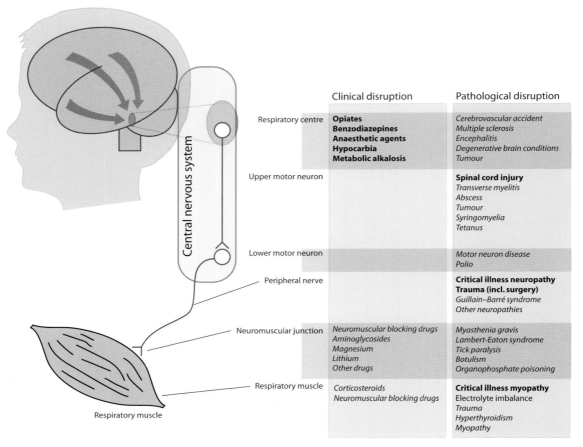

	Clinical disruption	Pathological disruption
Respiratory centre	**Opiates** **Benzodiazepines** **Anaesthetic agents** **Hypocarbia** **Metabolic alkalosis**	*Cerebrovascular accident* *Multiple sclerosis* *Encephalitis* *Degenerative brain conditions* *Tumour*
Upper motor neuron		**Spinal cord injury** *Transverse myelitis* *Abscess* *Tumour* *Syringomyelia* *Tetanus*
Lower motor neuron		*Motor neuron disease* *Polio*
Peripheral nerve		**Critical illness neuropathy** **Trauma (incl. surgery)** *Guillain–Barré syndrome* *Other neuropathies*
Neuromuscular junction	*Neuromuscular blocking drugs* *Aminoglycosides* *Magnesium* *Lithium* *Other drugs*	*Myasthenia gravis* *Lambert-Eaton syndrome* *Tick paralysis* *Botulism* *Organophosphate poisoning*
Respiratory muscle	*Corticosteroids* *Neuromuscular blocking drugs*	**Critical illness myopathy** Electrolyte imbalance *Trauma* *Hyperthyroidism* *Myopathy*

Figure 18.2 The neuromuscular control of ventilation.

The respiratory centre in the brain stem generates signals that are transmitted to the respiratory muscles (diaphragm and intercostals muscles) along upper motor neurons that run down the spinal cord, synapse with the cell bodies of lower motor neurons, then travel as peripheral nerves terminating at the neuromuscular junction. Failure to generate inspiratory effort can arise at any point between the respiratory centre in the brainstem and the neuromuscular junction, and the causes may be divided between those due to pathology or those due to clinical interference. Pathological causes are uncommon and in the vast majority of cases suppression of spontaneous respiratory effort arises from clinical manipulation, either deliberate or inadvertent. (*Italics* indicate least common causes, **bold** indicates most common causes.)

respiratory rhythm can be challenged in three ways:

1) Failure to generate *any* respiratory effort (primary post-ventilation apnoea)
2) Failure to sustain an acceptable minute ventilation
   a. Poor tidal volumes
   b. Failure to trigger – patient-ventilator dys-synchrony (PVD)
3) Repeated periods of apnoea (secondary apnoea).

Primary post-ventilation apnoea

If there was an absence of central or peripheral nervous system pathology at the time that mechanical ventilation was initiated, the most common cause of apnoea is central respiratory depression. This may be caused by sedatives and opiates given for

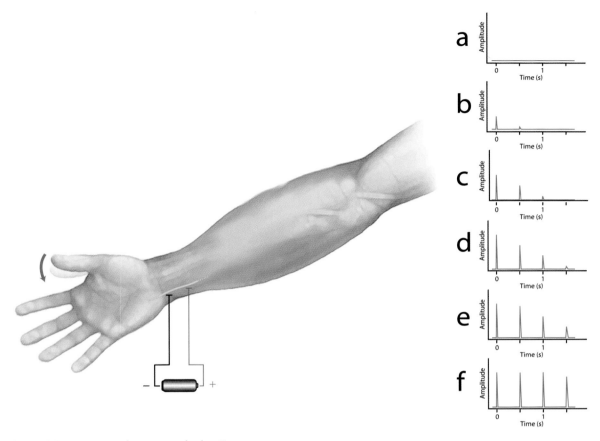

Figure 18.3 Assessment of neuromuscular function.

The usual method of peripheral nerve stimulation uses a battery-powered device which is applied over the ulnar nerve at the wrist with the cathode (negative electrode, black) positioned distal to the anode (positive electrode, red). The device applies a depolarizing voltage to the ulnar nerve at the cathode, which is transmitted both up and down the nerve. The depolarization terminates at the anode proximally and the neuromuscular junction distally, causing contraction of the thenar and hypothenar muscles, which causes the thumb to twitch towards the palm of the hand. A 'train-of-four' involves four discharges applied at 500-mS intervals. With complete blockade of the ulnar nerve, no twitches of the thumb can be felt (a). As the neuromuscular blockade fades, one (b), two (c), three (d) and four (e) twitches can be felt, with 'fade', and eventually four twitches without 'fade' (f).

patient comfort either alone, or together with a respiratory or metabolic alkalosis. If neuromuscular blocking drugs have been used or might have been used,[1] normal neuromuscular transmission should be demonstrated (Figure 18.3) before attempting to restore a respiratory rhythm. In the operating theatre, where rapid reversal of neuromuscular blockade is desirable, the process can be accelerated by the administration of an anticholinesterase, neostigmine, together with an anti-cholinergic, glycopyrrolate, to prevent bradycardia. This is not usually necessary in the ICU, where a brief delay in the return of neuromuscular conduction is less important. In the presence of normal neuromuscular transmission, respiratory drive can usually be restored by suspending or reducing the infusion of hypnotic and analgesic agents and reducing minute ventilation.

[1] For example, in a patient recently returned from the operating theatre.

Table 18.2 Causes of prolonged respiratory depression

Biologically advanced age
Liver or renal dysfunction
Prolonged continuous infusion of benzodiazepines (midazolam, diazepam, lorazepam) or *any* opiate (including remifentanil)
Poor neurological 'reserve' (pre-existing or acute CNS disease, e.g. dementia, head trauma, encephalitis, encephalopathy)
Hypothermia
Electrolyte imbalance, particularly abnormalities of plasma sodium

Table 18.3 Common causes of metabolic alkalosis in the patient weaning from mechanical ventilation

1) Chloride depletion
   a) Diuretics (furosemide, bumetanide, chlorothiazide, metolazone)
   b) Permissive hypercapnoea
   c) GI losses (stomach, large bowel)
2) Hypokalaemia
   a) Decreased intake or administration in fluids
   b) Increased urinary losses
3) Cationic antibiotics (ampicillin, penicillin)
4) Hypoalbuminaemia (modest effect, but very common)

In patients who have received mechanical ventilation for relatively short periods of time, up to 72 hours, return of a normal respiratory rhythm *should* occur within 30 to 60 minutes, depending on the magnitude of the reductions in minute ventilation, sedation, analgesia and the specific pharmacokinetics of the drugs used. Patients who have required full mechanical ventilation for more than 72 hours are at risk of prolonged respiratory depression (hours to days), particularly under some circumstances (Table 18.2). In the absence of any risk of acute cerebral injury, normal cranial nerve reflexes, and the presence of one or more of the factors in Table 18.2, brain computed tomography (CT) is unnecessary. Conversely, any focal neurological deficit, particularly involving the cranial nerves, deserves further investigation with cerebral CT, lumbar puncture and electro-encephalography (EEG). Respiratory depression caused by benzodiazepines or opiates can be present for many days in susceptible individuals and can be confirmed by the administration of small doses of flumazenil[2] or naloxone.[3] In the long term, the incidence of drug-related apnoea can be reduced with the use of targeted sedation using a rational and well validated measure such as the Richmond Agitation and Sedation Score (RASS),[2] daily sedation breaks and the use of intermittent opiate administration titrated to objective pain scores or, where possible, regional analgesia (see Chapter 8).

Metabolic alkalosis, a common biochemical abnormality in the ICU, may arise in a number of ways (Table 18.3) and buffers the respiratory stimulant effect of carbon dioxide on the respiratory centre. In the absence of central respiratory depression from other causes, metabolic alkalosis is not usually sufficient to cause primary apnoea, but may contribute to the delay in the return of normal respiratory drive. In patients who are also sodium and water depleted, the defect can be corrected by the administration of 0.9% sodium chloride, while in patients who are fluid overloaded, acetazolamide[4] will produce an alkaline diuresis.

Poor tidal volumes

Following the return of spontaneous respiratory effort by reductions in both mandatory minute ventilation and depth of sedation, most patients will tolerate the switch to a triggered mode, such as pressure support ventilation (PSV), which has no mandatory component. A few patients,

[2] Initially, 0.3 mg iv, repeated as necessary.
[3] Initially, 0.04 to 0.08 mg iv, repeated as necessary.

[4] 250 mg every eight hours via the nasogastric tube.

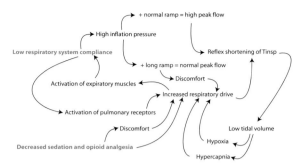

Figure 18.4 Factors in patients with low respiratory system compliance that interact to reduce the toleration for pressure-support ventilation.

however, do not tolerate this transition, becoming hypoxic, hypercapnic, agitated, tachycardic, hypertensive and sweaty – all signs of acute respiratory distress. Failure to tolerate PSV is usually the consequence of both low respiratory system compliance and discomfort (Figure 18.4). These patients require high inflation pressures to achieve reasonable tidal volumes, but at the expense of high peak inspiratory flow. Activation of pulmonary receptors as well as high peak flows lead to shortening of neural inspiratory time, shortening the duration of inspiration and reducing the inspiratory tidal volume. Significant increase in respiratory drive may also be accompanied by the recruitment of expiratory muscles, further reducing the compliance of the respiratory system, and consequently the inspiratory tidal volume. In addition, reduction or suspension of sedatives and opioids to reduce central respiratory depression can result in patient discomfort and anxiety. Occasionally, the patient can be stabilized in PSV by reducing the inflating pressure or prolonging the ramp to reduce the peak inspiratory flow, or both, reducing the flow threshold for expiratory cycling[5] to increase the duration of inspiration, increasing PEEP to improve oxygenation, and carefully re-introducing an opioid to reduce discomfort and respiratory drive. Most

patients in this situation, however, require the use of a hybrid mode, where the transition from mandatory to spontaneous ventilation can be achieved by gradual reductions in the mandatory ventilation rate.

Very occasionally, low tidal volumes are caused by inspiratory-flow induced cough. In such cases, reducing peak inspiratory flow or nebulized local anaesthetic[6] may help.

Patient–ventilator dys-synchrony (PVD)

Patients with abnormally small airways, such as those with asthma or emphysema, are at risk of developing intrinsic positive end-expiratory pressure (iPEEP, Box 18.2 and Figure 18.5). Before gas will flow into the lungs, which is necessary to trigger the ventilator, the patient has to generate a negative intrapleural pressure to counteract the iPEEP and must then generate *further* negative intrapleural pressure to create a pressure gradient from upper airway to alveoli in order to cause inspiratory gas flow (Figure 18.6). During acute exacerbations, these patients may also have weakened respiratory muscles. In addition, the process of trapping air flattens the diaphragm, putting it in a mechanically disadvantaged position and further compromising their inspiratory effort (Figure 18.7). Together, these effects can make it very difficult for patients with significant iPEEP to trigger the ventilator as often as they would like. This can be seen by careful inspection of the pressure profile on the ventilator where, between each patient-initiated breath, a number of unsuccessful inspiratory efforts can be seen as small downward deflections (Figure 18.8). As the ventilator is unable to meet the patient's ventilatory demand, both hypoxia and hypercapnia worsen. This then causes an increase in the patient's respiratory drive and (attempted) respiratory rate, often accompanied by signs of marked distress such as hypertension, tachycardia, sweating and agitation; this is recognized as the patient 'fighting'

[5] This is not possible on all makes or models of ventilator.

[6] 1 or 2 mL of 2% lidocaine or 0.5% bupivacaine.

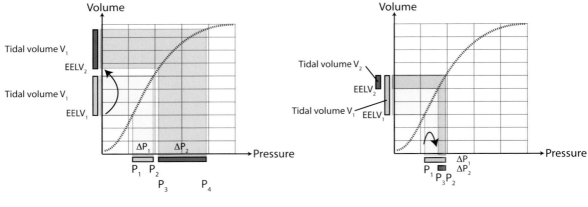

Volume-controlled ventilation

Pressure-controlled ventilation

Figure 18.5 The development of gas trapping in volume-targeted or pressure-targeted ventilation.

The figure shows the relationship between lung volume (shown on the y-axis) and airway pressure (x-axis) for a patient receiving either volume-volume (left) or pressure-volume (right) ventilation in whom gas trapping has occurred. In volume-targeted ventilation the inspiratory tidal volume remains constant (V_1), but there is a progressive increase in end-expiratory lung volume (EELV$_1$ to EELV$_2$) until the difference between end-inspiratory and end-expiratory pressure increases sufficiently (ΔP_1 to ΔP_2) to expel the inspired tidal volume in the time available. In pressure-volume ventilation, the inflating pressure remains constant (P_2), but there is a progressive increase in end-expiratory lung volume (EELV$_1$ to EELV$_2$) until the inspiratory tidal volume falls sufficiently to be expelled by the falling difference between end-inspiratory and end-expiratory alveolar pressure (ΔP_1 to ΔP_2). In both modes of ventilation, P_3 is the value of the intrinsic PEEP, not the end-expiratory pressure set on the ventilator.

the ventilator. In an acute situation where there is a significant risk of the patient coming to harm, the most effective remedy is to re-establish full control by deepening the sedation and re-instituting mandatory mechanical ventilation. Occasionally a single dose of muscle relaxant might also be required. Where the situation is judged not to be quite so dangerous, a number of approaches can be used to reduce the degree of gas trapping (Table 18.4).

Box 18.2

The expiratory phase of the ventilatory cycle is passive, but even with high respiratory rates, expiratory gas flow is normally complete before the onset of the next breath. The duration of exhalation is determined by (1) the elastic recoil of the lungs and chest wall, (2) the diameter of the small airways, (3) the resistance to expiratory gas flow (laminar versus turbulent) and (4) the volume of gas to be exhaled. The time available for expiratory gas flow is determined by (1) the respiratory rate and (2) the I:E ratio. Emphysema reduces the natural elasticity of lung tissue, and both emphysema and asthma cause a narrowing of the small airways. These factors combine to make exhalation in these conditions *slower* than in normal individuals. The result is that there is insufficient time to expel all of the inhaled gas at normal lung volumes, before the start of the next breath, resulting in a phenomenon known as 'gas trapping'. This process results in a progressive increase in the end-expiratory lung volume (called *dynamic hyperinflation*). The increased end-expiratory volume indicates significant residual end-expiratory intra-alveolar pressure, which is known as *intrinsic PEEP* or *auto-PEEP*. This situation is exacerbated by high respiratory rates[8, 9] and a short I:E ratio.

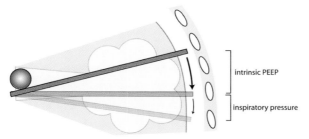

Figure 18.6 Effect of intrinsic positive end-expiratory pressure on ventilator triggering.

Illustration depicting the pressure gradient (represented by the brown plank) between the upper airway and alveoli in a patient with significant intrinsic positive end-expiratory pressure (PEEP). At the onset of inspiration the patient *first* has to generate a negative pleural pressure of the same magnitude as the intrinsic PEEP to bring alveolar pressure down to the upper airway pressure. *Then* the patient has to generate further negative pleural pressure to create a pressure gradient between the upper airway and the alveoli in order to draw gas (represented by the blue ball) into the lungs in order to trigger the ventilator.

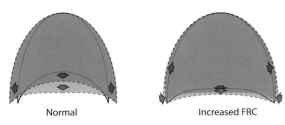

Figure 18.7 Effect of increased functional residual capacity (end-expiratory lung volume) on the disposition of the diaphragm.

In the normal lung (left), inspiration results in a widening of both the front-to-back and side-to-side diameter of the thorax, which pulls the diaphragm down a little into the abdomen (blue arrows). In this position, diaphragmatic contraction (red arrow) results in a further increase in thoracic volume.

In lungs with a significant increase in functional residual capacity (right), inspiration causes a modest increase in thoracic diameter and a draws the diaphragm even flatter (blue arrows). In this position contraction of the diaphragm (red arrows) makes a small additional increase in vertical thoracic volume, but now *reduces* the front-to-back and side-to-side diameter of the lower thorax.

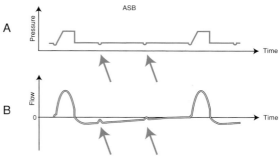

Figure 18.8 Pressure (A) and flow (B) waveforms on the ventilator during patient–ventilator dys-synchrony (PVD) in a triggered mode of ventilation.

At the beginning of the trace, an inspiratory effort, indicated by a negative deflection in the pressure profile and a positive deflection in the flow profile, triggers inspiratory pressure support. The expiratory flow (negative) from this breath is prolonged and shallow, indicating significant obstruction to expiratory flow. During expiration, the patient makes a further two inspiratory efforts (red arrows) which do not trigger inspiratory support. The patient is only able to trigger the ventilator at the third attempt, when expiratory flow has returned to zero.

SECONDARY APNOEA

The respiratory centre, based on information received from both central and peripheral[7] receptors, governs tidal volume and respiratory rate which, in turn, influence arterial $PaCO_2$, pH and PaO_2. This forms a chemical feedback system in which natural oscillations are minimized by regulation of the gain at each point in the cycle and by ensuring that under normal circumstances the signal and its feedback are never completely out of phase. When the signal and its feedback are 180° out of phase, a *negative* feedback system becomes a *positive* feedback one, exaggerating oscillations rather than damping them. In the respiratory system, this is recognized as periodic respiration, or *Cheyne-Stokes breathing* (Figure 18.9). The respiratory centre controls alveolar minute volume by modulating tidal volume when awake but respiratory rate

[7] Carotid bodies.

Table 18.4 Manoeuvres for reducing airtrapping

1) Measures to increase the diameter of the small airways
   a. Relax airway smooth muscle with β_2-adrenergic agonists or methylxanthines.
   b. Reduce airway inflammation with either intravenous or inhaled corticosteroids.
2) Measures to reduce the resistance to expiratory gas flow
   a. Reduce the expiratory pressure gradient by matching intrinsic PEEP with extrinsic (ventilator applied) PEEP.
   b. Convert turbulent to laminar flow by using a gas mixture with a lower density such as a helium/oxygen mixture.
3) Measures to improve the mechanics of respiration
   a. Increase respiratory muscle contractility with methylxanthines.
   b. Increase the elastic recoil of the chest wall with an elasticated corset.
4) Measures to increase the trigger sensitivity of the ventilator to the patient's inspiratory efforts
   a. Use flow trigger instead of pressure trigger.
5) Measures to increase the time for the expiratory phase
   a. Reduce the patient's respiratory rate with drugs that cause respiratory centre depression, such as opiates.
   b. Shorten the duration of inspiration by using a short ramp time and a high threshold for expiratory cycling.

Table 18.5 Strategies for reducing or eliminating secondary apnoeas

1) Reduce system gain
   a. Reduce inflation pressure
2) Reduce CNS response time
   a. Avoid nocturnal use of drugs which depress respiratory drive
   b. Use respiratory stimulants at night
3) Shorten circulation time
   a. Ino-dilators (milrinone)

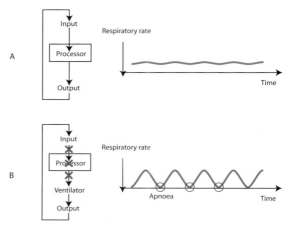

Figure 18.9 Periodic respiration in mechanically ventilated patients.

A: The respiratory rate (output) is normally controlled by the respiratory centre (processor) based on feedback signals (input) from sensors in the floor of the fourth ventricle responding to the pH of cerebrospinal fluid. Although there are small delays at each of these three steps, feedback occurs sufficiently rapidly to minimize the oscillations in respiratory rate.

B: When processing at any or all of the three steps in the loop is slowed, either by drugs or damage, and the loop is further prolonged by the interposition of the ventilator, feedback can become 'out of phase' with the signal being processed. Rather than damping oscillations in the system, this actually amplifies the oscillations in the system, resulting in 'periodic respiration' or Cheyne-Stokes breathing.

during sleep, and it is therefore particularly during sleep or when conscious input is limited by sedation or CNS dysfunction that apnoeas may occur. In patients with congestive cardiac failure daytime periodic breathing has a worse prognosis than if it occurs at night, although both indicate significant impairment of left-ventricular function. Patients receiving support in a triggered mode are protected from significant hypoxia by an apnoea-generated switch to a mandatory or hybrid mode. A number of strategies may reduce or eliminate the incidence of apnoeas (Table 18.5). These are worth pursuing because repeated apnoeas will result in the patient spending prolonged periods of time in 'apnoea ventilation', which will suppress spontaneous respiratory effort and result in VIDD and delayed recovery.

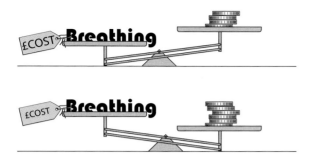

£COST **Breathing**

£COST **Breathing**

Figure 18.10 Balance between the work (cost) of breathing and the work (money) available.

What is the second stage of weaning?

Having re-established a normal respiratory rhythm, the second stage of weaning involves transferring the work of breathing from the ventilator back to the patient. In the majority of patients admitted to intensive care who require ventilatory support for less than three or four days, this process can be completed in minutes, because it is unlikely that there has been any *detectable* deterioration in respiratory muscle function in this short time. This does not necessarily apply to patients whose capacity to self-ventilate was at its limit beforehand and in whom even tiny deteriorations can render them ventilator dependent until this loss of function has been regained. The critical balance is that between the work[8] *required* to self-ventilate and the work *available* to do so (Figure 18.10). In order to restore a patient's capacity to self-ventilate, it is necessary to understand the factors that increase the work of breathing on the one hand (the cost) and, on the other hand, the patient's ability to do this work. These factors can then be manipulated, where possible, to the patient's benefit.

---

[8] Strictly speaking the rate at which work is done is referred to as *power*, and therefore the balance is between the power required and the power available. The word *work* is used here because clinicians frequently refer to the 'work of breathing'.

Determinants of the work of breathing

There are six components to the work of breathing. Five determine the work required per breath: the elastic properties of the lungs and chest wall (elastance), the resistance to inspiratory gas flow, the inertia of the lungs and chest wall, the friction of tissue deformation (Figure 18.11), and the tidal volume. The sixth, the respiratory rate, determines the rate at which this work is done.

INCREASED ELASTANCE

The lungs have elastic properties that are derived from (1) the lung tissue itself and (2) the effect of alveolar surface tension. Coating the alveolar surface is a special mix of phospholipids ('surfactant'), synthesized by type II alveolar cells, which reduces alveolar surface tension in a concentration-dependent manner. This means that as the surface area of the alveolus falls (for example during exhalation), the concentration of the surfactant on the surface *increases* and surface tension is reduced even further. This combined source of lung elastance means that lung elastance varies with lung volume (Figure 18.5), being high (stiff) at lung volumes near functional residual capacity, falling with an increase in lung volume, and then increasing again as the lung approaches vital capacity. Lung elastance increases with any process that (1) increases the tissue stiffness of the lungs or chest wall, (2) increases the end-expiratory lung volume to a less compliant part of the lung's pressure/volume or (3) reduces surfactant activity (Table 18.6). A separate source of elastance arises from the work that needs to be done in expanding the chest and pushing away the abdominal contents during inspiration. The majority of this elastance arises from static properties of the chest wall and abdomen, such as the weight and elasticity of the tissues, but some may arise from the contraction of chest wall and abdominal muscles during inspiration either as a response to pain or through dys-coordination. Some of the determinants

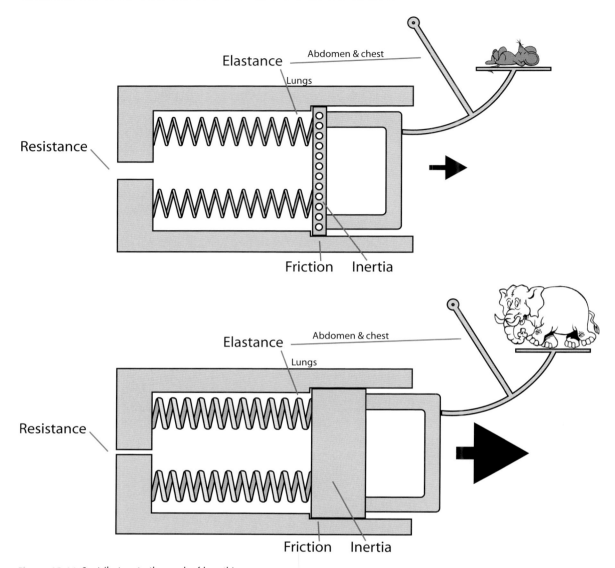

Figure 18.11 Contributors to the work of breathing.

An illustration of the work of breathing using an analogy between the respiratory system and a pump constructed of a cylinder and piston. Outward movement of the piston draws gas into the cylinder (inspiration) which is made more or less difficult depending in the size of the orifice through which gas is sucked in (resistance), the stiffness of the springs within the cylinder (elastance), the mass of the piston (inertia) and the friction between the piston and the cylinder.

of increased respiratory system elastance, such as lung fibrosis, are not easily reversed and some, such as alveolar consolidation, resolve with time. There remain, however, a number of opportunities to reduce total respiratory system elastance. The methods for doing so are described next.

Pulmonary vascular congestion, interstitial pulmonary oedema and alveolar oedema. Fluid movement in and out of capillaries (flux) is governed by the 'leakiness' of the capillary wall to fluid (the filtration coefficient, k_{fc}) and colloid (called the reflectance coefficient, σ) and the balance between two

Table 18.6 Causes of increased elastance of the lungs, pleura, chest wall and abdomen

	Problem	Solution
Increased tissue elastance of lungs and pleura	Fibrotic lung disease[9]	Corticosteroids
	Alveolar collapse or consolidation	Positive end-expiratory pressure, sighs or bi-level ventilation
		Even or negative fluid balance
	Interstitial and alveolar pulmonary oedema	Inotropes (dopamine, dobutamine, milrinone, enoximone, amrinone)
		After-load reduction (nitrates, angiotensin converting enzyme inhibitors, angiotensin II receptor antagonists, α-adrenergic receptor antagonists)
		Pre-load reduction (nitrates, diuretics)
		Colloid
		Diuretics
		Increased alveolar fluid clearance (β_2-adrenergic receptor agonists)
	Pleural effusion, thickening, scarring or calcification	Thoracocentesis
		Surgical decortication
	Low respiratory rate	(Respiratory stimulants)
Increased tissue elastance of chest wall and abdomen	Skeletal deformity (scoliosis, ankylosing spondylitis)	None, other than corrective surgery
	Increased weight/volume (obesity, ascites, oedema, bowel obstruction, ileus)	Manage ileus aggressively Drain ascites
	Supine or prone position	Nurse in head-up position
	Decreased tissue elasticity (scar tissue, fibrosing conditions of the skin[10], ectopic calcification)	Escharotomies
	Pain-induced muscle contraction (peritonitis, abdominal incisions, fractured ribs, pleurisy)	Good analgesia, preferably regional
Increased end-expiratory lung volume	Asthma, emphysema, bronchospasm	Bronchodilators
	Short expiratory time	(See also Table 18.4) Opiates to reduce respiratory drive
Loss of surfactant activity	Damage to type II pneumocytes	
	Degradation of surfactant by plasma proteins	

opposing forces: (1) the net hydrostatic pressure between inside (P_i) and outside (P_o) the capillary and (2) the net osmotic pressure inside (π_i) and outside (π_o) the capillary, summarized in the Starling

[9] Fibrosing alveolitis, usual interstitial pneumonia, viral pneumonitis, rheumatoid lung disease, polymyositis/dermatomyositis, extrinsic allergic alveolitis, radiation damage, bleomycin toxicity.

[10] Nephrogenic fibrosing dermopathy/nephrogenic systemic fibrosis, systemic sclerosis.

equation:

$$Flux = [k_{fc}(P_i - P_o) - \sigma(\pi_i - \pi_o)]. \qquad (18.1)$$

Under normal circumstances, fluid continuously seeps out of the pulmonary capillaries into the pulmonary interstitial space where it returns to the circulation via the pulmonary capillaries and lymphatics. A little fluid also seeps into the air spaces, but these are kept dry by Na^+-K^+-ATPase pumps on the basal membrane of type I and type II alveolar cells that create a sodium gradient between the alveolar fluid and cell interior. Sodium is drawn into the alveolar cells through apical sodium channels down its concentration gradient, followed electrostatically by chloride ions and osmotically by water. When the rate of pulmonary capillary leak exceeds the capacity of the drainage system, fluid accumulates in the interstitial space as interstitial pulmonary oedema. Eventually it spills into the alveolar air spaces as alveolar pulmonary oedema.

The causes of oedema can therefore be divided into those related to (1) increased capillary hydrostatic pressure, (2) a fall in the capillary reflectance coefficient (i.e. increased leakiness) or (3) changes in plasma oncotic pressure (Table 18.7). Regardless of aetiology, pulmonary oedema causes a significant increase in lung elastance. A conservative fluid regime[3] or a negative fluid balance[4] have been shown to reduce the duration of mechanical ventilation[3, 4] and improve outcome.[5] In the absence of overt alveolar pulmonary oedema associated with hypoxaemia or radiographic changes, it is difficult to know whether pulmonary vascular congestion is contributing to the work of breathing. Trans-pulmonary thermal dilution provides information on the extravascular lung water (EVLW) and total intrathoracic blood volume (TIBV) and has been used to examine the relationship between EVLW and outcome, but it has not been used to examine the effect of EVLW on the duration of weaning. A potentially attractive alternative would be measurement of plasma

Table 18.7 Causes of increased fluid efflux from the pulmonary capillaries

1) Increased pulmonary capillary hydrostatic pressure
   a) Fluid overload
      - Iatrogenic
      - Fluid retention (cardiac, hepatic or renal failure)
   b) Diastolic heart failure
   c) Mitral valve dysfunction
   d) Hypertension
      i. Acute, endocrine-mediated (phaeochromocytoma, thyroid storm)
      ii. Head injury
      iii. Renal artery stenosis
2) Decreased pulmonary capillary reflectance coefficient
   a) Systemic inflammation
      i. Sepsis
      ii. Pancreatitis
      iii. Multiple
      iv. Transfusion reaction
      v. Drug reaction
      vi. Drug overdose
      vii. Envenomation
   b) Pulmonary inflammation
      i. Pulmonary infection
      ii. Chemical damage (aspiration of acid, chemicals, smoke, amniotic fluid embolus)
      iii. Immune-mediated damage
      iv. Physical damage (ventilation-induced lung injury)
3) Decreased plasma oncotic pressure

concentrations of B-type natriuretic peptide (BNP), which can help to discriminate between respiratory and cardiogenic dyspnoea in the emergency room setting. Although in acutely ill patients BNP concentrations were not correlated with pulmonary artery wedge pressure, they were significantly higher in patients who failed a weaning trial,[6] as was dynamic pulmonary elastance. In practice, where pulmonary vascular congestion is thought to be contributing to the work of breathing, a therapeutic trial of agents to improve cardiac function,[11]

---

[11] For example, digoxin, dopamine, dobutamine, milrinone.

reduce after-load[12] and reduce pre-load,[13] is warranted. In patients with ARDS, the combination of albumin supplementation *and* diuretics was more effective than diuretics alone in reducing EVLW, and this is likely to apply to patients who are weaning. More recently, it has been shown that intravenous infusion of β_2-agonist (salbutamol), which up-regulates the epithelial basal sodium pump, is effective in reducing EVLW in patients with ARDS,[7] and this may be a useful additional manoeuvre.

Pleural disease. By reducing end-expiratory lung volume and reducing the compliance of the thoracic cage, pleural effusions serve to increase the elastance of the respiratory system, which is reversed by thoracentesis. Pleural effusion may also be a sign of significant pulmonary vascular congestion that may benefit from therapy. Infected and organized pleural effusions which have formed an empyema and which are hindering the weaning process require surgical clearance, either with open or videoscopically assisted decortication.

Pain relief. If inspiration causes the patient discomfort because of fractures of the ribs or sternum, pleural inflammation, recent abdominal surgery, or other painful abdominal pathology, then this will have two significant effects. First, reflex contraction of *expiratory* muscles during inspiration will cause significant increases in respiratory system elastance. Second, distress and anxiety will cause activation of the sympathetic nervous system, increases in blood pressure, heart rate and respiratory rate, as well as agitation and restlessness. All these responses result in increased carbon dioxide production and consequently the alveolar minute volume necessary to maintain a constant $PaCO_2$. These effects work together to increase significantly the work of breathing and, in some patients, can cause respiratory failure or even cardiac failure. Whenever possible, regional nerve blocks or epidural analgesia are

preferable, because these have the combined benefit of providing the best quality of pain relief as well as avoiding the need for systemic opiates. Unfortunately, these techniques require skill to site, effort to maintain and are all too often neglected in favour of systemic analgesics, especially opiates.

Reduction of abdominal distension. When increased abdominal girth and raised intra-abdominal pressure are not due to obesity or compounded by other contributing factors, these can be corrected and will result in worthwhile reductions in the elastance of the respiratory system. Constipation, for example, which is associated with weaning problems, should be identified early and treated aggressively, ascites should be drained, and other causes of abdominal distension sought and treated.

Correct posture. The benefit of nursing patients with the head of the bed elevated to 30 degrees or more for reducing the risk of ventilator-associated pneumonia is well recognized (see Chapter 14), but seems difficult to translate into clinical practice. Posture is particularly relevant for patients with a large abdominal girth, in whom the work of breathing needs to be minimized. In these patients, elevating the head of the bed can significantly improve respiratory system mechanics, but only provided that the patient is not allowed to slide down the bed so that the axis of elevation rises to the thoraco-lumbar region (Figure 18.12).

Alveolar recruitment. Alveolar collapse reduces respiratory system compliance that can be recovered by an alveolar recruitment manoeuvre (Figure 18.13). While the ideal recruitment manoeuvre for any given situation remains to be identified, it is more commonly applied to patients with severe hypoxic respiratory failure who are paralysed or deeply sedated. In patients with minimal or no sedation in whom recruitment manoeuvres are unlikely to be well tolerated, alveolar collapse can be reduced by appropriate levels of PEEP, attention to the management of secretions,

---

[12] For example, angiotensin-converting enzyme (ACE) inhibitors or α-adrenergic receptor antagonists.

[13] For example, diuretics or nitrates.

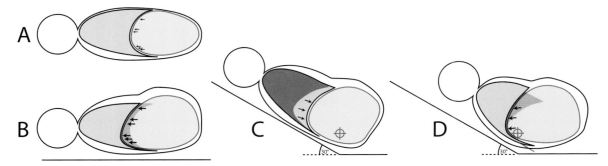

Figure 18.12 Effect of enlarged abdominal girth and posture on respiratory system elastance.

For the sake of simplicity, the abdominal contents can be considered to consist of water, which exerts an increasing pressure against the diaphragm the further from the anterior abdominal wall this is measured (A). With an enlarged abdominal girth (obesity, oedema, ascites), this pressure is increased (B), causing a reduction in end-expiratory lung volume and adding to the load on the diaphragm during inspiration. Elevation of the head of the bed reduces the pressure on the diaphragm and thereby the respiratory system elastance (C). Changing the axis of elevation from the hips (C) to the thoraco-lumbar region (D), which is where the axis tends to end up when the patient slides down the bed, results in respiratory system embarrassment that is even worse than when the patient was flat.

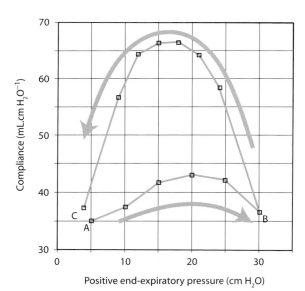

Figure 18.13 Change in lung compliance with alveolar recruitment.

While receiving pressure-targeted mechanical ventilation with an inflating pressure of 15 cm H_2O during an open cholecystectomy, PEEP was increased from 5 to 30 cm H_2O in steps of 5 cm H_2O and then reduced from 24 to 3 in steps of 3 cm H_2O. The graph shows the mean compliance at each PEEP value during both incremental (A to B) and decremental (B to C) PEEP changes and shows the effect on compliance of alveolar recruitment.

correct posture and the appropriate management of abdominal distension.

Gas trapping. Gas trapping (see Box 18.1) results in an increase in end-expiratory lung volume (EELV) and intrinsic PEEP. Gas trapping contributes to the work of breathing by increasing EELV, pushing the respiratory cycle onto a less compliant portion of the lung's pressure/volume curve (Figure 18.5), while narrowed airways increase the work of breathing by increasing the resistance to gas flow. The management of narrowed airways and gas trapping is discussed later.

INCREASED RESISTANCE

When gas flow is laminar, the resistance to flow is proportional to the length of the tube and the viscosity of the gas, but inversely proportional to the radius of the tube, raised to the power of 4:

$$\text{Resistance} = \frac{8 \times l \times \mu}{\pi \times r^4}, \tag{18.2}$$

where l = length, μ = viscosity and r = radius. This equation is useful because it emphasizes the dramatic effect that changes in airway have on resistance. For example, a 10% reduction in the diameter of an airway causes the resistance to increase by just over 50%. However, when gas flow is turbulent, the resistance to gas flow actually increases with *flow*:

$$\Delta P = 2.4 \times (flow)^{1.3} . \tag{18.3}$$

Whether gas flow is laminar or turbulent depends on the Reynolds number:

$$\text{Reynolds number} \propto \frac{velocity \times \rho}{\mu}, \tag{18.4}$$

where ρ = gas density, and μ = gas viscosity. With a Reynolds number above 1500, flow is entirely turbulent; with a Reynolds number under 1000, flow is entirely laminar, while between 1000 and 1500, flow is a mixture of the two. Equation 18.4 indicates that turbulence becomes more likely with increasing gas flow rates and density, but less likely with increasing viscosity.

Resistance to laminar gas flow can be minimized by maximally dilating the small airways, while replacing the nitrogen in inspired gas with helium can reduce the risk of flow becoming turbulent and has been shown to reduce significantly the work of breathing. Turbulence-related resistance can be minimized by reducing both the flow and velocity of gas movement, maximizing the diameter of the airways and, where possible, reducing the gas density.

INERTIA AND FRICTION

The power consumption required to overcome inertia is related to the weight of the lungs, the average speed of lung tissue movement and lung acceleration (see Box 18.3) and in adults with normal lungs, which only weigh about 125 g each, is traditionally regarded to be negligible. Patients who are having trouble weaning from mechanical ventilation are likely to have considerably increased inertial power consumption because each of the contributory factors is altered to the patient's disadvantage. Lung weight, for example, may be increased by anything up to ten- or twenty-fold. The lungs of patients dying of acute respiratory distress syndrome (ARDS) usually weigh in *excess* of 1000 g

---

Box 18.3

The force (F) required to accelerate an object is given by the mass of the object (m) multiplied by the acceleration (a) – Newton's first law:

$$F = m \times a. \tag{18.5}$$

The average power ($\bar{P}$) consumed is given by the force (F) multiplied by the average velocity ($\bar{v}$):

$$\bar{P} = F \times \bar{v}. \tag{18.6}$$

By combining Equations 18.5 and 18.6 we get an equation of the average power consumption required to overcome lung inertia:

$$\bar{P} = m \times a \times \bar{v}. \tag{18.7}$$

---

each. In addition, these patients tend to have high respiratory drive, with associated elevations of both respiratory rate and peak inspiratory flow, increasing both the average speed of lung movement and lung acceleration. In a patient in whom the latter two factors each increase only two-fold, and assuming a modest five-fold increase in lung weight, the inertial power consumption would increase by *no less* than twenty-fold, making it likely that inertial power consumption is important in patients weaning from mechanical ventilation.

RESPIRATORY RATE AND TIDAL VOLUME

Removal of carbon dioxide by the lungs is principally determined by the alveolar minute volume ($\dot{V}_A$), which is a function of the respiratory rate (f), tidal volume (V_T) and dead space (V_D):

$$\dot{V}_A = f \times (V_T - V_D). \tag{18.8}$$

Under normal circumstances, the respiratory centre determines the rate and depth of breathing so that the rate of carbon dioxide clearance in exhaled gas matches its rate of production in the tissues, thus maintaining the steady state. The respiratory centre is only indirectly sensitive to the arterial partial

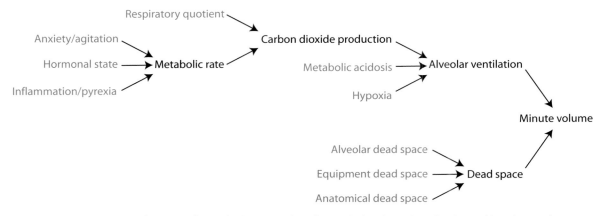

Figure 18.14 Determinants of minute volume. The items in red can be manipulated to reduce the *demand* for minute volume whilst the items in blue can be manipulated to increase the *supply* minute volume.

pressure of carbon dioxide; in fact, it responds primarily to the hydrogen ion (pH) concentration of the cerebrospinal fluid and secondarily to the partial pressure of oxygen detected by the carotid bodies. The alveolar minute volume necessary to achieve homeostasis is determined in the first instance by the rate of carbon dioxide production, though it may also be driven by metabolic acidosis or even, occasionally, hypoxia (Figure 18.14). Both rate and tidal volume contribute to the work of breathing but by different mechanisms, the former through resistance and the latter through elastance. Regardless of the relationship between tidal volume and respiratory rate, a decrease in the demand for minute volume will decrease the work of breathing, and therefore presents an opportunity to optimize the situation in the patient's favour.

Respiratory quotient. Metabolic energy (measured by ATP) is largely generated aerobically by the oxidation of carbohydrates and fats, with carbon dioxide and water as by-products. In the metabolism of carbohydrate, one mole of carbon dioxide is generated for each mole of oxygen consumed, giving a respiratory quotient[14] of 1. Fat, however, has a different

molecular structure and a respiratory quotient of about 0.6, depending on the type of fat in question. Clinical trials comparing isocaloric diets with a normal fat:carbohydrate ratio against one with a high fat:carbohydrate ratio have shown that this is an effective way of reducing carbon dioxide production, but whether this translates into more rapid weaning is unknown. In selected patients with borderline respiratory reserve, this may be a reasonable additional strategy.

Agitation and anxiety. With the discontinuation or lightening of sedation, delirium is found in up to 83% of patients depending on case mix and diagnostic methodology, with a minority of delirious patients (40%) having normal levels of arousal. Many of the risk factors for delirium in elderly general medical patients are shared by patients in intensive care (Table 18.8). Targeted interventions significantly reduce the incidence and duration of delirium in elderly general medical patients.[8] It is possible that the same might be true of ICU patients. While delirium has been shown to increase the duration of ICU stay as well as both morbidity and mortality, few intensive care units routinely look for it, despite current recommendations. Agitated delirium is likely to result in a number of complications that delay weaning, including a requirement for

---

[14] Respiratory quotient = moles of carbon dioxide produced/ moles of oxygen consumed.

Table 18.8 Risk factors for delirium

Age
Cognitive impairment
Severity of illness
Drug administration (especially sedatives and
    opioids)
Drug withdrawal (tobacco, alcohol, sedatives,
    analgesics, anxiolytics)
Dehydration
Visual impairment
Auditory impairment
Sepsis
Pain
Hypoxia
Liver or renal dysfunction
Poor glycaemic control
Sleep deprivation

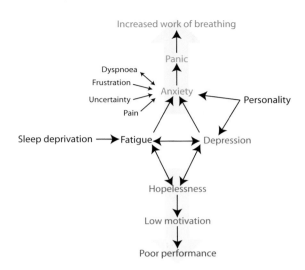

Figure 18.15 Emotional factors contributing to both the work of breathing (red) and the patient's capacity to perform work (blue).

further sedation, self-extubation, poor co-operation and increased energy expenditure.

With the return of cognitive function the vast majority (75% to 85%) of patients report anxiety,[9] with 60% to 80% rating this as moderate and up to 20% as severe.[9] Dyspnoea and tachypnoea are generated by fear and anxiety as well as being signs of task failure in the weaning patient, creating a vicious cycle in susceptible patients that culminates in weaning failure before objective muscular fatigue can be detected.[10] A number of stressors make patients vulnerable to fear and anxiety in this setting, including a high prevalence of fatigue, depression and disturbed sleep (Figure 18.15). Cognitive behaviour therapy is not a realistic option and treatment, if any, usually relies on benzodiazepines (diazepam, lorazepam) or antidepressants.[15] There is no information on the efficacy

of newer drugs such as pregabalin[16] or buspirone[17] in the ICU setting or atypical antidepressants such as tianeptine. More recently, a number of other potential targets have been identified for the treatment of anxiety, including receptors for glutamate, GABA-A, corticotropin-releasing factor 1 (CRF-1) and the endo-cannabinoids, as well as neuronal voltage-gated potassium channels.[18] Somatic symptoms of anxiety respond to adrenergic receptor antagonists, and, while β-blockers are the drug of choice in an outpatient setting, in critically ill patients labetolol offers the combined advantages of heart rate control and after-load reduction, and is probably underutilized. Psychological support in the form of biofeedback or hypnosis have been shown in specific cases to accelerate weaning, while a number of studies have shown that music therapy is effective in reducing anxiety in ventilator-dependent patients. Depression and

---

[15] For example, selective serotonin re-uptake inhibitors (SSRI) such as sertraline, citalopram, paroxetine or fluoxetine; selective noradrenaline re-uptake inhibitors (SNRI) such as venlafaxine; tricyclic antidepressant drugs such as amitriptylline or monoamine oxidase inhibitors (MAOI) such as phenelzine or tranylcypromine.

[16] An anticonvulsant which inhibits the release of excitatory neurotransmitters by binding to the α_2-δ sub-unit of the voltage-gated calcium channel which is also licensed in the UK for the treatment of generalized anxiety disorder.
[17] An agonist at the 5-HT1A receptor.
[18] Retigabine.

Table 18.9 Causes of hyper-metabolism

1) Over-feeding
2) Systemic inflammation
   a. Burns
   b. Sepsis
   c. Erythroderma (drug rash, psoriasis, eczema, Sezary syndrome)
3) Hyperthyroidism
4) Catecholamines
   - Exogenous (i.e. therapeutic administration)
   - Endogenous (phaeochromocytoma)
5) Hyper-pyrexial disorders
   - Malignant hyperthermia
   - Neuroleptic malignant syndrome
   - Serotonin syndrome
   - Central anti-cholinergic syndrome
6) Seizures
7) Drugs
   - Amphetamines and ecstasy
   - Theophylline
8) Mania
9) Hyperactive delirium

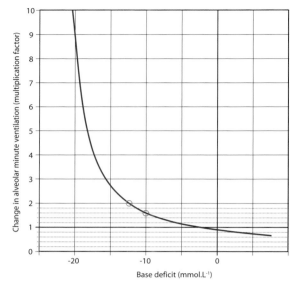

Figure 18.16 Increase in alveolar minute ventilation required to maintain a pH of 7.35 as the base deficit increases.

In the absence of a metabolic acidosis (base excess of zero) the alveolar ventilation only needs to be 0.9 of the normal (i.e. modest hypoventilation) to maintain a pH of 7.35, which is at the bottom end of the normal range. Once the base deficit has fallen to −10 mmol.L^{-1}, which represents a significant metabolic acidosis, alveolar ventilation has to increase to 1.6 times normal (i.e. a 60% increase) to maintain this pH. When the base deficit has fallen to −12.4 mmol.L^{-1}, alveolar ventilation needs to double to maintain this pH.

The graph is calculated on the basis of an adult producing 200 mL.minute^{-1} of carbon dioxide, a normal plasma bicarbonate concentration of 22.4 mmol.L^{-1}, a normal pH of 7.4 and a normal arterial partial pressure of carbon dioxide of 5 kPa.

hopelessness respond more quickly to psychostimulants[19] than traditional antidepressants. Sleep disturbance is associated with loss of both a normal sleep/wake cycle and circadian patterns of melatonin secretion, as well as a significant reduction of rapid eye movement (REM) sleep. Both the intensive care unit environment and drugs contribute to sleep disturbance. This may be amenable to exogenous melatonin supplementation, although a recent placebo-controlled evaluation showed no benefit.[11]

Hormonal state or inflammation. An increased metabolic rate can be caused in a number of ways (Table 18.9) and will impose an additional burden on the respiratory system. With the exception of over-feeding, sepsis, and exogenous catecholamines, most are uncommon and, if present, unlikely to be overlooked.

---

[19] Such as methylphenidate.

Metabolic acidosis. Non-respiratory acidosis in the ICU patient usually arises in one of two ways, tissue hypoperfusion or renal impairment. Patients with a metabolic acidosis from tissue hypoperfusion are usually too unwell for this phase of weaning. The vast majority of patients in this situation will have a metabolic acidosis from renal impairment. This adds considerably to the patient's respiratory workload (Figure 18.16). In patients who remain dependent on renal replacement therapy (RRT), the acidosis can be treated by increasing the duration or frequency of RRT or by using a more efficient technique, such as dialysis. For patients recovering from a renal insult and in whom there may be reasons for wanting to avoid RRT, the acidosis can be buffered by the administration of alkali, for example sodium bicarbonate.

Dead space. The proportion of each breath that does not come into contact with gas-exchanging tissue is called dead space. It is composed of gas that enters alveoli with no blood supply (physiological dead space), gas that sits in conducting airways such as the bronchi and distal trachea (anatomical dead space), and gas that sits in any equipment distal to the Y-piece of the ventilator circuit such as the tracheal tube and catheter mount (equipment dead space). Because dead space does not contribute to gas exchange, it is compensated for by an increase in either tidal volume or respiratory rate, either of which will add to the work of breathing. Relatively small apparent changes in equipment dead space, for example, in changing from ventilation through a tracheostomy tube to ventilation through the normal anatomical airway, can have significant (+30%) effects on the work of breathing.[12] Unnecessary increases in equipment dead-space, such as heat-and-moisture exchange filters or extended catheter mounts, should be avoided in patients who are difficult to wean.

For a given minute volume ($\dot{V} = V_T \times f$), tidal volume and respiratory rate are inversely related (Figure 18.17), and with increasing respiratory rate the work of breathing due to resistance increases, while that due to elastance (tidal volume) falls. Total work of breathing, which is the sum of the two components, thus describes a U-shaped curve with a minimum value in normal individuals falling between 12 and 15 breaths per minute (Figure 18.18, Panel A). An increase in resistance has the effect of causing the most efficient respiratory rate to drop (Figure 18.18, Panel B), while an increase in elastance has the opposite effect (Figure 18.18, Panel C).

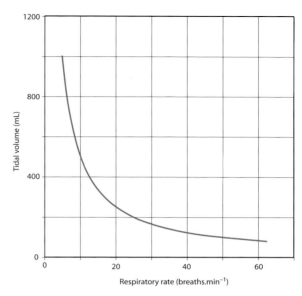

Figure 18.17 Relationship between respiratory rate and tidal volume with a constant minute volume.

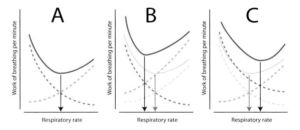

Figure 18.18 Relationship between respiratory rate (x axis) and total work of breathing (red line) for a given alveolar minute volume.

Total work is composed of elastance work (tidal volume, blue dotted line) which falls as the respiratory rate increases and resistance work (respiratory rate, yellow dotted line) which rises with the respiratory rate. The most efficient respiratory rate depends on the balance between resistance and elastance work (see text for details).

Determinants of the capacity to supply the work of breathing

In simple terms, the capacity to supply the work of breathing depends on two factors: the *strength* of the respiratory muscles to provide the desired tidal volume and the *endurance* to provide this tidal volume

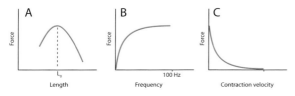

Figure 18.19 Relationship between force generated by a single muscle fibre and pre-contraction length, stimulation frequency and contraction velocity.

repeatedly at a rate that can provide the required alveolar minute volume.

Like nerves, muscle cells at rest are normally polarized, with the inside of the cell about 70 mV more negative than the outside. The arrival of a neural impulse at the motor end-plate causes the release of acetylcholine which rapidly diffuses across the neuromuscular junction to bind with acetylcholine receptors in the post-synaptic membrane of the muscle fibre. Activation of the acetylcholine receptors causes sodium channels in the muscle cell membrane to open briefly, allowing sodium to rush in to the muscle fibre. If enough acetylcholine receptors have been activated, enough sodium is able to enter the muscle cell to cause the intracellular voltage to rise above the trigger threshold, which then causes voltage-gated calcium channels to open in the membrane surrounding an intracellular calcium store (the sarcoplasmic reticulum), allowing calcium ions to flood into the muscle cell. The rise in free intracellular calcium concentration activates the actin-myosin complex, resulting in muscular contraction, though it is limited by the rapid re-uptake of free intracellular calcium back into sarcoplasmic reticulum. The force (Newtons, N) that a single muscle fibre is able to generate naturally depends on its cross-sectional area (m^2), but thereafter depends on the overlap between actin and myosin (pre-contraction length), the frequency with which the nerve impulses arrive (impulses per second, Hz), and the velocity of contraction ($m.s^{-1}$; see Figure 18.19), as well as its intrinsic contractility

(strength). In *whole* muscles, which are composed of groups of muscle fibres that share a common motor neuron (motor units), the strength of contraction is further controlled by the sequential recruitment of *additional* motor units under both reflex and voluntary control, a process termed 'recruitment' (Figure 18.20). While *complete* disruption of any of the links in the neuromuscular chain of command (Figure 18.2) will prevent any patient-initiated respiratory effort at all, *partial* disruption at any point will reduce the patient's capacity to supply the work of breathing and will appear as respiratory muscle weakness and effort intolerance.

CENTRAL NERVOUS SYSTEM

In practice *previously unrecognized* central nervous system pathology (CNS; Figure 18.2) is very unusual as a cause of impaired respiratory performance following a period of mechanical ventilation, although it should not be overlooked in patients for whom no other cause can be found. In most patients CNS pathology is recognized *prior* to the onset of mechanical ventilation and, in cases where this is the cause of the respiratory failure, the decision whether or not to institute respiratory support is made very difficult because of the irreversibility of the majority of these conditions and the low probability of successful extubation (4% in motor neuron disease, 20% in dense hemispheric infarction, 50% in multiple sclerosis). Covert high cervical cord trauma either where the presenting clinical problem distracts the clinicians from looking for cervical trauma (see Box 18.4), or where the injury is sustained by a patient with unknown or overlooked atlanto-axial instability during tracheal intubation, is an unusual cause of acquired CNS damage resulting in respiratory muscle weakness.

Late recovery of respiratory function has been reported following some forms of CNS damage but for the majority of patients this is an irreversible cause of respiratory failure

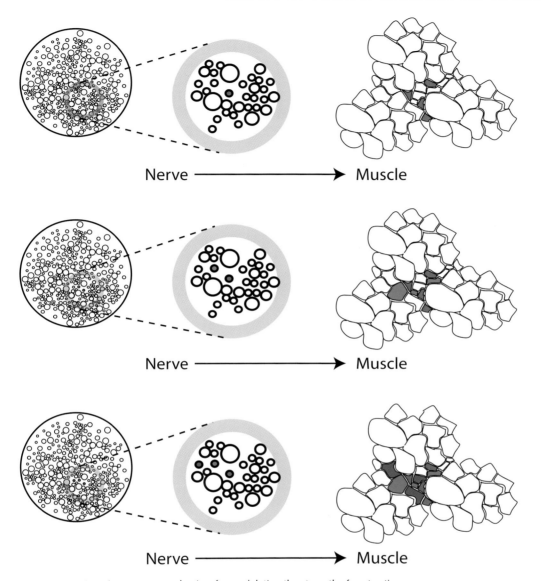

Figure 18.20 Recruitment as a mechanism for modulating the strength of contraction.

The diagram represents a motor nerve (left) with a section of the motor neurones shown in detail (pink circle), and the muscle that this nerve supplies (right). Increasing strength of contraction from top to bottom is mediated, in part, by the recruitment of additional motor neurones (red, then green, then blue) and their associated motor units.

requiring long-term mechanical support (see Chapter 19).

PERIPHERAL NERVE

As with pathology of the central nervous system, pre-existing pathology of the peripheral nerves, which can cause difficulty with weaning, is not common, although modest degrees of neuropathy may be a contributory factor in some patients with diabetes, malnutrition or alcohol abuse. With the exception of Guillain–Barré, other causes of peripheral neuropathy (Table 18.10) that cause or

Box 18.4

A 56-year-old man was admitted to the intensive care unit following an out-of-hospital cardiac arrest associated with a myocardial infarction. After 2 days of mechanical ventilation all sedative medication was discontinued, but after a further 48 hours the patient remained completely unresponsive to peripheral stimuli and showed no signs of respiratory effort. Initially, it was assumed that the man had suffered a severe hypoxic brain injury. Later, a neurological examination revealed that the patient had intact cranial nerve reflexes associated with flaccid tetraplegia, highly suggestive of a cervical cord lesion. A lateral radiograph of the patient's neck revealed a fracture-dislocation of C5 on C6. Review of the ambulance records showed that the man had been found on the floor at the bottom of a flight of stairs.

Table 18.10 Peripheral motor (± sensory) neuropathy associated with respiratory failure present before the institution of mechanical ventilation

Trauma – Neck stabbing, chiropractic manipulation, blunt neck trauma.

Viral infections – Herpes zoster, West Nile virus

Bacterial infections – Diphtheria, Lyme disease

Vasculitis – Systemic lupus erythematosus, Wegener's disease, polymyositis

Immune-mediated – Guillain–Barré, neuralgic amyotrophy, paraneoplastic, chronic idiopathic demyelinating polyradiculoneuropathy

Other – Diabetes, alcoholism, malnutrition, lead poisoning, porphyria, sarcoidosis

contribute to respiratory failure are rare. In contrast, neuropathy, acquired *after* the onset of mechanical ventilation, is much more common, has the potential to be overlooked, and falls into two main categories: physical injury to the phrenic nerves and critical illness polyneuropathy.

Injury to the phrenic nerves has been reported following surgery to the neck or thoracic inlet, inter-scalene nerve block and central line insertion, but by far the commonest setting is following cardiac surgery, where the incidence may be as high as 10%. The commonest mechanism during cardiothoracic surgery is thermal injury from the ice slush used to cool the heart during cardiac bypass, although direct damage may occur during the harvesting of the internal mammary arteries for coronary artery grafting or in the removal of tumours involving the nerves. Sensitive detection of phrenic nerve damage requires special techniques such a diaphragmatic electromyography, phrenic nerve conduction studies or diaphragmatic ultrasonography: this is because traditional techniques such as plain radiography[20] or paradoxical diaphragm movement demonstrated by fluoroscopy during a sniff, are neither sensitive nor specific. The impact that phrenic nerve dysfunction has on the capacity to self-ventilate depends on the degree of dysfunction (partial versus complete or unilateral versus bilateral) and the presence of co-existing pulmonary pathology, and can range from very modest prolongation of the weaning process to long-term dependence on ventilatory support.

Neuropathy acquired during the course of critical illness was originally described in 1983 as a mixed[13] or pure motor[14] axonal polyneuropathy. Prospective studies on patients requiring mechanical ventilation for more than 7 days suggest that this 'critical illness polyneuropathy' (CIP) occurs in up to 41% of patients, while in patients selected on the basis of sepsis and multiple organ failure an incidence of between 53% and 100% has been reported. In high-risk patients CIP has been detected within a few days of ICU admission and is found in up to 78% of patients who are difficult to wean. There is reasonable evidence that the risk of CIP appears

---

[20] Looking for a raised hemi-diaphragm in unilateral phrenic nerve palsy.

to increase with both the duration and severity of illness, while the role of neuromuscular-blocking drugs, corticosteroids, aminoglycosides, hypoalbuminaemia and female sex is less clear. A role for hyperglycaemia in precipitating CIP has been suggested both directly and indirectly, which is supported by the finding that intensive glycaemic control significantly reduces the incidence of CIP.[15]

The severity and duration of weakness secondary to immune-mediated demyelinating neuropathies, such as Guillain–Barré syndrome, can be reduced by early aggressive immunosuppression with plasma exchange and methylprednisolone. Established demylination and axonal neuropathies have no specific therapy, but do improve with the passage of time. Traumatic neuropathies related to cardiac surgery are best avoided by avoiding the use of ice slush for cardioprotection.

NEUROMUSCULAR CONDUCTION

Although occasionally reported, the chance of a previously undiagnosed neuromuscular disorder, such as myasthenia gravis or Eaton–Lambert syndrome, causing difficulty weaning is very small. Similarly, patients presenting with a respiratory failure associated with botulism, tick paralysis or organophosphate poisoning are likely to present with a history that suggests the diagnosis. Prolonged post-operative neuromuscular blockade can occur in patients who are unable to metabolize these drugs, either through deficiency of plasma cholinesterase (suxamethonium, mivacurium), or impaired hepatic (vecuronium, rocuronium, pancuronium) or renal function (vecuronium), but normal neuromuscular function usually returns within a day or two at the most. Neuromuscular transmission can also be reduced by therapeutic use of magnesium and other drugs including gentamicin, procainamide, neomycin and quinine. In general, however, impaired neuromuscular transmission is not a significant cause of prolonged weaning.

The synthesis of antibodies directed at components of the pre-synaptic (Eaton–Lambert), or post-synaptic (myasthenia) apparatus, which interfere with neuromuscular conduction, can sometimes be reduced by removal of the inciting tumour or by immunosuppression with corticosteroids, with residual impairment often responding to treatment with long-acting anti-cholinesterases such as pyridostigmine. Drug-mediated interference with neuromuscular conduction resolves as these drugs are metabolized, providing that continued administration is avoided.

MUSCLE FUNCTION

The majority of inherited disorders of muscle function, such as the myopathies, muscular dystrophies[21] or myotonic[22] disorders, present during childhood or early adulthood and in a similar way to the progressive neurological disorders may present ethical dilemmas when respiratory failure supervenes. These are only very rarely diagnosed in the course of prolonged weaning. Late-onset acid maltase deficiency and facio scapulo humeral dystrophy are unusual causes of respiratory failure arising in middle-aged adults. None of these myopathies have specific treatments. Acquired myopathies that can result in respiratory failure include polymyositis and dermatomyositis, as well as those caused by electrolyte imbalance (hypokalaemia, hypophosphataemia, hypocalcaemia, hypermagnesaemia or hypomagnesaemia), endocrine disorders (hyperthyroidism and hypothyroidism, hypercortisolism and Addison's disease), and drug-related myopathies. Although not reported as a cause of respiratory failure, it is likely that systemic causes of myositis and rhabdomyolysis will involve the respiratory muscles and in some cases contribute to respiratory muscle weakness. This would apply to patients

---

[21] Duchenne, Becker, facioscapulohumeral limb-girdle
[22] Myotonic dystrophy.

requiring mechanical ventilation with heat stroke, viral[23] or bacterial[24] myositis and toxic rhabdomyolysis. All of these problems are much more likely to present with weakness rather than arising as insidious causes of weakness following ICU admission. There are, however, two distinct conditions that are acquired during periods of critical illness requiring mechanical ventilation that specifically interfere with respiratory muscle function, namely ventilator-induced diaphragmatic dysfunction and critical illness myopathy.

Ventilator-induced diaphragmatic dysfunction (VIDD). Diaphragm inactivity caused by mechanical ventilation results in a significant reduction in diaphragmatic strength that worsens with the duration of mechanical ventilation and which is reduced by the use of a triggered mode of ventilation rather than continuous mandatory ventilation. See Chapter 14 for further details.

Critical illness myopathy (CIM). A number of myopathies have been described under the general rubric of CIM, and it is currently unclear whether these are distinct disorders or different views of the same condition that reflect a selection bias in the patients studied. Given that critically ill patients are almost certain to receive the support of mechanical ventilation, it is highly likely that most patients will develop some degree of VIDD (see earlier). In addition to this, but completely independently of VIDD, systemic inflammation results in significant reductions in diaphragm strength and endurance. A reduction in diaphragmatic function is also seen in hyperoxia. Attenuation of this phenomenon by a range of free radical scavengers indicates a significant causative role for the oxidant damage. This is also the mechanism suspected in VIDD. Mechanical unloading of the diaphragm by artificial ventilation abrogates, to some extent, the damage under these circumstances perhaps by reducing oxygen influx.

Either as an exaggerated form of this myopathy, or as a distinct entity, others have described a form associated with rises in creatine kinase concentrations in patients receiving high doses of corticosteroids either with or without non-depolarizing muscle relaxants, the so-called *acute necrotizing myopathy.* Finally, a third form, the *thick filament myopathy,* has been described where electron microscopy reveals loss of myosin.

Clinical features cannot distinguish between the variants of CIM, or even between CIM and CIP. All of these conditions are characterized by flaccid weakness. Deep tendon reflexes may be normal or depressed. In contrast to myositis, myalgia is unusual in CIM, and the plasma concentration of creatine kinase may be normal. In contrast, a modest increase in the plasma concentration of creatine kinase, not unusual in critically ill patients, may be found in patients with CIP. Finally, needle electromyography cannot distinguish between CIP and CIM in unconscious or sedated patients in whom the distinction can only be made by muscle biopsy or measurement of compound muscle action potentials from direct muscle stimulation. Studies which have used these more invasive techniques suggest that CIM is even more common than CIP.[16]

Fatigue. Fatigue is defined as the inability to sustain a muscular work rate (power output) and is limited by features of the entire chain of command illustrated in Figure 18.2, from brain to muscle. In normal subjects the maximum sustainable muscular power output is limited in three specific ways. First, it is limited by the sustainable power output of the muscle itself, referred to here as *intrinsic* fatigue.[25] Second, it is limited by the capacity of the neuromuscular junction to transmit impulses,

---

[23] Influenza, coxsackie, dengue, cytomegalovirus, West Nile virus, HIV.

[24] Leptospirosis, mycoplasma.

[25] In the literature, this has usually been termed *low-frequency fatigue,* but for the non-expert this term is confusing for two reasons. First, it might be interpreted to suggest that the loss of force generation is the result of a fall in the frequency of action potentials arriving from the spinal cord, which is in fact the mechanism of spinal fatigue. Second, and based on

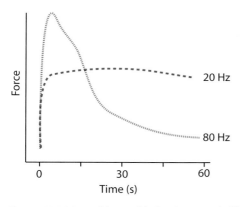

Force

20 Hz

80 Hz

0   30   60
Time (s)

Figure 18.21 Loss of force with time in a muscle fibre stimulated at 80 Hz (red) or 20 Hz (blue).

referred to here as *neuromuscular transmission* fatigue. Third, it is limited by *neural* fatigue which has two components, (1) the number of motor units that are activated and the rate of motor neuron firing (Figure 18.19, panel B), referred to here as *spinal* fatigue, and (2) central nervous system drive, which is a function of complex emotional factors, and which is referred to here as *central* fatigue.

Intrinsic fatigue can be differentiated into high- and low-frequency types on the basis of the stimulation frequency that results in contractile failure (Figure 18.21). High-frequency fatigue arises rapidly, recovers rapidly, and is caused by a failure of t-tubule depolarization, decreased calcium release from the sarcoplasmic reticulum and failure of excitation-contraction coupling. Low-frequency fatigue arises more slowly, requires prolonged rest for recovery and was thought to arise from the inhibition of actin-myosin interaction by intracellular lactic acidosis and elevated concentrations of inorganic phosphate, a view based on experiments performed at room temperature. More recently, it has been shown that the effects of both acidosis and inorganic phosphate are

the first misunderstanding, it might lead the non-expert into believing that the reduction in action potential frequency explains the left-shift of the surface EMG power spectrum that has been shown to occur just prior to the onset of fatigue.

markedly attenuated at $37\,°C$ but that reductions in myofibrillar calcium sensitivity are caused by reactive oxygen species. Low-frequency, but not high-frequency, fatigue can be reduced in both skeletal and respiratory muscles by prior administration of N-acetylcysteine, which enhances the availability of intracellular cysteine and glutathione (Figure 18.22).

There is no question that the normal human diaphragm can become *intrinsically* fatigued under experimental conditions, that it occurs when tidal forces above 40% of the maximum inspiratory force are required, and that recovery to normal contractility takes many hours. However, in the clinical situation, intrinsic fatigue of respiratory muscles does not appear to contribute to weaning failure[10] because of the intervention of more proximal mechanisms.

Spinal fatigue is thought to arise from a fall in the frequency of action potentials generated by the anterior horn cells of the spinal cord as a reflex to prevent complete contraction failure. Although the force of muscle fibre contraction is determined by the frequency of stimulation (Figure 18.19 panel B), the sustainability of a contraction is inversely proportional to firing frequency (Figure 18.21). On the basis that the pattern of force loss in peripheral skeletal muscle during a maximal voluntary contraction can be mimicked by stimulating the motor nerve with a gradually reducing stimulating frequency, it has been assumed that this phenomenon is mediated centrally (perhaps at spinal level) in order to prevent fatigue arising from high-frequency stimulation, a phenomenon referred to as 'central wisdom'.[17] *Central* fatigue describes an involuntary and subconscious reduction of motor drive that has been shown to account in some studies,[18] but not in others,[19] for a significant proportion of the fall in diaphragmatic force during prolonged inspiratory loading. In the clinical situation, it has been suggested that central fatigue protects against the development of intrinsic fatigue in patients whose

10 Hz

40 Hz

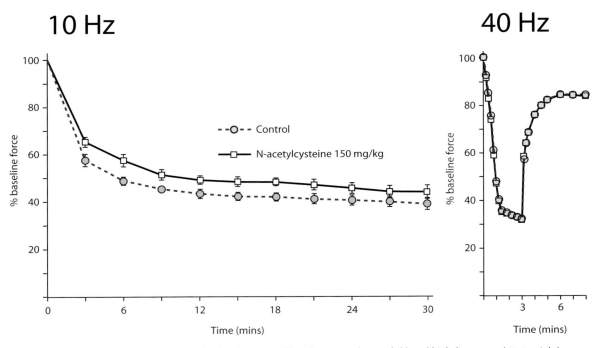

Figure 18.22 Effect of N-acetylcysteine on the development of low-frequency (10 Hz, left) and high-frequency (40 Hz, right) fatigue in tibialis anterior muscle in man.

Derived from data in Reid MB, Stokic DS, Koch SM *et al. J Clin Invest.* 1994;94(6):2468–74.

work of breathing is excessive.[10] Both central and spinal fatigue appear to be mechanisms designed to protect the organism from developing either intrinsic fatigue or exceeding the cardiovascular system's ability to supply substrate. So, for example, limited exercise tolerance in patients with stable congestive cardiac failure was *not* associated with intrinsic diaphragmatic fatigue, despite significant functional limitation. The central governor is therefore able to limit neural drive to ensure a balance between demand and supply, even where the latter has been compromised by hypoxia, anaemia or heart failure. Respiratory fatigue, by whatever mechanism, is accompanied by an increase in sympathetic drive and even more so if accompanied by hypoxia. The increased cardiac after-load and heart rate increase myocardial oxygen demand just when the oxygen supply may be limited by hypoxaemia and global oxygen consumption increased, causing

the mixed venous saturation to fall. Compromised left ventricular function causes left atrial pressure to rise, leading to a fall in pulmonary compliance and an increase in the work of breathing. This is a potentially fatal downward spiral. Acute myocardial ischaemia during weaning is associated with weaning failure which has been reversed by inotropes, angioplasty and coronary artery bypass surgery.

IMPROVING RESPIRATORY MUSCLE FUNCTION

Having established that weakness is due to myopathy by consideration of the history, appropriate clinical examination, laboratory and neurophysiological investigations, the differentiation between VIDD and CIM with muscle biopsy does not provide additional information that might benefit the patient. What is required are strategies for enhancing muscle bulk, contractility (strength), endurance and effort

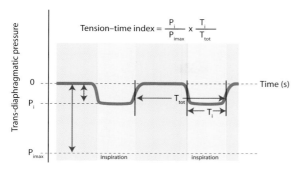

Figure 18.23 Calculation of the diaphragmatic tension–time index as a measure of respiratory system work-load or power output.

Tension–time index $= \dfrac{P_i}{P_{imax}} \times \dfrac{T_i}{T_{tot}}$

Table 18.11 Non-training strategies for enhancing physical performance

1) Increase muscle mass
   a. Anabolic steroids (nandrolone, testosterone, dihydrotestosterone, andostenedione, dehydroepiandrostenedione, clostebol)
   b. Human chorionic gonadrotrophin (males only)
   c. Luteinizing hormone (males only)
   d. Growth hormone
   e. Insulin
   f. Insulin-like growth factor
2) Increase contractility
   a. Methylxanthines (e.g. caffeine)
   b. Amphetamines
   c. Cocaine
   d. β-adrenergic agonists
3) Increasing oxygen delivery
   a. Erythropoeitin
   b. Blood transfusion
4) Psychological approaches
   a. Stress reduction (alcohol, cannabinoids, hypnotism, music therapy)
   b. Motivation

tolerance in order to improve respiratory muscle performance.

In the first instance, as discussed earlier under 'When should weaning be initiated?', VIDD and respiratory muscle wasting should be minimized by converting to a patient-triggered mode of ventilation as soon as possible.

Training. Muscle training occurs as a physiological adaptation to stress, with the pattern of adaptation (strength or endurance) being determined by characteristics of the stress imposed. Respiratory muscle responds to training in exactly the same way as skeletal muscle, resulting in significant performance enhancement in both normal individuals and patients alike, and has been successfully used to aid weaning from mechanical ventilation. The normal principles of muscular training established by sports physiologists apply to the respiratory system and require that an adequate load is applied for a sufficient length of time and that sufficient rest is allowed. However, there is evidence that loads capable of inducing *intrinsic* fatigue can induce muscle damage with the extent of damage being proportional to the load. Respiratory system load (power output) may be expressed as the tension–time index (Figure 18.23), which is a function of the maximum inspiratory pressure with respiratory fatigue occurring with a tension–time index above 0.15.[20] Clinical training sessions have generally only lasted 10

to 30 minutes, been performed on 5 to 7 days per week, and required an estimated tension–time index of between 0.1 to 0.3. The world of elite competitive sport has had a long-standing interest in the use of strategies *in addition to* training for enhancing performance (Table 18.11), but only some of these have been used to assist in the weaning process.

Muscle mass. Male patients requiring prolonged mechanical ventilation have been shown to have low blood concentrations of testosterone, with the potential that this might be interfering with muscle function. Androgen therapy in the presence of documented hypogonadism is not controversial. Supraphysiological doses of androgens increase muscle mass and strength in normal men, with an effect that is mediated through insulin-like growth factor 1 (IGF-1). Pharmacological androgen therapy has been used with some success in patients with chronic wasting disorders, such as the acquired immunodeficiency syndrome (AIDS), but in a small trial in surgical ventilator-dependent patients, androgen therapy was associated with increased mortality.[21] Reversal of muscle catabolism with growth hormone has been attempted, but despite being able to promote a positive nitrogen balance, the use of synthetic growth hormone appears to increase mortality.[22] Growth hormone therapy is associated with a significant deterioration in glycaemic control and evidence that this alone might increase mortality in critically ill patients is accumulating.[15, 23] It is quite possible, therefore, that with adequate glycaemic control growth hormone therapy may be beneficial.

Contractility. The methylxanthines, and in particular aminophylline, have been used clinically for the relief of bronchospasm since the mid-1950s. Suspicion that the clinical benefits of aminophylline seemed disproportionate to its potency as a bronchodilator prompted an investigation into the effects of aminophylline on diaphragmatic contractility. Aminophylline improves diaphragmatic contractility both in vitro and in vivo and a number of other studies have shown a significant effect in both volunteers[24] and patients.[25] Successful weaning has been credited to aminophylline-induced improvement of diaphragmatic function.[26] Despite the lack of evidence, the use of methylxanthines may be warranted in selected patients.

Oxygen delivery. Exercise tolerance and performance is related to haemoglobin concentration in patients with heart failure just as much as in elite athletes, and correction of anaemia may allow some patients to wean successfully.

Motivation. The effect of motivation on physical performance is beyond question, and motivation, or lack of it, is an integral component of the psychological response to weaning (Figure 18.15). Motivation is a complex psychological phenomenon[27] and optimizing a patient's motivation is unlikely to be achieved simply by exhortations to 'try harder'.

This is an area that is in desperate need of further work.

CONDUCTING THE SECOND STAGE

The second stage of weaning can start when 100% of the patient's minute-volume is generated by patient-triggered breaths in either a hybrid or triggered mode of mechanical ventilation. At this point, the balance between load and capacity is unknown. Investigators have used a huge range of static and dynamic tests of lung mechanics and respiratory muscle strength, either singly or in combination, in order to try to predict which patients can tolerate unassisted ventilation,[26] but unfortunately none of these work well enough. The conclusion, therefore, from recent consensus guidelines[28] is this point can only be determined by daily assessments using a spontaneous breathing trial (SBT) of between 30 and 120 minutes where 'failure' is measured by a combination of objective and subjective criteria (Table 18.12). It does not appear to make any difference whether the SBT is conducted with a T-piece, a CPAP circuit ($5\,cm\,H_2O$) or pressure support ($<7\,cm\,H_2O$) and PEEP, but there does not appear to be any benefit from conducting more than one SBT per day.[29] Failure of the first SBT should prompt a systematic evaluation and correction of factors that might be contributing to the work of breathing or to neuromuscular weakness, while failure of a further two or three should lead to consideration of tracheostomy.

Hesitation about the timing of tracheostomy has, to some extent, been based on the perception that a surgical procedure of this nature is not a trivial undertaking and the benefits need to clearly outweigh the risks. The increasing popularity of percutaneous techniques together with careful patient selection and a better appreciation of the risks and

---

[26] Unfortunately, a number of these studies have used successful extubation as the end-point, overlooking the fact that a patient might be perfectly capable of self-ventilating without being able to tolerate extubation or de-cannulation.

Table 18.12 Criteria used to terminate a spontaneous breathing trial

	Brochard, 1994[48]	Ely, 1996[49]	Kollef, 1997[50]	Valverrdu, 1998[51]
SpO2		<90%	<90%	
PaO2	<6.7 kPa			
pH	<7.32			
HR	+20%	>140 or ±20%	≥140	>140 or ±20% or arrhythmias
BP	+20%	<90 or >180	<90 or >180	<80 or >160
RR	>35 min⁻¹ or +50%	>35 min	>35	>35 min or +50%
Mental condition	Agitation or ↓LOC	Anxiety	Agitation, anxiety or ↓LOC	Agitation or ↓LOC
Discomfort			Chest pain	
Sweating	Yes	Yes	Yes	Yes

benefits (see Chapter 17), such as reductions in the work of breathing, sedation requirements, risk of ventilator-associated pneumonia and the duration of mechanical ventilation, have made early tracheostomy a much more acceptable option.

Between each daily SBT, the patient should be returned either to a non-fatiguing mode of ventilation with either a constant level of support or support that is only slowly and modestly reduced.

A number of ventilator manufacturers offer modes of ventilation that are automatic in the sense of providing a variable level of pressure support depending on patient effort, for example Adaptive Support Ventilation (Hamilton Medical) and SmartCare (Draeger). The latter has recently been evaluated in a prospective multicentre randomized controlled trial[30] and was shown to result in more rapid weaning than traditional physician-guided weaning.

PROTOCOLS

Failure to wean efficiently may be caused either by a failure to pursue the *best* strategy or to pursue an *agreed* strategy. These failings are minimized in units that are managed by specialists in intensive care medicine and when steps are taken to promote continuity of management. The extent to which the introduction of a protocol is able to acceler-

Table 18.13 Factors that determine a physician's clinical management strategy

1) Training and education
   Undergraduate
   Post-qualification
2) Experience
   Length of service
   Primary specialty
3) Personality and outlook

ate the weaning process is therefore a measure of the deficiencies of the existing clinical management system as well as the ability of the particular protocol to correct them. Of the four prospective randomized trials of protocol-driven weaning, which were all conducted in the US, three showed significant reductions in the duration of mechanical ventilation[31, 32, 33] and one did not,[34] with the latter conducted in a 'closed', academic and highly protocol-driven unit. The benefit of protocols, which have been endorsed by the American College of Chest Physicians, the American Association of Respiratory Care and the American College of Critical Care Medicine,[28] are likely to be most significant in units in which patients are primarily managed by doctors who are not intensive care specialists or where the continuity of care is jeopardized by frequent changes in leadership and in the absence of a commonly agreed-upon approach.

Table 18.14 Criteria for extubation or de-cannulation

1) An artificial airway is not required to maintain the patency of the patient's upper airway.
2) The patient has sufficient neurological function to protect their airway and any increased risk to the airway has subsided or has been treated.
3) The patient has the strength, coordination and laryngeal function to expectorate their pulmonary secretions.
4) The patient has the strength and endurance to breathe on their own.

There are, however, significant obstacles to the introduction and implementation of clinical protocols which have been recognized by those with internationally recognized expertise in the subject, and which have met reluctance by clinicians to accept the need for change or to adapt to changes following implementation. Successful implementation is assisted by the provision of feedback and by locally obtained evidence of the impact of the protocol on relevant outcomes. Furthermore, it is accepted that protocols should not be considered as static constructs, but should be adapted or improved as part of a continuous Plan-Do-Study-Act (PDSA) cycle.

Extubation and de-cannulation

Removal of the endotracheal tube, *extubation*, or tracheostomy tube, *de-cannulation*, is appropriate provided that four conditions are met (Table 18.14).

AIRWAY PATENCY

Upper airway obstruction from external compression,[27] intrinsic inflammation[28] or a mass[29] is an uncommon indication for intubation or tracheostomy (Figure 18.24). In these cases, neurological or muscular dysfunction is almost never an issue. Extubation or de-cannulation can only be contemplated when the airway obstruction has resolved, which may require surgical intervention or some other form of treatment such as antibiotics, steroids, topical vasoconstrictors, chemotherapy or radiotherapy. If definitive relief of the obstruction with surgery is not appropriate, resolution of the obstruction must be gauged clinically and radiologically. If the cuff of the tracheal tube is at the site of the obstruction, an increase in airway diameter will be heralded by a spontaneous cuff leak. However, if the cuff of the tracheal tube is distal to the site of the obstruction, resolution will occur without generating a cuff leak (Figure 18.25). In this situation, the condition of the airway can be intermittently tested by listening for the presence of a leak around the tracheal tube during complete deflation of the cuff. Once a cuff leak has been detected, resolution of the airway obstruction can be assessed more accurately by computerized tomography. If this confirms sufficient resolution to contemplate extubation, this is best performed in the operating theatre under deep inhalational anaesthesia and in the presence of an experienced ENT surgeon.

Upper airway narrowing can also arise as a *consequence* of intubation and occurs in 5% to 10% of patients. Post-extubation stridor is more common in females, patients who have been intubated for more than 36 hours and in patients who have been intubated with an oversized tube.[35] Assessment of the degree of laryngeal swelling can be made by quantitative measurement of the cuff leak, which can be expressed either as an absolute volume or as a proportion of the tidal volume. In a recent study, only 2.7% of patients with a cuff leak greater than 110 mL per breath required treatment for post-extubation stridor, making this quite a useful test for ruling out the presence of significant laryngeal oedema.[35] However, only 13.8% of

---

27 Mediastinal lymph nodes, thyroid mass.
28 Acute tracheitis, bacterial epiglottitis, pharyngitis, tonsillitis Ludwig's angina, Vincent's angina, burns, anaphylaxis, angioneurotic oedema.
29 Tumour, abscess or haematoma within the tissues of the airway wall (trachea, larynx, pharynx, tongue).

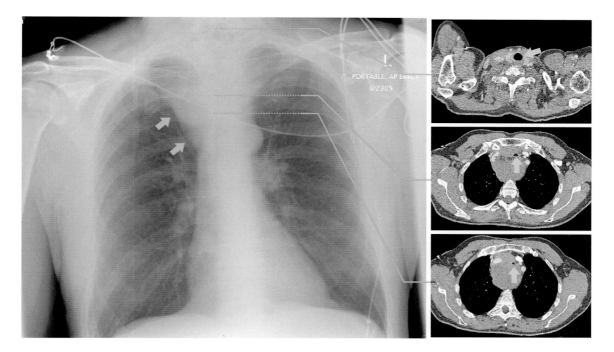

Figure 18.24 Airway compression by mediastinal lymphoma.

The antero-posterior chest radiograph (left) shows a large upper mediastinal mass (blue arrows). Computerized tomography (CT) shows a normal tracheal diameter in the neck above the clavicles (right, top) indicated by the yellow arrow. CT slices just below the clavicles (right, middle) and just above the aortic arch (right, bottom) show progressive narrowing of the trachea (yellow arrows).

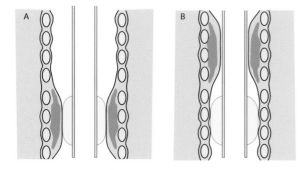

Figure 18.25 The position of upper airway obstruction in relation to the cuff of the tracheal tube.

A: Cuff sited at the point of airway obstruction.

B: Cuff sited below the point of airway obstruction.

those with a cuff leak less than 110 mL had stridor, making this test a weak predictor of post-extubation stridor.[35] A number of studies have examined the value of corticosteroids in reducing the incidence of post-extubation stridor in adults. In three studies, in which a single pre-extubation dose was given, this did not reduce the incidence of either stridor or re-intubation (Figure 18.26). In three more recent studies in which corticosteroids were given every 4 to 6 hours for between 12 and 24 hours prior to extubation, there was a significant reduction in the incidence of both stridor and re-intubation (Figure 18.27). Of these three later studies, two were performed in 'high risk' patients selected on the basis of cuff leak criteria. In these two studies, the re-intubation rate in control patients was 12%. The largest of the three studies was performed in unselected patients ventilated for at least 36 hours, and the re-intubation rate in control patients was only 7.5%. These data suggest that patients intubated for over 36 hours who have a cuff leak less than 110 mL or 24% of the tidal volume should be treated

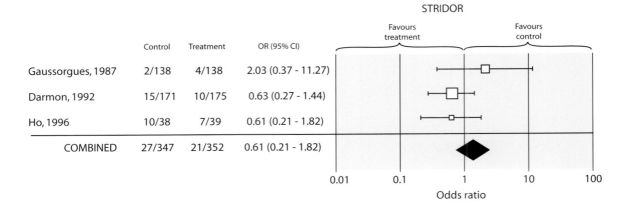

Figure 18.26 Forest plot for three studies of single-dose corticosteroid prior to extubation.

Data from Gaussorgues P, Boyer F, Piperno D *et al. Presse Med.* 1987;16(31):1531–2.

Darmon JY, Rauss A, Dreyfuss D *et al. Anesthesiology.* 1992;77(2):245–51

Ho LI, Harn HJ, Lien TC *et al. Intensive Care Med.* 1996;22(9):933–6.

with corticosteroids for 12 to 24 hours prior to extubation. In those in whom post-extubation stridor develops, nebulized adrenaline may prevent the need for re-intubation. The value of heliox in this setting has yet to be established.

AIRWAY PROTECTION

Tracheal intubation to prevent airway contamination arises in a limited number of situations (Table 18.15). With the exception of those associated with brain dysfunction (brain injury, variceal haemorrhage) airway protection is only needed in the short

term and the patients can be safely extubated with the return of consciousness, or once the bleeding has been controlled. Tracheostomy is indicated in those with neurological dysfunction that may resolve only slowly, if at all.

SECRETION CLEARANCE

Without an effective cough to expectorate pulmonary secretions they accumulate in the tracheobronchial tree and result in a number of complications. These include partial or complete bronchial obstruction, increased work of breathing, infection

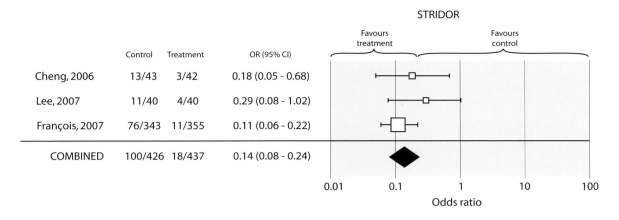

Figure 18.27 Forest plot for three studies of multiple dose corticosteroids for at least 12 hours prior to extubation.

Data from Cheng KC, Hou CC, Huang HC *et al. Crit Care Med.* 2006;34(5):1345–50.

Lee CH, Peng MJ, Wu CL. *Crit Care.* 2007;11(4):R72.

Francois B, Bellissant E, Gissot V *et al. Lancet.* 2007;369(9567):1083–9.

Table 18.15 Indications for acute airway protection

1) Acute reduction in conscious level
   a. Drug overdose
   b. Seizures
   c. Acute brain injury (cerebrovascular accident, traumatic brain injury, cardiac arrest)
2) Acute aspiration risk
   a. Massive upper gastrointestinal bleed
   b. Massive epistaxis
3) 1 and 2 together
   a. Variceal haemorrhage

and ultimately hypoxia and acute respiratory failure. A patient's capacity to prevent the accumulation of pulmonary secretions depends on three main factors (Table 18.16). First, it depends on the ability to appreciate that the airway needs to be cleared. Second, it depends on the strength to expectorate the secretions. Third, it depends on the endurance to prevent the accumulation of airway secretions or aspirated material in the airway.

The effect of impaired airway sensation has yet to be studied, but patients with impaired neurological function are much more likely to require re-intubation. In one study, a Glasgow Coma Score

Table 18.16 Factors required for clearing respiratory secretions

1) Appreciation of the need to cough
   a. Intact upper airway sensation
   b. Intact cortical processing
2) Strength to cough the secretions out of the airway

Patient	Secretions
a. Closed abdominal cavity	d. Viscosity
b. Intact abdominal muscle function	e. Viscidity
Neuromuscular conduction	
Muscle strength	
Uninhibited by pain	
c. Ability to close glottis.	

3) Endurance to cough the volume of secretions produced

Patient	Secretions
a. Endurance	b. Volume

(GCS) under 8 increased the risk three-fold[36] (95% confidence interval 1.8 to 4.7) while in a separate investigation the inability to obey four simple commands[30] increased the risk by 4.3 times[37] (1.8 to 10.4).

Successful expectoration not only depends on the patient's ability to cough, but is also determined by the physical characteristics of the sputum. Cough 'strength' can be estimated in intubated patients either quantitatively, by measuring the peak expiratory flow rate (PEFR), semi-quantitatively with the 'white card test', or qualitatively. A peak expiratory flow rate of 60 L.min^{-1} or less increases the risk of re-intubation 4.8- to 5.1-fold.[37, 38] The 'white card test' simply involves holding a piece of card 1 to 2 cm from the end of the patient's tracheal tube and asking them to cough. The patient is deemed to have passed the test if they can project airway secretions onto the card. A negative white card test increases the risk of re-intubation three-fold[39] (95% confidence interval 1.3 to 6.7), while the qualitatitive assessment of a poor or absent cough increased

the risk 3.9-fold[39] (95% confidence interval 1.8 to 8.9). In de-cannulated patients cough strength is also critically dependant on airtight closure of the tracheostomy stoma. A stoma dressing that bulges or leaks when the patient coughs is *inadequate*, and puts the patient at risk of needing re-cannulation. In patients with large stomas, it may be necessary to use a series of progressively smaller stoma stents[31] to help to keep the stoma plugged as it closes. A weak cough may also be caused by laryngeal dysfunction. Although this is more likely to occur in patients who have been extubated rather then de-cannulated, the actual incidence in either group of patients is unknown. Besides cough strength, sputum viscosity and viscidity also determine the effort required to clear secretions. Mucus management is discussed in Chapter 4.

Over time, the patient's ability to maintain their airway clear of secretions depends on the balance between, on the one hand, their endurance, and on the other, the volume of secretions produced. As discussed above, anaemia impairs stamina, and in one study the risk of re-intubation was over 5.3-fold higher[39] in patients with a haemoglobin under 10 gm.dL^{-1}. Unfavourable respiratory system mechanics are often associated with a high respiratory rate and a small tidal volume, which can be expressed as f/Vт, otherwise known as the rapid shallow breathing index[40] (RSBI). A number of studies have shown that a high RSBI is associated with the risk of re-intubation, with thresholds for failure varying from 100[38] or 105[40] to as little as 57.[41] Respiratory system mechanics improve naturally during the diuretic phase of recovery from acute illness, which heralds the return of a normal capillary reflectance co-efficient and the mobilization of tissue fluid. Patients who are in this phase and

---

30 Open your eyes, follow my hand with your eyes, squeeze my hand, stick out your tongue.

31 These are available in a range of designs from a number of companies including Hood Laboratories (Pembroke, Massachusetts), Natus Medical (San Carlos, California), Bentec Medical (Woodland, California), Boston Medical Products (Westborough, Massachusetts), and Koken (Tokyo).

passing more than 500 mL of urine per six hours[42] or have a negative fluid balance over the preceding 24 hours[41] have a significantly reduced risk of re-intubation. Conversely, a number of studies have confirmed that the volume of secretions is important. For example, moderate or copious secretion production, as judged by the nurse, was associated with an 8.7-fold increased risk of re-intubation[39] (95% confidence interval 2.1 to 35.7). In another study, the production of more than 2.5 mL.hr^{-1} of sputum was associated with three-fold increased risk of re-intubation[37] (95% confidence interval 1 to 8.8). Finally, using suction frequency as a proxy measure for the volume of sputum production it has been shown that patients who require to be suctioned more than once every two hours are 16-fold more likely to require re-intubation[39] (95% confidence interval 2.2 to 116).

INDEPENDENT VENTILATION

Successful completion of a spontaneous breathing trial (SBT) is currently the best evidence that a patient is capable of supplying the work of breathing, as discussed earlier.

EXTUBATION

Extubation is most commonly performed during the earlier part of the day for a number of reasons. First, this is a time when there are plenty of staff available, especially medical staff, who can help to manage any problem that may arise. Second, visibility is high, which means that the patient's post-extubation progress can be easily monitored from a distance. Third, it gives the patient plenty of time to deteriorate during 'office hours' when staff and visibility are at a premium. In case the patient should need immediate re-intubation, steps should be taken to ensure that the patient's stomach is empty at the time of extubation. Patients receiving enteral nutrition via a small-bore tube should have this discontinued four to six hours prior to extubation. Patients being fed through a large-bore

nasogastric tube (12 Fr or more) whose stomachs can be emptied by suction can probably continue to be fed up to one or two hours prior to extubation, although the safety of this approach has not been tested. Facilities for re-intubation should be at hand and an appropriate face mask for delivering oxygen should be assembled ready for use. The extubation procedure should be explained to the patient clearly and calmly. The head of the bed should then be elevated to 30 to 45 degrees and the patient's mouth gently but thoroughly suctioned. If a large-bore nasogastric tube is present, this too should be suctioned to ensure that the stomach is empty. The upper airway should also be cleared of secretions by suction. Finally, the tracheal tube tie should be released, the tracheal cuff slowly deflated while the suction catheter is in the trachea to catch sub-glottic material and the tracheal tube removed smoothly in one movement.

DE-CANNULATION

Unlike extubation, the process of de-cannulation is frequently performed using a number of intermediate steps (Table 18.17) over a number of days, although the appropriate sequence and specific advantages are un-documented. While some of these steps may appear to be sensible, they are in fact associated with significant increases in the work of breathing, either through effects on inspiratory or expiratory resistance or by interfering with cough strength. For most patients, these intermediate steps do not in themselves cause any problems other than for delaying definitive de-cannulation by a couple of days. For some patients, however, the additional burden imposed can precipitate respiratory distress, with an inevitable return to mechanical ventilation. Without careful, consistent and courageous management these patients may spend prolonged periods cycling between low levels of supported ventilation in a triggered mode and an intermediary form of de-cannulation. These patients are then put at significant risk of developing a ventilator-associated

Table 18.17 Characteristics of intermediate steps in de-cannulation

	Inspiratory resistance	Expiratory resistance	Dead space	Cough strength	Speech
Plain tube, cuff down	−	−	−	−	No
Plain tube, cuff down + speaking valve	−	++	−	+	Yes
Fenestrated tube, cuff up + speaking valve	−	+	−	++	Yes
Fenestrated tube, cuff down + speaking valve	−	±	−	+++	Yes
Plain tube, cuff down, capped	+++	+++	−	+	Yes
Small un-cuffed tube, capped	+	+	−	++	Yes
Stoma button	−	−	+	+++	Yes
De-cannulation	−	−	+	+±	Yes

pneumonia. This cycle can be broken by appreciating the significant physiological advantage of proceeding more directly to full de-cannulation or de-cannulation with placement of stoma button.

FAILED EXTUBATION

Between 5% and 15% of patients require re-intubation because of respiratory difficulties. Patients who require re-intubation are significantly more likely to develop ventilator-associated pneumonia (OR 5.94, 95% confidence interval 1.27 to 22.71), spend longer in both the ICU and hospital, and are significantly less likely to survive. Two studies have looked at the value of non-invasive ventilation (NIV) to 'rescue' patients who develop respiratory distress following extubation. In the first study, which randomized 39 patients to NIV and 42 patients to standard medical therapy, there was no significant difference in re-intubation rate (72% versus 69%), duration of ICU stay, or either ICU or hospital survival.[43] In the more recent study, which randomized 114 patients to NIV and 107 patients to standard medical therapy, there was no difference in the re-intubation rate (48% in both) but there was a significantly increased ICU mortality in patients randomized to NIV[44] (25% versus 14%). One explanation for this difference was that the delay to re-intubation was significantly longer in patients randomized to NIV. A number of studies have looked at early transition to NIV in patients

with acute-on-chronic respiratory failure who fail one or more SBTs. A meta-analysis of five such trials in adults concluded that this approach resulted in a significantly shorter duration of mechanical support, a reduced incidence of ventilator-associated pneumonia, reduced ICU and hospital length-of-stay and, perhaps most importantly, reduced mortality[45] (relative risk 0.41, 95% confidence interval 0.22 to 0.76). Finally, two trials have evaluated the use of NIV in reducing the incidence of failed extubation in high-risk patients who *pass* their SBT.[46, 47] Combined, these two studies show a significant reduction in the risk of re-intubation (odds ratio 0.36, 95% CI 0.18 to 0.72) and in the ICU mortality (odds ratio 0.22, 95% CI 0.08 to 0.59).

REFERENCES

1. Esteban A, Alia I, Ibanez J. Modes of mechanical ventilation and weaning: a national survey of Spanish hospitals. *Chest.* 1994;106:1188−93.

2. Ely EW, Truman B, Shintani A *et al.* Monitoring sedation status over time in ICU patients: reliability and validity of the Richmond Agitation-Sedation Scale (RASS). *JAMA.* 2003;289(22):2983−91.

3. Wiedemann HP, Wheeler AP, Bernard GR, *et al.* Comparison of two fluid-management strategies in acute lung injury. *N Engl J Med.* 2006;354(24):2564−75.

4. Epstein CD, Peerless JR. Weaning readiness and fluid balance in older critically ill surgical patients. *Am J Crit Care*. 2006;15(1):54–64.

5. Mitchell JP, Schuller D, Calandrino FS *et al*. Improved outcome based on fluid management in critically ill patients requiring pulmonary artery catheterization. *Am Rev Respir Dis*. 1992;145(5):990–8.

6. Mekontso-Dessap A, de Prost N, Girou E *et al*. B-type natriuretic peptide and weaning from mechanical ventilation. *Intensive Care Med*. 2006;32(10):1529–36.

7. Perkins GD, McAuley DF, Thickett DR *et al*. The beta-agonist lung injury trial (BALTI): a randomized placebo-controlled clinical trial. *Am J Respir Crit Care Med*. 2006;173(3): 281–7.

8. Inouye SK, Bogardus ST, Charpentier PA *et al*. A multicomponent intervention to prevent delirium in hospitalized older patients. *N Engl J Med*. 1999;340:669–76.

9. Chlan LL. Relationship between two anxiety instruments in patients receiving mechanical ventilatory support. *J Adv Nurs*. 2004;48(5): 493–9.

10. Laghi F, Cattapan SE, Jubran A *et al*. Is weaning failure caused by low-frequency fatigue of the diaphragm? *Am J Respir Crit Care Med*. 2003;167(2):120–7.

11. Ibrahim MG, Bellomo R, Hart GK *et al*. A double-blind placebo-controlled randomized pilot study of nocturnal melatonin in tracheostomised patients. *Crit Care Resusc*. 2006;8(3):187–91.

12. Chadda K, Louis B, Benaissa L *et al*. Physiological effects of decannulation in tracheostomized patients. *Intensive Care Med*. 2002;28(12):1761–7.

13. Bolton CF, Brown JD, Sibbald WJ. The electrophysiologic investigation of respiratory paralysis in critically ill patients. *Neurology*. 1983;33 (suppl 2):186.

14. Roelefs RI, Cerra F, Bielka N *et al*. Prolonged respiratory insufficiency due to acute motor neuropathy: a new syndrome? *Neurology*. 1983;33 (suppl 2):240.

15. Van den Berghe G, Wouters P, Weekers F *et al*. Intensive insulin therapy in critically ill patients. *N Engl J Med*. 2001;345(19): 1359–67.

16. Trojaborg W, Weimer LH, Hays AP. Electrophysiologic studies in critical illness associated weakness: myopathy or neuropathy–a reappraisal. *Clin Neurophysiol*. 2001;112(9):1586–93.

17. Moxham J. Respiratory muscle fatigue: mechanisms, evaluation and therapy. *Br J Anaesth*. 1990;65:43–53.

18. Bellemare F, Bigland-Ritchie B. Central components of diaphragmatic fatigue assessed by phrenic nerve stimulation. *J Appl Physiol*. 1987;62(3):1307–16.

19. McKenzie DK, Bigland-Ritchie B, Gorman RB *et al*. Central and peripheral fatigue of human diaphragm and limb muscles assessed by twitch interpolation. *J Physiol*. 1992;454: 643–56.

20. Vassilakopoulos T, Zakynthinos S, Roussos C. The tension-time index and the frequency/tidal volume ratio are the major pathophysiologic determinants of weaning failure and success. *Am J Respir Crit Care Med*. 1998;158(2):378–85.

21. Bulger EM, Jurkovich GJ, Farver CL *et al*. Oxandrolone does not improve outcome of ventilator dependent surgical patients. *Ann Surg*. 2004;240(3):472–8; discussion 478–80.

22. Takala J, Ruokonen E, Webster NR *et al*. Increased mortality associated with growth hormone treatment in critically ill adults. *N Engl J Med*. 1999;341(11):785–92.

23. Krinsley JS. Effect of an intensive glucose management protocol on the mortality of

critically ill adult patients. *Mayo Clic Proc.* 2004;79(8):992–1000.

24. Ide T, Nichols DG, Buck JR *et al.* Effect of aminophylline on high-energy phosphate metabolism and fatigue in the diaphragm. *Anesthesiology.* 1995;83(3):557–67.

25. Murciano D, Auclair MH, Pariente R *et al.* A randomized, controlled trial of theophylline in patients with severe chronic obstructive pulmonary disease. *N Engl J Med.* 1989; 320(23):1521–5.

26. Bascom AT, Lattin CD, Aboussouan LS *et al.* Effect of acute aminophylline administration on diaphragm function in high cervical tetraplegia: a case report. *Chest.* 2005; 127(2):658–61.

27. Ryan RM, Deci EL. Self-determination theory and the facilitation of intrinsic motivation, social development, and well-being. *Am Psychol.* 2000;55(1):68–78.

28. MacIntyre NR, Cook DJ, Ely EW, Jr. *et al.* Evidence-based guidelines for weaning and discontinuing ventilatory support: a collective task force facilitated by the American College of Chest Physicians; the American Association for Respiratory Care; and the American College of Critical Care Medicine. *Chest.* 2001;120(6 Suppl): 375S-95S.

29. Esteban A, Frutos F, Tobin MJ *et al.* A comparison of four methods of weaning patients from mechanical ventilation. Spanish Lung Failure Collaborative Group. *N Engl J Med.* 1995;332(6): 345–50.

30. Lellouche F, Mancebo J, Jolliet P *et al.* A multicenter randomized trial of computer-driven protocolized weaning from mechanical ventilation. *Am J Respir Crit Care Med.* 2006;174(8):894–900.

31. Ely EW, Baker AM, Dunagan DP *et al.* Effect on the duration of mechanical ventilation of

identifying patients capable of breathing spontaneously. *N Engl J Med.* 1996; 335(25):1864–9.

32. Kollef MH, Shapiro SD, Silver P *et al.* A randomized, controlled trial of protocol directed versus physician-directed weaning from mechanical ventilation. *Crit Care Med.* 1997;25(4):567–74.

33. Marelich GP, Murin S, Battistella F *et al.* Protocol weaning of mechanical ventilation in medical and surgical patients by respiratory care practitioners and nurses. *Chest.* 2000;118:459–67.

34. Krishnan JA, Moore D, Robeson C *et al.* A prospective, controlled trial of a protocol-based strategy to discontinue mechanical ventilation. *Am J Respir Crit Care Med.* 2004;169(6):673–8.

35. Kriner EJ, Shafazand S, Colice GL. The endotracheal tube cuff-leak test as a predictor for postextubation stridor. *Respir Care.* 2005;50(12):1632–8.

36. Namen AM, Ely EW, Tatter SB *et al.* Predictors of successful extubation in neurosurgical patients. *Am J Respir Crit Care Med.* 2001;163(3 Pt 1):658–64.

37. Salam A, Tilluckdharry L, Amoateng-Adjepong Y *et al.* Neurologic status, cough, secretions and extubation outcomes. *Intensive Care Med.* 2004;30(7):1334–9.

38. Smina M, Salam A, Khamiees M, Gada P *et al.* Cough peak flows and extubation outcomes. *Chest.* 2003;124(1):262–8.

39. Khamiees M, Raju P, DeGirolamo A *et al.* Predictors of extubation outcome in patients who have succesfully completed a spontaneous breathing trial. *Chest.* 2001; 120:1262–70.

40. Yang KL, Tobin MJ. A prospective study on indexes predicting the outcome of trials of weaning from mechanical ventilation. *N Engl J Med.* 1991;324(21):1445–50.

41. Frutos-Vivar F, Ferguson ND, Esteban A *et al.* Risk factors for extubation failure in patients following a successful spontaneous breathing trial. *Chest.* 2006;130(6):1664–71.

42. Tahvanainen J, Salmenpera M, Nikki P. Extubation criteria after weaning from intermittent mandatory ventilation and continuous positive airway pressure. *Crit Care Med.* 1983;11(9):702–7.

43. Keenan SP, Powers C, McCormack DG *et al.* Noninvasive positive-pressure ventilation for postextubation respiratory distress: a randomized controlled trial. *JAMA.* 2002; 287(24):3238–44.

44. Esteban A, Frutos-Vivar F, Ferguson ND *et al.* Noninvasive positive-pressure ventilation for respiratory failure after extubation. *N Engl J Med.* 2004;350(24):2452–60.

45. Burns KE, Adhikari NK, Meade MO. A meta-analysis of noninvasive weaning to facilitate liberation from mechanical ventilation. *Can J Anaesth.* 2006;53(3): 305–15.

46. Ferrer M, Valencia M, Nicolas JM *et al.* Early noninvasive ventilation averts extubation failure in patients at risk: a randomized trial. *Am J Respir Crit Care Med.* 2006;173(2): 164–70.

47. Nava S, Gregoretti C, Fanfulla F *et al.* Noninvasive ventilation to prevent respiratory failure after extubation in high-risk patients. *Crit Care Med.* 2005;33(11):2465–70.

48. Brochard L, Rauss A, Benito S *et al.* Comparison of three methods of gradual withdrawal from ventilatory support during weaning from mechanical ventilation. *Am J Respir Crit Care Med.* 1994;150(4): 896–903.

49. Ely EW, Baker AM, Dunagan DP *et al.* Effect on the duration of mechanical ventilation of identifying patients capable of breathing spontaneously. *N Engl J Med.* 1996; 335(25):1864–9.

50. Kollef MH, Shapiro SD, Silver P *et al.* A randomized controlled trial of protocol-directed versus physician-directed weaning from mechanical ventilation. *Crit Care Med.* 1997;25(4): 567–74.

51. Vallverdu I, Calaf N, Subirana M *et al.* Clinical characteristics, respiratory functional parameters, and outcome of two-hour T-piece trial in patients weaning from mechanical ventilation. *Am J Respir Crit Care Med.* 1998; 158(6):1855–62.

Chapter 19

Long-term ventilatory support

CRAIG DAVIDSON

Historical introduction

The polio outbreaks that affected the developed world in the early and mid-twentieth century are of particular historical importance. They acted as an impetus to the development of intensive care as a place where 'life support' could be provided while awaiting recovery from critical illness. Second, as survival in those who developed respiratory failure occurred, particularly following the introduction of positive pressure ventilation, significant numbers then required long-term respiratory support.

Depending upon the severity of an outbreak, there was the need to provide artificial ventilation to relatively large numbers of polio patients. Most at risk were children and young adults, who had not acquired 'herd' immunity. Providing such emergency care was to present major logistic problems for the hospitals at that time. Few ventilators were available before 1940, and even in the 1950s hospitals could easily be overwhelmed. In the healthcare service of today, it is easy to forget the devastating impact of the polio epidemics. Throughout the 1950s, over 3000 died in the US each year and, in the 1952–3 Copenhagen outbreak, one hospital was required to provide mechanical ventilation for 31 patients over the course of 3 weeks. Today, nearly 60 years after effective vaccination brought the epidemics under control, over 100 000 long-term survivors remain alive in the US and up to 30 000 in the UK.

The ability of negative pressure ventilation to sustain life had been established in animal experiments as early as 1670. When redeveloped in the early twentieth century for use in man, ventilation was achieved by encasing the chest and abdomen in a cuirass or, alternatively, the whole body was enclosed in a tank ventilator with air being drawn into the lungs by leaving the head outside of the tank. The demonstration that the provision of artificial ventilation during the peak paralytic phase was life saving led to the rapid manufacture of 'iron lungs' in the US and, by the late 1930s, elsewhere in the world. The images of converted school halls with 30 or 40 polio patients treated in rows of iron lungs is iconic of this era (Figure 19.1). However, the mortality rate in bulbar cases was still around 80%. Lassen and colleagues in Sweden are credited with appreciating the reason for failure was negative pressure ventilation.[1] While the cuirass or tank was effective in spinal polio, those with bulbar involvement were at risk from both inadequate support of breathing and from aspiration. The former arose because of collapse of the upper airway, the result of a combination of bulbar muscle weakness and negative intrathoracic pressure promoting upper airway obstruction in similar fashion to the pathophysiology

Core Topics in Mechanical Ventilation, ed. Iain Mackenzie. Published by Cambridge University Press.
© Cambridge University Press 2008.

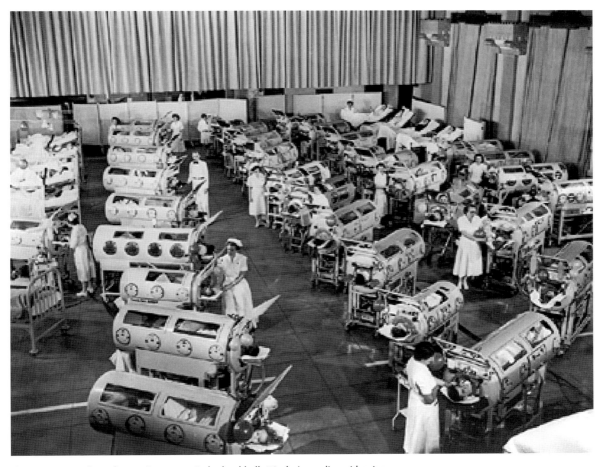

Figure 19.1 Iron lung therapy in a converted school hall, US, during polio epidemics.

of obstructive sleep apnoea. Aspiration was an additional complication, especially as tank ventilation necessitated lying supine. If a tracheostomy with positive pressure ventilation was employed, aspiration still remained a risk until cuffed tubes were developed.

In 1952–1953, during a particularly severe outbreak in Copenhagen, the superiority of positive-pressure ventilation was established with additional protection from aspiration with the innovation of the cuffed tracheal tube. This was an exciting and important time in the history of mechanical ventilation. The developments necessary for treating polio patients led on to the concept of care being pro-

vided in specialized areas of a hospital, the predecessor of the modern intensive care unit (ICU). For more historical details on these developments, see Chapter 20.

The concept of intermittent respiratory support

During the Copenhagen outbreak, overwhelmed by the number of patients requiring mechanical ventilation, medical students were organized into teams to ventilate patients continuously by hand for up to 24 hours a day. The technique of cuffed tube positive-pressure ventilation dramatically reduced the fatality rate in spino-bulbar disease. It was rapidly introduced throughout the world and was to produce survivors with very limited respiratory reserve who would previously have died. Many, however, regained respiratory muscle function within weeks and the first description of ventilatory weaning date from this era. It was also appreciated that spontaneous ventilation might be inadequate at night, even if sufficient by day. However, for some survivors sufficient recovery of respiratory muscle function failed to occur. Such individuals were destined to remain in hospital for many years, because only here was it possible to provide sufficient expertise in the use of iron lungs and other devices.

Accordingly, before effective vaccination reduced the impact of polio, the epidemics were to produce an increasing number of individuals with 'stable' neuromuscular disease dependent on long-term ventilatory support. Even if recovery occurred, those affected by polio in infancy might again develop respiratory failure as scoliosis developed during adolescent growth. For these patients, and increasingly for others with different causes for respiratory pump failure, sleep began to be recognized as associated with a reduction in alveolar ventilation and the potential to develop chronic respiratory failure. Importantly, it became appreciated that such patients could be treated by intermittent ventilatory support. By providing intermittent treatment ('tanking at night'), chronic hypercapnia could be controlled, leaving the affected person independent of ventilatory support by day.

The mechanisms by which intermittent support can restore health, correct abnormalities in blood gases and reverse both the pulmonary hypertension and the associated episodes of cor pulmonale continue to be investigated. Of prime importance is the restoration of central respiratory drive.[2] By reducing the compensatory renal retention of bicarbonate, any tendency to hypoventilation will result in a greater stimulus to the brain stem chemoreceptors. More recently, the restorative effect of improved

sleep quality and quantity has come to be recognized.[3] An effect upon the pulmonary mechanics, with an increase in residual lung volume, may contribute by reducing the load upon the respiratory pump.[4] Changes in pulmonary haemodynamics and a reduction in the degree of pulmonary hypertension are probably dependent upon correction of severe nocturnal hypoxia.[5] Although sleep is the obvious risk period, it may not be critical that alveolar ventilation is protected during *sleep*. For instance, Schonhofer and colleagues have suggested that if hypercapnia is adequately corrected at any stage in the day, similar benefit is obtained whether provided in sleep or when awake.[6]

Whatever the mechanisms involved, the recognition that intermittent support was effective led to the application of overnight ventilatory support in a variety of causes of chronic respiratory failure. This was most commonly achieved with non-invasive negative pressure devices and, as ventilation units were established to manage such dependent polio patients, those with other causes of 'pump' failure became users of non-invasive ventilation. These included idiopathic scoliosis, patients with surgical thoracoplasty in the treatment of tuberculosis and the 'stable' or slowly progressive neuromuscular conditions such as the adult onset muscular dystrophies.

The early development of home mechanical ventilation (HMV)

Throughout the latter half of the twentieth century, centres with expertise in providing long-term ventilation were established in Europe, Australasia and America. Development was largely haphazard and dependent upon enthusiasts. Treatment was largely by negative pressure devices and the units were often established in or near isolation hospitals. Alternative negative pressure techniques, such as the thoraco-abdominal cuirass (Figure 19.2) or the poncho wrap were less technically demanding and could therefore be used more easily in the

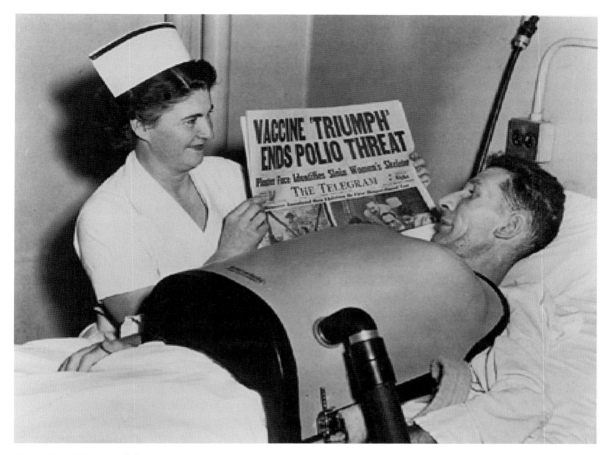

Figure 19.2 Cuirass ventilation.

home. The rocking bed, which exploits gravitational pull on the abdominal organs to 'drive' respiration, had the attraction of minimal technology[7] while glossopharyngeal breathing ('frog breathing') gave patients additional independence from machines. The latter involves repeated 'swallowing' or 'gulping' of small packets of air and progressive retention by intermittent glottic closure. In the experienced patient, frog breathing can more than double vital capacity and provide a sufficiently augmented inspiration to allow an effective cough. Simple mandatory positive pressure volume-controlled ventilators could also be used to 'breath stack' and were often employed as physiotherapy aids. Negative pressure and the physical methods are less effective

than non-invasive positive pressure at augmenting tidal volume, and early on, progression to invasive tracheostomy ventilation was necessary as muscle weakness or spinal deformity progressed.[8]

In the UK, Geoffrey Spencer was one of the pioneers in the provision of home ventilation. He had trained in anaesthesia and was involved in the early establishment of critical care. Recognizing the needs of ventilator-dependent patients, he developed the Phipps Respiratory Unit as a long stay facility at St. Thomas' Hospital in 1968. He went on to develop the concept of home care for what was coined 'responauts'. These were ventilator-dependent individuals whose return to home was enabled by the provision of trained carers. Through

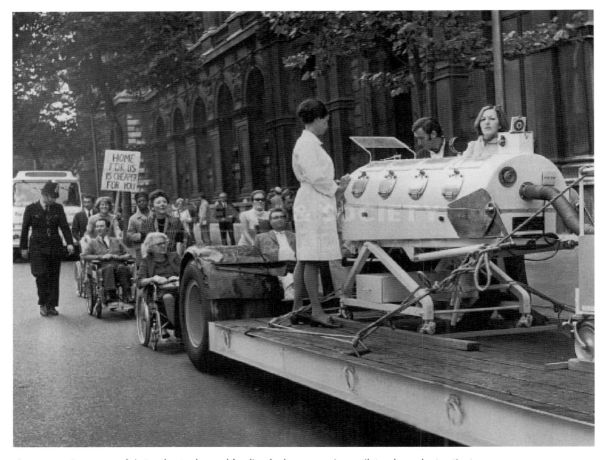

Figure 19.3 Protest march in London to demand funding for home care in ventilator-dependent patients.

a landmark initiative, funded by the Department of Health, carers were trained to look after patients at home. The demonstration that this was both desired by patients and cost effective established the case. Given the era of protest in the 1960s and the need to grab political attention and stimulate media interest, marches were organized to secure the rights of ventilated individuals to live at home (Figure 19.3). Similar developments were to occur elsewhere in the world, such as at the Austin unit in Melbourne and the Rancho Los Amigos in California.

By the end of the twentieth century, many countries in Europe had established ventilator units to support home care. Usually, this was through central government funding. In France, Antadir had been established as a national charitable organization during the polio period. Subsequently, it was contracted by the French government to organize a service for home mechanical ventilation (HMV). Antadir employs medical and nursing staff and, with the support of technicians, is able to give comprehensive care for patients at home. The organization provides routine and emergency home visits and, because it also supervises the provision of oxygen and nebulizer services, it is able to provide a comprehensive system of care for the ventilator-dependent individual. HMV patients are able to

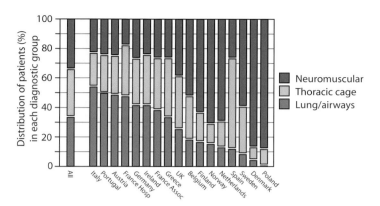

Figure 19.4 Home mechanical ventilation in Europe: Diagnostic groups. Lloyd Owen *et al. Eur Respir J*, 2005.

travel within France and get support from the local centre wherever they are in the country. Antadir defined the conditions that qualify for treatment, deals with the ventilator manufacturers, sets the standards for care and provides holiday centres for patients and their families.[1] Similar organizations exist in Germany, Switzerland and the Scandinavian countries but have yet to be established in the UK and some other European countries. Acting as patient advocate, these national ventilator organizations have been able to promote the expansion of HMV, leading to a growth of paediatric provision and the treatment by both NIV and tracheostomy ventilation of progressive neuromuscular diseases such as Duchenne muscular dystrophy (DMD) and motor neuron disease (MND).[8] In contrast, the development in other countries has been less well organized. The provision of HMV in the European Union has recently been audited with interesting variation in both the number of patients treated and the relative proportion of different disease categories.[9] In northern European countries, where national HMV organizations are common, more patients are treated, but there is a lower proportion in whom chronic obstructive pulmonary disease (COPD) is the cause of respiratory failure (Figure 19.4).

_____
1 See http:www.antadir.com.

The positive pressure revolution

The initial use of non-invasive positive pressure ventilation (originally termed NIPPV but now conventionally shortened to the abbreviation NIV) was in acute episodes of respiratory failure complicating COPD. As such patients can outnumber the availability of ICU provision, the widespread uptake of NIV in hospitals was assured when shown to reduce progression to the need for intubation and, in more severe cases, reduce mortality compared with conventional intubation.

It was quickly appreciated that the HMV patient using physical or negative pressure devices could benefit from the new technology. The new ventilators were lightweight and portable, powered by electrical turbines that needed little servicing and, compared with negative pressure machines, more easily applicable to those with skeletal deformity. With a general expansion of interest and experience of non-invasive positive-pressure ventilation, there was a further expansion of provision and a widening of the indications for HMV treatment throughout the 1990s. This was because the new technology was more acceptable to patients, because the cost was lower and because of a change in medical and societal perception. In particular, those patients with progressive neuromuscular disease, formerly not considered for treatment, began to be treated.

There was, therefore, an expansion in the use of NIV to diseases such as MND, spinal muscular atrophy and the childhood metabolic syndromes. HMV was also extended to patients with intrinsic lung disease such as COPD, bronchiectasis and cystic fibrosis.

The development of NIPPV was dependent on the technology used to treat obstructive sleep apnoea (OSA). Instead of using continuous positive pressure (CPAP), ventilators capable of sensing inspiration, and providing pressure support to spontaneous breathing, were developed. Positive pressure during inspiration is often combined with a lower level of expiratory pressure (EPAP) to provide bi-level pressure support (BiPAP). Such ventilators employ single ventilator tubing and are interfaced with the patient through a face or nose mask. Exhalation valves to reduce re-breathing of exhaled carbon dioxide are therefore necessary, the additional value of expiratory pressure being to flush exhaled air through an exhalation port.

While detecting inspiration and augmenting tidal volume with pressure support is effective in patients with adequate respiratory effort, such triggered modes may be ineffective in patients with profound respiratory muscle weakness. Furthermore, significant mask leak interferes with detection of inspiration. In these circumstances, a timed (or assist control) mode is required in which a mandatory number of breaths are delivered. As with invasive ventilation, such mandatory breaths can be synchronized with spontaneous breathing. Most modern NIV ventilators employed in non-dependent patients (conventionally defined as a need for support for less than 14 to 18 hours per day) therefore now use a triggered mode with a back-up rate of mandatory breaths should triggering be undetected or true apnoea occur. Conventionally, volume-controlled ventilators were employed, particularly in mainland Europe. The advantage of pressure-controlled devices, when used non-invasively, is a more consistent augmentation of spontaneous breathing. This will be relatively independent of

mask leak (so-called 'leak compensation') unless excessive. Additionally, the technical simplicity of microprocessor-controlled turbines accounted for a rapid switch to pressure rather than volume-controlled devices when used non-invasively. It was, however, argued that in patients with high respiratory impedance (those with chest wall disease or the morbidly obese) volume-controlled ventilation would be required as pressure generators would be unable to produce the high pressure and flow rates required. As the power of modern turbines has increased, volume ventilators are no longer necessary when used non-invasively.[10, 11]

With triggered breathing, the glottis is open as the ventilator increases airway pressure. With mandatory ventilator delivered breaths, partial glottic closure, as occurs at the end of spontaneous expiration, will reduce the effectiveness of ventilatory support. While such asynchrony undoubtedly occurs, it rarely appears to be significant. In any case, ventilator and patient synchrony has markedly improved with better interface design, reducing leak and flow rather than pressure triggers. The need for controlled modes may therefore be questioned (except in the tracheostomy ventilated patient). Most patients can be treated by an appropriately adjusted pressure support mode with back-up mandatory breaths should apnoea occur (termed *S/T mode* on some machines). Patients seem to prefer pressure support. New modes that combine pressure with a volume guarantee (e.g. AVAPS, Respironics, USA) have been developed but it is unclear whether this will prove a useful mode or just an interesting technical gadget.[12]

For ventilator-dependent patients with a tracheostomy, either volume- or pressure-controlled machines can be employed. As spontaneous breathing is inadequate in such users, machine-timed (mandatory) breaths will be required and safer ventilator alarms are needed. Often, such patients have significant locomotor disability and are wheelchair-dependent. In these circumstances, the lower power requirement of a volume generator may be an advantage. A fuller description of these technical aspects is beyond the brief of this chapter.[8]

Who benefits from home mechanical ventilation?

The effectiveness of NIV might suggest the question should now be posed in reverse. In what disease or patient groups is it not now accepted practice to offer NIV when chronic respiratory failure develops? While the long-term value of domiciliary NIV in COPD and bronchiectasis remains uncertain, those with respiratory 'pump' failure resulting from chest wall or neuromuscular disease clearly gain benefit.[4, 8] This can be measured by reversal of abnormalities in blood gases, improved sleep quality and daytime cognition, the reversal of pulmonary hypertension and improved survival.[13] Remarkably few randomized studies have been conducted. Until recent years, studies have used an untreated historical cohort as the control group rather than being prospective. None has involved many patients, and a variety of diagnostic groups and of different methods of NIV provision have been employed. Despite suggestions that better randomized controlled trials (RCT) are necessary, the obvious benefit in chest wall and stable neuromuscular (NM) disease now make such studies unethical. The evidence for the effectiveness of NIV has instead been better investigated in the progressive NM diseases and in COPD.

Chest wall and neuromuscular causes of respiratory failure

Comparison between different medical conditions historically treated with HMV, using continued use as a surrogate for survival, have demonstrated greater benefit in chest wall disease (such as scoliosis, thoracoplasty and arthrogryphosis) and stable neuromuscular disease (such as old polio and the late onset myopathies e.g. acid maltase deficiency, myotonic dystrophy or limb girdle dystrophy) than in intrinsic lung disease or the more progressive NM diseases such as DMD.[4, 8, 13]

The use of NIV in progressive NM disease has been more contentious. Doubt was expressed that NIV would improve quality of life because of the technical difficulties of providing effective mask ventilation when there is facial muscle weakness (because of leak) or bulbar disease (because of glottic obstruction and aspiration). Interestingly, while bulbar involvement reduces the effectiveness of NIV in MND,[14] it is less of a problem in the muscular dystrophies when NIV usually remains effective even when bulbar dysfunction requires the institution of gastrostomy feeding.[8]

The timing of initiation of NIV is important. Delaying until daytime respiratory failure has developed, rather than starting treatment at an earlier stage when there might be evidence of nocturnal hypoventilation but the daytime arterial partial pressure of carbon dioxide ($PaCO_2$) remains normal, appears to make a difference. One study in DMD that employed NIV before the onset of daytime respiratory failure reported a higher mortality in the treated group.[15] Various explanations for this unexpected result have been made. For instance, patients on NIV and their families might have been falsely reassured at times of intercurrent illness and so remain at home while untreated patients were admitted to hospital. In a more recent study, patients were randomized to start NIV when there was evidence of nocturnal hypoventilation or NIV was delayed until daytime respiratory failure had developed.[16] Outcome was better in the former group as judged by emergency need for admission and the majority of patients in the delayed group required to start NIV within six months. The improved survival observed in recent decades in DMD is largely due to the impact of NIV,[8] although prophylactic spinal surgery before severe scoliosis develops will delay the onset of respiratory failure. The increasing use of angiotensin-converting enzyme (ACE) inhibitors and β-blockers in the treatment of cardiomyopathy is expected to further improve prognosis.

In MND, early studies suggested a better survival in NIV-treated patients and this has been confirmed by a recent RCT.[14] Patients with an early onset of diaphragm failure, as suggested by orthopnoea, or a history of sleep disturbance should be assessed for NIV, although this option may still not be being raised in discussion.[17] Unless evidence of sleep-disordered breathing is sought there is the danger of presentation with acute respiratory failure. Once intubated, such patients can rarely be successfully weaned with the resulting difficulty of returning such patients to home with tracheostomy ventilation.[18]

Chronic obstructive pulmonary disease

The use of NIV in managing episodes of acute respiratory failure in COPD is now well established. Problems remain in the provision of a high quality acute NIV service because this requires considerable investment in training. Indications include early use to prevent progression to the need for intubation, later use as an alternative to intubation, use as a bridge to support spontaneous breathing following extubation and proactive use to shorten the period of ventilatory weaning. Further details of acute NIV are considered in Chapter 3.

The value of NIV in the long-term management of stable chronic respiratory failure is more contentious.[19] Early trials of non-invasive ventilation employed negative pressure and were carried out in the 1980s, a time when the concept of chronic respiratory muscle fatigue through excessive workload was fashionable. No benefit was found and the suggestion that chronic respiratory muscle fatigue is important has largely been disproved.[20] Appreciation of the frequency of sleep disturbance, with recurrent nocturnal hypoventilation contributing to a reduction in respiratory drive during wakefulness, has led to a re-examination of NIV in stable COPD. Case series suggested benefit, such as reduced hos-

pitalization, and one crossover RCT found quality of life, daytime $PaCO_2$ and sleep quantity to be improved in comparison with overnight oxygen therapy.[21] Two recent larger RCTs have, however, been negative for the outcome measures of mortality and hospitalization rate. A recent meta-analysis of chronic NIV in COPD concluded that there was insufficient evidence to support its use.[22]

Despite such trial evidence, in a 2001 survey that identified more than 2000 HMV users in England and Wales, it was found that COPD was the most frequent indication particularly by units, or hospitals, that treated few home care patients (Figure 19.5). Similar findings were reported in a European-wide survey where COPD was a common indication particularly in southern countries (Figure 19.4). Why then are clinicians behaving differently from trial evidence? In the French and Italian RCTs, the trial design excluded patients with an overlap syndrome of COPD with OSA or COPD with obesity-hypoventilation syndrome (OHS). As a result, most patients enlisted had very advanced emphysema with significant daytime CO_2 retention but little in the way of sleep disordered symptoms. Clinicians, however, employ chronic NIV when the degree of respiratory failure (indicated by the $PaCO_2$) is out of proportion to the severity of airflow obstruction (that is, when an overlap syndrome is likely).

COPD patients are less compliant with home ventilation than in neuromuscular or chest wall disease.[23] Whether this relates to greater difficulty in adequately unloading the respiratory muscles without interfering with sleep is unclear. It is possible that greater care in titration of the EPAP and adjustment of the degree of pressure support, rise time and trigger sensitivity is required for effective HMV in COPD. These aspects remain to be explored.

In the absence of clear trial evidence in COPD, a consensus of expert opinion has proposed guidelines for the use of chronic NIV in the USA.[24] These have since been made more restrictive and require exclusion of OSA and evidence of both hypercapnia

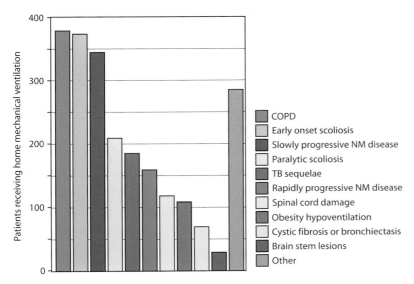

Figure 19.5 Results of the HMV-UK census of 2100 patients identified in England and Wales receiving home mechanical ventilation.

and significant oxygen desaturation, despite oxygen therapy, during the night. In addition a three-month trial of ventilatory assistance without a back-up rate i.e. using a triggered bi-level pressure support machine must exclude OSA as contributing to hypercapnia.[19] This process has been driven by reimbursement and, in particular, a lower charge for triggered mode ventilators. Nevertheless, they do provide some guide to treatment that is, at least, pragmatic.

Our own policy is to consider home NIV when severe COPD patients have

- recurrent admissions caused by acute hypercapnia correctable by NIV,
- overlap syndromes with symptoms of sleep disordered breathing, or
- symptomatic hypercapnia with long-term oxygen therapy.

A positive response to a trial of NIV at home should include evidence of effectiveness (better sleep quality, improved quality of life, and a fall in $PaCO_2$) and a reasonable degree of compliance, for example more than three hours use per night.

If commissioning of HMV develops in the UK, such outcome measures will be a minimum require-ment. Meanwhile, the result of further RCTs under way in Germany and Australia are eagerly awaited. Their importance is evidenced by the rapid increase in use of NIV in COPD in Europe and the fact that COPD is a much more common cause of chronic respiratory failure than neuromuscular and chest wall disease.

Obesity-hypoventilation syndrome (OHS)

Because obesity is a risk factor for both OSA and OHS, it is not surprisingly it has become an emerging cause for domiciliary NIV.[25] A combination of upper airway obstruction, hypoventilation through excessive load on the respiratory muscles in the recumbent position and central apnoea is often found. There may in addition be associated asthma or COPD.[26] An acute hypercapnic presentation following sedation for minor surgery or non-pneumonic respiratory tract infection is common.[27] NIV is effective therapy but can be subsequently switched to simple CPAP in many cases. Reversal of hypercapnia is also reported after weight loss, particularly the more significant weight reduction that follows bariatric surgery.[28] The pathophysiological role of the neuro-hormone

Table 19.1 Comparison of non-invasive ventilation (NIV) and invasive home mechanical ventilation		
	Non-invasive ventilation	Tracheostomy HMV
Advantages	Home care easily provided with relatively low cost equipment. Little training required. Relief of symptoms of sleep disordered breathing with better daytime functioning and improved sleep quality. Patient empowerment: disease 'ownership'. Ventilator portability (e.g. holidays, university or school). Reduced need for hospital admission (e.g. with respiratory infection).	Increased safety. Ability to access lower airways (suctioning).
Potential problems	No access to lower respiratory tract. Less effective if bulbar function poor. Interface problems when NIV need > 12 hours. Potential danger from non-specialist provision	Increased home care costs. Carer training and safety issues. Complications of tracheostomy. Suctioning and increase in sepsis. Disease progression: 'locked in' condition

leptin, in which central resistance to its normal appetite suppressing effect is seen, is also thought to contribute to respiratory failure. A fall in leptin in parallel with an increase in CO_2 drive has been reported.[29]

While simple bi-level pressure support is adequate when OSA predominates, the low total respiratory system compliance of the massively obese and the potential of volume assured ventilation[2] (AVAPS, Respironics, USA) to more effectively maintain tidal volume than conventional pressure support has been investigated. While trans-cutaneous PCO_2 control was better, this did not provide clinical benefit in terms of sleep quality or quantity, or quality of life scores.[12]

Comparison of invasive and non-invasive techniques

There are numerous advantages of NIV compared with invasive ventilation. As listed in Table 19.1, these are largely related to the lower requirement for specialist knowledge by carers or families and as a result lower cost.

A high quality of life is possible, despite total ventilator dependency, but requires the ability to direct personal care and to demand treatment despite disability (Figure 19.6). There are, however, some disadvantages with a high degree of ventilatory dependency. While NIV may still be capable of adequately supporting ventilation at times of intercurrent respiratory illness, impaired cough and an inability to clear secretions may result in the need for specialist physiotherapy in hospital. The recognition of this has led to the development of a variety of cough assist devices.[13, 30, 31] We have been using an insufflation-exsufflation device (Emerson, Massachusetts, USA) for acute hospital care for some years and our practice is to now provide this for home care following more than one admission if the patient's cough is ineffective. Unscheduled hospital admission has been reduced by such a policy.

In the patient with high ventilatory dependency, usually defined as the need for NIV >18 hours per day (although >12 hrs is very significant dependency), the use of NIV can become intrusive on quality of life. Facial skin ulceration may be avoided by rotating the use of interfaces (full face and

---

[2] Pressure-controlled, volume-targeted. See Chapter 5.

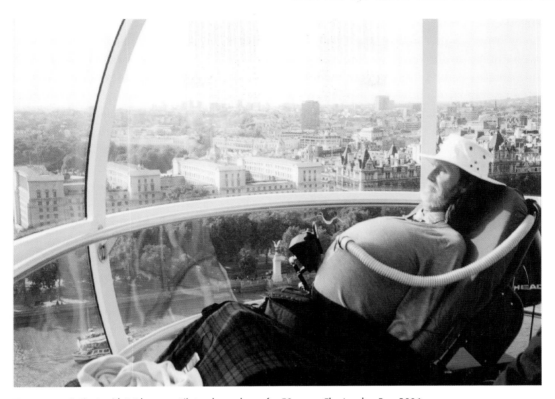

Figure 19.6 Patient with 24 hour ventilator dependency for 59 years. The London Eye, 2006.

nasal or different manufacturer) and by employing a combination of modes.[32] Air swallowing can become a problem and providing adequate nutrition may require a gastrostomy as nasogastric tubes will interfere with NIV delivery. Eventually, the question of conversion to tracheostomy MV arises in progressive NM disease. When considering this, apart from ensuring that patients are fully informed (as well as their relatives), it is important to involve the community service providers and to plan the training of carers. It is certainly better to arrange conversion as an elective procedure. We have found that a mini-tracheostomy, by allowing suctioning at times of crisis, can delay or even prevent the need to convert to invasive ventilation.

For the home user, an un-cuffed tracheostomy is preferred but may not be possible if bulbar function is poor. It makes tube changes easier and the absence of a cuff impairs swallow less than a cuffed

tube and probably causes less tracheal injury. It is also a safer option as spontaneous breathing is possible in the case of ventilator failure (another reason for patients to learn frog breathing). For additional safety such patients need a battery back-up for power failure and a spare ventilator.

Recurrent stomal infection and socially unacceptable leak is more likely with surgical tracheostomies, and we therefore use the dilator technique used in intensive care. The frequency of bronchial sepsis is higher in the months following tracheostomy, and this persists if care continues in hospital or intermediate facility, presumably because of the risk from the environment in such locations. Other complications, such as tracheal stenosis or minor bleeding (and major from innominate artery erosion), occur with long-term invasive ventilation.

An important consideration is progression of the associated NM disease to a point where life quality is unacceptable. This requires a considerable amount of sensitivity in discussion and time. Patients rate the ability to communicate effectively as of paramount importance. Insertion of a one-way valve (Passey Muir) in the ventilator tubing is often needed as the respiratory muscle weakness progresses. Increasing the pressure during expiration can also be effective. However, as bulbar function fails, voice quality deteriorates and aspiration increasingly occurs, which further impacts on quality of life with an increasing need for and frequency of invasive suctioning. Considerable ethical issues arise in progressive NM disease,[8, 13, 33] especially when intellect is impaired or competency is in doubt. Further consideration of these aspects, including advance directives and terminal care arrangements, are beyond the scope of this chapter.

What are the targets of therapy with HMV?

The initial reason for introducing NIV is symptom control. The onset and progression of symptoms is however gradual. Unlike OSA, where the Epworth sleepiness scale is a good indicator of the severity of sleep disturbance,[34] acclimatization to fatigue or assigning it to disease progression or depression may result in unrecognized hypoventilation. Following adjustment to nocturnal NIV, the majority of patients, who have developed daytime hypercapnia by the time they start, notice a marked improvement in daytime functioning and report more restorative sleep. Arterial blood gases improve with a return towards normal levels of carbon dioxide and normalization of arterial oxygen (shunt reversal and a fall in the alveolar–arterial oxygen tension gradient). Improved survival and lower morbidity are equally important goals, but it is unclear which surveillance indicators should be used to guide treatment. Some experts aim for simple symptom control plus satisfactory overnight oximetry, using the latter as a surrogate for adequate ventilatory support. Others aim for normalization of day-time $PaCO_2$ plus satisfactory overnight capnography, adjusting ventilatory pressures or mode accordingly. However, there is the danger of increasing daytime dyspnoea by lowering the $PaCO_2$ too far and we aim for a high normal value. In some European countries, polysomnography is employed to titrate NIV. Interestingly, more sleep disturbance seems to occur with too rigid a control of overnight capnography. Maximal unloading of the diaphragm by titrating the degree of pressure support and adjusting the expiratory pressure during sleep has been investigated.[35] Excessive EPAP was found to be a common problem in NM disease. Awake titration for maximal comfort is the more commonly used method with further investigation and adjustment if symptoms persist or oximetry is poor.

In COPD and the progressive neuromuscular diseases, symptom control remains the first priority and, as the benefit of NIV probably arises from provision of restorative sleep, these are simply measured. In obesity hypoventilation, reversal of 'disease' with weight loss following surgery has been demonstrated.[28] Providing NIV in this condition probably impacts on life expectancy, but unless it is offered within a total care package in this difficult 'life-style illness' it can only really be expected to ameliorate symptoms.

Organization of HMV

Different organizational systems have developed throughout the world, often as a result of local innovators and enthusiasts and depending upon the healthcare provision in the country. Across Europe, Lloyd-Owen et al.[9] have described marked variation in provision, partly influenced by political and medical restraints. As national organizations throughout the European Union become more regulated and centrally organized, there is the potential for linkage of provision and greater opportunities for patients to travel.

One issue is the convenience of local provision versus the advantages of specialist centres. With

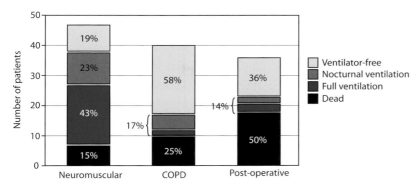

Figure 19.7 Weaning success and need for NIV or invasive ventilation in 154 patients referred because of weaning failure. Pilcher *et al.* Thorax, 2005.

greater familiarity in the use of NIV acutely, more hospitals are able to provide support to local HMV users. Larger specialist centres have the benefit of greater experience and of offering a wider range of equipment. They are better able to support patients with out-of-hours care, technical support and emergency admission. While many stable patients are best supported by shared care arrangements, those with progressive NM disease often require additional expertise in orthotics, wheelchair provision, environmental controls and communication aids. These can be best provided in ventilation centres. Co-morbidity and the occasional need for operative intervention may also require services that can only be coordinated through such units.

Emergency care is often the most difficult issue for patients who live at a distance from a ventilator unit. Clear guidelines for local hospitals are useful. Provision of emergency intubation as a life saving measure, and later transfer to the central unit for assisted extubation or tracheostomy weaning can then follow.

In recent years, the plight of the critical care patient that has failed to wean from respiratory support has increasingly been appreciated. Weaning centres have developed in the US for economic reasons while a weaning service running alongside the other activities of a home ventilation unit has been more common in Europe. Our own experience[36]

has been that many such patients need ongoing NIV at hospital discharge, usually because of underlying NM disease (Figure 19.7).

Future issues

As detailed earlier, the indications for HMV in COPD remain controversial. Surveys throughout Europe show this, and obesity hypoventilation, as the diagnostic groups associated with increased provision. The results of RCTs in COPD being carried out in Germany and Australia are eagerly awaited. The best balance between local versus specialist centre provision will require co-operation between providers. The value of national organizations to oversee service development has already been established. The outcome measures of primary importance remain uncertain. The question remains about the importance of $PaCO_2$ control versus improved sleep quality and the control of recurrent arousal and sympathetic stimulation. The value of additional oxygen therapy and the role of recurrent uncontrolled hypoxia in the development of accelerated pulmonary hypertension that may develop after years of apparent stability remain to be established. Greater emphasis on patient-centred care, the value of patient self-help groups and the provision of information through the internet will also shape future provision.

REFERENCES

1. Lassen HCA. A preliminary report on the 1952 epidemic of poliomyelitis in Copenhagen with special reference to the treatment of acute respiratory insufficiency. *Lancet*. 1953;1:37–41.

2. Annane D, Quera-Salva MA, Lofaso F *et al*. Mechanisms underlying effects of nocturnal ventilation on daytime blood gases in neuromuscular diseases. *Eur Respir J*. 1999; 13(1):157–62.

3. Schonhofer B, Kohler D. Effect of non-invasive mechanical ventilation on sleep and nocturnal ventilation in patients with chronic respiratory failure. *Thorax*. 2000; 55(4):308–13.

4. Shneerson JM, Simonds AK. Noninvasive ventilation for chest wall and neuromuscular disorders. *Eur Respir J*. 2002;20(2):480–7.

5. Schonhofer B, Barchfeld T, Wenzel M *et al*. Long term effects of non-invasive mechanical ventilation on pulmonary haemodynamics in patients with chronic respiratory failure. *Thorax*. 2001;56(7):524–8.

6. Schonhofer B, Geibel M, Sonneborn M *et al*. Daytime mechanical ventilation in chronic respiratory insufficiency. *Eur Respir J*. 1997; 10(12):2840–6.

7. Cormican LJ, Higgins S, Davidson AC *et al*. Rocking bed and prolonged independence from nocturnal non-invasive ventilation in neurogenic respiratory failure associated with limb weakness. *Postgrad Med J*. 2004;80 (944):360–2.

8. Simonds AK. Home ventilation. *Eur Respir J Suppl*. 2003;47:38S–46S.

9. Lloyd-Owen SJ, Donaldson GC, Ambrosino N *et al*. Patterns of home mechanical ventilation use in Europe: results from the Eurovent survey. *Eur Respir J*. 2005;25(6): 1025–31.

10. Schonhofer B, Sonneborn M, Haidl P *et al*. Comparison of two different modes for noninvasive mechanical ventilation in chronic respiratory failure: volume versus pressure controlled device. *Eur Respir J*. 1997;10(1):184–91.

11. Tuggey JM, Elliott MW. Randomized crossover study of pressure and volume non-invasive ventilation in chest wall deformity. *Thorax*. 2005;60(10):859–64.

12. Storre JH, Seuthe B, Fiechter R *et al*. Average volume-assured pressure support in obesity hypoventilation: A randomized crossover trial. *Chest*. 2006;130(3):815–21.

13. Howard RS, Davidson C. Long term ventilation in neurogenic respiratory failure. *J Neurol Neurosurg Psychiatry*. 2003;74 Suppl 3:iii24–30.

14. Bourke SC, Tomlinson M, Williams TL *et al*. Effects of non-invasive ventilation on survival and quality of life in patients with amyotrophic lateral sclerosis: a randomized controlled trial. *Lancet Neurol*. 2006;5(2): 140–7.

15. Raphael JC, Chevret S, Chastang C *et al*. Randomised trial of preventive nasal ventilation in Duchenne muscular dystrophy. French Multicentre Cooperative Group on Home Mechanical Ventilation Assistance in Duchenne de Boulogne Muscular Dystrophy. *Lancet*. 1994;343(8913):1600–4.

16. Ward S, Chatwin M, Heather S *et al*. Randomized controlled trial of non-invasive ventilation (NIV) for nocturnal hypoventilation in neuromuscular and chest wall disease patients with daytime normocapnia. *Thorax*. 2005;60(12):1019–24.

17. Bourke SC, Williams TL, Bullock RE *et al*. Non-invasive ventilation in motor neuron disease: current UK practice. *Amyotroph Lateral Scler Other Motor Neuron Disord*. 2002; 3(3):145–9.

18. Bradley MD, Orrell RW, Clarke J *et al.* Outcome of ventilatory support for acute respiratory failure in motor neurone disease. *J Neurol Neurosurg Psychiatry*. 2002;72(6): 752–6.

19. Hill NS. Noninvasive ventilation for chronic obstructive pulmonary disease. *Respir Care*. 2004;49(1):72–87; discussion 87–9.

20. Schonhofer B, Polkey MI, Suchi S *et al.* Effect of home mechanical ventilation on inspiratory muscle strength in COPD. *Chest*. 2006;130(6):1834–8.

21. Meecham Jones DJ, Paul EA *et al.* Nasal pressure support ventilation plus oxygen compared with oxygen therapy alone in hypercapnic COPD. *Am J Respir Crit Care Med*. 1995;152(2):538–44.

22. Wijkstra PJ, Lacasse Y, Guyatt GH *et al.* A meta-analysis of nocturnal noninvasive positive pressure ventilation in patients with stable COPD. *Chest*. 2003;124(1):337–43.

23. Criner GJ, Brennan K, Travaline JM *et al.* Efficacy and compliance with noninvasive positive pressure ventilation in patients with chronic respiratory failure. *Chest*. 1999; 116(3):667–75.

24. Clinical indications for noninvasive positive pressure ventilation in chronic respiratory failure due to restrictive lung disease, COPD, and nocturnal hypoventilation–a consensus conference report. *Chest*. 1999;116(2): 521–34.

25. Janssens JP, Derivaz S, Breitenstein E *et al.* Changing patterns in long-term noninvasive ventilation: a 7-year prospective study in the Geneva Lake area. *Chest*. 2003;123(1): 67–79.

26. Cuvelier A, Muir JF. Acute and chronic respiratory failure in patients with obesity-hypoventilation syndrome: a new challenge for noninvasive ventilation. *Chest*. 2005; 128(2):483–5.

27. Perez de Llano LA, Golpe R, Ortiz Piquer M *et al.* Short-term and long-term effects of nasal intermittent positive pressure ventilation in patients with obesity-hypoventilation syndrome. *Chest*. 2005;128(2):587–94.

28. Olson AL, Zwillich C. The obesity hypoventilation syndrome. *Am J Med*. 2005;118(9):948–56.

29. Yee BJ, Cheung J, Phipps P *et al.* Treatment of obesity hypoventilation syndrome and serum leptin. *Respiration*. 2006;73(2):209–12.

30. Chatwin M, Ross E, Hart N *et al.* Cough augmentation with mechanical insufflation/exsufflation in patients with neuromuscular weakness. *Eur Respir J*. 2003;21(3):502–8.

31. Mustfa N, Aiello M, Lyall RA *et al.* Cough augmentation in amyotrophic lateral sclerosis. *Neurology*. 2003;61(9): 1285–87.

32. Toussaint M, Steens M, Wasteels G *et al.* Diurnal ventilation via mouthpiece: survival in end-stage Duchenne patients. *Eur Respir J*. 2006;28(3):549–55.

33. Polkey MI, Lyall RA, Davidson AC *et al.* Ethical and clinical issues in the use of home non-invasive mechanical ventilation for the palliation of breathlessness in motor neurone disease. *Thorax*. 1999;54(4): 367–71.

34. Johns MW. A new method for measuring sleepiness: the Epworth sleepiness scale. *Sleep*. 1991;14:540–5.

35. Fanfulla F, Delmastro M, Berardinelli A *et al.* Effects of different ventilator settings on sleep and inspiratory effort in patients with neuromuscular disease. *Am J Respir Crit Care Med*. 2005;172(5):619–24.

36. Pilcher DV, Bailey MJ, Treacher DF *et al.* Outcomes, cost and long term survival of patients referred to a regional weaning centre. *Thorax*. 2005;60(3):187–92.

Chapter 20

The history of mechanical ventilation

IAIN MACKENZIE

Prehistory

The essential connection between breathing and life has been recognized since biblical times at least:

. . . the Lord God formed the man from the dust of the ground and breathed into his nostrils the breath of life, and the man became a living being.[1]

The importance of a clear airway in permitting breathing has also long been appreciated. There are, for example, possible illustrations of therapeutic tracheostomy in ancient Egyptian tablets dating from the First Dynasty (3600 BC) and the procedure is also mentioned in a book of Hindu medicine, the *Rig Veda*, which may have been written as early as 2000 BC.

Some authors have interpreted a passage from the Old Testament as a description of artificial expired air ventilation:

. . . And he went up and lay upon the child, and put his mouth upon his mouth, and his eyes upon his eyes, and his hands upon his hands: and he stretched himself upon the child; and the flesh of the child waxed warm . . .and the child opened his eyes . . .[2]

However, clear evidence of forced tidal ventilation as a means of sustaining or restoring life is lacking until the mid-sixteenth century when Andreas Vesalius (Figure 20.1), the Brussels-born anatomist and professor of medicine at Padua, clearly describes expired air ventilation through an intratracheal reed to keep a dog alive:[1]

But that life may in a manner of speaking be restored to the animal, an opening must be attempted in the trunk of the trachea, into which a tube of reed or cane should be put; you will then blow into this, so that the lung may arise again and the animal take in air. Indeed, with a slight breath in the case of this living animal the lung will swell to the full extent of the thoracic cavity, and the heart become strong and exhibit a wondrous variety of motions.

and later,

. . . and as I do this and take care that the lung is inflated at intervals, the motion of heart and arteries does not stop . . .

Credit for the first *mechanical* (rather than expired air) ventilation in order to sustain life goes to Robert Hooke, who used a pair of bellows to ventilate a dog via a tracheostomy during a demonstration to the Royal Society in London in 1664:

In prosecution of some enquiries into the nature of respiration in several animals, a dog was

[1] Genesis 2:6–8.
[2] Kings II 4:34–5.

Core Topics in Mechanical Ventilation, ed. Iain Mackenzie. Published by Cambridge University Press.
© Cambridge University Press 2008.

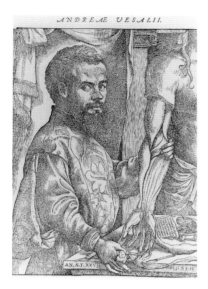

dissected, and by means of a pair of bellows, and a certain pipe thrust into the wind-pipe of the dog, the heart continued beating for a very long while after all the thorax and belly had been opened . . .

By this time, Harvey had largely corrected the Galenic concept of the circulation of the blood in his book *Exercitatio Anatomica de Mortu Cordis et Sanguinis in Animalibus* in 1628, and the work Hooke was performing, in association with Richard Lower, resulted in the latter publishing *Tractatus de Corde* in 1669, which more clearly explained the relationship between the lungs, the heart and the circulation. While progress continued to be made in an ever deeper *scientific* understanding of human form and function, the *rational* application of this knowledge in a clinical context lagged far behind. Nevertheless, attempts to use mechanical ventilation to restore (rather than sustain) life in *humans* began in the mid-eighteenth century on an empirical basis, slightly ahead of the discovery of carbon dioxide (Joseph Black, 1752), oxygen (Joseph

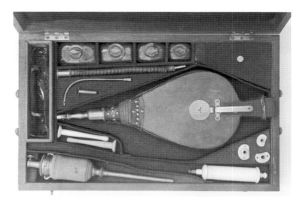

Priestley, 1774) and an explanation of the role of these two gases with respect to metabolism and the lungs by Antoine Lavoisier in 1789. Thus the first documented occurrence of effective mouth-to-mouth resuscitation was recorded by William Tossach in 1744,[2] later followed by descriptions of Hooke-style bellows mechanical ventilation by John Hunter in 1776[3] (Figure 20.2). This technique was still being recommended in medical texts of the early nineteenth century:

Dr Monro, for this purpose, recommends a wooden pipe fitted at one end for filling the nostril, and at the other end for being blown into by a person's mouth, or for receiving the pipe of a pair of bellows.[4]

Such resuscitation activities were encouraged and reported by the Humane Societies which sprang up throughout Europe between 1767 (Amsterdam) and 1790 (Glasgow) and which were dedicated to the assistance of victims of drowning and sudden death.[5] These philanthropic organizations reflected a growing social awareness that had begun in the earlier part of the century, driven by emerging industrialization and urban poverty and marked by the opening of numerous hospitals in London and the provinces[3] for the free treatment of the 'deserving' poor. It is in the context of unconscious victims of drowning or asphyxiation that the first attempts at orotracheal intubation are recorded, made desirable by the unfortunate complication of gastric inflation that accompanied enthusiastic use of bellows. John Hunter suggested that pressure on the larynx might prevent this problem (a manoeuvre described 200 years later by Sellick):

If during this operation the larynx be gently pressed against the oesophagus and spine, it will prevent the stomach and intestines being too much distended by the air . . .

These early attempts at mechanical ventilation were brought to an end in the 1830s by Leroy's studies in France[6] in which he showed in both animals and cadavers that overenthusiastic inflation, especially if exhalation was neglected in favour of inflation, resulted in serious lung damage or death. Based on these results and the report presented to the French Academy of Sciences in 1829, the French authorities counselled against positive-pressure ventilation – advice that was rapidly accepted throughout Europe. Thereafter, artificial ventilation in adults was attempted by a whole family of eponymous postural methods assisted by movement of the arms (the 'Sylvester' technique) or compression of the abdomen (the 'Leroy' technique), amongst many others. For neonates, however, the demise of positive-pressure ventilation for resuscitation from birth asphyxia was only short-lived, being itself revived in 1845 by the French obstetrician Depaul.

Even with the pioneering use of ether by Crawford Long (Figure 20.3) in Jefferson, Georgia, (1842) and William Morton in Boston (1846), which heralded

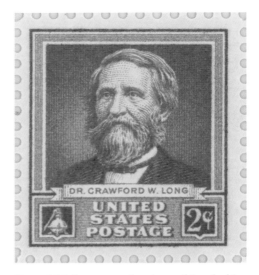

Figure 20.3 Commemorative stamp of Crawford Long. Image courtesy of the The Health Sciences Historical Collections, the University of Tennessee Health Sciences Library. Memphis, TN.

the birth of anaesthesia, the demand for methods to provide sustained support of ventilation in the nineteenth century were very limited.

Anaesthesia and the sealed airway

Until the introduction of the intravenous anaesthetic agent thiopentone in 1934, both anaesthesia and survival depended on spontaneous ventilation and a clear airway. Continued spontaneous ventilation was readily achieved providing the patient was not anaesthetised too deeply and the pleural space was left intact, page 392. Maintenance of a clear airway was also relatively easy, particularly for those who could position the patient to their advantage or who had no need to go near the face or airway. These conditions, however, discriminated against surgeons whose work involved the throat, mouth, nose or face and who had to use their ingenuity to keep their patients both anaesthetized and alive. Of the few who succeeded in this endeavour, each solved the problem for himself by developing tracheal tubes placed percutaneously[7] or orally[8, 9] and rendered water-tight by

---

3 Five hospitals in London (Westminster 1720, Guy's 1724, St George's 1733, the London 1740 and the Middlesex 1745) joined St Bartholomew's and St Thomas' which had been founded in the middle ages, and hospitals were founded in Edinburgh (1729), Winchester (1737), Bristol (1737), York (1740), Exeter (1741), Bath (1742), Northampton (1743), Cambridge (1766), Oxford (1770).

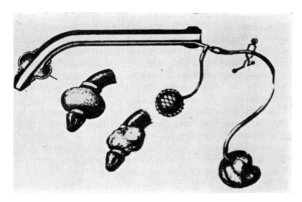

Figure 20.4 Eisenmenger's cuffed metal orotracheal tubes, 1893.

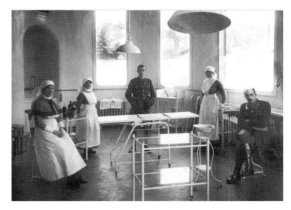

Figure 20.5 The operating theatre at the Queen's Hospital Sidcup, 1917.

The Plastic Theatre at the Queen's Hospital Sidcup, 1917. The officers are Rubens Wade (Gillies' first anaesthetist) standing; Gillies seated. Reproduced with permission from The Gillies Archives at Queen Mary's Hospital, Sidcup.

pharyngeal packing[8] or with an inflatable cuff[7, 9] (Figure 20.4). For the majority of surgeons, however, the anaesthetic technique was of little interest and was determined by the experience of the available assistant rather than a specifically trained and dedicated medically qualified practitioner.

As a consequence, aspects of orotracheal intubation were repeatedly re-invented during the early years of the twentieth century, such as the cuffed tube (Dorrance, 1910,[10] Guedel and Waters, 1928[11]), but these rigid wide-bore cuffed endotracheal tubes failed to become popular because in the hands of those recruited to administer the anaesthetic they were very hard to place, even with the help of Chevalier Jackson's laryngoscope. Instead, the technique of 'insufflation' anaesthesia held sway between 1910 and 1926. This involved the constant delivery of an anaesthetic gas mixture into the trachea via a thin flexible catheter. With the help of a laryngoscope and appropriately designed forceps, these insufflation catheters were much easier to place, and gas escaping from the laryngeal inlet prevented, to some extent, the ingress of material into the airway. This was therefore the prevailing technique in 1919 when an Irish graduate, Ivan Magill, started work as 'anaesthetist' to the Queen's Hospital in Sidcup, having given a handful of anaesthetics as a student and in his previous post at Barnet War (now General) Hospital (Figure 20.5). He and

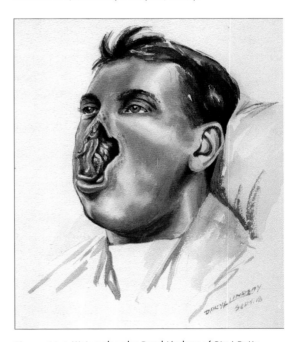

Figure 20.6 Watercolour by Daryl Lindsay of Pte J Potts, Borders Regiment, wounded 22 August 1918. Reproduced with permission.

his fellow anaesthetist Stanley Rowbotham were immediately faced with the problem of maintaining anaesthesia in patients whose faces were in the surgical field (Figure 20.6). With insufflation anaesthesia, they found that both the surgeon and the operative field were sprayed with blood and debris blown out of the pharynx, and so adapted to a technique involving two translaryngeal catheters, one for fresh gas, and the second for exhaled gas, an arrangement which also allowed the pharynx to be packed. Although an improvement, this two-catheter arrangement was cumbersome, and with the later adoption of nitrous oxide and oxygen for the maintenance of anaesthesia (which resulted in a much better post-operative condition of the patients), it was also expensive. Accordingly, Magill and Rowbotham substituted a single wide intratracheal catheter placed blindly through the nose, and sealed in the trachea with either pharyngeal packing or an inflatable cuff, together with a low-flow, semi-closed to-and-fro breathing circuit.

The complete demise of the insufflation technique was eventually precipitated by the introduction of cyclopropane as an anaesthetic agent in 1934. With vastly superior properties, it rapidly replaced both ether and chloroform, but its expense demanded the adoption of very low gas flows to minimize cost. Such a technique was already in existence, having been described by Waters in 1924,[12] but required a completely sealed airway. Thus by the mid-1930s, Magill had developed the techniques, specialization in anaesthesia had provided the skill base, and cyclopropane had provided the impetus to establish endotracheal intubation with a cuffed tube (the sealed airway) as a standard anaesthetic technique.

Anaesthesia and the pneumothorax problem

Although from inception anaesthesia significantly improved the conditions for surgery (for both patient and surgeon), it depended, as mentioned earlier, on the patient being able to self-ventilate. Incursion into the chest was inevitably accompanied by the collapse of one or both lungs, respiratory compromise, and almost invariably death.

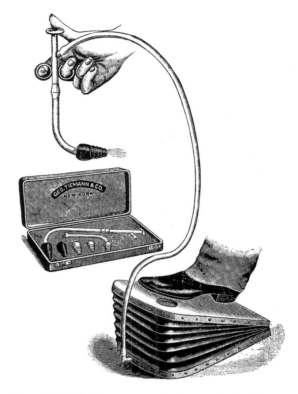

Figure 20.7 Fell-O'Dwyer apparatus for anaesthesia with positive-pressure ventilation.

This was referred to as the 'pneumothorax problem', which for the majority of surgeons rendered the chest an absolute 'no-go' zone. As with the sealed airway, a few surgeons with a specific interest in thoracic surgery successfully addressed the 'pneumothorax problem' as early as 1896.[13] The technique described in the United States by Rudolf Matas[4] was an adaptation of the Fell-O'Dwyer apparatus, which was originally designed to provide respiratory support for victims of opiate overdose. The Fell-O'Dwyer apparatus (Figure 20.7) was O'Dwyer's combination, in 1893, of his intralaryngeal tube, which he described in 1880[5] as a

---

4 Matas R. Intralaryngeal insufflation for the relief of acute surgical pneumothorax. Its history and methods with a description of the latest devices for this purpose. *JAMA* 1900; 34:1371–5, 1468–73.

5 Reported as O'Dwyer J. Intubation of the larynx. *NY Med J* 1885;8:145–7 in Goerig M, Filos K, Ayisi KW. George Fell and

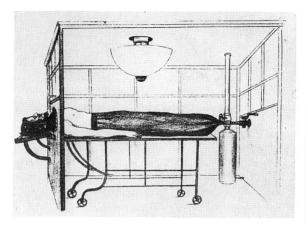 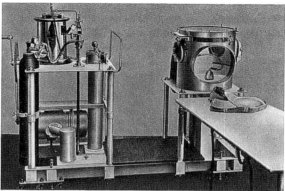

Figure 20.8 Left: Sauerbruch's differential pressure ventilating chamber. Right: Brauer's positive-pressure ventilating head container.

means of providing an airway in cases of laryngeal obstruction (most commonly caused by diphtheria), with Fell's bellows-powered positive-pressure ventilator.

However, these techniques were not widely adopted for exactly the same reasons that endotracheal intubation remained a peculiar art – there were no specifically trained practitioners and little need. For most operations, muscular relaxation was not required, the patient's own ventilation was maintained, and even for intra-abdominal surgery the abdominal muscles could be adequately relaxed with spinal anaesthesia, or deep inhalational or insufflation anaesthesia. In Europe, thoracic surgeons were drawn to Sauerbruch's solution to the 'pneumothorax problem' because it did not depend on skilled assistance, but used a negative-pressure chamber similar to a giant 'iron lung' to ventilate the patient. The patient was placed in an airtight operating chamber positioned with the head through an opening, which was sealed around the patient's neck. Outside the chamber an assistant at the patient's head administered the anaesthetic,

the development of respiratory machines. Ch 20.1 in *The History of Anaesthesia*. Atkinson RS and Boulton TB (eds). Parthenon Publishing Group, Casterton Hall.

while the surgeon was in the chamber with the rest of the patient (Figure 20.8). On exactly the same principle as an iron lung, ventilation was achieved by rhythmic changes in the air pressure within the chamber, effected by a large set of bellows. Brauer described a slightly less cumbersome version the following year (1905), in which the arrangement was reversed, the patient lying with the head enclosed in a positive-pressure ventilating chamber, and Tiegel's subsequent arrangement remained the most popular solution until the end of the 1930s. Even in the United States, Matas' combination of intubation and positive-pressure ventilation was supplanted by insufflation anaesthesia as described by Meltzer and Auer in 1909.[14]

This left positive-pressure ventilation to the physiologists and the Swedish surgeon KH Giertz, one of Sauerbruch's assistants at Breslau,[6] who was dissatisfied by the differential-pressure method and was convinced by his experimental work in animals that artificial ventilation was a significantly better technique. Under the influence of Giertz, Paul Frenckner, a university lecturer in ENT surgery, developed a range of cuffed endotracheal tubes and, together with Anderson, an engineer from

[6] Now Wroclaw, Poland.

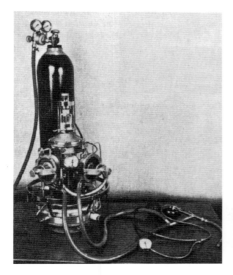 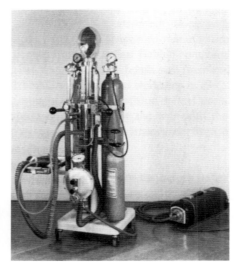

Figure 20.9 Left: Frenckner's 1934 Spiropulsator. Right: The commercially produced Spiropulsator of 1940 designed by Frenckner, Anderson and Crafoord.

the Swedish gas company AGA, developed the first positive-pressure mechanical ventilator in 1934[7] – the Spiropulsator (Figure 20.9). Later, the thoracic surgeon Clarence Crafoord joined the project and contributed to the design of the first commercial model in 1940. Positive-pressure mechanical ventilation with a cuffed endotracheal tube thus became established in Scandinavia but was vigorously resisted in North America for many years, so much so that in 1952 Henry Beecher, wrote

It has been repeatedly advocated that respiratory failure be produced by deliberate overventilation of patients under anesthesia and that this be followed by artificial ('controlled') respiration by the anesthetist . . . For several reasons we do not believe that this technic [sic] is usually necessary or advisable[8] . . .

In the UK, where low-flow anaesthesia using cuffed endotracheal tubes was commonplace after the mid-1930s, manual hyperventilation and apnoea were easily achieved and introduced into clinical practice in 1936. The replacement of *manual* by *mechanical* ventilation required the intervention of a man who was neither medically qualified nor formally trained in anaesthesia.

John Blease (1906–1985)

Born on the Wirral in 1906, John Blease (Figure 20.10) left school at the age of 14 and started his working life as a butcher's boy. His mechanical deftness soon led him to repairing tractors before eventually setting up a car repair business with his brother in the mid 1920s. His self-taught engineering skills and sharp mind are reflected in the fact that in the 1930s he was able to build his own 1000cc motorcycle with which he won many amateur races competing against commercial machines. His neighbour at that time,

[7] Almqvist E. *Technological changes in a company: AGA – the first 80 years*. This branch of the AGA Corporation later became part of Siemens-Elema.
[8] Page 37 in Beecher, H. K. *Principles, Problems, and Practices of Anesthesia for Thoracic Surgery*. Publication no. 129 in the

series, American Lectures in Anesthesia, Adriani, J (ed). Charles C Thomas, Springfield, Illinois. 1952. 65pp.

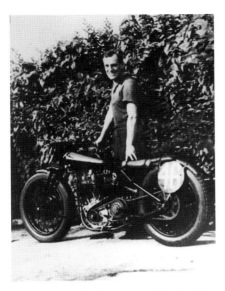

Figure 20.10 John Blease. Reproduced with permission from Spacelabs Healthcare Ltd, Chesham, Buckinghamshire.

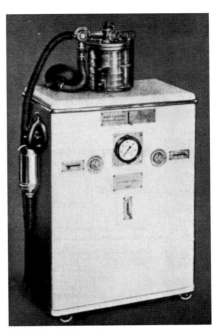

Figure 20.11 The Blease Pulmoflator.

Dr Henry Roberts, who as a general practitioner provided anaesthetic services to the Liverpool Dental Hospital, commissioned the production of some pieces of anaesthetic equipment from Blease. Rather bizarrely, Blease, following Roberts' sudden death in 1937, took over his anaesthetic duties at the Liverpool Dental Hospital and was therefore quite a proficient anaesthetist when he was pressed into service as an anaesthetist at Birkenhead General Hospital, following the heavy air raids on Merseyside in the first week of May 1941. It was during this period that Blease conceived of the idea of a mechanical device to provide the 'controlled ventilation' required during prolonged thoracic surgery, producing a prototype that was demonstrated in 1947 and produced commercially in 1950 – the Blease Pulmoflator. By the beginning of the 1950s, there was sufficient demand for mechanical ventilation during anaesthesia to support four commercial producers – The Blease Anaesthetic Equipment Company and Schonander Elema in Europe and Puritan-Bennett and Emerson in the United States (Figure 20.11).

Negative-pressure ventilation by physicians

The realization that tidal ventilation could be achieved by reducing the extrathoracic pressure, rather than increasing the intrathoracic pressure, is credited to John Mayow in the early 1670s, but a serious attempt to apply this to man did not occur for over 150 years. In 1832, the Scottish physician John Dalziel developed an upright box to provide negative-pressure ventilation (NPV), and although the device was warmly praised by one observer,[15] the concept never caught on. Barrington Baker[16] has suggested that Dalziel's invention was a victim of the medical establishment's reaction to Leroy's studies,[6] as mentioned previously, but a more pragmatic reason might be the difficulty in demonstrating the efficacy of a resuscitation device which could not be taken to those requiring it and for which the need was modest and unpredictable. With the same purposes in mind, Dalziel's tank NPV was repeatedly 're-invented' in the last quarter of the nineteenth century by others, including Alfred Jones in 1864, Ignez von Hauke in 1874 and Eugene Woillez in 1876. An alternative to the tank was a negative-pressure ventilator that only covered the abdomen and chest, a design which came to be known as a *cuirass*. The first cuirass NPV was designed by Waldenberg[17] in 1880 and as with the tank NPV suffered numerous re-inventions (Alexander Graham Bell, Eisenmenger) until its eventual adoption into clinical practice in a number of commercially available guises, such as the Stille, Kifa, Fairchild-Huxley, London County Council and Monaghan.

During the course of the nineteenth century, however, circumstances gradually changed. The impact of the Industrial Revolution had a profound effect on urban demographics, with London expanding from a population of 600 000 in 1700 to 1 million in 1800 and over 2 million by 1850. The population explosion and changing socio-political environment increased awareness of, and concern for, the un-sanitary conditions of the urban poor, saw life expectancy at birth increase from 36 years in 1801 to 47 in 1900. An ironic and unexpected consequence of the improved living conditions was the emergence of polio as a much-feared disease of childhood. Possibly described as early as 1789,[18] poliomyelitis became much more easily recognized during the latter part of the nineteenth century and early twentieth century. Acquired in infancy, the impact of the disease was imperceptible against a background of an appallingly high infant mortality, but with more sanitary conditions reducing environmental exposure to the virus in infancy, acquisition of the disease was delayed to childhood and early adulthood when a paralytic illness was much more difficult to overlook. During the first half of the twentieth century, large epidemics of poliomyelitis culminated in the final re-inventions of the tank NPV by Stewart and Rogoff in 1918 and then by Philip

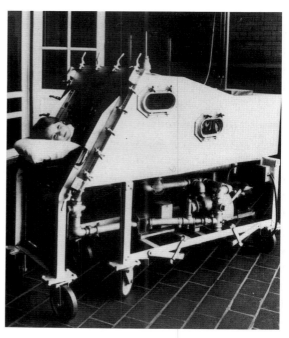

Figure 20.12 Drinker and Shaw's 'iron lung'.

Drinker and Louis Shaw in 1927 (Figure 20.12). Evidence confirming the clinical success of long-term negative-pressure ventilation was published in 1929,[19] and by 1931 there were over 70 adult-sized and 12 infant-sized Drinker Respirators across North America, which had been used in the respiratory support of 198 patients, including 100 cases of poliomyelitis.[20]

In the UK, Siebe Gorman and Company in London manufactured the Drinker Respirator and the first of these 'iron lungs' was installed at Great Ormond Street in 1934. Unfortunately, the Drinker Respirator was very expensive, and during the polio epidemic of 1937–8, the need for these machines far exceeded their supply. In Australia, Edward and Donald Both who ran a small business making scientific and medical equipment were commissioned to design and build a cheap, lightweight version of the Drinker respirator at their small Adelaide factory. The following year, Edward Both was in

London promoting a portable electrocardiograph when he heard a plea on BBC radio for a respirator for a patient with poliomyelitis. Edward contacted the South Australian Agent-General and within a week or two had constructed a Both respirator in a hired garage which was accepted by the health department of the London County Council. Edward made two other respirators, one put on display in London and the second lent to the Radcliffe Infirmary in Oxford where a film was made of it in operation. Lord Nuffield, whose wealth from the manufacture of Morris motor cars at Oxford had allowed him to endow the chair of anaesthesia at Oxford, was shown the film by Robert Macintosh, the first Professor of Anaesthesia at Oxford. In November 1938, Lord Nuffield agreed to manufacture the Both Respirator in Oxford and offered to donate a Both Respirator to any hospital in the commonwealth that wanted one. Despite fierce criticism from some quarters (having been described as a 'wanton waste of private benevolence'),[21] by March 1939 there were 965 Both Respirators in use which formed the nucleus of respiratory units across the UK and elsewhere, dealing for the most part with patients paralysed by polio.

Scandinavia 1949 to 1952

During an epidemic of poliomyelitis in Stockholm in 1949 and 1950, Carl-Gunnar Engström, an epidemiologist at the Stockholm Hospital for Contagious Diseases, observed a series of patients with respiratory failure treated with tracheostomy and negative-pressure ventilation, a technique recently imported from the US by Sjöberg.[22] Although this treatment was life saving for many, for the unfortunate minority with both respiratory and bulbar paralysis, survival was rare. Engström's study of respiratory function in these patients, which included blood gas analysis, led him to conclude that these patients were dying of inadequate ventilation[23] rather than the poliomyelitis itself, as was

believed at the time. He therefore designed and had built a prototype of a mechanical positive-pressure ventilator, which guaranteed the delivery of a set tidal volume rather than inspiratory pressure. This device was presented at conferences in both Copenhagen and Stockholm[24] in the autumn of 1951 and in December was successfully used in the treatment of a patient with polio-related chronic respiratory failure.

The following autumn, Copenhagen was struck by a polio epidemic that was unprecedented in three respects: the number of victims, the proportion of victims developing paralysis, and the unusually high proportion developing both respiratory and bulbar paralysis. Patients with poliomyelitis in the metropolitan area of the Danish capital were admitted to the 500-bed Blegdam Hospital for communicable diseases, which possessed one tank and six cuirass respirators. In the period between 1934 and 1944, this hospital had managed 76 cases of acute respiratory failure from poliomyelitis in cuirass ventilators, with a mortality of 80%.[25] In contrast, in the first three weeks of the 1952 epidemic 31 patients with polio required respiratory support (of just over 80 admissions), of whom 27 died – a mortality rate of 87%. Concerned by the flood of admissions, the unusually high proportion and pattern of paralytic cases and the appalling mortality, Henry Lassen, the chief of the service and Professor of Epidemiology, sought advice. Mogens Bjørneboe suggested they involve Bjørn Ibsen, a young anaesthetist who had helped Bjørneboe manage a case of tetanus neonatorum earlier in the year. On that occasion, Ibsen had used curare for muscle relaxation and positive-pressure ventilation via a tracheostomy, and, although the infant eventually died, this did not occur until they returned to the traditional management for these cases using intravenous barbiturate. Reluctantly, Lassen called a meeting in his office on Monday August 25 which included Bjørneboe, Ibsen, and the head of the clinical chemistry laboratory, Poul Astrup, amongst others. Reviewing one of the fatalities up to that point, Lassen and the other physicians were puzzled by the normal appearance of the 12-year-old boy's lungs together with ante-mortem hypertension and a serum bicarbonate of 44 mmol.L^{-1}, the hallmarks of hypercapnia. It suddenly occurred to Ibsen that the cause of death must have been chronic hypoventilation, the same conclusion that Engström had reached the year before in Stockholm. Despite receiving tracheostomies, which were cannulated with un-cuffed metal tubes, the accumulation of tracheobronchial secretions was preventing the negative-pressure ventilators from delivering adequate tidal volumes. The hypoventilation was occult because the accompanying hypoxia responded to the administration of additional oxygen. Despite reservations from Lassen and the other physicians, it was eventually agreed to let Ibsen take over the management of one of the patients. The following day Ibsen, Bjørneboe and Astrup met at the laboratory to agree a plan and collect the equipment required. On Wednesday, August 27, they took over the care of Vivi, a 12-year-old girl who was in extremis and not expected to survive. A tracheostomy was performed at her bedside under local anaesthetic, but despite the presence of a cuffed tracheostomy tube, the combination of bronchospasm and atelectasis made it almost impossible for Ibsen to ventilate her with the Waters circuit. He gave her 100 mg of thiopentone, allowing him to suction her airway and ventilate her properly. Measurements of exhaled carbon dioxide using a Brinkman carbovisor and oximetry using a Millikan oximeter allowed him to demonstrate the simultaneous presence of severe hypercapnia and normal arterial saturation, as well as the disappearance of the signs of hypercapnia (hypertension, sweating) with positive-pressure ventilation. With the rapid reduction in arterial carbon dioxide content, Vivi became quite hypotensive but responded

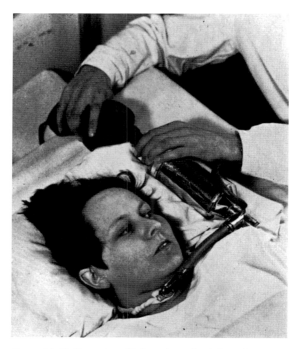

Figure 20.13 Manual ventilation of a polio victim using a Water's circuit.

to a blood transfusion, and she was then placed in a cuirass ventilator. Almost immediately, the signs of hypoventilation returned, accompanied by a rise in blood carbon dioxide content. Convinced by this demonstration, Lassen directed that the management of respiratory failure was to change immediately, but because there were no commercially available positive-pressure ventilators, the work had to be done by hand. All 26 or so of Copenhagen's anaesthetists were recruited to the task, and they in turn trained and supervised about 450 medical and dental students who worked in teams of 4 to 6, each team hand-ventilating a patient around the clock (Figure 20.13). With this new strategy, the case-fatality rate plummeted during September, despite a sharp rise in the number of new cases.

On hearing of the epidemic in Copenhagen, Engström sent his ventilator to the Blegdams Hospital, where it underwent successful clinical evaluation. With a certain degree of foresight, the Swedish

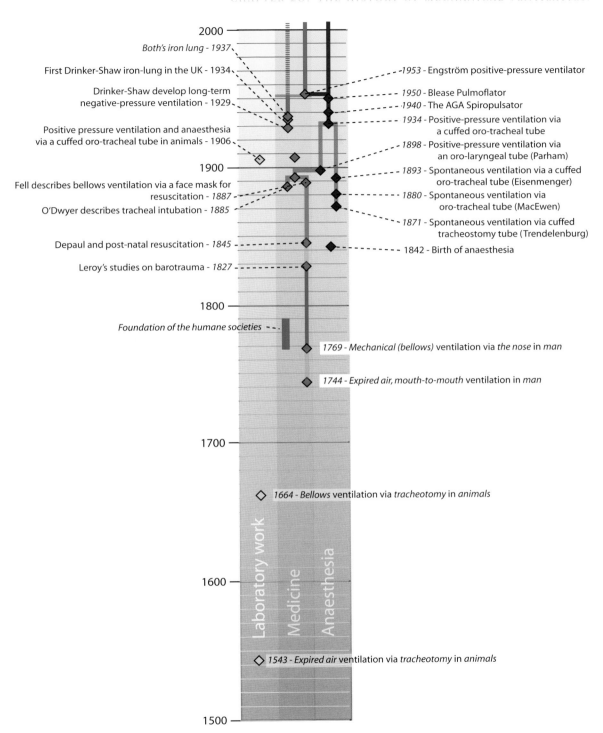

Both's iron lung - 1937

First Drinker-Shaw iron-lung in the UK - 1934

Drinker-Shaw develop long-term
negative-pressure ventilation - 1929

Positive pressure ventilation and anaesthesia
via a cuffed oro-tracheal tube in animals - 1906

Fell describes bellows ventilation via a face mask for
resuscitation - 1887

O'Dwyer describes tracheal intubation - 1885

Depaul and post-natal resuscitation - 1845

Leroy's studies on barotrauma - 1827

Foundation of the humane societies

1953 - Engström positive-pressure ventilator

1950 - Blease Pulmoflator

1940 - The AGA Spiropulsator

1934 - Positive-pressure ventilation via
a cuffed oro-tracheal tube

1898 - Positive-pressure ventilation via
an oro-laryngeal tube (Parham)

1893 - Spontaneous ventilation via a cuffed
oro-tracheal tube (Eisenmenger)

1880 - Spontaneous ventilation via
oro-tracheal tube (MacEwen)

1871 - Spontaneous ventilation via cuffed
tracheostomy tube (Trendelenburg)

1842 - Birth of anaesthesia

1769 - Mechanical (bellows) ventilation via the nose in man

1744 - Expired air, mouth-to-mouth ventilation in man

1664 - Bellows ventilation via tracheotomy in animals

Laboratory work

Medicine

Anaesthesia

1543 - Expired air ventilation via tracheotomy in animals

Figure 20.14 Time-line of the development of mechanical ventilation.

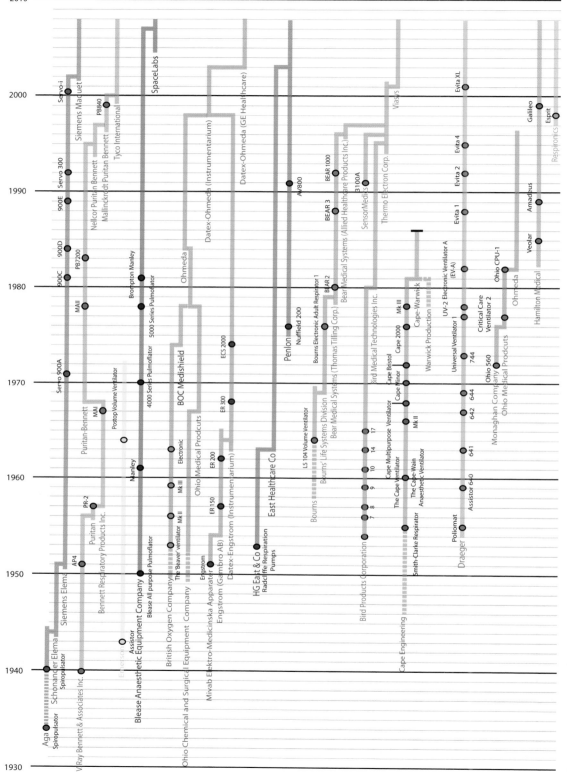

Figure 20.15 Commercial development of ventilator technology.

health authorities decided to have the Engström ventilator commercially manufactured by Mivab Elektro-Medicinska Apparater in Stockholm, just in time for their own polio epidemic the following year. Bjorn Ibsen went on to become chief anaesthetist at the Kommune-hospital in Copenhagen in 1954 where he established the first intensive care unit in a general hospital.

The last 50 years

Given the events of 1952, it is not surprising that there was an explosion in the number of positive-pressure ventilators designed in 1953, including the Bang,[26] Clevedon,[27] Beaver[28] (manufactured by BOC), Pask[29] and Radcliffe[30] (later Penlon) in anticipation of further polio epidemics. Respiratory support units were established in large hospitals throughout Europe to cope with these patients, as well as the small numbers with other causes of respiratory failure. During the decade, however, the incidence of polio was dramatically reduced by the introduction of mass vaccination programmes resulting from the work of, first, Salk in 1955 and then Sabin in 1956. As the numbers of polio patients plummeted through the second half of the decade, many of the respiratory units in the US were closed, while in Europe they continued to operate as general intensive care units.

The events in Copenhagen in 1952 mark the real beginning of mechanical ventilation in that the technique had become sufficiently accepted to support commercial production of the machines, at least in Europe. The market for intensive care ventilators in Europe was shared by a number of manufacturers, including Mivab Elektro-Medicinska Apparater (Engstrom) and Aga Medical Division (Pulmospirator) in Scandinavia, and Blease, the British Oxygen Company (Beaver) and East & Co (East-Radcliffe) in the UK (Figure 20.15). The European bias was for machines that were volume targeted

and would provide a guaranteed tidal volume in the face of variable pulmonary compliance, the basis of Engstrom's life-saving hypothesis. In contrast, adoption of non-anaesthetic mechanical ventilation in the United States was both delayed and short-lived. When the demand for non-anaesthetic mechanical ventilation eventually materialized in the US in the early 1960s, the machines were based on technology developed during the war for high-altitude bombing and were therefore largely pressure controlled (Emerson, Bird, and Bennett Respiratory Products).

Early machines were mechanical or electromechanical, could only deliver either volume-targeted or pressure-targeted breaths – depending on how they were constructed, and lacked alarm systems. Subsequent developments of the mechanical ventilator have largely been driven by the combination of advances in technology and commercial pressure, without substantial departure from the original concepts. The exceptions to this generalization are the forms of high-frequency ventilation that were developed in the 1970s and the brief interest in ventilators controlled by fluidics.

The first major evolutionary step of the purely pneumatic and mechanical ventilators of the 1950s and 1960s came with release of Bennet's MA1 in 1967, which controlled the mechanical gas delivery using electronics. This division between electronic 'control' and mechanical 'muscle' was then taken a step further in 1971 with the Servo 900 series. The final step into the current generation of ventilators was the development in the 1980s of microprocessor-controlled machines such as the Siemen's 900C (1981), the Ohmeda CPU-1 (1982) and the Puritan-Bennett 7200 (1983). With these machines, the intrinsic link to the mechanism driving inflation was broken completely with the ability to target breaths to either volume or pressure using a flow profile that could be finely controlled, together with a sophisticated array of alarms.

REFERENCES

1. Vesalius A. *De Humani Corporis Fabrica*. Basle, Oporini, I. 1542.

2. Tossach W. A man, dead in appearance recovered by distending the lungs with air. *Med Essays Obs (Edinburgh)*. 1744;5(2): 605.

3. Hunter J. Proposals for the recovery of people apparently drowned. *Philos Trans R Soc London*. 1776;66:412.

4. Buchan W. *Domestic Medicine; or, A Treatise on the Prevention and Cure of Diseases, by Regimen and Simple Medicines*. Edinburgh, Thomas Nelson. 1814.

5. Sternbach GL, Varon J, Fromm R *et al*. The humane societies. *Resuscitation*. 2000; 45:71–5.

6. Leroy J. Recherches sur l'asphyxie. *J Physiol* (Paris). 1827;7:45–65.

7. Trendelenburg F. Tamponnade der Trachea. *Archiv f Klin Chirurg*. 1871;12:121–33.

8. MacEwen W. General observations on the introduction of tracheal tubes by the mouth, instead of performing tracheotomy or laryngotomy. *BMJ*. 1880;2:122–4.

9. Eisenmenger V. Zur tamponade des larynx nach Prof. Maydl. *Wien Med Woch*. 1893;43: 199–210.

10. Dorrance GM. On the treatment of traumatic injuries of the lungs and pleurae. *Surg Gynecol Obstet*. 1910;11:160–92.

11. Guedel AE, Waters RM. A new intratracheal catheter. *Curr Res Anesth Analg*. 1928;7: 238–9.

12. Waters RM. *Curr Res Anesth Analg*. 1924; 3:20.

13. Tuffier T, Hallion L. Intrathoracic operations with artificial respiration by insufflation. *Comp Ren Soc Biologie*. 1896;48:951.

14. Meltzer SJ, Auer J. *Exp Med*. 1909;11:622.

15. Lewins R. Apparatus for promoting respiration in cases of suspended animation. *Edinburgh Med Surg J*. 1840;54:255–6

16. Baker AB. Artificial respiration, the history of an idea. *Med Hist*. 1971;15(4):336–51.

17. Waldenburg L. *Die Pneumatische Behandlung der Respirations und Circulationskrankheitien im Anschluss an die Pneumatometrie und Spirometrie*. Berlin, Hirschwald. 1880.

18. Underwood M. *A Treatise on the Diseases of Children, with General Directions for the Management of Infants from the Birth. A New Edition, Revised and Enlarged*, etc. ed. London, J. Matthews. 1789.

19. Drinker P, McKhann CF. The Use of a New Apparatus for the Prolonged Administration of Artificial Respiration: I. A Fatal Case of Poliomyelitis. *JAMA*. 1929;92:1658.

20. Drinker P. Prolonged administration of artificial respiration. *Lancet*. 1931;1:1186.

21. Menzies F. Mechanical respirators. *BMJ*. 1939;1:35.

22. Sjöberg A. Mechanism of suffocation in spinobulbar poliomyelitis and experiences with operative treatment. *Arch Oto-laryngol*. 1950;52:323.

23. Engström C-G. Om CO_2-retentionens betydelse vid respirationsinsufficiens. *Sven Läkartidn*. 1950;47:3007.

24. Sjöberg A, Engstöm C-G, Svanborg N. Diagnostiska och kliniska rön vid behandling av bulbospinal poliomyelit (Svenska Läkaresällskapet. Sammankomst den 16 okt. 1951). *Nord Med*. 1952;47:536.

25. Lassen HCA. A preliminary report on the 1952 epidemic of poliomyelitis in Copenhagen with special reference to the treatment of acute respiratory insufficiency. *Lancet*. 1953;1:37–41.

26. Bang C. A new respirator. *Lancet*. 1953;i: 723–6.

27. Macrae J, McKendrick GDW, Claremont JM *et al*. The Clevedon positive-pressure respirator. *Lancet*. 1953;ii:971–2.

28. Beaver RA. Pneumoflator for treatment of respiratory paralysis. *Lancet*. 1953;1:977–8.

29. Pask EA. A simple respirator. *Lancet*. 1953;2: 141.

30. Ritchie Russell W, Schuster E. Respiration pump for poliomyelitis. *Lancet*. 1953;2: 707–9.

Glossary

$\triangle P.$ See *Inflating pressure*.

A. Physiological symbol for alveolar gas.

a. Physiological symbol for arterial blood.

Aa gradient. The calculated difference between the alveolar and arterial partial pressure of oxygen, i.e. $P_{A_{O_2}} - P_{a_{O_2}}$, with units of kPa or mm Hg. This is a more rigorous but much less user-friendly gauge of the lung's capacity to take up oxygen than the 'PF ratio' (see $P_{a_{O_2}} / F_{I_{O_2}}$ *ratio*), which tends to be used clinically.

Airway pressure-release ventilation (APRV). A *hybrid mode* of ventilation in which the airway pressure intermittently drops from a higher level to a lower level. Two distinctions can be drawn between APRV and *bi-level ventilation*. First, in APRV much longer time is spent in P_{high} than P_{low}, effectively reversing the I:E ratio. Second, in APRV the mandatory breaths are interspersed with *triggered* (e.g. supported) breaths, while in *bi-level ventilation* mandatory breaths are interspersed with *spontaneous* (e.g. unsupported) breaths.

APRV. See *Airway pressure-release ventilation*.

Apnoea. The absence of spontaneous respiratory effort. **Primary:** Failure to develop a spontaneous respiratory rhythm following a period of mandatory mechanical ventilation. **Secondary:** The development of apnoeic episodes, usually during sleep, arising after the restoration of a spontaneous respiratory rhythm in patients who have received mechanical ventilation.

Assist-control ventilation (ACV). A *hybrid mode* of ventilation in which the mandatory breaths, traditionally volume-controlled (V-ACV), are supressed by patient-triggered breaths that receive the same support. If the mandatory rate is set below the patient's own respiratory rate then all the breaths delivered are triggered. On some more recent ventilators, this mode can be set to deliver pressure-controlled breaths (pressure assist-control ventilation, P-ACV).

Atmospheric pressure. Synonym: *barometric pressure*. Pressure exerted by the air, which at sea level is defined as one atmosphere (= 101.325 kPa or 100 mbar). Atmospheric pressure falls with increasing altitude.

Auto-PEEP. See *Intrinsic PEEP*.

Barometric pressure. See *Atmospheric pressure*.

Bi-level ventilation. A form of ventilation in which the airway pressure cycles between two levels of CPAP. The patient can breath *spontaneously* during both P_{high} and P_{low} phases, and only receives inspiratory assistance during the low–high transition. When the term 'bi-level ventilation' is applied correctly, the rate of phase cycling only contributes minimally to the patient's minute volume, which is mainly determined by the patient's spontaneous breaths.

Bi-level positive airway pressure (BiPAP™). Synonym: *variable positive airway pressure*. A proprietary term owned by Respironics describing non-invasive ventilation with some similarities to *bi-level ventilation*. In contrast to true bi-level ventilation, BiPAP™ phase cycling accounts entirely for the patient's minute volume. In BiPAP™ P_{low} is referred to as the expiratory positive airway pressure (EPAP) and P_{high} is referred to as the inspiratory positive airway pressure (IPAP). The inflating pressure is calculated as IPAP−EPAP.

Biphasic Positive Airway Pressure (BIPAP). A proprietary term used by Draeger to refer to a *hybrid mode* of ventilation with pressure-controlled mandatory breaths. When supplemented by pressure-controlled *triggered* breaths, this mode becomes 'BIPAP plus'.

BIPAP. see *Biphasic Positive Airway Pressure*.

BIPAP Plus. see *Biphasic Positive Airway Pressure*.

BiPAP™. see *Bi-level Positive Airway Pressure*.

Bradypnoea. An abnormally slow respiratory rate.

Closing volume. The expiratory lung volume at which terminal airways begin to collapse, preventing the expiration of any more alveolar gas from the lung units distal to the collapse. The closing volume increases with age, as the lung loses its elasticity. In children and young to middle-aged adults the normal pulmonary end-expiratory lung volume exceeds the closing volume. In middle- to old-age, the closing volume exceeds the end-expiratory lung volume.

Continuous Positive Airway Pressure (CPAP). Externally applied positive end-expiratory pressure during spontaneous breathing where the inspiratory breaths are not supported is traditionally called 'continuous positive airway pressure' (CPAP). This is in contrast to externally applied positive end-expiratory pressure during

triggered (supported) or mandatory breaths, which is traditionally referred to as 'positive end-expiratory pressure' (PEEP). The distinction between the two terms is less significant, and indeed confusing, in modes of ventilation in which spontaneous, triggered and mandatory breaths co-exist, such as in some forms of APRV.

CMV. *Control(led)-mode ventilation* or *continuous mandatory ventilation*, see also *Intermittent Positive Pressure Ventilation*.

Compliance. Describes the ease with which a material can be stretched (floppy, stretchy, elastic, expandable). In mathematical terms, it is expressed as the volume change per unit change in pressure: $C = \dfrac{\Delta V}{\Delta P}$. Compliance is the opposite (reciprocal) of *elastance*.

Continuous Mandatory Ventilation (CMV). See *Intermittent Positive-Pressure Ventilation*.

Controlled ventilation. See *Intermittent Positive-Pressure Ventilation*.

Control-mode ventilation (CMV). See *Intermittent Positive Pressure Ventilation*.

Cycle time (Tc). The time between the start of inspiration of two consecutive breaths, which is the sum of the inspiratory time (T_I) and expiratory time (T_E):

$$T_C = T_I + T_E. \tag{1}$$

The cycle time is also determined by the respiratory rate (f):

$$T_C = \frac{60}{f}. \tag{2}$$

Combining Equations (1) and (2), you get

$$T_I + T_E = \frac{60}{f}. \tag{3}$$

Dead space (VD). The volume of gas in each breath that does not participate in gas exchange, either because the gas enters non-perfused alveoli (alveolar dead space, V_{D_A}), or remains in either the conducting airways (anatomical dead space, VD_{anat}) or airway equipment (equipment dead space, VD_{eqpt}):

$$VD = VD_A + VD_{anat} + VD_{eqpt}.$$

The sum of the alveolar and anatomical dead spaces are referred to as the *physiological dead space*.

De-cannulation. The process of removing a tracheostomy tube (see also *extubation*).

Delta P (ΔP). See *Inflating pressure*.

DUOPAP. A proprietary term used by Hamilton to refer to a *hybrid mode* of ventilation with pressure-controlled mandatory breaths which may, if desired, be supplemented by pressure-controlled triggered breaths.

Duty cycle. The inspiratory time expressed as a proportion of the cycle time:

$$\text{Duty cycle} = \frac{T_I}{T_C} = \frac{T_I}{T_I + T_E}.$$

Elastance. Describes the difficulty with which a material can be stretched (stiffness, inelasticity, rigidity). In mathematical terms, it is expressed as the pressure change per unit change in volume: $E = \dfrac{\Delta P}{\Delta V}$. Elastance is the opposite (reciprocal) of *compliance*.

ECCO2R. See *Extracorporeal CO_2 removal*.

ECMO. See *Extracorporeal membrane oxygenation*.

End-expiratory lung volume. See *Functional residual capacity*.

Endotracheal tube. See *trans-laryngeal tube*.

EPAP. Expiratory positive airway pressure. See *Bi-level positive airway pressure*.

Exhaled minute volume ($\dot{V}_e$). The total volume of gas exhaled by the patient in one minute, measured at body temperature, sea level, and fully saturated with water vapour.

Expiratory time (T_E). The time between the onset of expiratory gas flow and the start of the next breath.

Extracorporeal CO_2 removal. A system which removes carbon dioxide from either venous or arterial blood using an extracorporeal semi-permeable membrane and then returns

the treated blood to the patient. The systems can either be pumped (veno-venous or veno-arterial) or pumpless (arterio-venous). Due to the relatively small surface area of the membrane and oxygen's poor solubility, these systems are unable to effectively oxygenate the blood, in contrast to extracorporeal membrane oxygenation (ECMO) systems.

Extracorporeal membrane oxygenation (ECMO). A system which draws venous blood from the patient and pumps it past a semi-permeable membrane with a very large surface area. This membrane allows carbon dioxide to diffuse out of the blood and oxygen to diffuse into the blood, exactly mimicking the lungs. The blood is then returned to the patient's arterial system under pressure.

Extubation. The process of removing a trans-laryngeal tube, as opposed to *de-cannulation*, which refers to the removal of a tracheostomy tube. **Accidental**: Unplanned extubation arising from actions taken by members of staff. **Self-**: Unplanned extubation effected by the patient themselves, either voluntarily or involuntarily. **Unplanned**: Inadvertent removal of the endotracheal tube either by the patient (self-extubation) or staff (accidental extubation).

f. See *Respiratory rate*.

Functional residual capacity. The physiological term for the volume of gas that remains in the lung immediately prior to the onset of inspiration. This is also called the end-expiratory lung volume.

Gas-trapping. See *Hyperinflation*.

Glottic opening (also *glottis opening*). The space bounded by the vocal cords.

HFOV. See *High-frequency oscillatory ventilation*.

High-frequency oscillatory ventilation. (HFOV) A system of ventilation which uses respiratory rates between 300 and 900 breaths per minute.

Hybrid mode. A ventilator mode that combines ventilator-initiated (mandatory) breaths and patient-initiated (triggered) breaths. In some forms of hybrid mode, the mandatory breaths may be suppressed by triggered breaths.

Hydrophilic. A molecule, or section of a molecule, that readily associates with an aqueous environment by possession of electrically charged ions or radicals at its surface. At the macroscopic level, a hydrophilic substance will either dissolve in pure water (solids) or mix evenly with water (liquids).

Hydrophobic. A molecule, or part of a molecule, that repels water by lacking any surface charge. At the macroscopic level, a hydrophobic substance will not dissolve in water (solids) or will not mix with water (liquids).

Hypercarbia. See *Hypercapnia*.

Hypercapnia. A partial pressure of carbon dioxide that is above the upper limit of the reference range. Synonymous with, but preferred to, *hypercarbia*.

Hyperinflation. Synonym: *gas-trapping*. An increase in the end-expiratory lung volume caused by a loss of the lung's elasticity and narrowing of the small airways. **Dynamic**:. An increase in the end-expiratory lung volume caused by tachynpoea, which reduces the expiratory time and prevents the completion of expiration before the onset of the next inspiration.

I:E ratio. The ratio between inspiratory time (T_I) and expiratory time (T_E), which as a ratio has no units. The normal I:E ratio is 1:2. If absolute value of either component is required, this must be calculated as follows:

$$T_I = \frac{T_I}{T_I + T_E} \times T_C \qquad (4)$$

$$T_E = \frac{T_E}{T_I + T_E} \times T_C, \qquad (5)$$

where T_C is the cycle time, and which itself can be calculated from the respiratory rate (see *Cycle time*).

Inflating pressure. Synonyms: *Delta P, ΔP; Pressure-support above PEEP, PSAP*. In a pressure-controlled breath, the inflating pressure is the difference between the end-expiratory or baseline airway pressure and the end-inspiratory airway pressure. All other things being equal, the inflating pressure in a pressure-controlled breath determines the inspiratory tidal volume. Care must be taken when setting the parameters for pressure-controlled breaths. The user-determined variables for pressure-controlled breaths may either be set as the PEEP and the inflating pressure, or alternatively as the PEEP and the end-inspiratory pressure. In high-frequency oscillatory ventilation with the SensorMedics machines, delta P refers to the amplitude of the pressure excursions above and below the mean airway pressure.

Inspiratory time (T_I). The time in seconds between the start of inspiration and the start of exhalation.

Intermittent Positive-Pressure Ventilation (IPPV). Synonyms: *control(led)-mode* or *continuous mandatory ventilation, CMV; intermittent positive-pressure breathing, IPPB*. A mandatory volume-controlled mode of ventilation.

Intrinsic PEEP. Synonyms: *auto-PEEP, gas-trapping*. Alveolar pressure is positive relative to atmospheric pressure during expiration, and normally falls to atmospheric pressure prior to the onset of the next inspiratory phase. If the flow of expiratory gas is limited, alveolar pressure is still positive at the start of the next inspiratory phase, thus constituting intrinsic positive end-expiratory pressure (PEEP).

Intubation. The process of placing a tube into the trachea either via the nose (nasotracheal intubation) or the mouth (orotracheal intubation).

Inverse-ratio ventilation. (IRV). Synonym: *pressure-controlled inverse-ratio ventilation (PCIRV)*. Ventilation in which the inspiratory time exceeds the expiratory, in contrast to normal ventilation in which the opposite pertains.

IPAP. Inspiratory positive airway pressure. See *Bi-level positive airway pressure.*

IPPB. Intermittent Positive-Pressure Breathing (anachr.) see *Intermittent Positive-Pressure Ventilation.*

IPPV. See *Intermittent Positive Pressure Ventilation.*

IRV. See *Inverse-ratio ventilation.*

Laryngeal inlet. The space bounded anteriorly by the epiglottis, posteriorly by the arytenoid and corniculate cartilages and between them the interarytenoid notch, and laterally by the aryepiglottic folds.

Mandatory. ~breath. A ventilator-initiated breath; ~ **mode.** A ventilator mode in which all the *supported* breaths are ventilator-initiated. In some mandatory modes, the patient may take their own breaths, but these are not supported by the ventilator and are termed *spontaneous* breaths.

Maximum airway pressure. Synonyms; P_{Peak}, *peak airway pressure*), the maximum <u>measured</u> pressure in the ventilator circuit during volume-controlled ventilation. P_{max} is attained at the end of inspiration and is generated by the combination of tidal volume, pulmonary compliance and airway resistance. In the presence of an end-inspiratory pause, the resistive component of P_{max} dissipates, allowing the airway pressure to fall to the component that is solely due to tidal volume and pulmonary compliance, known as the *plateau pressure*. In pressure-controlled breaths, the maximum airway pressure, which is a parameter <u>set</u> by the operator, is referred to as P_{high} or P_{insp}.

Mean airway pressure ($P_{\overline{aw}}$). The time-averaged airway pressure.

Minute volume. The volume of gas delivered to the patient each minute, calculated by multiplying the tidal volume by the respiratory rate. See also *Exhaled minute volume.* **Alveolar:** The volume of gas delivered to the alveoli each minute.

Nasotracheal tube. An endotracheal tube that passes through the nose, nasopharynx and oropharynx to enter the upper trachea through the glottic opening.

NIV. See *Non-invasive ventilation.*

Neural respiratory rate. The respiratory rate generated by the respiratory centre in the brain stem, as opposed to the observed respiratory rate.

Non-invasive ventilation. (NIV). Ventilatory support that partially or totally supplies the work of breathing but without the use of a tracheal tube. Most commonly, the patient interface involves a tight-fitting facial or nasal mask, but the term NIV can equally well be applied to forms of ventilatory support that have no patient interface, such as negative-pressure ventilation ('iron lung'), cuirass ventilation or rocker beds.

Orotracheal tube. An endotracheal tube that passes through the mouth and oropharynx to enter the upper trachea through the glottic opening.

$P_{A_{CO_2}}$. The partial pressure of carbon dioxide in alveolar gas.

$P_{A_{O_2}}$. The partial pressure of oxygen in alveolar gas.

Pa_{CO_2}. The partial pressure of carbon dioxide in arterial blood.

Pa_{O_2}. The partial pressure of oxygen in arterial blood.

$Pa_{O_2}/F_{I_{O_2}}$ ratio. This is not, strictly speaking, a ratio because the numerator and the denominator have different units. The arterial partial pressure of oxygen (in kPa or mmHg) divided by the fractional inspired oxygen concentration is used by clinicians as a rough gauge of the lung's capacity to take up oxygen and is often referred to in speech as the 'PF ratio'. A more accurate but more cumbersome way of expressing the same concept is to calculate the difference between the alveolar and arterial partial pressures of oxygen, i.e. $P_{A_{O_2}} - P_{a_{O_2}}$ expressed in kPa or mmHg. See also *Aa gradient*.

$P_{\overline{aw}}$. See *Mean airway pressure*.

P_{High}. See *Maximum airway pressure*.

P_{Insp}. See *Maximum airway pressure*.

P_{max}. See *Maximum airway pressure*.

P_{peak}. See *Maximum airway pressure*.

$P_{plateau}$. See *Maximum airway pressure*.

PAV. Proportional assist ventilation. See also *Proportional pressure support*.

PCIRV. Pressure-controlled inverse-ratio ventilation. See also *Inverse-ratio ventilation*.

Partial. ~pressure. The fraction of total gas pressure (P_{tot}) that is contributed by one gas in a mixture of gases, which is determined by the proportional concentration of that gas in the mixture. Thus where P_{tot} is the total gas pressure in a mixture of 3 gases (x, y and z) with volumes of Vol_x, Vol_y and Vol_z, the partial pressure of gas y (P_y) is given by the following:

$$P_y = \left(\frac{Vol_y}{Vol_x + Vol_y + Vol_z} \right) \times P_{tot}.$$

~ ventilation or ~ ventilatory support. A *hybrid mode* of ventilation.

Peak pressure. See *Maximum airway pressure*.

PEEP. See *Positive end-expiratory pressure*.

$PEEP_i$. See *intrinsic PEEP*.

PF ratio. See $P_{a_{O_2}}/F_{I_{O_2}}$ ratio.

Plateau (airway) pressure ($P_{plateau}$). In volume-controlled breaths with an end-inspiratory pause, the plateau airway pressure is the end-inspiratory pressure that remains when the resistive component has dissipated. See also *Maximum airway pressure*.

Positive end-expiratory pressure (PEEP). Externally applied pressure that maintains a positive airway pressure during expiration in patients receiving ventilatory support with *triggered* and *mandatory* breaths. During *spontaneous* breaths this is called continuous positive airway pressure (CPAP).

PPS. See *Proportional Pressure Support*.

Pressure-controlled inverse-ratio ventilation (PCIRV). See *Inverse-ratio ventilation*.

Proportional Assist Ventilation (PAV). Proprietary term owned by the University of Manitoba. See *Proportional pressure support*.

Proportional Pressure Support (PPS). Synonyms: *proportional assist ventilation*. A triggered mode similar to pressure support except that the degree of support varies according to patient effort such that with increasing patient effort more support is provided.

Ramp. See *Rise time*.

Respiratory rate (f). The number of breaths in one minute. See also *neural respiratory rate*.

Rise time. Synonym; *ramp*. The time taken from the start of inflation for airway pressure or flow to reach the maximum. This is normally about 200 ms in adults. In some make/models of ventilator rise time is also expressed as a percentage of the cycle time.

SIMV. Synchronized Intermittent Mandatory Ventilation.

Spontaneous. ~ breath. A breath in which inspiration is determined solely by the patient and for which the patient receives no inspiratory support. Compare with *triggered breath*. ~mode. A ventilator mode in which the patient initiates all inspiratory activity and receives no inspiratory assistance with the work of breathing. Compare with *triggered mode*.

Supported. ~ breaths; ~ mode. See under *triggered*, which is the preferred term.

T_I. See *Inspiratory time*.

T$_E$. See *Expiratory time*.

Tachypnoea. An abnormally fast respiratory rate.

Tracheal tube. A tubular airway that provides a conduit for ventilatory gases that terminates in the trachea, passing either through the larynx (trans-laryngeal tube), or entering the trachea through a tracheostomy (tracheostomy tube).

Trans-laryngeal intubation. See *Intubation*.

Trans-laryngeal tube. A tube designed to provide respiratory gases to a patient's lungs by passing through the nose (nasotracheal tube) or mouth (orotracheal tube), passing through the patient's larynx, and ending in the mid-trachea. The distal end may have an inflatable cuff with which to provide an air-tight seal with the trachea, in which case this is referred to as a 'cuffed' tube. Trans-laryngeal tubes are commonly referred to as 'endotracheal' tubes, but this term fails to distinguish this type of tube from a tracheostomy tube, which also sits within (endo-) the trachea (-tracheal).

Tidal volume (V$_T$). The volume of gas that is either inhaled, or exhaled in one breath. Inspiratory tidal volume is rarely the same as expiratory tidal volume because, (i) gas is inspired at room temperature, but in the body is warmed to body temperature and therefore expands, (ii) inspired gas may not necessarily be fully saturated with water vapour, but exhaled gas is, (iii) the composition of inspiratory and expiratory gases are not the same.

Triggered. ∼ breath. A patient-initiated breath which receives inspiratory support, either pressure-controlled (pressure support ventilation, PSV; pressure assist-control ventilation, P-ACV), or volume-controlled (assist-control ventilation). Triggered breaths can be part of a *hybrid mode*, where they are permitted in the interval between mandatory breaths (SIMV, PCV, IPPV+) and either suppress, (SIMV, IPPV+) or occur in addition to (PCV), the mandatory component. Triggered breaths should be distinguished from *spontaneous* breaths, which do not receive inspiratory assistance; ∼ **mode**. A mode of ventilation in which all the breaths are triggered, that is patient-initiated and each receives inspiratory assistance with the work of breathing. Compare *spontaneous*.

V$_E$. See *Exhaled minute volume*.

V$_T$. See *Tidal volume*.

Ventilating pressure. See *inflating pressure*.

Ventilatory rate. The rate that is set on a ventilator at which mechanical breaths are delivered to the patient in either a *mandatory* or *hybrid mode*.

Weaning. The process of transferring the work of breathing from the mechanical ventilator to the patient, defined as starting when the patient is able to initiate inspiratory effort.

Index